To Rosal

Thanks for everything!

All best!

Laurinda Dixon

THE DOCUMENTED IMAGE

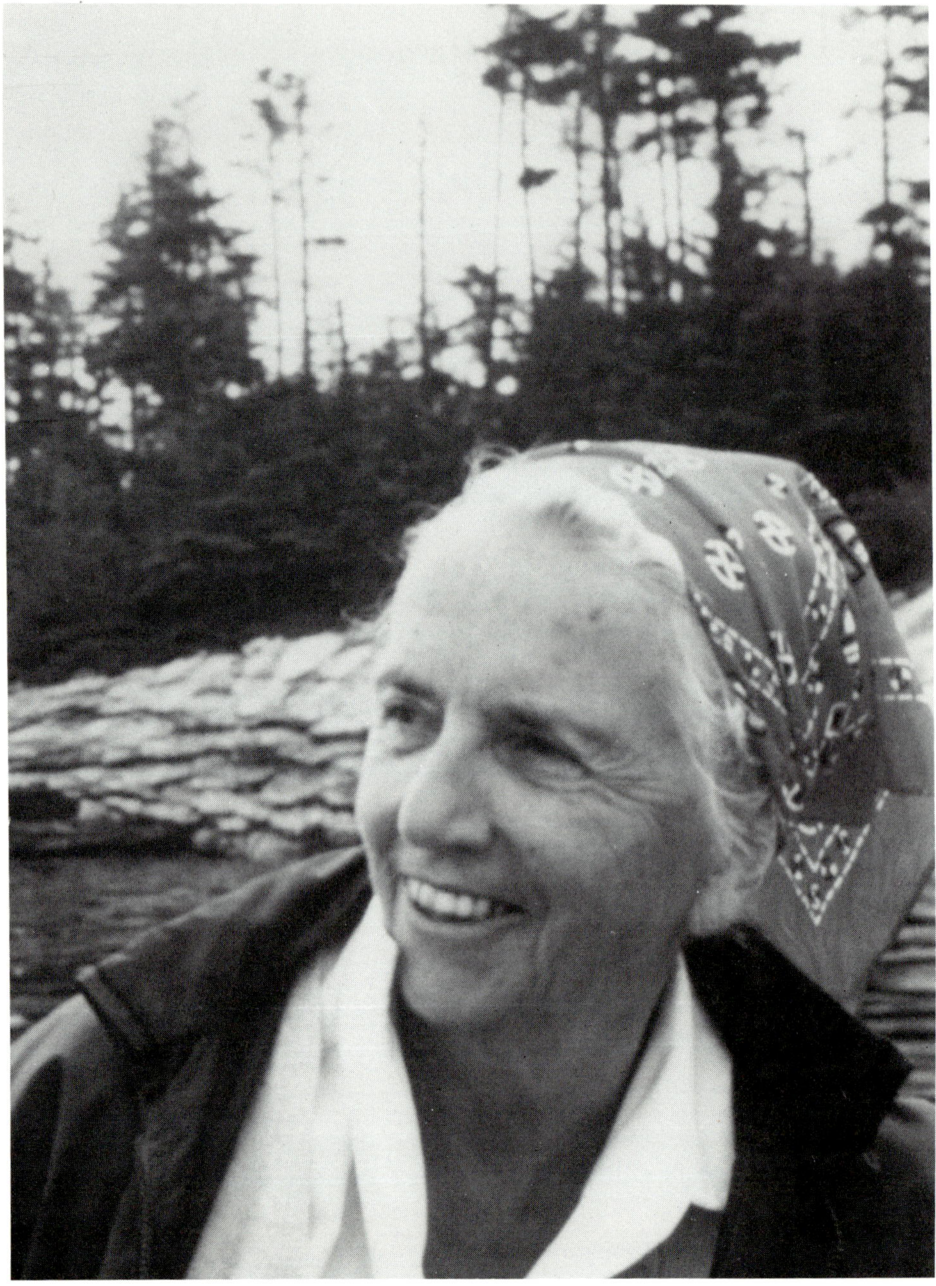

Dedicated to the memory of ELIZABETH GILMORE HOLT, 1905–1987

THE DOCUMENTED IMAGE

Visions in Art History

Edited by

GABRIEL P. WEISBERG

LAURINDA S. DIXON

with the assistance of

ANTJE BULTMANN LEMKE

SYRACUSE UNIVERSITY PRESS

Syracuse, New York 13244-5160

First published 1987

First Edition
93 92 91 90 89 88 87 5 4 3 2 1

The paper used in this publication meets the minimum requirements of American National Standard for Information Sciences—Permanence of Paper for Printed Library Materials, ANSI Z39.48-1984. ∞™

Library of Congress Cataloging-in-Publication Data

The Documented image.

Bibliography: p.
Includes index.
1. Art—Historiography. 2. Art criticism—Methodology. I. Weisberg, Gabriel P. II. Dixon, Laurinda S. III. Lemke, Antje Bultmann.
N7480.D63 1987 707′.2 87-17960
ISBN 0-8156-2410-7 (alk. paper)

Manufactured in the United States of America

CONTENTS

ILLUSTRATIONS

CONTRIBUTORS

ROBERT L. ALEXANDER is Professor Emeritus of the School of Art and Art History at the University of Iowa.

JACQUELYNN BAAS is the Director of the Hood Museum of Art at Dartmouth College.

JANE BLOCK is a member of the staff of the Department of Art and Archaeology Library at Princeton University.

RUTH BUTLER is a Professor in the Art Department at the University of Massachusetts in Boston.

GEORGIA BRADY BUMGARDNER is Curator of Graphic Arts at the American Antiquarian Society in Worcester, Massachusetts.

PETRA TEN-DOESSCHATE CHU is a Professor in the Department of Art and Music at Seton Hall University.

LAURINDA S. DIXON is an Associate Professor in the Fine Arts Department at Syracuse University.

WOLFGANG M. FREITAG is Librarian at the Fine Arts Library of the Fogg Art Museum at Harvard University.

CREIGHTON GILBERT is a Professor in the Department of the History of Art at Yale University.

E. H. GOMBRICH is Professor Emeritus of the University of London; he served as Director of the Warburg Institute from 1959 to 1976.

SHARON HIRSH is an Associate Professor in the Fine Arts Department at Dickinson College.

GENEVIÈVE LACAMBRE is the *Conservateur en chef* at the Musée d'Orsay in Paris.

ANTJE BULTMANN LEMKE is Professor Emeritus of the School of Information Studies at Syracuse University.

CHRISTINA LODDER is a Lecturer in the Department of Art History at the University of St. Andrews, Scotland.

HANS LÜTHY is the Director of the *Schweizerisches Institut für Kunstwissenschaft* in Zürich, Switzerland.

ROBIN SPENCER is Senior Lecturer in the Department of Art History at the University of St. Andrews, Scotland.

DAVID TATHAM is a Professor in the Fine Arts Department at Syracuse University.

JANE VAN NIMMEN is the Curator of the Sarah G. and Lionel C. Epstein Collection in Washington, D.C.

GABRIEL P. WEISBERG is Professor and Chair of the Department of Art History at the University of Minnesota.

PEG WEISS is a Research Associate Professor in the Fine Arts Department at Syracuse University.

INTRODUCTION

The Legacy of Elizabeth Gilmore Holt, 1905–1987

The LEGACY of ELIZABETH GILMORE HOLT

GABRIEL P. WEISBERG AND LAURINDA S. DIXON

The *writings of Elizabeth Gilmore Holt* as well as her staunch personal advocacy of populist concepts continually serve as beacons that have had a pronounced impact on generations of art historians, art students, and members of the general public. Whether examining her *Literary Sources of Art History* (Princeton, 1947) or using *A Documentary History of Art* (1957, 1958), the message has been apparent: the field of art history must democratize, must pay attention to field documents, must examine figures behind the scenes as much as the "name players," and should continually assess the writings of a period—in whatever form they appear—if that era and the concepts it espoused are to be fully contextualized.

In her more recent books—*The Triumph of Art for the Public* and *The Art of All Nations 1850–1873*—these principles have been put to more specific use in the study of the nineteenth century. With the focus on art critics, art dealers, and public and private exhibitions, Holt has contrasted the ideals of the artistic world with the concerns and interests of the reality of everyday life. Often the documents she has carefully translated and the personalities she has exhumed from the past are figures whose seminal ideas illuminated the varied aspects of the art and cultural world.

While aware of the cosmic forces of art history through the centuries, she was mesmerized by the nineteenth century—as the era of rebellion and democratic growth. The nineteenth century became her century; no figure was too obscure for examination and no writing too mundane for study if they contained *ideas* that would shed light on the ways in which the arts flourished and interacted with the public.

Since Elizabeth Holt refused to accept conventional answers to traditional problems, she sought her solutions in unusual locations. Much of her time was spent traveling throughout the world where she gained access to untapped archives and libraries. Her methodology was often built up from the painstaking school of "trial and error" and from her own excellent European training in art history and the history of culture. Never one to separate art history from larger societal issues and ideas, Elizabeth Holt followed a series of underlying concepts that are important to illuminate if we are to arrive at a clearer understanding of her lasting contribution to the field of art history, in general, and more specifically to nineteenth-century studies. Each of these concepts is an outgrowth of her own personal credo, and, hence, she has become a force in the field by following personal beliefs that are transmitted through her writings.

She stressed the importance of locating actual documents in reconstructing lost historical contexts for works of art. Continually aware of the growing indifference to the accuracy of the historical past as a means of understanding the present, Dr. Holt's working philosophy has painstakingly tried to reconstruct how art works were seen and appreciated within their own time frames. In this way, she has tried to set the record straight, eliminating the heavy reliance on speculation and generalization, which has plagued the work of hundreds of younger scholars within our own era. In locating documents in archives or in republishing insightful critical reviews of a painting published at the time of an exhibition, Dr. Holt has provided a clear means by which the importance of a work could be assessed for an audience in the past.

The response of long-neglected critics to a work of art also provides clues that demonstrate that a work could have meant something different for its time period than what we have been led to believe it meant through the writings of more contemporary authors who did not return to period sources with as strong degree of accuracy. History and the historical period have been her foundation; the insightful assessment of documents has been her process, leading a student—at no matter what level—to value the close reading of documents and texts as a means of getting closer to the historical truth of a period. It is a methodology grounded on the love of language that also demonstrates how the archivist has a place in helping the art historian achieve a fuller picture of an art object within context.

Dr. Holt sought the contemporary public's perception and reaction to works of art as revealed in documents. Closely associated with her interest and ability in reconstructing lost contexts and meaning through the utilization of documents has been her assessment of what the contemporary public (the public from the period in which the object was created) knew or recognized in the work of art exhibited or discussed. Quite often the general public might have been more sophisticated in its understanding of an art object than we have realized, since a review of a work may have appeared in a widely accessible journal that reached a broad audience. In this sense, the use of documents (or texts) must be seen as educational tools that helped a contemporary audience see a work of art in a specific context—or a specific way—at the time it was exhibited. The educational role of a writer was often quite pronounced and the work of art, examined in this way, often became a vehicle for educating the masses and reaching the broadest audience. It was not only the avant-garde that was touched by the art work and its explanation, it was also the general public of the city or country that found itself debating the merits of an art work because the discussion of the object had been aired in a magazine or newspaper that had visibility. In a sense, the role of the art critic—and the power of an art object to elicit emotions in a viewer—was seminal in the nineteenth century. It is just this impact that Elizabeth Holt has reconstructed so that we can have a clearer understanding of how history was made and came alive in the past by affecting the public.

The role that the display and merchandising of art played in the public perception of art is an important ingredient. Since the critics and documents Holt used were often tied to the visibility and accessibility of art works for the public, the location where art objects were shown became critical in her studies. She recognized that private shows, public exhibitions, official salons, group exhibitions, and independent efforts had not been systematically examined or chronicled. Too often past art historians had concentrated on the traditional patronage system—the nobility or the government—failing to see how things had radically changed within the nineteenth century. The new exhibition areas often attracted hordes of people—quite often uneducated, to be sure, but at least interested enough to attend the event. This signified that there was a public that was ready to be reached, and if the exhibitions were properly packaged and discussions held about their merits in the press, then the exhibitions (and their aims) would become as significant as the types of art work that was shown in them. Locating documents or texts that also spoke about the exhibition and its actual display meant that works of art would be assessed with a public in mind. The publicity, location, attraction, and sponsorship of exhibitions became areas for her fecund imagination; in the process, a whole new way of assessing and examining art—through its actual process of exhibition and marketing—became fair game. A new use had been found for documents to help explain the varied aspects of the nineteenth century.

Dr. Holt realized the importance of the artistic "symbol," based upon societal conventions, to the understanding of human history. Although documents and texts have been foremost in her mind as a means of examining history, Elizabeth Holt early on recognized that the actual object under discussion had to be examined and studied against what the texts had to say. One could not exist without the other. If only texts were studied without an attempt to see the work of art, then a false picture of the past could be constructed. She wanted to avoid this current dilemma at all costs. Accordingly, the close reading of documents meant that an art work had also to be read against what the author had to say; if a work of art was not easily accessible (or lost) and only the text remained, then it was imperative that images—often engravings—had to be located so that the writings of an author could be tested and examined against the image. In this way, the contextual reading of the image was enlarged, and the work under discussion was directly related to the concerns of the historical moment. Dr. Holt did not want objects to go unexamined. She believed that deeper insights and meanings could be detected if the image became a symbol for the text and, in a larger context, for the society that actually produced it.

She believed that connoisseurship separated from context modifies a discipline that belongs to the common experience of all people. But, if there were one principle that she valued above all others it was that solely a formalistic examination of art objects was useless. By divorcing art objects from the period in which they were created, by establishing false or too general principles, or by emphasizing too carefully the look of a work of art without a historical framework to hinge it on, this examination meant the elevation of superficiality. It also signified that the discipline of art history could be constructed with only a small audience in mind—the specialist and the connoisseur. She saw these figures as enemies in the democratization process. They wanted to contain the objects within a schema constructed solely for the small world of specialists—for individuals who spoke solely to each other or a few associates. In rebelling against this attitude, Elizabeth Holt returned to the historical roots of the discipline of art history demonstrating that the art works had often been created with an eye toward the largest possible audience. In turn, this audience had always been seen as existing outside the object as a spectator, and it was through the use of documents and texts from the period in which the object was created that one could see that art became an experience for all people from all nations. This democratizing, populist belief permeates all her writings, and this methodology has reached the pupils who have followed her ideals in their own work. It is a process that is also at work in this volume underscoring the writings of all the authors' contributions to which we shall now turn.

THE ESSAYS

The authors in the present volume, aware of the themes and interests of Elizabeth Holt, have expanded on her approach by selecting topics close to their own interests. There are also essays that touch only tangentially some of the concepts of Dr. Holt, but they have also been included in this publication since they demonstrate a further examination of her methodology. They also provide further credence for this commemorative volume by presenting art history as a discipline with its own history, writers, and point of view. Since some of them suggest what the discipline may become in the future, they are a worthy addition to Dr. Holt's philosophy. Grouped under the general rubric of the historiography of art history and placed toward the end of the book, they provide a fitting conclusion and evolution of the populist viewpoint that underlies so many of the articles.

The MERCHANDISING of ART for the PUBLIC

The theme tackled by the writers in the first part refers to the merchandising of art for the public and the resultant effect on public taste and the demand for art objects caused by this phenomenon. The four articles that best examine these issues are those by Robin Spencer, David Tatham, Georgia Brady Bumgardner, and Gabriel P. Weisberg. Each will be discussed in turn.

In Robin Spencer's "Whistler's First One-Man Exhibition Reconstructed," the author is intuitively aware of the significance of art exhibitions in framing art work and making them palatable for the public. Spencer recreates every nuance of the look of the exhibition, documents how Whistler worked to stimulate the sale of his art objects through the appearance of the pieces in the show, and demonstrates how the actual exhibition space became an extension of the artist's studio or the client's home. In this way, the exhibition took on a personal dimension: the artist arranged the works according to his own inclination, and the potential client examined the pieces with an eye toward how the objects would look in his own constructed environment. While Spencer isolates the activity of Whistler in promoting his own work—demonstrating that the progressive creator had to think of himself as an entrepreneur who had to promote his own pictures—in a subsidiary theme, he explores the role of commercial galleries in orchestrating public taste. Since the public did not always know what it wanted in the world of art and since the public was asserting control of the art market toward the end of the nineteenth century (much as it is today), the sensitive artist had to be cognizant of the dangers to true creativity if this was allowed to continue unchecked. Whistler was interested in charting his own future, and Spencer presents unknown documents about Whistler's challenging authority by decorating the exhibition space itself; the will of the independent artist becomes the main ingredient for controlling his own destiny while manipulating the artistic exhibition (and hoped-for clients) to his own ends. It is a challenging thesis. It forcefully demonstrates how all types of exhibitions and exhibition spaces must be assessed. Spencer demonstrates that the tastes of the public were not always the taste of the artist involved, underscoring the importance of accurately reconstructing the past in order to arrive at the truth.

In "Abraham Tuthill at Mrs. Trollope's Bazaar: Three Pictures at an Exhibition in Cincinnati in 1830," David Tatham examines how an "ordinary" artist merchandised his work in frontier America. He provides an unusual contrast to the sophistication of Whistler and his European public described in Spencer's article. In the process of unfolding his tale, Tatham demonstrates the importance of a single document that establishes the role of an early American picture gallery (one that was also significant as a work of period architecture). But the most important aspect of Tatham's essay is his ability to reconstruct the machinations of Abraham Tuthill in revealing himself as a forward-looking representative of "high culture" to attract an impressionable following, sell his objects, and provide Americans with a dream that they had acquired something truly "civilized" with his works, while in reality he was selling them much less. The essay is both a study in the importance of artistic showmanship and a comment on the vagaries of public taste. Since Tuthill was clearly an itinerant painter with little natural brilliance to recommend him, his ability to advertise his work to a public eager to be ensnared by any semblance of "culture" helps Tatham reconstruct a picture of the American frontier and the early vestiges of collecting art from contemporary creators. It underscores the importance of the artist as his own entrepreneur (much as Spencer has done in his essay) and provides a droll picture of the democratization process in the United States.

Georgia Brady Bumgardner in "The Popularization of Gentility: Illustrations in American Literary Annuals" continues to examine a theme presented in Tatham's article—the emergence of popular taste when it is manipulated by the artistic establishment. Her theme—nineteenth-century literary annuals geared to the educated middle class permits her to explore the impact these annuals had upon public awareness and the receptivity to certain types of art work. She carefully notes that these literary annuals became extremely significant vehicles for disseminating art, increasing the reputation of American art, and heightening the importance of the old masters as a means of presenting a viable art history for the masses. She emphasizes, in conclusion, that by cultivating a popular interest in works of art, visual sophistication became one way to recognize the presence of gentility.

In "S. Bing in America" Gabriel P. Weisberg further examines the duping of the American public by revealing that one of the major proponents of *Japonisme*—an international movement of Japanese culture and the arts—was quite capable of using personal wiles in order to achieve a materialistic gain. Sensing that Americans were eager to be involved in the collection of fashionable objects supposedly of exquisite quality, Bing utilized the salesroom, independent exhibitions, and personal contacts to spread the taste for Japanese objects in America. Often his American clients were untutored in their responses (similar to what Tatham has revealed in his essay), allowing the entrepreneurial dealer to sell whatever the traffic would bear in Japanese objects. Perhaps it was even possible for the French dealer to dispose of items that were not what they were supposed to be, since he recognized that art could be merchandised for the public and that advertisements and press campaigns could make many believe they had something quite substantial when in reality they had nothing of the sort. As an outgrowth of the chauvinistic French position and the methods utilized by a clever (and still quite well-reputed dealer), "S. Bing in America" exposes the business side of a famed art dealer who often did much to foster the better interests in Japanese art and art nouveau but who was not without his venal side, especially when it came to business dealings with American taste for *Japonisme*. In this sense, the democratization of this movement through exhibitions and sales, while seemingly helpful for many, demonstrates that dealers, artists, and promoters recognized the fickleness of public taste and response. All wanted to channel it to their own needs and Bing emerged as, most likely, the most successful in this regard, since he was not a practicing artist and he could manipulate the exhibitions and salesrooms to an even greater degree than others.

The IMPORTANCE of EXHIBITIONS in the PROMOTION of ART and ARTISTS

Japonisme, as a source of study, also serves as the focus of another article: "Hokusai and the French Diplomats: Some Remarks on the Collection of Baron de Chassiron" by Geneviève Lacambre. In this illuminating essay the author further establishes how Japanese art objects were known in France and focuses on the validity of the Chassiron collection (first established in Paris in 1871) as a means of demonstrating what precise objects were available to collectors and artists. While the collection may not have been widely known, its existence today manages to convince a reader that untapped resources and documents can further enlarge knowledge about a well-explored theme.

Closely linked to the importance of exhibitions in promoting or merchandising a style or artist were those public shows that had a more educational, rather than monetary, role to play in fostering an awareness of an artist's style. Two essays in this volume are particularly appropriate: Ruth Butler's study of "Rodin and His American Collectors" and Petra ten-Doesschate Chu's essay "Nineteenth-Century Visitors to the Frans Hals Museum." Both essays also contain aspects that are strongly revisionist, expressing noticeably independent viewpoints similar to the philosophical position often taken by Holt.

In "Rodin and His American Collectors," Butler painstakingly documents the roles of collectors and exhibitions in creating the earliest public appreciation of Rodin's work at a time when America was dominated by a strong Victorian sensibility that revealed an aversion to blatant erotic themes. Since Butler also isolates the importance of the personality of Loie Fuller, herself an artist and collector with a strong sense of independence, Butler reconstructs how Loie Fuller's influence on the American public helped create a commercial interest in Rodin's sculpture. Most importantly, Butler isolates the strain of "artistic freedom" that dominates Rodin's pieces and suggests that it was this content that created a lasting influence on American art. It was possible for American collectors and artists to be trained, to get over their innate gullibility (as pointed up in earlier essays), and to understand a contemporary creator through first-rate examples. Butler correctly reveals that America's early enthusiastic appreciation of Rodin pushed France out of its lethargy. Because the Americans engaged in a fervent campaign of promotion, they pushed the French toward the establishment of an official museum to honor Rodin's genius. Butler's carefully crafted essay reveals the reverse of the traditional perception of the American art scene as following that of Europe.

Through an examination of a hitherto unexplored issue, Butler has revised our knowledge of history by demonstrating that the general public of a given country (in this case, the United States) could help make the career of a given creator by enthusiastically embracing his work at a time when a career had not been fully canonized in its own country.

Petra ten-Doesschate Chu's "Nineteenth-Century Visitors to the Frans Hals Museum" further perceptively examines the significance of a public exhibition—in this case an entire museum display—in fostering an awareness of a master from a former time. In this way it is possible, even permissible to see, how Frans Hals's paintings and personality were visible reminders of what this artist had to offer contemporary painters. Chu's assessment of the role of the Frans Hals Museum in Haarlem, Holland, reveals that visitors to this museum caused an important reversal in public opinion about the artist and a revision in the often low opinion of his bourgeois subject matter. Significantly, the entire article hinges upon an important document—one that Elizabeth Holt would be happy to see properly used—the visitor's register book, which was signed by all of the prominent collectors and artists who came to the museum throughout the nineteenth century. The assessment of this document permits the author to demonstrate that Hals's impact on nineteenth-century art was international in scope. Impressive visitors from France, Russia, Germany, and the United States came to the museum and often incorporated elements of Hals's style into their own compositions. The appreciation of Hals can be subdivided into time frames: during the 1860s Hals was seen as an artist celebrating bourgeois republican culture and as a positive force on realism; in the 1870s and 1880s he was appreciated for his virtuoso technique that foreshadowed Manet and the Impressionists; by the turn of the century, Hals was seen as a painter who understood the commonplace, who made a virtue out of studying the banal. Thus, by carefully utilizing an existing but neglected document, Chu has shown that the Hals museum had an astounding impact on artists everywhere. It is one of the strongest cases in the present volume for the full use of documents within context, as it provides the means by which to assess an entire tradition; it, therefore, unlocks an unknown theme while relating to the general issue of how art exhibitions (even permanent ones housed within museums) can have a long lasting influence on a public.

DOCUMENTS as SOURCES for REVISIONIST ART HISTORY

Petra ten-Doesschate Chu's essay provides a natural bridge to the consideration of documents or unknown historical facts that provide a new—often revisionist—view of the influence of art on the general public. In this section of the volume, three art historians—Jane Block, Laurinda S. Dixon, and Peg Weiss—examine issues pertinent to this theme. In Jane Block's "A Neglected Collaboration: Van de Velde, Lemmen, and the Diffusion of the Belgian Style," the author effectively documents the largely unacknowledged impact of the artist/designer Georges Lemmen on the far more visible creator Henri van de Velde. Block suggests, in the development of her thesis, that both should be given equal credit for founding the "new style" that swept the decorative arts in Belgium at the turn of the century.

The essay traces van de Velde's and Lemmen's often intersecting careers through published and unpublished sources, examining their relationship until it fell apart around 1902. The article provides a balanced view of the evolution of the Belgian arts and crafts movement, offering insights into how it came about and demonstrating how both men worked toward the same ends at the time. Both men are seen as benefiting from their mutual friendship and from their ties with significant patrons of the movement including S. Bing and J. Meier-Graefe. Their mutual association is presented as a paradigm of artistic collaboration and reciprocal influence demonstrating that they can be studied in tandem in the future. Block also provides convincing reasons why Lemmen has been slighted in studies of Belgian art nouveau, ascribing the low esteem in which his works are held to his early, almost untimely death and the extremely long and vigorous career of van de Velde. The essay, with its avowed purpose to rectify a historical oversight, also puts into practice Elizabeth Holt's philosophy of examining the neglected figures from the past whose contribution has either been forgotten or overshadowed.

A similar fascination with the neglected and obscure aspects of nineteenth-century fin-de-siècle creativity dominates Laurinda Dixon's essay, "Art and Music at the Salons de la Rose + Croix, 1892–1897." Dixon carefully posits the theory that the Rose + Croix mentality and exhibition coincided with a far deeper end-of-century malaise that emphasized the fatalistic while simultaneously espousing dynamic optimism. Most importantly, the essay demonstrates that the Rose + Croix group believed in synesthesia—the correspondences between the arts—for art and music are noted as having been related through a system of shared values and mutual ideas. The examination of the Rose + Croix fascination with music parallels Elizabeth Holt's interests in other fields of discourse as sources of significant clues and influences for art history. The music that was intended to be heard in the presence of actual art objects provides a further dimension for art historical consideration. Since art exhibitions, expecially those of the Rose + Croix, have been studied solely for the types of art objects that were exhibited, this approach provides an added dimension more appropriate to the period under examination and one in keeping with the avowed method of contextualizing art works. The Rose + Croix salons, because of this study, will be seen as key areas for artistic innovation as supported by the composer Erik Satie's creation of a school for French nationalist music derived from the Germanic concept of the Wagnerian *Gesamtkunstwerk*. The domain of art historical inquiry is further enlarged by this essay, which is in keeping with Holt's own conceptual framework.

Peg Weiss's "Kandinsky and 'Old Russia'—An Ethnographic Exploration" further enlarges on a revisionist tack by uncovering a nationalistic and personal strain of abstract iconography in Kandinsky's work. This direction is based on the artist's previous serious historical and cultural study of the Zyrian people of northern Russia, providing the opportunity for a little-known consideration to become absolutely crucial for the study of the artist. Weiss reads into Kandinsky's "ethnological" works a most specific iconography based upon the artist's own commitment to the Zyrian shamanistic religion. She documents through specific examples Kandinsky's adoption of these motifs, which form an intricate, personal statement. Since Weiss focuses on Kandinsky's early training and his promising career in ethnology, she uses a series of unknown articles that he wrote as part of a professional research trip sponsored by the Russian Imperial Society of Natural History, Anthropology, and Ethnography. Similar to Dixon's ability to move beyond the narrowly defined confines of art history, Weiss has demonstrated how anthropology and ethnology functioned as significant ingredients to the makeup of the artist. This early training in ethnology echoed/resonated throughout Kandinsky's career. Elements of folk culture (and folklore) can be recognized in many of the abstract paintings for which he has achieved international fame. In revealing this material, Weiss provides a seminal ingredient for future study of Kandinsky, while at the same time, she makes an extremely strong case for the art historian's consideration of all areas of influence on a creator in order to expand the boundaries of discourse and research.

The interests of Peg Weiss bring the reader very close to the next major theme of the articles in this volume: the consideration of the art work as a symbol that arises from a historical context but which often has its starting point in the need to serve the public. Four essays address this theme.

The WORK of ART as SYMBOL ARISING from a HISTORICAL CONTEXT

In "The Special Orders of Robert Mills," Robert L. Alexander focuses on the architecture of Robert Mills, especially his creation of an "American Order" of the classical column. Obviously the order was derived from the long-standing classical tradition, but it was modified to fit the context of the fitful struggle to visualize the new republic in the United States. In combining Greco-Roman architectural elements derived from Vitruvius, aspects that were generally understood by the American public, Mills presented a personal architecture that evoked a symbolic message. The new American Order emphasized the strength, independence, and moral integrity of the new country. It is a carefully structured essay that makes these points most tellingly.

The meaning of works of art, even those concepts that have been lost for centuries, is the theme of the next essay by Creighton Gilbert, "Boccaccio Looking at Actual Frescoes." This study imaginatively isolates the symbolic elements of Boccaccio's description of a lost fresco series by Giotto, and it establishes their importance for the "man in the street" of the fourteenth century. Gilbert's approach demonstrates that the images were powerful reminders for the common man, thus removing examination of the fresco cycle from the realm of abstract consideration. In this way he effectively recreates a political, social, historical, and literary context for Giotto's work. The essay fully reminds us that sources for art history can, once again, come from all disciplines, thereby underscoring the universalist literary approach that Elizabeth Holt first used in *The Literary Sources of Art History.* Gilbert's ability to reconstruct a lost fresco cycle through the use of documents, albeit documents from the Renaissance, also reiterates the usefulness of this approach for all periods. He most tellingly demonstrates that the meaning of Giotto's image could be explained increasing the accessibility of the lost images.

The two remaining essays in this section, those by Sharon Hirsh and Christina Lodder, follow a slightly different methodology than the others. In both cases the authors examine one work in depth hoping to arrive at a deeper understanding of the importance of the objects both in the context of the history of the period and of the evolution of the artist's work. While they don't explore a decidedly revisionist posture, they do examine the symbolic implications of an icon through the use of pertinent documents and by a close reading of the objects in question. Somewhat more traditional in their viewpoints and methods than others, both authors do arrive at a holistic statement. In the case of Hirsh's "Le Chemin Symbolique: Ferdinand Hodler's Symbolic Path of *Autumn Evening*," a stylistic analysis of Hodler's *Autumn Evening* demonstrates that the forms and colors of his native Switzerland were personal symbols of the artist's philosophy of life and death. The painting is seen as representative of Hodler's belief in the underlying order of nature, a study of the "parallelism" of human existence that was closely linked to the forms and rhythms of nature. The author effectively examines Hodler's notebooks to isolate the evolution of the symbol, demonstrating how integral this was to the artist. Christina Lodder's "Tatlin's Monument to the Third International as a Symbol of Revolution" explores one significant object in terms of its importance to the social and political contexts of the time. The author reveals how the work had much more than a personal importance; it became a symbolic icon for an entire epoch, drawing upon common contemporary experience and unique visual conventions for a specific public response. Lodder reveals that the materials of construction, its spiral shape, and its revolving motion around a central core (an axis) had significant iconographic implications understood by the Russian public of the time. She elucidates her theory by referring to documents outside the realm of art history: Russian utopian philosophy, the writings of Lenin, and finally, the works of the futurist poet Velimir Khlebnikov. Both authors achieve similar ends—a deeper understanding of one work—and while they rely on the use of documents (to a certain degree), their approaches may not appear as radical as other essayists in this volume. This is not to say that their work is any less effective, only that they have been evolving from a different methodological base in order to achieve their goals—a base that is, most likely, allied with well-established traditions in art history.

The HISTORIOGRAPHY of ART HISTORY

Another group of essays in this book are related to another area of concern held by Elizabeth Holt: the historiography of art history. Always cognizant of the fact that the discipline needed to be encouraged—enlarged—so that it would not remain the fiefdom of the few, these essayists have approached this area from a variety of issues. E. H. Gombrich in his "The Values of the Byzantine Tradition" examines Goethe's resistance, as an old man, to change in the face of evolving public taste and the persuasiveness of new, often previously unavailable, art historical documentation. The essay further examines Goethe's confrontation with the emerging Romantic School that favored painters of the Northern Renaissance above the traditional classic Greek models. Gombrich shows that the growing fascination with medievalism was a concerted reaction against the anticlericalism of the French Revolution combined with the growth of an emergent Germanic nationalism. The resultant dispersal of monastic art caused the beginning of collecting medieval art as well as the first attempts to construct a historical picture of the makings of medieval art. The author notes that the Boisserée brothers, though persuasive in their attempt to convert Goethe toward an appreciation of their rediscovered art, were not successful. Goethe held fast. He remained in the old generation of die-hard neoclassicists opposed to the mysticism and vagueness of the tradition that medieval art then represented. In this essay Gombrich effectively concentrates on the debate between the old and the new, the traditional and the rediscovered; he demonstrates that old orders and faiths don't change quickly and are often inflexible. This historical essay has much of relevance for the debates running throughout the discipline of art history both in the past and in some of the essays in this book.

Hans Lüthy's "Charles Clément and the French Landscape" can be nicely contrasted with Gombrich's assessment of Goethe. Although a largely overlooked critic of certain aspects of nineteenth-century art, Charles Clément tried to define (through isolation) a nineteenth-century school of landscape painters. His method, based on historical objectivity and distance, helped project the positive worth of the examination as a new area of painting. Clément's essay on landscape painting was also an early example of an art historical method—one of the earliest that can be recorded. The critic compared the "old school" of neoclassical landscape painting with the "modern school," developing a theory of romantic image making where spirit and emotion were valued over precise finish, over technique. Clément also established some fundamental concerns that art historians in their own writings must consider: first, he tried to develop an objective, historic viewpoint by which he could assess works from the past and those from his own time; second, he wanted the writer's personality to remain secondary, in the background, so that what was being written about would be more important than the style in which it was being expressed. Clément can, therefore, serve as a paradigm of what it takes to be open to new ideas (in a contemporary sense as a critic) and in a historical context. His ability to positively recognize the validity of a new style makes him a critic to examine, and it distinguishes his writings from the subjective statements of his more poetic contemporaries.

The validity of the art historical approach to past masters was also found in the writings of Friedrich Schlegel, whom Jane Van Nimmen analyzes in her "Friedrich Schlegel's Response to Raphael in Paris." Here the change from examining the mature works of Raphael's approach to a study of his earliest works is found in an examination of an exhibition of Raphael's work at the Louvre where his compositions were chronologically arranged. While the exhibition fostered a study of Raphael, it was Schlegel's ability to comment on the evolution of Raphael's approach that gave rise to the concept of a stylistic analysis of a Renaissance painter's imagery. Since Schlegel was impressed by the early works of Raphael, he used the exhibition and his own writings to mold public perceptions. Although Schlegel dethroned Raphael from supreme importance, an examination of his writings serves as a case study—further evidence of the power of an art historian to mold taste and set the course for future investigation and appreciation. When this is done with an open approach, it would seem quite fair; when this method emphasized a closed canonization of only the great names studied without compassion or context, then art history would become a stultifying experience.

NINETEENTH-CENTURY ART HISTORICAL IMPLICATIONS in TWENTIETH-CENTURY CONTEXT

The last two essays in the book, Jacquelynn Baas's "Reconsidering Walter Benjamin: 'The Age of Mechanical Reproduction' in Retrospect" and Wolfgang M. Freitag's "Art Reproductions in the Library," underscore implications for the field that are appropriate for the twentieth century. Baas examines Walter Benjamin's assumption that the invention of photography in the first half of the nineteenth century greatly changed the nature and reception of the visual arts in our own period where mechanical reproduction of art images has been a dominant mode. In noting that Benjamin was incorrect about his history of mechanical reproduction, Baas attacks the belief that photography was the key for creation aimed at a mass audience. While film and television still must be seen as influential stimulants on an audience, the author notes that museum attendance and the fundamental interest in studying graphic arts, painting, and sculpture has made art works per se more deeply valued in an "age of mechanical reproduction." Her essay is one of the advocacy of the original object, a position held by Elizabeth Holt as long as the object can be substantially explained and understood by the masses.

Wolfgang Freitag takes us along another path through his consideration of the importance of the visual reproduction for the teaching of art history to young students. Since he places the copies of art works (from Roman copies of Greek sculpture to laser discs in our time) within a historical context, he tries to come to grips with the way in which copies have affected perceptions of art works and molded the discipline of art history. Since Freitag is not at all sure just what the appropriate function of the artificial image should be in the study of the history of art he opens a "Pandora's box," raising issues that art historians have not adequately addressed in our time or in the past. Freitag also sees art libraries as difficult places to work, locales that don't always foster a populist approach to the discipline, and he questions what the future will hold. In this he really appears not alone, as several of the authors in this section are interested in what young students should study, or how they should be trained, or what their method should be. Freitag's basic validity is his ability to take the issues up to our own time; he demonstrates that art history is still an evolving discipline that has much thinking to do about itself and how it functions, especially if it is going to survive as a legitimate humanities discourse with a goal of truly educating the public—at all levels.

In a sense, all the writers in this volume have understood the varied approaches and methods that Elizabeth Holt has helped instill in the discipline of art history. Their varied messages and their selection of various "trial cases" must be seen as methodological studies whereby they have placed their ideas before an ever-changing public. In turn, members of this public will be able to judge from the wide variety of examples reproduced in this volume how these methods can influence them and help mold their thinking and future perceptions. What is equally significant is that quite often these ideologies have been conditioned by the beliefs of one art historian—Elizabeth Gilmore Holt—whose teaching and writings have helped raise these approaches as legitimate areas of study, making the field of art history ever more open and varied in the process. There can be little doubt that an examination of past traditions and methods can now lead to a revised examination of the present and to the use of new study methods that will open the field of art history ever further to true humanistic discourse.

I
The Merchandising of Art for the Public

1

ABRAHAM TUTHILL at MRS. TROLLOPE'S BAZAAR

Three Pictures at an Exhibition in Cincinnati in 1830

DAVID TATHAM

On Thursday, 23 September 1830, the *Daily Cincinnati Gazette* carried this notice in its columns:

> Sale of Oil Paintings at the Bazaar; by A. B. Roff, Auct'r, on Saturday afternoon, at 3 o'clock. Executed by A. G. Tuthill, pupil of the celebrated Benj. West; consisting of a beautiful collection of splendid oil paintings, among which are a full length portrait of DeWitt Clinton, with a view of Lockport on the grand canal, who is represented as congratulating the people upon the completion of that important work. A portrait of Sir Benjamin West, the distinguished artist of our country, who presided over the academy of fine arts in England. A view of Madison Barracks at Sackets Harbour, together with several fancy pieces. Our citizens are respectfully invited to call at the Bazaar and see them previous to the sale.[1]

The significance of the notice is twofold. Despite its brevity, it offers perhaps the fullest documentation yet unearthed of an art exhibition in the early years of the Bazaar in Cincinnati, one of the most interesting buildings of Jacksonian America and one meant from the outset to house, among other things, a public picture gallery. The notice also offers a glimpse of how Abraham Guglielmus Dominey Tuthill (1776–1843), an itinerant artist who has long had the dubious distinction of being the least known of Benjamin West's American students, went about merchandising his work. Of the three paintings described in the notice, at least two are extant.

The Bazaar was the creation of its original proprietor, the Englishwoman Frances Milton Trollope (1779–1863). Mrs. Trollope later enjoyed much success as a travel writer and novelist, but at the time of her adventure with the Bazaar she had published nothing. She had left England late in 1827 with three of her children and their drawing master, the French artist Auguste Jean Jacques Hervieu (1794–1858), to seek her family's fortune in America. Two of her children, including Anthony, the future novelist, remained in England with their father. Soon after arriving in Cincinnati in 1828, she met with success in devising theatrical spectacles for the fledgling Western Museum. Encouraged by this and with her husband's constant support, she designed and erected the Bazaar in 1829, investing in it all of her family's available capital. Though it was meant to be primarily a commercial building, it included space for the arts and entertainments.[2]

Within a plan of about 37 by 100 feet, the building housed her retail shop (the Bazaar proper), a coffeehouse, a barroom, a ballroom, public parlors, a residential

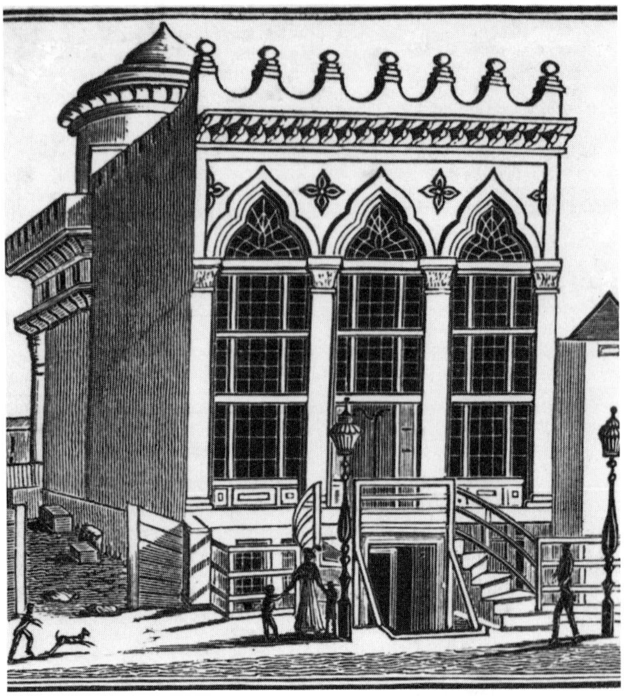

Fig. 1.1. *The Bazaar,* wood engraving published in *The Cincinnati Mirror and Western Gazette of Literature and Science,* vol. 3, 1833. The "Chinese" elements were on the rear façade. Courtesy of the American Antiquarian Society.

suite for Mrs. Trollope and her family, and, in an annex, a picture gallery. An onion-domed rotunda surmounted the building; its castellated promenade overlooked the city and its river, as well as the sugar refinery, steam engine factory, and distillery, which were among its close neighbors. She expected that the Bazaar's extraordinary appearance (fig. 1.1), which a contemporary described as "Graeco-Moresco-Gothic-Chinese," would draw and fix the admiring attention of townsfolk, river travelers, and visiting backwoodsmen, but it did not. She also believed that the uplifting tone of the lectures, musicales, and exhibitions she planned (but during her brief proprietorship had little opportunity to stage), as well as the refined taste of the fancy goods she imported for sale, would elevate the level of culture in a community that was scarcely a generation beyond frontier life. Here too, she was wrong. The Bazaar failed in the spring of 1830, only a few months after it had opened. Though virtually impoverished, she managed to tour parts of the eastern United States before returning to England in 1831. The building, which passed through the hands of several owners in succeeding years, housed the exhibits of the Ohio Mechanics' Institute later in the 1830s. When Anthony Trollope visited it in 1861, he was dismayed to find a run-down medical institute of questionable repute. The Bazaar was demolished in 1881.[3]

In 1832, Mrs. Trollope's first book, the *Domestic Manners of the Americans,* recounted her years in the United States but remained silent about the Bazaar. Hervieu's illustrations for the volume contained no picture of it, though it had been the center of his activity as an artist for many months. His plan to paint a panorama for the Bazaar's rotunda apparently came to nothing, but his decorations for the ballroom, reportedly based on those of the Alhambra, were much admired locally in 1829.[4] In the

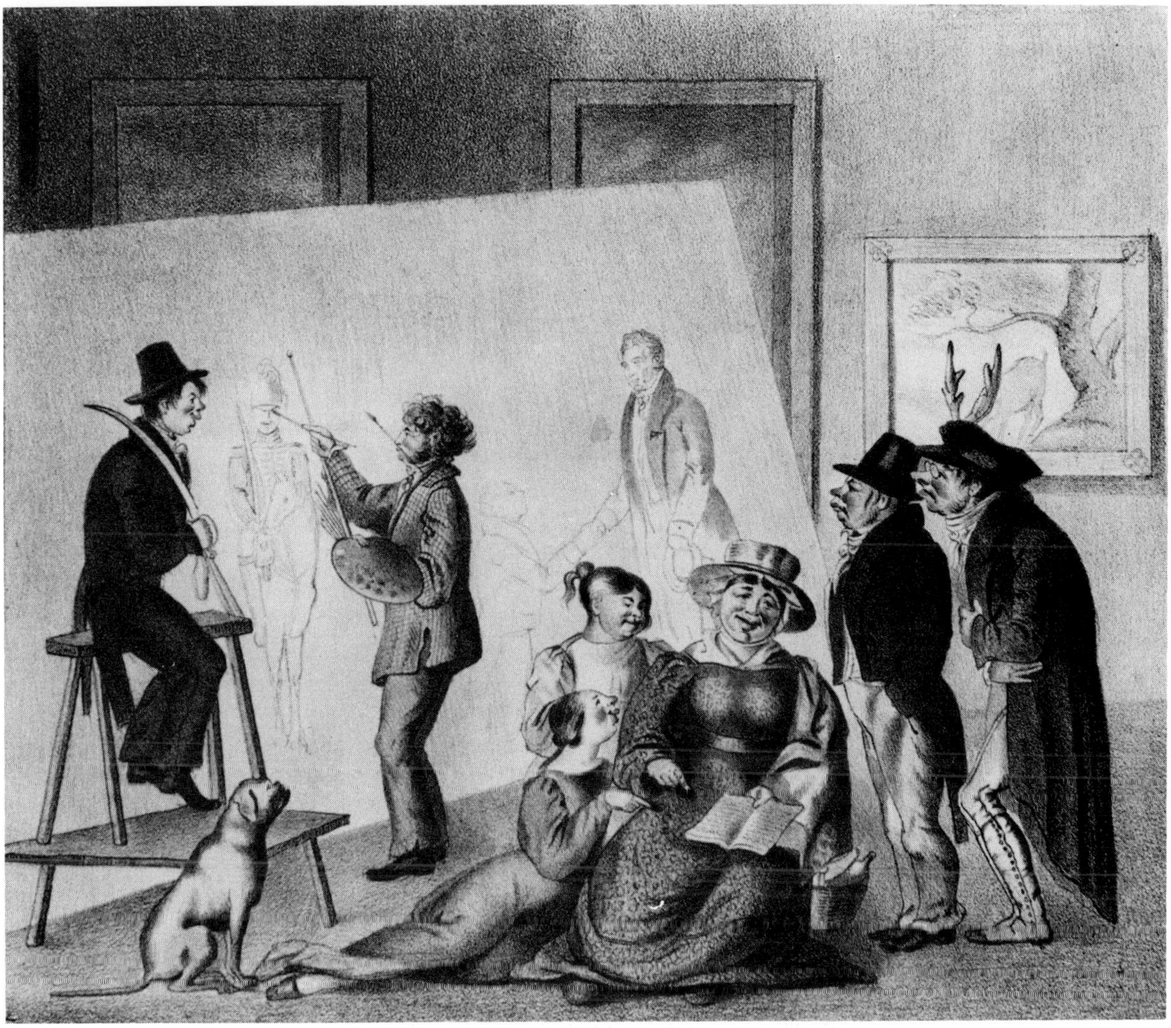

Fig. 1.2. Unknown artist, *The Trollope Family,* 1832. Lithograph, 8½ × 10⅜ in. Courtesy of the New-York Historical Society, New York City.

same year, he painted on a scale of twelve by sixteen feet a depiction of the Marquis de Lafayette's landing at Cincinnati during his grand tour of the United States in 1825, an event that had preceded Hervieu's visit by three years. Mrs. Trollope was acquainted with Lafayette; he had entertained her and her husband at La Grange in 1823 and had encouraged her to visit the United States. The painting hung in the Bazaar until Hervieu carried it away with him when he and his patron left the city. They may have taken it to England. If it remains in existence, its present whereabouts are unrecorded.[5]

When the publication of *Domestic Manners,* with its uncharitable views on American life, made Mrs. Trollope a popular subject of satire in the United States, fun was poked at Hervieu as well. We see them caricatured in the lithograph *The Trollope Family* (fig. 1.2), published in Philadelphia in 1832 by the firm of Childs & Inman.

The print is unsigned, and no evidence of its authorship has surfaced. Behind a blissfully domestic Mrs. Trollope, Hervieu works on his picture of Lafayette, transforming a local bumpkin into a splendidly uniformed guard of honor. If the lithographic artist had actually seen the painting, which he could have done not only in Cincinnati but also in Washington and Philadelphia when Hervieu exhibited it in those cities in the spring of 1830, then we may have some notion of the pictorial source Hervieu used for his likeness of Lafayette. The figure sketchily shown at the right of Hervieu's canvas seems to have been adapted from Ary Scheffer's full-length portrait of 1823, probably by way of Jean Marie Leroux's engraving after it.[6]

Although Abraham Tuthill's exhibition at the Bazaar occurred six months after Mrs. Trollope and Hervieu had left Cincinnati, he may have planned the event with them in advance of their departure. Alternatively, the news of Hervieu's move from the area may have encouraged Tuthill to try to fill the artistic vacuum. Certainly, he knew the city well, having painted there as early as 1815, and had good reason to suppose that the Bazaar would offer the most prestigious site for an exhibition in the westerly lands. He was, in any event, not likely to have transported a sizable group of paintings by land, by lake, and by river more than 500 miles without some kind of prior arrangement for a showing. He may have visited Cincinnati in 1828 or 1829 (his travels in these years are poorly documented), and if he did he almost certainly would have met Mrs. Trollope and Hervieu. The three had much in common, not least the fact that each had lived in both England and France. It is even remotely possible that Tuthill had known Mrs. Trollope during his years in England early in the century.

The few known facts of Tuthill's life are easily summarized. He was born at Oyster Ponds (now Orient), Long Island. After painting a few naive portraits, he moved to New York City in 1799 and attempted in vain to become a pupil of Gilbert Stuart in Philadelphia. On Stuart's advice, he set out for England to study with West, but his ship took him first to Bordeaux, where he spent three months with an American family. By August 1800, he was in London. He seems to have remained in England for seven years, but how much of this time was spent in association with West is unknown. Among West's other American students in these years were Washington Allston, who arrived in 1801, and Rembrandt Peale, who arrived a year later. After another visit to France, Tuthill sailed back to America, probably in 1808. He apparently attempted to establish himself as a portrait painter in New York, but with so little success that in 1812 or 1813 he set out to ply his trade in places where he would have less competition.[7]

William Dunlap, the painter, playwright, and chronicler of American art, who had traveled to England to study with West in the 1780s, first met Tuthill in New York in 1812. He later recalled that Tuthill "told me that he had been to London to study the art [of portrait painting], but his works bore little indication of that school. He likewise claimed to be a pupil of Mr. West's."[8] The few examples of Tuthill's work for the period 1808–12 that have come to light justify the skepticism implicit in Dunlap's remarks. They are surprisingly primitive for an artist who had spent eight years in Europe presumably studying and practicing the art of painting likenesses. When Dunlap next met Tuthill, some years later but certainly before 1830, he was painting in upstate New York. Dunlap found him "much improved in manner, appearance, and painting," praise that is undermined by what it implies about the past. Dunlap then added, ungenerously, that Tuthill "had been successful as an itinerant . . . by presenting smooth and well-varnished pictures, with some resemblance to his sitters."[9]

In his travels throughout the hinterlands of the United States, Tuthill used as a home base first Montpelier, Vermont (where several of his relatives had settled), and then Buffalo, New York. From Vermont, he ranged westward across New York State and beyond into Ohio as early as 1815. By 1820, he had traversed the top of New York State from Lake Champlain to Lake Ontario a few times, leaving behind him portraits in Plattsburgh, Watertown, Sackets Harbor, and elsewhere. With the opening of the Erie and Champlain canals in 1825, he visited the booming canal towns of Utica, Syracuse, Rochester, Lockport, and Buffalo. From Buffalo, he traveled to Detroit in 1825 and to Cincinnati in 1830. His route to Cincinnati was by lake boat to Erie, Pennsylvania, overland a dozen or so miles to French Creek, a tributary of the Allegheny, and then by riverboat and steamer to the Ohio and the Queen City. He moved about constantly until his retirement to Montpelier in 1840. The extent of his travels may well be unmatched by any other itinerant artist of his day.

Like other itinerants, Tuthill advertised his presence in local newspapers, but the *Gazette* notice is far more elaborate than most. The text is surely Tuthill's own; who else could have have praised the works and their maker so skillfully? The notice emphasizes Tuthill's pedigree as a student of West, as well it should, for no other itinerant painter in America could then claim such a distinguished association. Study with West promised a certain level of artistic prowess, more, it must be said, than Tuthill's paintings delivered, though few of his customers would have had an adequate basis for judging the disparity. His notice also played on the residue of anti-British feeling remaining from the War of 1812. It did so by reminding (or informing) Tuthill's audience that his teacher had been the American who "presided over the academy of fine arts in England," referring to West's near-unbroken tenure as president of the Royal Academy from 1792 until his death in 1820. Any claim of American superiority over the English in a matter of culture was rare enough in Ohio in 1830 to be relished; this one gilded Tuthill's credentials. In an attempt to make West even more important than he was, Tuthill endowed him with the knighthood that he had in fact declined in 1792.

The notice states that an auctioneer would conduct the sale, but it does not say that the sale would be an auction. We may be confident that it was not, if for no other reason than that in 1843, Tuthill still owned two of the three paintings described in the *Gazette*. The hint of an auction was perhaps meant to encourage the casual reader to think that a bargain might be had at the Bazaar. Tuthill's ultimate objective was to gain portrait commissions, but we may suppose that he was quite willing to sell any or all of the works he exhibited. If, in addition to the subjects mentioned in the notice—two portraits of illustrious persons, a view, and "several fancy pieces"—he also showed a few examples of his stock-in-trade, domestic portraiture, then at least nine paintings were on view. There seems to be no way of knowing precisely where he hung them—whether in the picture gallery or a parlor—or what other attractions the Bazaar then offered to the public.

The three paintings Tuthill selected for mention in the notice are of three different subject types. They demonstrated that he had a greater range than most other itinerant artists. *Benjamin West* (fig. 1.3) is a simple bust portrait. *DeWitt Clinton Opening the Erie Canal* (fig. 1.5) is a full-length portrait in the grand manner. *Madison Barracks* (unlocated, but see fig. 1.6) is a view. Any visitor to the Bazaar would have known a good deal about all three subjects, for they were of recent national interest. We may suppose that Tuthill needed little encouragement to tell his viewers about his own association with each of the three subjects.

Tuthill's portrait of his old mentor West, was, for more than a century,

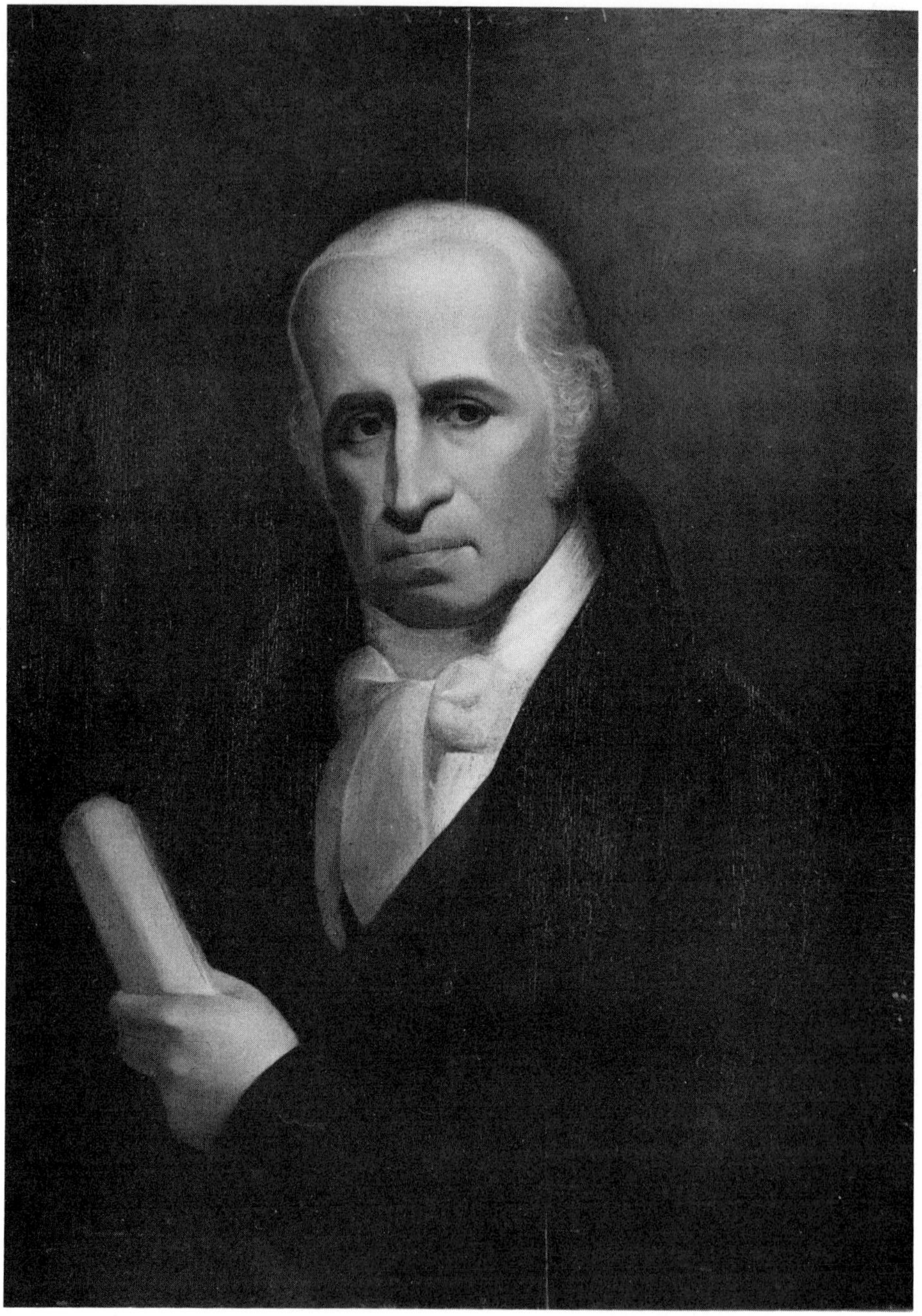

Fig. 1.3. Abraham G. D. Tuthill, *Benjamin West,* c. 1812–15. Oil on wood, 28 × 21⅜ in. Courtesy of the Shelburne Museum, Shelburne, Vermont.

assumed to be from life and was accordingly assigned to Tuthill's years in England, 1800–07. A second version of the portrait exists in a private collection; it lacks the hand and scroll and gives West a slightly milder visage. It is not known which of the two is the earlier or which was exhibited at the Bazaar. Tuthill owned both versions at the end

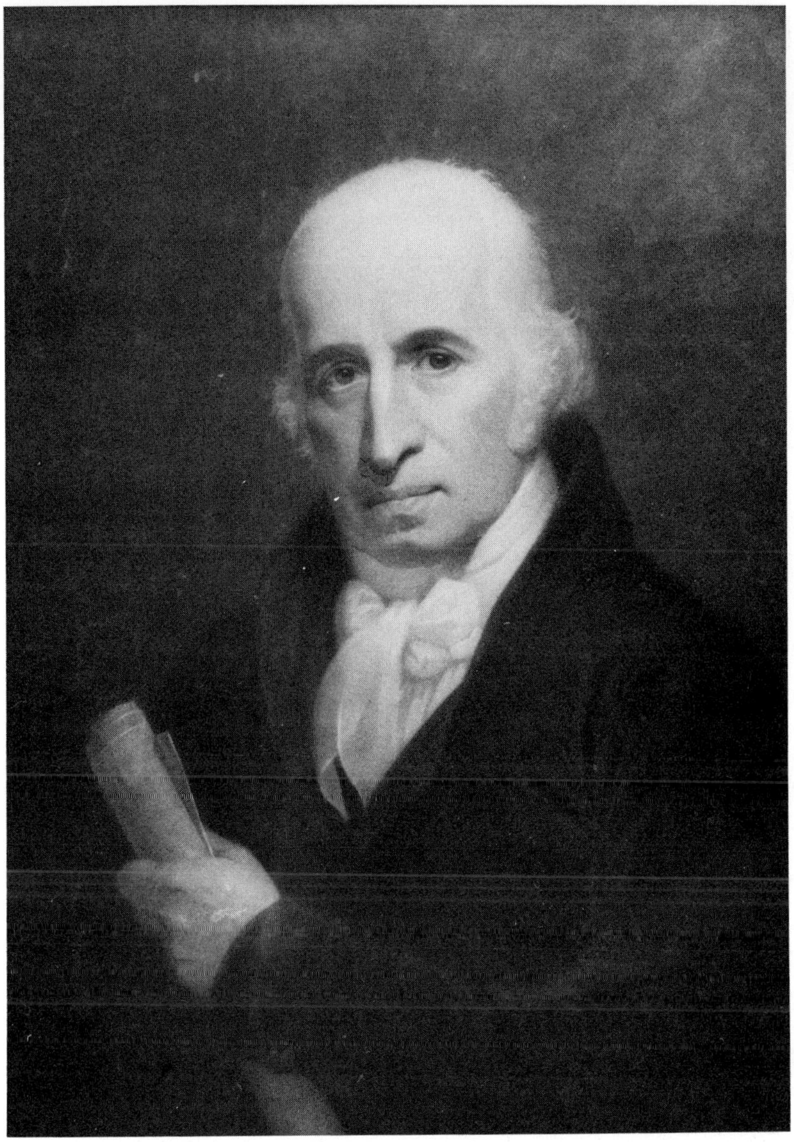

Fig. 1.4. George Dawe, after Andrew Robertson, *Benjamin West,* 1804. Mezzotint, 12 × 9⅝ in. © British Museum.

of his life. The Shelburne Museum version, shown here, is inscribed on the verso, "Benjamin West painted from life by his pupil Abraham G. D. Tuthill." Another inscription in a different hand follows, reading, "Probably in 1798 while studying with West in London." The inscriptions, which were apparently added by descendants of Tuthill's sister, are factually incorrect.

As Dorinda Evans has recently shown, Tuthill did not paint either version from life.[10] Rather, he adapted his likeness of West from George Dawe's mezzotint of 1804 (fig. 1.4) after Andrew Robertson's miniature. It seems reasonable to assume that Tuthill painted both versions in America when West was no longer available to sit for

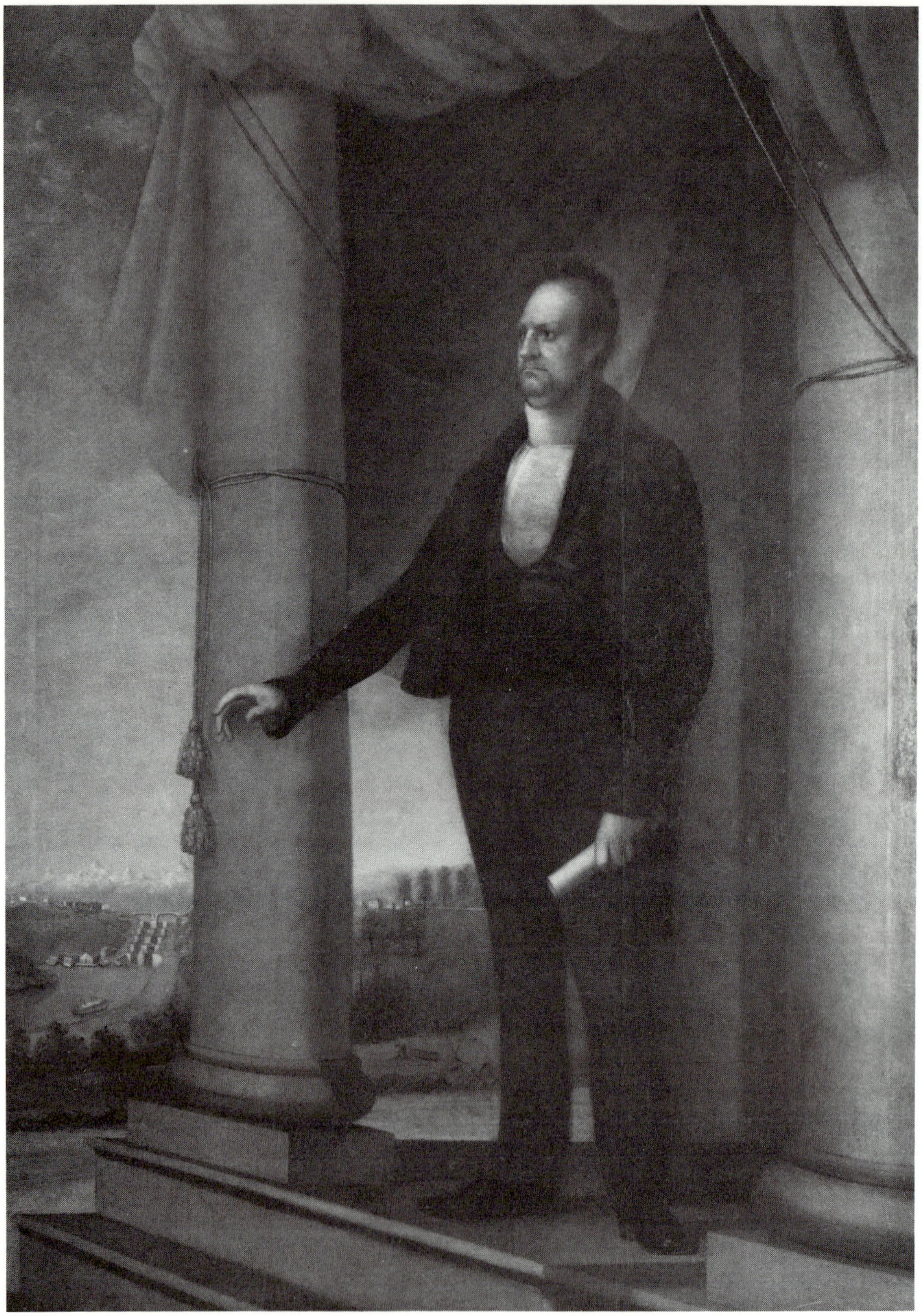

Fig. 1.5. Abraham G. D. Tuthill, *DeWitt Clinton Opening the Erie Canal,* c. 1825–26. Oil on canvas, 91 × 67½ in. Courtesy of the Shelburne Museum, Shelburne, Vermont.

him. The primitiveness of the rendering encourages the assignment of both versions to the years 1808–12, though it may also reflect a difficulty in working from an engraving rather than from a living sitter. Tuthill may indeed have painted West in England between 1800 and 1807—but certainly not as early as 1798, when Tuthill was still in America. If such a portrait once existed, he no longer had access to it when he undertook the likeness he exhibited at the Bazaar. To resurrect his master's countenance, he turned to the Robertson/Dawe image.

Tuthill's life-size portrait of Governor DeWitt Clinton (fig. 1.5), probably painted in 1825, is a much more interesting piece. It shows the artist struggling to work in the grand manner. Clinton satisfied that style's requirement that its subject be a person of true historical importance. He had been mayor of New York City, United States senator, lieutenant governor and was, in 1825, governor of the state of New York. His role in promoting the concept of a canal linking the Hudson River with the Great Lakes and bringing it into being had made him a national hero. The importance of the canal to westward expansion and to the economic and cultural development of vast areas of the United States was understood well before the waterway was completed. By 1830, its success had exceeded the most optimistic expectations. Even so distant a place as Cincinnati profited from the canal-induced growth of trade and settlement around the Great Lakes.

To open the canal officially, Clinton and his party led a flotilla of canal boats on the first through-passage from Buffalo to New York harbor, a trip of two weeks. Festive civic ceremonies greeted the dignitaries at every sizable town along the way. After leaving Buffalo on the morning of the 26th of October, 1825, Clinton's first important stop was at Lockport that evening. Tuthill portrays Clinton at Lockport, specifying the location by showing in the background the step-like series of five double-combined locks that were hailed as one of the great engineering feats of Jacksonian America. Below the locks, figures stand on the deck and cabin of a canal boat, its towline taut but its source of motive power, a mule, hidden by foliage. The portico is presumably contrived; none so grand then existed in Lockport. Close by it runs the canal or another body of water. Clinton sternly congratulates the people. The stumps in the middle ground and the buildings of Lockport signify the taming of nature. Distant clouds billow on the horizon.

Though Tuthill's concept was sound, his execution of it was, for a pupil of West, lamentably inadequate. The perspective of the canal boat and the portico floor, the fit of the base of the Tuscan column on its plinth, the length of Clinton's extended arm—these are merely the most obvious pictorial faults of the picture. Clinton's paunchy figure is a far cry from the idealization expected in the grand manner. Still, it was a good "news" picture, and interest in the occasion it depicts may have deflected attention from its shortcomings. Clinton's trousers make him, along with Lafayette in Samuel F. B. Morse's full-length portrait of 1825, among the first in America to be painted in the newly fashionable mode of dress.[11]

An inscription on a piece of paper attached to the back of the canvas reads in part, "Gov. DeWitt Clinton supposed to be delivering address at opening of Erie Canal (in background) painted from life by Abraham G. D. Tuthill, born 1781 [sic]; died 1848 [sic]. . . . " This inscription by a descendant of Tuthill's sister was added long after the artist's death. It is unlikely that Tuthill painted Clinton from life on the occasion of his address at Lockport—there was no time for it. Tuthill may well have been

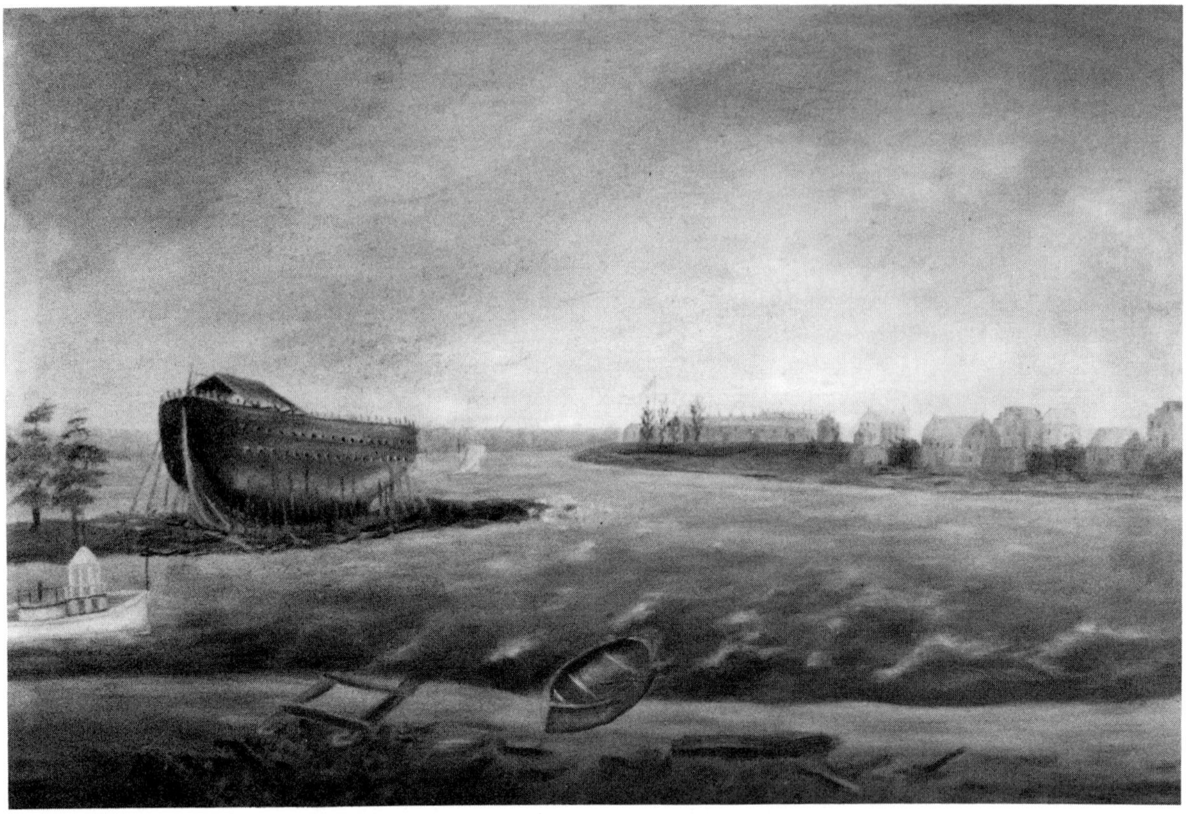

Fig. 1.6. Unknown artist, *View of Madison Barracks, Sackets Harbor, with the Partly Built New Orleans,* c. 1816–20. Oil on canvas, 11¾ × 18 in. Jefferson County (N.Y.) Historical Society. Photo North-South Photography.

present, however. A second likeness of Clinton by Tuthill, a bust portrait also owned by the Shelburne Museum, is a sufficiently different image to have precluded its use as a source for the Lockport painting.

Two creases run from top to bottom on the full length portrait, dividing the picture in three. They may document Tuthill's means of transporting the painting to Cincinnati by removing the canvas from its stretcher, folding it into thirds, and rolling it up for carriage in a tube.

The third painting mentioned in the notice, Tuthill's unlocated view of Madison Barracks at Sackets Harbor, almost certainly offered visitors to the Bazaar not only a depiction of one of the nation's most important military outposts but also one of its most bizarre curiosities. The small village of Sackets Harbor on Lake Ontario in northern New York State became a military station in 1808 for purposes of enforcing the Embargo Act of 1807. With the outbreak of the War of 1812, its strategic location in relation to Canada and the St. Lawrence River made it a major fortified naval station and the locus of much extended and costly warfare. In October 1814, its shipyard began work on the *New Orleans,* a large warship with a keel of 187 feet, a beam of 57 feet, and a depth of hold of 30 feet. In March 1815, following the end of the war, work on the

New Orleans was discontinued but the capacious, virtually complete hull of the ship was preserved in the yard, fitted up with offices and quarters for use as a government building. It remained on the site until the 1880s. Between 1816 and 1819 the federal government erected Madison Barracks nearby to house a regiment of troops. Though the military importance of Sackets Harbor declined following the opening of the Erie Canal, it remained an army outpost into the twentieth century.

An unsigned painting of Madison Barracks ca. 1816–20 (fig. 1.6) in the collections of the Jefferson County Historical Society of Watertown, New York, shows the looming hulk of the *New Orleans* and contrasts this never-to-be-launched piece of naval architecture with the long, trim row of the barracks. Other contemporary depictions of the barracks also include the *New Orleans* as a prominent feature. Tuthill must certainly have done so as well, for he knew this oddity from his visits to Sackets Harbor ca. 1819–20 and knew how it cried out for explanation.

One of the functions of the paintings Tuthill showed—West, Clinton, and the barracks alike—was to provide a basis for story-telling, to give the artist a means of verbally ensnaring the attention of his viewers and establishing with them the kind of rapport that any good tradesman seeks. Itinerant painters needed to be effective salesmen; Tuthill's palaver was sufficiently adequate to bring him success on the road for a quarter of a century. The Bazaar provided him with an uncommonly grand salesroom. It may also have elicited uncommon eloquence from him as he described his pictures. It hardly needs saying that there was little enough eloquence in the paintings themselves.

What Tuthill's career reveals about the practices that worked to "civilize" Ohio, Michigan, western Pennsylvania, and upstate New York between 1815 and 1840 is in some ways more interesting and more important than his achievements as a painter. Like Mrs. Trollope, he claimed, with at least a modicum of justification, to be a representative of high culture and, like her, he attempted to sell semblances of that culture to a provincial public that hankered after a taste of it. She failed in the effort and took her revenge in *Domestic Manners*. He succeeded and left in more than a hundred paintings scattered from Ohio to Vermont a late, faint, distorted echo of Benjamin West, barely audible in the clamor of Jacksonian America.

NOTES

This essay is offered in honor of Elizabeth Gilmore Holt's interest in, and contributions to the study of, the popular culture of Jacksonian America. I thank Alyce Jordan for assistance in research.

1. *Daily Cincinnati Gazette*, 30 Nov. 1830, p. 3. I have found no subsequent mention of the sale.

2. The best brief introduction to Mrs. Trollope's years in the United States and to Hervieu's career as an artist is Donald Smalley's introduction and extensive notes to his edition of her *Domestic Manners of the Americans* (New York: Alfred A. Knopf, 1949).

3. Carl Abbott, "The Location and External Appearance of Mrs. Trollope's Bazaar," *Journal of the Society of Architectural Historians* 29 (1970): 256–60; Clay Lancaster, "The Egyptian Hall and Mrs. Trollope's Bazaar," *Magazine of Art* 43 (March 1950): 94–99. The description "Graeco-Moresco-Gothic-Chinese" comes from Thomas Hamilton, *Men and Manners in America* (London: T. Cadell, 1833), 169–70.

4. Lancaster, "Egyptian Hall," 98.

5. For *The Landing of Lafayette* see Smalley in Trollope, *Domestic Manners*, xlix–li; and John Francis McDermott, "Mrs. Trollope's Illustrator: Auguste Hervieu in America," *Gazette des beaux-arts* s.6 51 (1958): 169–90.

6. The Scheffer portrait is at the United States Capitol, Washington, D.C. The Leroux engraving and adaptations of it were circulated widely in advance of and during Lafayette's tour of 1824–25.

7. Alfred Frankenstein and Arthur K. D. Healy, "Two Journeymen Painters," *Art in America* 38 (February 1950): 47–63; Margaret W. M. Shaeffer, "Tracing Artist Tuthill's Steps through the North," *Jefferson County Historical Society Bulletin* 15 (1974): 2–9; Helen Wortis, "Abraham G. D. Tuthill of Oyster Ponds," *Long Island Forum* 39 (October 1976): 218–22, and "The Letters of Abraham G. D. Tuthill to Sylvester Dering," *Journal of Long Island History* 15 (1979): 45–69; and David Tatham, *Abraham Tuthill: Portrait Painter in the Young Republic*, exhibition catalogue (Watertown, NY: Jefferson County Historical Society, 1983), 5–24.

8. William Dunlap, *A History of the Rise and Progress of the Arts of Design in the United States* (New York: George P. Scott, 1834), 2:149–50.

9. Ibid.

10. Dorinda Evans, *Benjamin West and His American Students* (Washington, D.C.: Smithsonian Institution Press, 1980), 144–45.

11. Trousers are shown in numerous American genre subjects between 1820 and 1825 and perhaps in a few portraits, but Morse's *Lafayette* surely deserves its reputation as the first portrait of a trousered person of major importance by a leading American painter.

2

The POPULARIZATION of GENTILITY

Illustrations in American Literary Annuals

GEORGIA BRADY BUMGARDNER

BETWEEN 1825 AND THE OUTBREAK OF THE CIVIL WAR, literary annuals—compilations of prose and poetry frequently of a sentimental and romantic nature and often elegantly bound and profusely illustrated—were a fixture on the American publishing scene. Their antecedents were the almanac, which first became popular in Germany and France, and the first English annual published by Rudolph Ackerman in London in November 1822. Copies were sent to America, and its success on both sides of the Atlantic was immediate.[1] Three years later the American market generated its own version of the literary annual. Called the *Atlantic Souvenir*, its first issue appeared in Philadelphia published by the firm of Carey & Lea in time for Christmas 1825. Others soon followed, and at the peak of their popularity in the late 1840s thirty annuals were vying for readers and selling in editions of as many as ten thousand copies each.

The vogue for the literary annual can be attributed to an expanding educated middle-class public that delighted in deluxe illustrated editions of genteel literature. Regarded as in every way "tasteful," they made ideal gifts for women, because they could be counted on to be polite, free from vulgarity, and genteel in manner and appearance, though seldom brilliant in content. In many of the extant copies affectionate inscriptions testify to their function as gifts from men to fiancées, wives, sisters, and mothers.

From the very first, expectations for the literary annuals were high. A reviewer wrote of the first *Atlantic Souvenir* (1826):

> The plan of this work is calculated to have so good an effect on the taste of the community, that we hope the publishers will be encouraged to continue it annually. Their aim should be, as far as possible, to enlist the best writers in different parts of the country, to procure articles on American topics, and designs of American scenery. It will thus have a character and a value to itself, not to be found in any other works of a similar kind.[2]

The illustrations were integral to the literary annual format; if anything it was the literature that was given second rank. Pictures were either found or commissioned and then authors were hired to write the stories and poems. This in part explains both why so much critical attention was devoted to the illustrations and why the annuals favored particular themes. Between 1835 and 1845 they show a shift in subject matter from landscape to genre to romantic scenes, as editors and writers naturally leaned toward subjects that could easily find a literary companion.

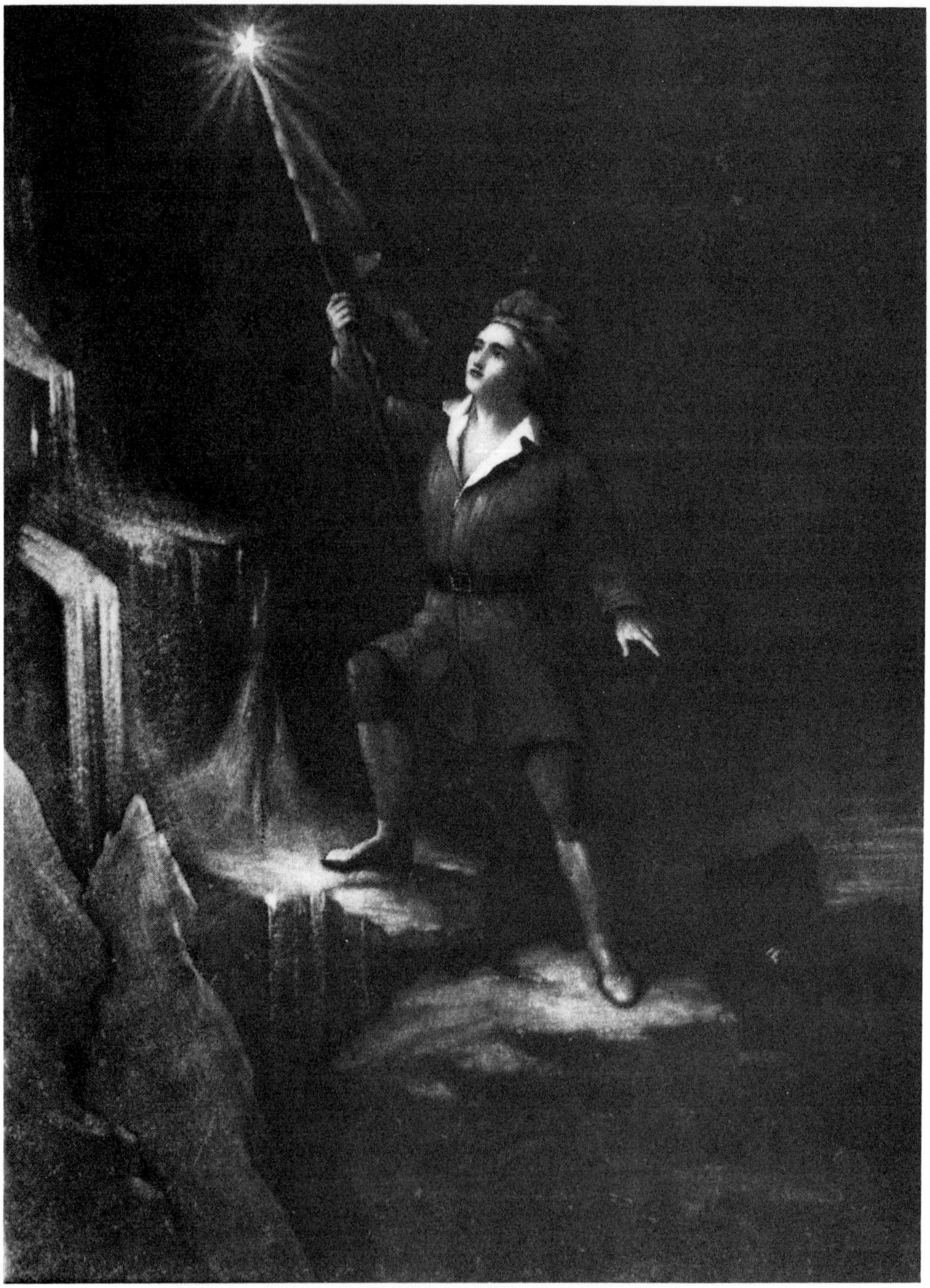

Fig. 2.1. *Excelsior,* engraved by John Sartain (1808–97), after a painting by Thomas Buchanan Read (1822–72), in *The Rose of Sharon* for 1845 (Boston, 1844). Courtesy of the American Antiquarian Society.

Though the result was a decline in artistic merit and eventually a lapse into over-sentimentality, the quality of reproduction improved, thanks to advances in technology, especially steel engraving, which began to replace copper as the predominant medium for reproduction just as these publications appeared in the market. Although it has been suggested that the literary annuals, beginning with the *Atlantic Souvenir,* were the first to use engraved reproductions of original paintings and drawings,[3] this is not the case. Engraved reproductions of American paintings and watercolors—landscapes, genre scenes, portraits, and literary subjects—had been illustrating magazines since the late 1780s.[4] They were primitive in technique, however, until around 1820 when an American engraver and inventor, Jacob Perkins, patented a process which involved decarbonizing steel to make it soft enough to receive impressions from dies for bank-note engraving. The steel was then hardened through another process,[5] and engravers and copperplate printers soon adapted the process to the production of illustrations in both Great Britain and the United States. John Sartain, a prolific engraver, describes in his *Brief Sketch of the History of Engraving* how the steel-engraving technique could be combined with etching to create strong, dark lines, which would withstand the printing of large editions.[6]

Lithography was rarely used. Its grainy texture was unsuited to the fine line work that had become the accepted norm for most publications, and the octavo format of the literary annual was too small for lithography to be used to advantage in them. Mezzotint, on the other hand, was popular. It underwent something of a revival in the mid-nineteenth century, and many engravers of illustrations for literary annuals used it. John Sartain was its foremost practitioner, and over four hundred of his mezzotints appear in some sixty-five annuals.[7] Sartain simplified the technique by etching the outlines and areas of deep shadow, an innovation that facilitated the work (fig. 2.1).

As the century progressed, technical innovations were eagerly adopted by the publishers of annuals as they appeared. A color plate printed in London by George Baxter was described as a "rare and most effective" frontispiece for the *Missionary Memorial* for 1846 (fig. 2.2).[8] When chromolithography was introduced a critic wrote:

> The publishers of this most beautiful Annual [the *Iris*] have certainly surpassed themselves in the liberal quantity and gorgeous finish of the illustrations. The designs are by Captain Eastman and the plates are in Duval's best style of coloring. In all that relates to artistic effect, The Iris certainly has the highest claims to admiration; and the subjects being for the most part American, give a value and freshness to the volume particularly desirable in these days of old designs and worn-out engravings.[9]

The subject matter was also new—the lives and legends of American Indians (fig. 2.3).

As a result of the high standards the annuals were able to achieve, technical mediocrity was also quickly recognized and invited the critics' scorn. *The Pearl* and *The Offering* for December 1833 ran afoul of critical opinion for poor reproductions: "As works of art, neither of these Annuals are worthy of notice. We have the illustrations of Rogers' Italy, and some other well-known prints served up to us in a style of inferior mezzotint, and palmed upon the public as the superb embellishments of an expensive Annual. It is almost too bad."[10] John Gadsby Chapman, the illustrator of Harper's Bible, supplied nine works for the *Opal* for 1844, of which a reviewer wrote,

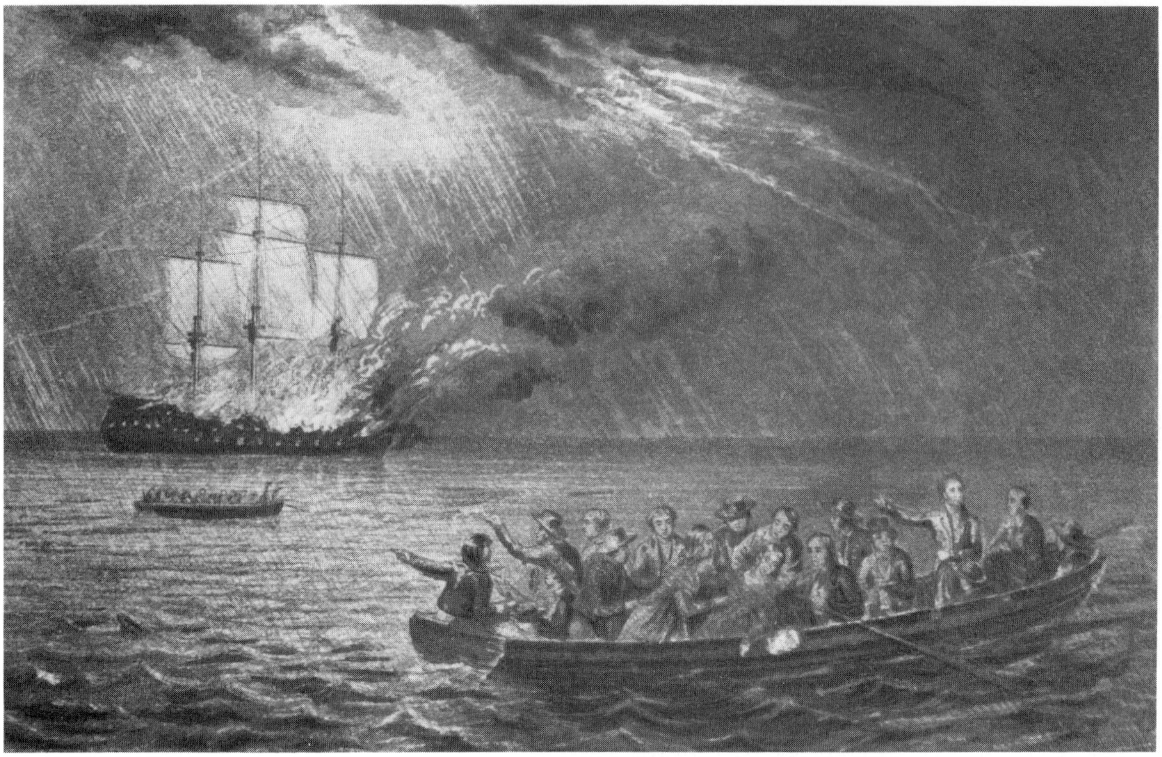

Fig. 2.2. *Destruction of the Tanjore by Lightning off Ceylon*, printed by George Baxter (1804–67) in *The Missionary Memorial* (New York, 1845). Courtesy of the American Antiquarian Society.

"Some of the engravings are handsome, and others quite ordinary," but generally speaking the volume "will be an ornament on the centre-table of any purchaser."[11] Undaunted by the rather faint praise, the publisher commissioned Chapman to supply designs for the next three years.

For a while the use of these reproductive techniques remained restricted by the relatively few original works of art available for reproduction. More than one publisher had earlier complained about the dearth of original paintings, the difficulty of locating them, and the unwillingness of their owners to grant permission to reproduce them. But beginning in 1825, the literary annuals began rapidly to become the major vehicle for disseminating at least a certain kind of art,[12] and the output of American painters began to increase as well.

In the first issue of the *Atlantic Souvenir* only two of the seven illustrations had American subjects; one of them was *Montmorenci* engraved by Cephas G. Childs after a painting by Thomas Doughty (fig. 2.4). A year later, in January 1827, the *North American Review* critic noted with pleasure more engravings of American scenery: there was a view of New York (fig. 2.5), engraved by Peter Maverick after a painting by William Guy Wall, which was "engraved as well as we could wish," and views of Trenton Falls and Passaic Falls. The other six illustrations, though of European subjects, were competently engraved by Americans. Wrote the critic:

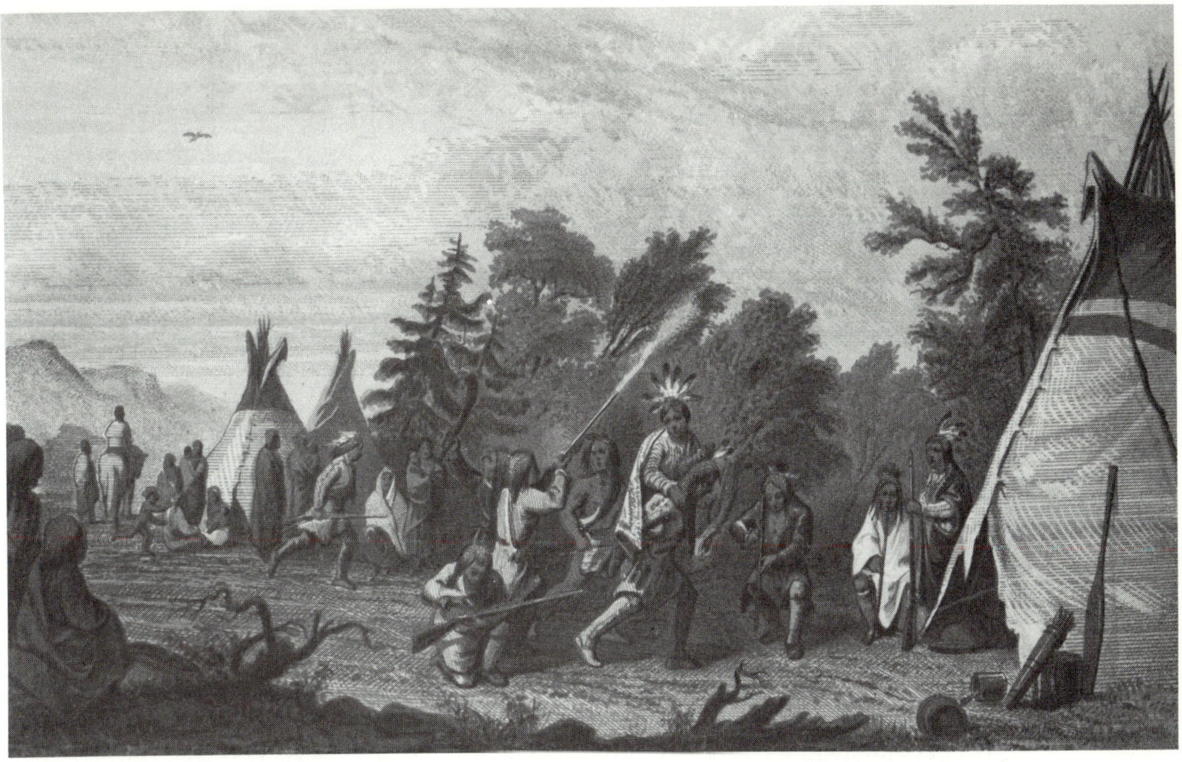

Fig. 2.3. *Marriage Custom of the Indians*, drawn on stone by Christian Schussele (c. 1824–79) after Seth Eastman (1808–75); lithographed by Peter S. Duval in *The Iris* for 1852 (Philadelphia, 1851). Courtesy of the American Antiquarian Society.

> The Souvenir [is] not merely [to be regarded] as a pretty book for a New Year's present to one's friend, but as a means of exciting public attention to the fine arts, as an encouragement to our painters and engravers, and as a pledge of future excellence in a department of art which has hitherto been greatly neglected. . . . It is time that correct and finished illustrations of our scenery were published. It is time that our wealthy men encouraged such designs, and that a public taste for them was cultivated. . . . Let the tools of the engraver be employed on something else besides door plates and visiting cards. It is chiefly on account of our desire to see the improvement of art and taste among us, that we hope that the publishers of the Souvenir . . . may always receive ample remuneration from the public, so that they in turn may amply remunerate the artists in their employment, and stimulate them to a cheerful and vigorous exertion of their powers.[13]

In fact they apparently were well paid. Carey & Lea in Philadelphia paid engravers an average of $225 per plate; Carey's average payment to Sully was $200 for a painting. These were substantial amounts at a time when many wage earners made only one to two dollars per day.[14] If a painting to be reproduced were privately owned, the owner in addition to being noted in the list of illustrations (or "embellishments," as they were often then called) was sometimes also paid for the privilege of copying and publishing his property.

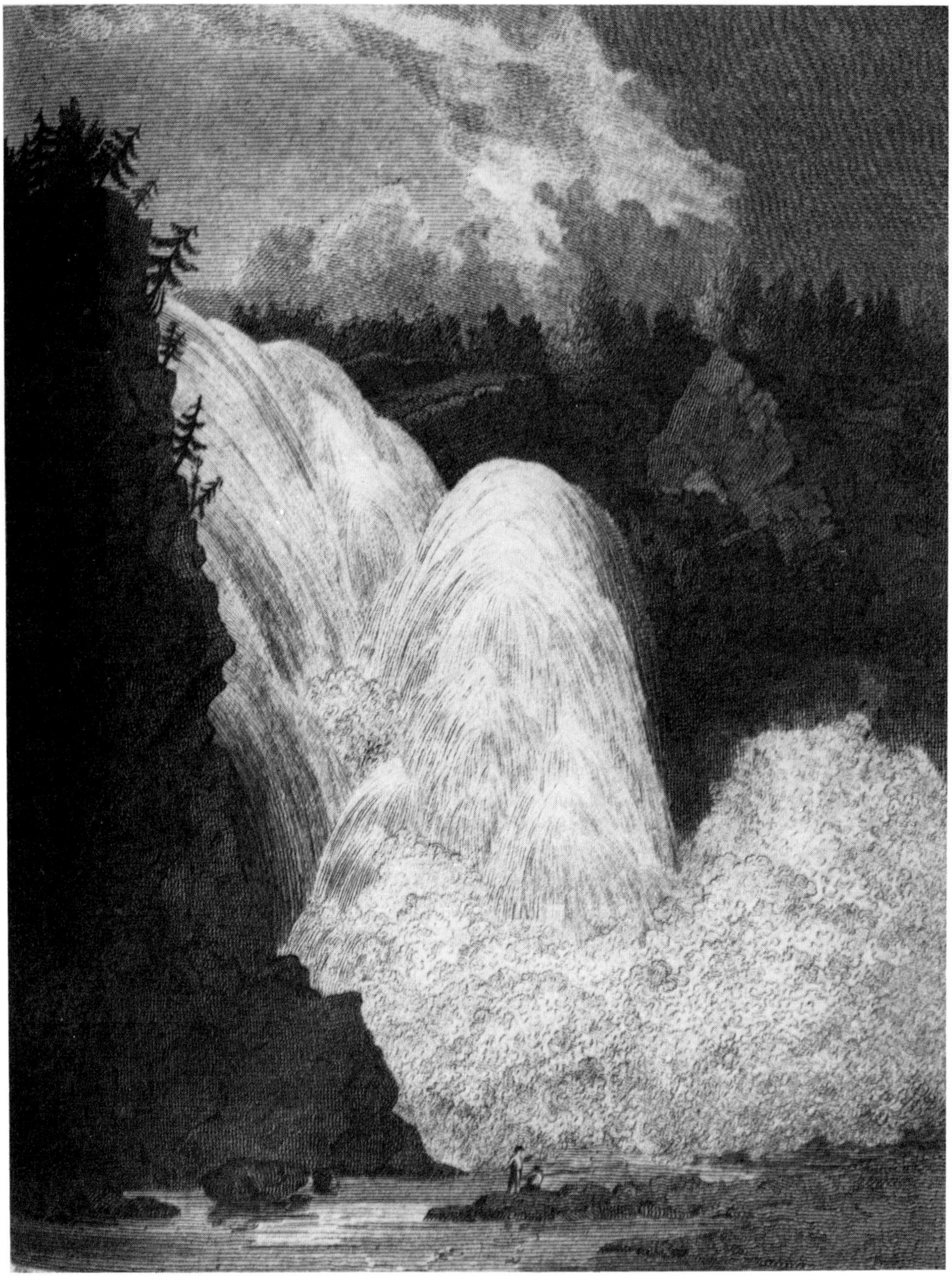

Fig. 2.4. *Montmorenci,* engraved by Cephas G. Childs (1793–1871) after Thomas Doughty (1793–1856) in *The Atlantic Souvenir* for 1826 (Philadelphia, 1825). Courtesy of the American Antiquarian Society.

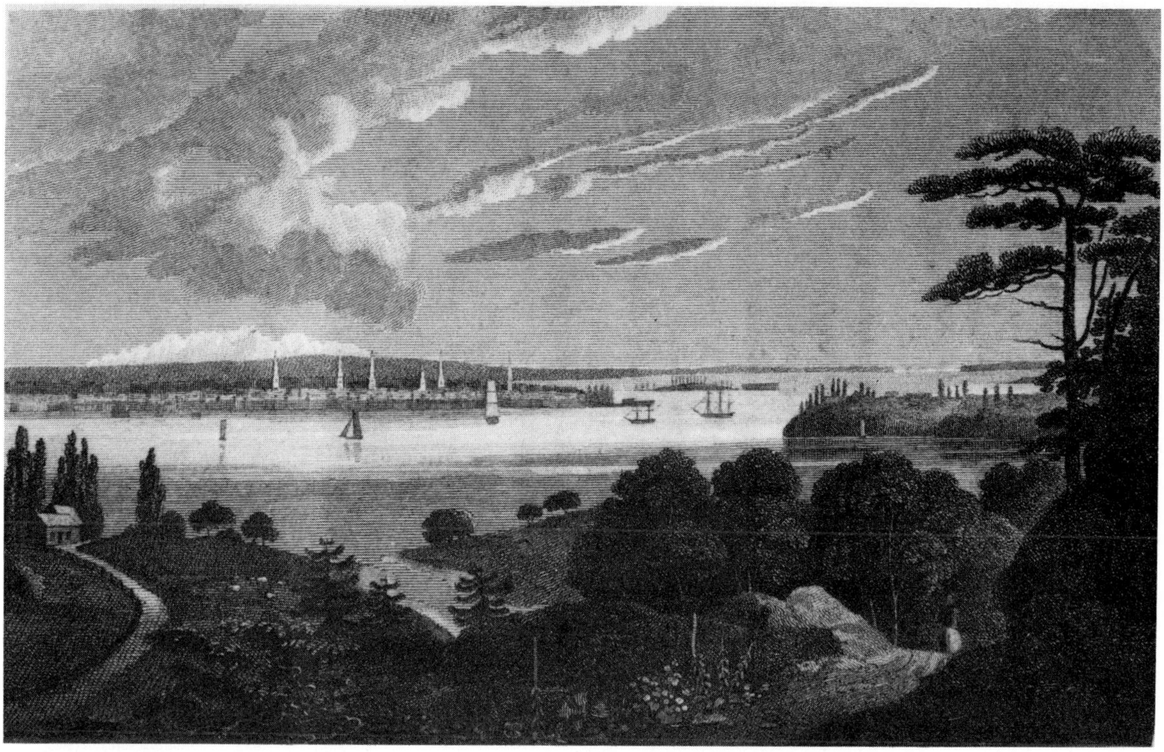

Fig. 2.5. *New York*, engraved by Peter Maverick (1780–1831) after William Guy Wall (1792–?) in *The Atlantic Souvenir* for 1827 (Philadelphia, 1826). Courtesy of the American Antiquarian Society.

Particularly during the decade 1825–35, when the vogue for landscape painting was at its zenith, the demand for landscapes so exceeded the supply that even amateur artists were allowed to compete in the market. Henry Inman wrote to the engraver Cephas G. Childs in 1829: "The landscape drawing which accompanies this note is the one I spoke of to you and upon which you are to expend all the skill you can spare for the credit of our N[ew] York *Talisman*. It is done by an amateur friend of mine, John Neilson Jr. by name and should you have the good fortune to meet him face to face, you will find him to be a good fellow by nature."[15] In another letter, Inman explained that Childs would receive $150 for engraving the illustration on steel. The publisher's schedule required that the engraving be completed by the middle of July if the finished volumes were to be ready in time for Christmas.[16] Neilson supplied two other landscapes for the same publisher.

By commissioning and reproducing paintings by men like Thomas Cole, Alvan Fisher, William Guy Wall, and Thomas Doughty, the annuals both encouraged American artists and interested the public in their work. In the thirteen years that Samuel G. Goodrich edited and published the *Token*, he employed forty American engravers and reproduced many American paintings, including some from his own collection.[17] Exhibition records indicate that a few publishers and editors purchased and exhibited the paintings reproduced in their annuals. Samuel G. Goodrich owned several paintings that he both exhibited and published, including Alvan Fisher's *Prairie on Fire,* which was exhibited at the Boston Athenaeum and published in the *Token* for 1829 and the *Garland* for 1830.[18] Edward L. Carey of the Philadelphia publishing firm, Carey & Hart, purchased fourteen paintings from Thomas Sully between 1833 and 1845. Several of these, including the portrait of the actress Fanny Kemble, were displayed before they were published.[19]

After the mid-1830s the vogue for landscapes receded. A critic for the *North American Review* wrote in January 1834 that pictures "should not only gratify the eye of taste by the beauty of their embellishments, but should be made the vehicle of good principles and valuable information."[20] A review of *The Whirlwind,* engraved by Edward Gallaudet after a drawing by Thomas Cole, said: "Like a picture of a waterfall, it cannot satisfy the mind. True, there are the twisted tree—the prostrate forest—the black and frowning sky; but we lack the 'rushing of a mighty wind'—the motion of the storm clouds—the all-pervading roar of the elements. The scene is beyond the blazon of the pencil." (fig. 2.6)[21] The critic seemed to want all nature's wrath to be portrayed in the small space of an engraved illustration. A decade earlier, critics were praising illustrations of American scenery and begging for more. After the mid-1830s, illustrations were expected to express lofty ideals, not just a realistic and factual rendering of a view.

The engraved landscapes were soon replaced by reproductions of genre and narrative paintings. No landscapes by Alvan Fisher appear in the literary annuals after 1832; none by Thomas Cole after 1837; and none by Thomas Doughty after 1839. Reproductions of paintings by landscape artists who reached their maturity in the 1830s are even rarer. For example, only one reproduction of Kensett's works—and that one engraved by Kensett himself—can be found.[22] Aside from the new demand for "lofty themes," one reason for this loss of popularity was that landscape lent itself rather poorly to the purposes of a literary publication; it offered only very limited possibilities to the writers whose job it was to weave stories around the illustrations that the editors of the literary annuals chose to reproduce. Genre offered a far greater variety of options, although even a genre painting could occasionally baffle the writer's skill. One William E. Burton was commissioned by Carey to write a story around a painting by William Sidney Mount called *The Long Story* (or sometimes *The Tough Story*), owned by the Baltimore collector Robert Gilmore (fig. 2.7). Carey described it as a "wounded man inflicting a long yarn upon his listeners," but Burton decided to write to Mount himself asking for guidance as to its meaning. "The completeness and graphic nature of your designs in general forbids the idea of a want of purpose in the group in question. May I ask you the favor of your opinions on the subject?"[23] Burton never wrote the story for Carey. The reproduction of Mount's painting appeared in *The Gift* for 1842 accompanied by a story that the humorist Seba Smith had provided. The editor of *Graham's Magazine* wrote about the engraving:

> Mr. Mount's merits are those of acute observation and fidelity. These merits, although not of the highest order, have the advantage of being universally appreciable. This is an advantage which he secures—clinches—by dealing only in homely subjects. If he has ideality (a question which as yet we have had no means of deciding) and would employ his peculiar talents upon loftier themes, he might attain a very desirable eminence indeed.... Nothing could be more true to nature than the picture before us; but the painter has sacrificed to this truth (at some

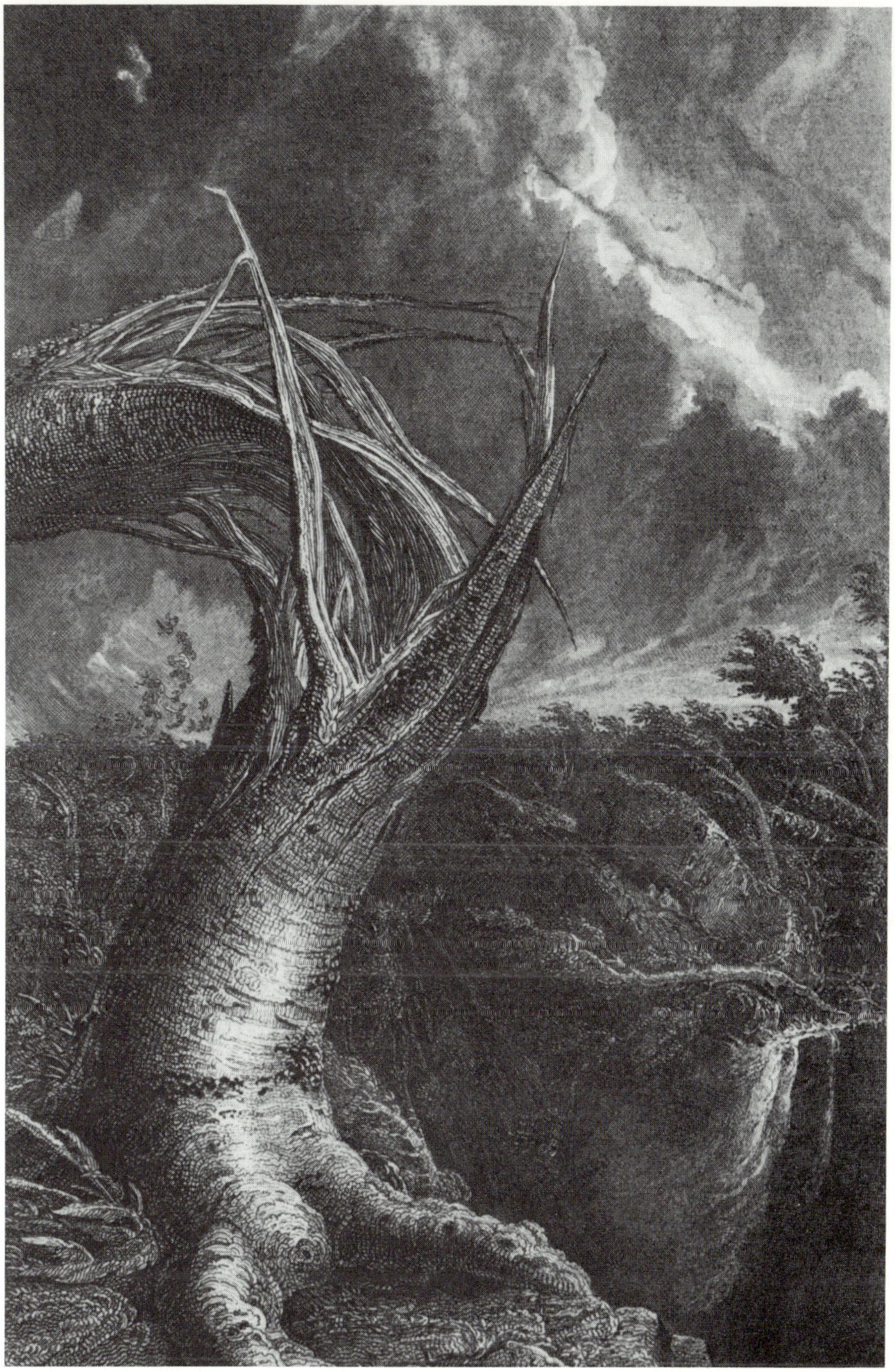

Fig. 2.6. *The Whirlwind*, engraved by Edward Gallaudet (1809–47) after Thomas Cole (1801–48) in *The Token and Atlantic Souvenir* for 1837 (Boston, 1836). Courtesy of the American Antiquarian Society.

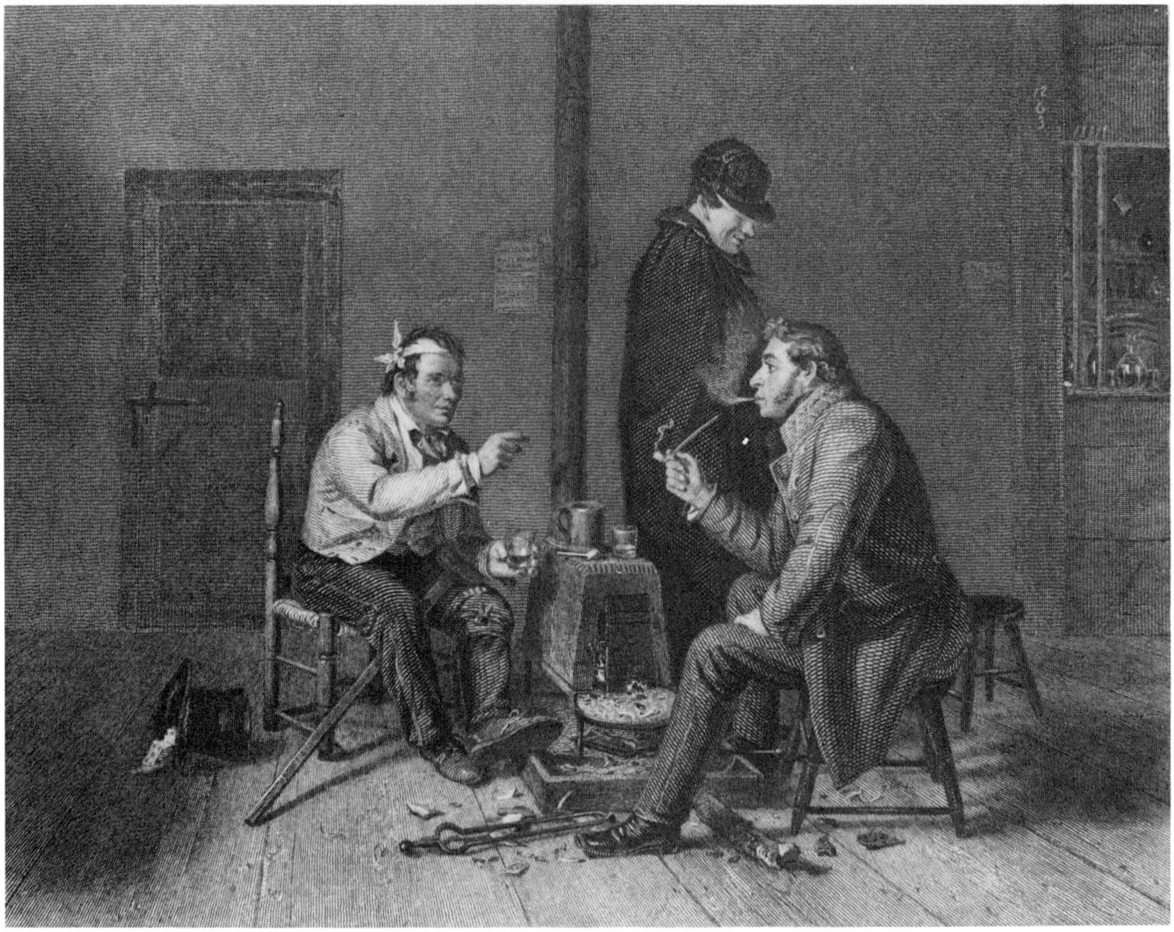

Fig. 2.7. *The Tough Story,* engraved by Joseph Ives Pease (1809–83) after William Sidney Mount (1807–68) in *The Gift* for 1842 (Philadelphia, 1841). Courtesy of the American Antiquarian Society.

> points) artistical effects of superior value. What can be more displeasing, for example, than the unrelieved nakedness of the wall in the background, or the situation of the group precisely in the centre of the design, or, especially than the tall regular stove pipe, running up parrallel [sic] with the back of the standing figure, and dividing the apartment exactly in two?[24]

Had the critic had his way, the background would have been filled with objects or perhaps with a window looking onto the outside world. The stove and its pipe would have been moved, and the composition thereby weakened. In Barbara Novak's view, Mount was a "sophisticated designer, a thoughtful painter, whose best works can be measured formally against other works of quality in the history of art."[25] The wall was blank and the stovepipe was in the middle because that arrangement was integral to the composition. Burton had apparently recognized this, even if he could not fathom the painter's message.

If the critics did not like Mount's work, what did they like? The same writer who criticized Mount's composition wrote of *The Sled,* engraved by W. E. Tucker after a painting by John Gadsby Chapman, that it was "a most effective design, evincing the well-educated artist. The idea of rapid motion is skillfully embodied in the countenance of the boy, in the peculiar falling curve of the hill, and exquisitely corroborated in the whirl of the clouds. This is the true artistic keeping,"[26] a description that reflects the middle-class taste for sentimental prints on parlor walls (fig. 2.8). A mezzotint by John Sartain after a painting by Thomas Sully was called "a perfect gem" and a "master-piece of the art of engraving in mezzotint."[27] In December 1844 another critic wrote of an engraving by John Cheney after a painting by Gilbert Stuart, "There is an inexpressible sweetness and grace in this little vignette, an idea of which is impossible to convey in words."[28] It is not surprising then that Mount's work was not greeted by these proponents of middle-class sensibility with more enthusiasm. Sweetness and grace were notably absent from *The Long Story.*

Considering this reaction, why was Mount singled out for the distinction of being the only significant genre painter of his generation whose works appeared more than once in the annuals? Apparently, along with Sully, he was a particular favorite of the publisher Carey, who had at least four of his paintings in his private collection. Together with Abraham Hart, Carey published the *Gift* from 1836 to 1845 and also issued other annuals in which he reproduced Mount paintings, including *The Long Story,* nine times. In spite of the criticism, incidentally, Mount was apparently pleased to have reproductions of his paintings appear in them.[29]

Fortunately the annuals were not the only medium for the dissemination of American painting. By mid-century exhibitions had become common in the cities, and some sophisticated print publishers reproduced works of major artists—George Caleb Bingham, David G. Blythe, Martin Johnson Heade, John F. Kensett, Fitz Hugh Lane, and Robert Salmon—whose lack of "gentility" or devotion to landscape made their work inappropriate for middle-class female eyes or difficult to integrate into the literary annual.

But whatever their shortcomings, the annuals made high quality reproductions of both American and several centuries of European art readily available to a generation of Americans that might otherwise never been exposed to it at all. English artists Edmund Thomas Parris, William Henry Bartlett, Joseph M. W. Turner, Richard Westall, and Thomas Gainsborough were popular; among the old master painters reproduced were Domenichino, Baroccio, Raphael, Holbein, Claude Lorrain, Murillo, Rubens, and Watteau. Van Dyke's portrait of Charles IV was reproduced in the *Gallery of Mezzotints* by John Sartain, and Rembrandt's *Peasant Girl* was engraved by J. Pease. Religiously oriented literary annuals relied almost exclusively on old master paintings, for American religious paintings were rare. Correggio's *Ecce Homo* was issued in the *Mayflower* for 1847, and Gaspard Poussin's *Landscape with Abraham and Isaac* and Annibale Caracci's *St. John in the Desert* were reproduced for the pages of the *Rose of Sharon* in 1852.

In subject matter they were conservative: first, landscapes by artists of the Hudson River School because they were unlikely to violate the canons of middle-class taste; then, genre paintings of a sentimental sort and acceptable religious subjects that avoided themes that might be regarded as lacking in gentility—one will seek in vain for a Saint Sebastian pierced by arrows or other topics that would provide the artist with an excuse to paint a sensuous nude.

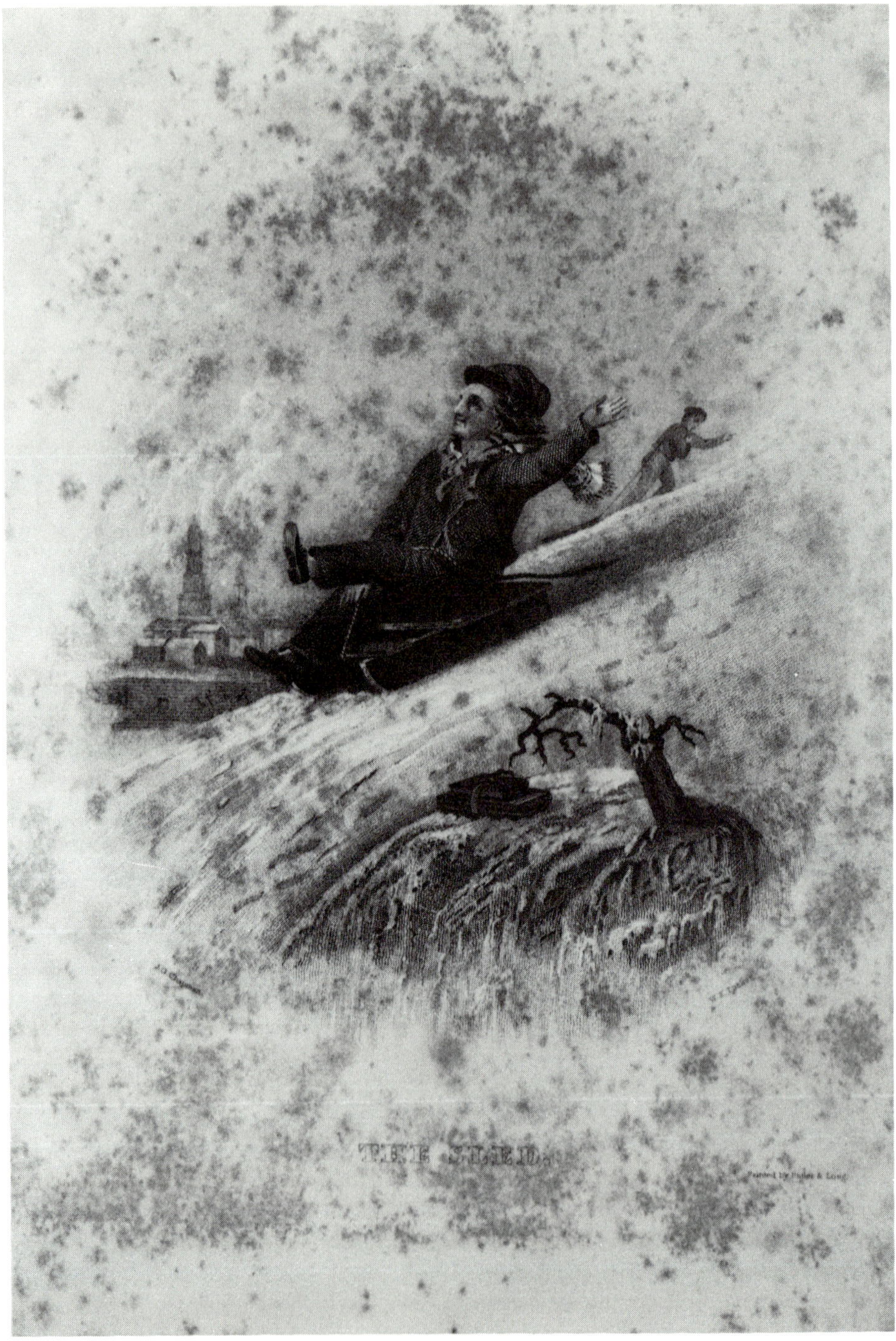

Fig. 2.8. *The Sled,* engraved by William E. Tucker (1801–57) after John Gadsby Chapman (1808–89) in *The Gift* for 1842 (Philadelphia, 1841). Courtesy of the American Antiquarian Society.

Reproductions of old master paintings were not derived directly from the originals but were copied from European engraved reproductions available in the United States or smaller reproductions found in imported publications or, less frequently, painted copies of old master canvases in public and private collections. Neither the choice nor the method invariably met with critical approval. A critic of the *Token* and the *Atlantic Souvenir* wrote:

> They disappoint us. Have we no original talent, no original subjects, in our great and glorious country, that in our choice repositories of the arts of design and engraving we must exhibit copies of foreign skill—and old copies, too, of prints which have gathered dust and yellowness during the summer in the windows of all the print-sellers in our principal cities? Must we depend forever on transatlantic genius and foreign talent? No less than eleven out of the thirteen embellishments to the work are of this character. . . . We do not find fault with their execution—for it is in the main, creditable—but we blame this truckling dependence upon foreign imagination. It is high time that our annuals should exhibit something like originality in their embellishments.[30]

In the mid-1850s, Samuel Griswold Goodrich, editor (and occasionally publisher) of the *Token* between 1828 and 1841 wrote: "At last the race of Annuals [draws] near to the end of its career, yet not without having produced a certain revolution in public taste. . . . These charming works scattered the very gems of art far and wide, making the reading mass familiar with the finest specimens of engraving, and not only cultivating an appetite for this species of luxury, but in fact exalting the general standard of taste all over the civilized world."[31]

NOTES

1. The history of the production of literary annuals is found in Ralph Thompson, *American Literary Annuals & Gift Books 1825–1865* (New York: H. W. Wilson Company, 1936).

2. *North American Review* 22 (1826): 446.

3. Grunewald Center for the Graphic Arts, *The American Personality: The Artist-Illustrator of Life in the United States, 1860–1930* (Los Angeles, 1976), 13.

4. See Peter J. Parker and Stefanie Munsing Winkelbauer, "Embellishments for Practical Repositories: Eighteenth-Century American Magazine Illustration," in *Eighteenth-Century Prints in Colonial America*, ed. Joan D. Dometsch (Williamsburg, Va., 1979), 71–97; and Benjamin Lewis, *A Guide to Engravings in American Magazines 1744–1810* (New York: New York Public Library, 1959).

5. Frederick W. Faxon, *Literary Annuals and Gift Books: A Bibliography 1823–1903* (Pinner, Middlesex, U.K.: Private Libraries Association, 1973), 19.

6. John Sartain, *A Brief Sketch of the History and Practice of Engraving* (Philadelphia, 1880), 12.

7. One means of access to the body of illustrations in literary annuals is the engraver index of E. Bruce Kirkham and John W. Fink, *Indices to American Literary Annuals and Gift Books, 1825–1865* (New Haven: Research Publications, 1975).

8. *The Knickerbocker* 26 (1845): 589.

9. *Graham's Magazine* 39 (1851): 380.

10. *The Knickerbocker* 2 (1833): 470–71.

11. *Graham's Magazine* 25 (1844): 48.

12. The dissemination of fine art in literary annuals has been described by David S. Lovejoy in "American Painting in Early Nineteenth-Century Gift Books," *American Quarterly* 7 (1955): 345–61; and by Benjamin Rowland in "Popular Romanticism: Art and the Gift Books," *Art Quarterly* 20 (1957): 365–81. I am indebted to Lovejoy's study for leading me to the reviews in contemporary literary journals.

13. *North American Review* 24 (1827): 229–30.

14. David Kaser, ed., *The Cost Book of Carey & Lea, 1825–1838* (Philadelphia: University of Pennsylvania Press, 1963), 275–84; figures for 1840 taken from Carroll D. Wright, *History of Wages and Prices in Massachusetts: 1752–1883* (Boston: Wright & Potter Printing Co., 1885), 120.

15. Letter dated 27 May 1829 in the Henry Inman Collection, Manuscript Department, American Antiquarian Society, Worcester, Mass.

16. Letter dated 27 April 1829, Inman Collection (cited above).

17. Daniel Roselle, *Samuel Griswold Goodrich, Creator of Peter Parley* (Albany, N.Y.: SUNY Press, 1968), 102–4.

18. Robert F. Perkins Jr. and William J. Gavin III, eds., *Boston Athenaeum Art Exhibition Index, 1827–1874* (Boston: Library of the Boston Athenaeum, 1980).

19. Anna Wells Rutledge, *Cumulative Record of Exhibition Catalogues, The Pennsylvania Academy of the Fine Arts, 1807–1870* (Philadelphia: American Philosophical Society, 1955).

20. *North American Review* 38 (1834): 198.

21. *The Knickerbocker* 8 (1836): 484.

22. This engraving is reproduced in John Paul Driscoll and John K. Howat, *John Frederick Kensett: An American Master* (New York: W. W. Norton, 1985), 16.

23. This letter and others concerning the reproductions of Mount's works are published in Alfred Frankenstein, *William Sidney Mount* (New York: Harry N. Abrams, 1975), 74–78.

24. *Graham's Magazine* 19 (1841): 250.

25. Barbara Novak, *American Painting of the Nineteenth Century* (New York: Praeger, 1969), 149.

26. *Graham's Magazine* 19 (1841): 250.

27. *The Knickerbocker* 24 (1844): 593.

28. *Graham's Magazine* 26 (1844): 295.

29. Letter from William S. Mount to Edward L. Carey, 9 January 1842; Gratz Collection, Case 8, Box 2, Historical Society of Pennsylvania, and Frankenstein, *William Sidney Mount*, 76–77.

30. *The Knickerbocker* 4 (1834): 318–19.

31. Samuel Griswold Goodrich, *Recollections of a Lifetime* (New York: Miller, Orton & Mulligan, 1856), p. 261.

3

WHISTLER'S FIRST ONE-MAN EXHIBITION RECONSTRUCTED

ROBIN SPENCER

IN THE DEVELOPMENT OF MODERNISM, 1874 represents an *annus mirabilis* for the history of art. On 15 April, on second-floor premises off the Boulevard des Capucines, Paris, recently vacated by the photographer Nadar, the *Société anonyme des artistes peintres, sculpteurs, graveurs etc.* held their first group exhibition and were soon to be collectively known as the Impressionists. Within weeks, in a leased and specially designed gallery on Pall Mall, London, the Paris-trained American expatriate Whistler was drawing the public to a carefully chosen exhibition of his own work. Both manifestations, one a group show and the other a one-man exhibition, had arisen in answer to the prevailing conditions for the public exhibition of pictures as the rise of an independent, modern art began to outgrow the loosening control exercised by the academic systems in both capital cities. Whistler had benefited from the independent exhibition of his pictures as early as 1859, when he showed recent work in François Bonvin's studio where it was seen by Gustave Courbet. With Edouard Manet, Henri Fantin-Latour, and other realist painters of the 1860s, he had experienced the critical hostility of the French *Salon* and its juries. In the spring of 1867, Whistler was in Paris when Courbet and Manet held their one-man exhibitions in opposition to the official exhibitions of the state.[1]

In London the dissatisfaction of artists with the Royal Academy had increased in the 1860s. The official government inquiry into the organization of the Royal Academy and its membership in 1863 and the move from Trafalgar Square to Burlington House in 1868 to allow more space for exhibitors had not done enough to appease complaints from artists, especially those like Whistler with more independent styles of painting; in spite of the abolition of the "crinoline" and "sky top" lines.[2] A number of commercial galleries, such as the Dudley Gallery and Ernest Gambart's French Gallery, handled Whistler's pictures and those of his friends Thomas Armstrong, Frederic Leighton, Edward Poynter, Val Prinsep, Albert Moore, Frederick Sandys and G. F. Watts. For many years, Dante Gabriel Rossetti, William Holman Hunt, Edward Burne-Jones and other Pre-Raphaelite followers had preferred not to exhibit at the Academy but arranged their affairs through a network of private patrons and dealers. About 1872, the dealer Murray Marks proposed to start a fine art company with the Anglo-Greek collector Alexander Ionides, and Rossetti, Burne-Jones and William Morris. Its aim was to supply the demand Morris's firm, "Morris, Marshall, Faulkener and Company," had created and to deal in pictures, prints, and blue and white china, which were the natural complement to Morris's designs. They had the exclusive right to sell pictures by Watts, Burne-Jones, and Rossetti, and Whistler's etchings and possibly also his paintings.[3] Ventures such as these were intended to benefit the practising artist and to undercut the growing industry of the art world, which was largely in the hands of the bigger commercial dealers.

William Holman Hunt chose to take on the art dealers on his own terms with the help of his friend Frederick Stephens, the art critic of the *Athenaeum.* In November 1873, Hunt allowed his *The Shadow of Death* to be shown at a one-picture exhibition at the New British Institution. Its exhibition attracted Whistler's attention because he pasted the *Athenaeum's* notice of Hunt's showing in a book of press cuttings.[4] Sale of *The Shadow of Death* by Hunt to the dealer Agnews for £10,500 together with a share in future profits from its reproduction by engraving (which was to raise £20,000 from proofs alone) was described by William Michael Rossetti as "a colossal price indeed"; Gerald Reitlinger in 1961 called it "possibly the fourth most expensive picture that had ever been sold in the history of collecting."[5]

In contrast to Hunt, Whistler's prices were comparatively modest. In 1873, he asked £600 for a full-length portrait of Mrs. Louis Huth (Y125), ventured "6 or 7 hundred" for a "Venus" (Y93), and "at least 8 hundred or a thousand" for a picture with two figures, from the sitter's husband. For a Thames scene, *Variations in Pink and Grey* (Y105), Whistler received £250 from Huth at this time.[6] Whistler's prices for the two proposed pictures may have been optimistic. They never seem to have been commissioned, and doubtless Whistler hoped to secure himself financially in the coming years. The last year in which Whistler exhibited a painting at the Royal Academy was 1872, when *Arrangement in Grey and Black: Portrait of the Painter's Mother* (Y101) was reluctantly shown only after Sir William Boxall R.A. had threatened to resign if it was not.

Although Whistler had been asked, by Degas, to exhibit with the *Société anonyme* in 1874, he was, understandably, reluctant to do so. An exhibition of his recent work, shown in the rue Lafitte gallery of Durand-Ruel early in 1873 found no buyers and received little public attention.[7] Even his friend Fantin-Latour expressed incomprehension in front of the nocturnes of the river Thames, as he did when he saw works by Renoir and Monet the following year.[8] In London, Whistler had found a small but sympathetic audience. He had hoped to be able to complete two full-length portraits of Frederick Leyland and his wife in time for the Academy exhibition of 1873, but they were not ready until the end of the year. The following May, Dante Gabriel Rossetti wrote to Ford Madox Brown:

> I see Whistler is getting up an exhibition! I think I twig the motive power. He must have finished the Leyland portraits, and persuaded L. that they were sure to be hung badly if sent to the R.A.—whereupon L., rather than see himself hoisted, paid bang out for an independent show of them. I have no doubt at this juncture it will send Whistler sky-high, and Leyland will probably buy no one else any more! I believe Leyland's picture will set the fashion in frills and buckles.[9]

While it seems unlikely that Leyland's generosity extended to paying "bang out" for Whistler's exhibition held at 48 Pall Mall in June 1874, Rossetti, who had introduced Whistler to Leyland in 1864, was no doubt otherwise correct in his perceptive account of Whistler's "motive power." But unlike his French colleagues, who seem to have had neither the resources nor the inclination to modify radically the exhibiting conditions of Nadar's studios in 1874, Whistler's intention from the start was to display his work as it might ultimately be seen on the walls of his patron's private homes. Whistler's critics were to be as quick to notice the setting he designed for his work as they were to describe individual pictures. Because Whistler incurred a lawsuit from its owner for not returning the Pall Mall gallery to its original condition, which included the rehanging of a maroon wall cloth, we possess a well-documented testimony of the stages in the preparation for the exhibition.[10]

On 19 January 1874, Whistler entered into an agreement with E. Clifton Griffith to lease the gallery known as the Flemish Gallery at the rear of the ground floor of 48 Pall Mall "for the term of one year or thereabouts ... terminating on the thirty first day of December 1874 at the rent or sum of Three hundred and fifteen pounds," and to "agree to keep the Interior of the said gallery together with the walls and all fixtures in good order & condition and to leave the same in as good condition as they now are." The rent was to be paid in four equal instalments of £78 15s. 9d. at three monthly intervals.[11]

The Flemish Gallery does not seem to have been a prosperous concern, nor E. Clifton Griffith a professional art dealer.[12] Tucked behind the elegant frontage of Pall Mall, from where at No. 120 Gambart's French Gallery had operated until 1867, the Flemish Gallery's last exhibition seems to have been in the summer of 1872, when a display of foreign pictures including works by Portaels, Escosura, and Sier attracted a notice in the *Art Journal.*[13] Whistler's exhibition opened on 4 June and coincided with the time when most art critics directed their attention to the annual Royal Academy exhibition. The long-term planning involved in preparing for June indicates that Whistler intended to mount a premeditated and well-considered challenge to the art world.

> In April 1874 Fredk Fox 418 Britannia Terrace Kings Road Chelsea Frame Maker & Decorator was instructed by Mr Whistler to inspect & see what repairs were necessary to the Gallery & to decorate same according to his designs— Found the rain had come thro' & destroyed the ceiling & thro' the skylight at the end & destroyed the papering on the skylight— The wall of the Gallery had been some time back roughly distempered & covered with a maroon cloth The cloth was in bad condition dirty & full of nail holes
>
> Took the cloth down—thoroughly washed & distempered the walls afresh—repaired the damaged paper in the sky light—The wainscotting had several coats of rough distemper on—dark brown—very unsightly. The wall was uncovered about 6 feet above the cloth—& having been frequently washed & distempered had run down the wall behind the cloth & on to the wainscot & presented a very unsightly appearance—The walls & wainscotts all had to be washed & pummis stoned & with difficulty were removed—
>
> The wall had to be sized & red leaded as was necessary to have a body before coloring to prevent the stains of the distemper coming thro—
>
> Mr Fox then colored the walls with 2 coats of Pink distemper & the Ceiling with 1 coat & afterwds Mr Whistler did not like the effect the color being too light— The ceiling was then done with 1 coat of brown distemper & the wall with 2 coats of pink grey distemper— The skylight was washed & had one coat of white paint—the panels underneath the skylight had 2 coats of paint—the panels grey pink—the styles (round the panels) pink—they were the mouldings round the panels were formerly gilt—but Mr Fox put 2 coats of color on the gilt (gilt color—he forgets)—Mr Fox had to stop the wainscotting before painting

> & the upper part of the division he painted in 4 coats of white paint—& the lower division he formed into 20 odd panels formed of 1½ inch moulding—he painted it with 3 coats of paint—grey white with grey mouldings—(forgets) The stairs in the Gallery were all washed & had 3 coats of white paint—The room at the back of the Gallery—with skylight—had two coats of paint—primrose & the paper on the walls distempered—The paint in the room was formerly in middling condition—stone color—but the paper was dirty—the skylight had only formerly been white washed & was cracked & peeling off & very dirty— The door panel beneath the skylight had also to be scraped & painted with 2 coats of paint—The pay box walls were also distempered by Mr Fox pink—They were formerly whitewashed & were very dirty—
>
> The repair & painting occupied 2 months from 4 April to 4 June—on & off—& all Fox's bill came to £30 odd pounds—
>
> Mr Fox could have reinstated the cloth as it was with 3 men in a day & that would have cost about 18/—or £1 outside—that was to replace the cloth—hang 2 small doors that were taken down—& put some bolts on that were removed—There was no fitting to do but simply to put back the things in their places—
>
> The condition of the Gallery & the other parts all considerably improved—Mr Fox saw Mr Griffith in the Gallery on several occasions—three or four times while the work was proceeding—but he never made any remarks to Mr Fox about the painting—& indeed he never spoke to Mr Fox & Mr Fox never heard Mr Griffith make any remarks to anybody else about it—
>
> The Lobby under the stairs was also washed & had 1 coat of white paint
>
> The whole place was left in thorough repair—the only damage done was what was done by the wet coming thro' the roof again—& that Griffith has repainted himself.[14]

Shortly before 4 June, Whistler issued invitation cards for Thursday the 4th, Friday the 5th, and Saturday June 6th, "on which days the gallery will be open for Private view from 10 to 6." Walter Greaves, Whistler's pupil, later recalled that he, Whistler's mother, and family were "all making Butterflies as hard as we could," rushing out and posting the cards until the letter boxes of Chelsea were in a state of congestion unprecedented in that quiet corner of London.[15] The private view on Saturday the 6th was attended by the actress Isobel Bateman, the manager of Durand-Ruel's *Society of French Artists*' gallery Charles Deschamps, Thomas Carlyle, his brother, his niece Mary Aitken, and "a pleasant company of artists, art critics, literary personages and others."[16]

Whistler hung a representative selection of his work in all media. It included several recently finished full-length portraits, the *Arrangement in Black* (Y97) and *Symphony in Flesh Color and Pink* (Y106) (fig. 3.1) (the portraits of Mr. and Mrs. Leyland); the portrait of Cicely Alexander, *Harmony in Grey and Green* (Y129); *Arrangement in Black, No. 2* (Mrs. Louis Huth) (Y125); *Portrait of Thomas Carlyle, Arrangement in Grey and Black, No. 2* (Y137); *Arrangement in Grey and Black, Portrait of the Painter's Mother* (Y101); and *Harmony in Grey and Peach Color* (Y131). Earlier work was represented by the marine *Blue Waves* (Y41) from 1862; a *Harmony in Grey, No.* [*sic*] priced at 100 guineas in an annotated catalogue, which may have been *Symphony in Grey and Green: The Ocean* (Y72) painted on Whistler's visit to Valparaiso in 1866; a *Nocturne in Grey and Gold* (Y117), probably that of Southampton Water;

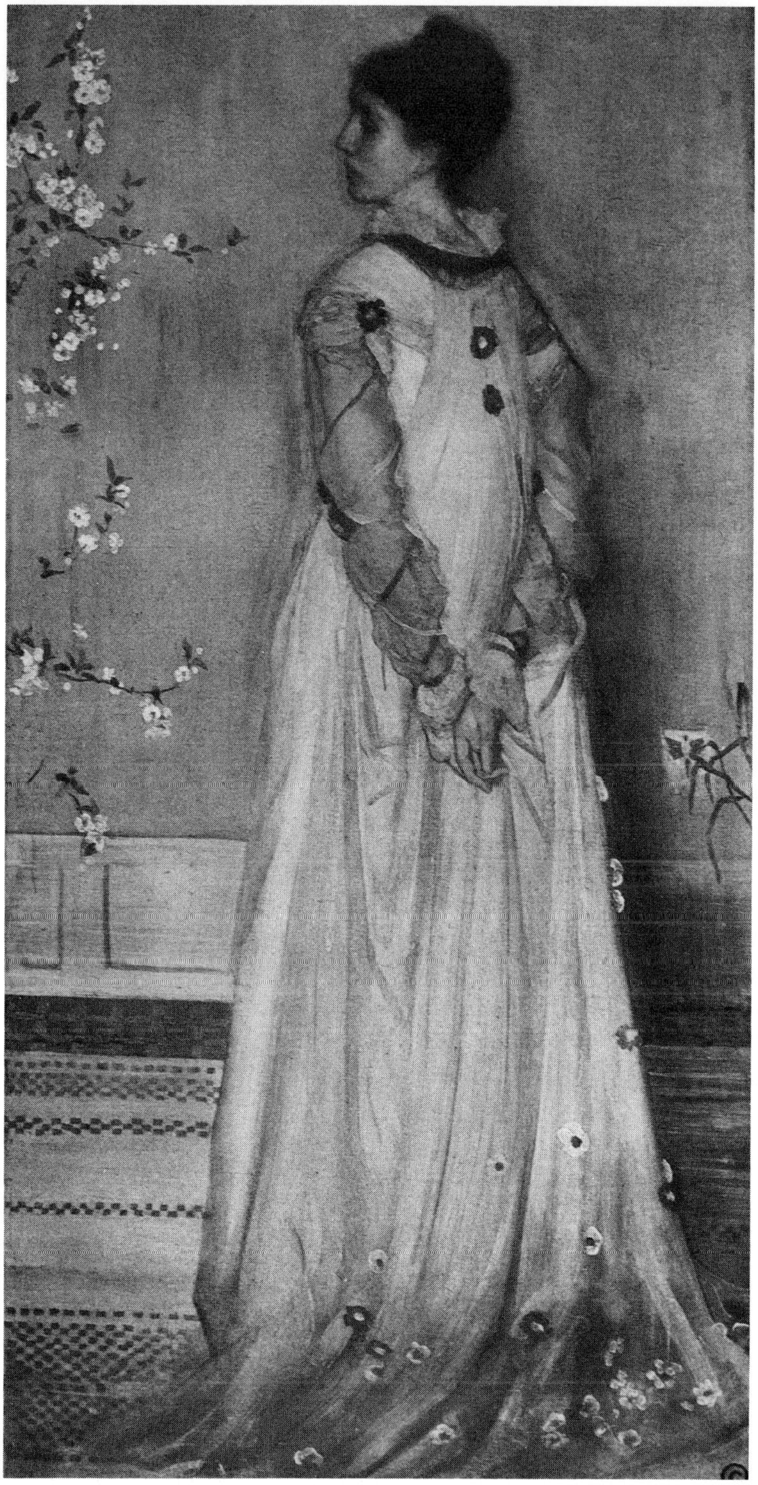

Fig. 3.1. James A. McN. Whistler, *Symphony in Flesh Colour and Pink: Portrait of Mrs. Frances Leyland,* 1871–74 (exhibited 1874). Canvas, 77⅛ × 40¼ in. © The Frick Collection, New York.

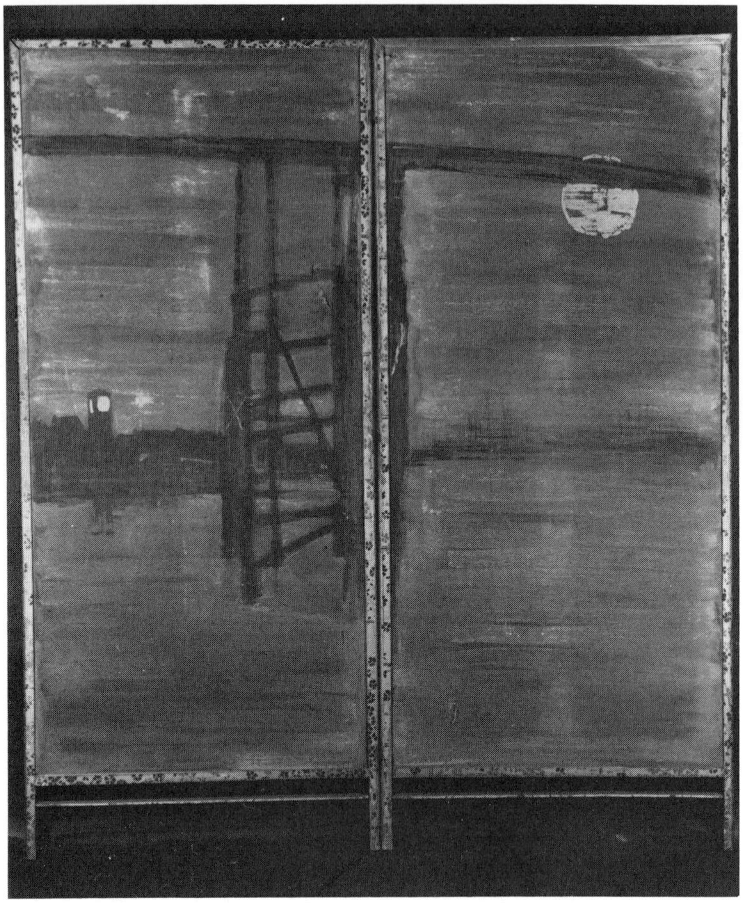

Fig. 3.2. James A. McN. Whistler, *Blue and Silver: Screen with Old Battersea Bridge,* 1872. Brown paper laid on canvas, 76¾ × 71¾ in. (fully opened). Exhibited 1874. Birnie Philip Bequest, University of Glasgow.

and three Sketches for Large Paintings from the "Six Projects" planned as a decorative scheme for Leyland in 1868—*Symphony in Blue and Pink* (Y86), *Variations in Blue and Green* (Y84), and *Symphony in White and Red* (Y87). Also included in the exhibition were fifty etchings and drypoints, thirty-six drawings, and the freestanding *Screen—Blue and Silver* (Y139), (see fig. 3.2), which had also been painted for Leyland in 1872.[17]

The appearance of the exhibition can be reconstructed with a fair degree of accuracy from reports in the press.[18] Along one of the long walls the four full-length portraits were hung, from left to right, those of Mrs. Leyland, Mr. Leyland, *Harmony in Grey and Peach Color,* and last that of Mrs. Louis Huth. Beneath them were hung the three sketches for large paintings and next to the floor were chalk drawings. In a line round the room were the etchings and drypoints, interspersed between the paintings. On the opposite wall hung the portrait of Carlyle next to that of Cicely Alexander. On the short end wall was Whistler's *Portrait of the Painter's Mother,* with an etching of "an interior" hung "directly under."[19]

Assuming that the etchings were hung for maximum visual convenience at eye level above a wainscoting, which would have been between two and three feet in height (as recommended by Charles Eastlake's *Hints on Household Taste*), the four full-length portraits on one of the long walls must have been placed at least five feet above the ground, thereby dominating the arrangement and providing four alternating vertical accents: flesh color (Mrs. Leyland), black (Mr. Leyland), gray and peach, and last black again (Mrs. Louis Huth). In order to accommodate such a display, the length of the gallery, eighteen feet from floor to ceiling, exceeded forty feet. By hanging paintings and drawings beneath the portraits, a vertical/horizontal rhythm AB AB AB AB was created along the wall, which was softened by the passages of brilliant complementary color in the smaller three sketches for large paintings. These hanging arrangements necessitated constant visual stimulation for the spectator from two distinct viewpoints: close up to the wall for detailed inspection of etchings and chalk drawings, and further back near the center of the gallery for viewing the medium-sized (18″ × 24″) but less finished three sketches, and further back still for the large full-length portraits. This unity of color and alternating visual rhythm was a system of hanging favored by Whistler with ever increasing elaboration for future exhibitions (see figs. 3.3; 3.4).

On the floor of the gallery was spread a "glaring yellow matting, striped in two shades" (fig. 3.5), and in the room were "finely formed couches and chairs . . . covered with rich light maroon cloth."[20] Blue pots with growing flowers and plants stood on steps and ledges, while the light from the roof was subdued and mellowed by passing through thin white blinds. The lighting arrangements duplicated the conditions in which Whistler painted in his studio. His desire that paintings should be viewed alike in studio, gallery, and ultimately the patron's home was also shared by Rossetti.[21] The practice of softening top light with white paint on the skylight and a blind was to be further developed when Whistler designed and patented a velarium for the Society of British Artists' exhibition in 1888 (see fig. 3.6).

Sidney Colvin, writing in *The Academy,* was one of the first critics to appreciate Whistler's decision to mount a one-man exhibition.

> But the excuse for private exhibition is that our great annual shows, in the present state of public taste, do not really provide a genial element for works of art; that what makes most figure there is work of such common-place, misdirected, unpleasurable kind as has little right to be called art at all; and that the same traditions which cause work of this kind to prevail, often cause grave injustice to be done to work answering to truer instincts. If there is any case in which an artist is justified in opening a gallery of his own, it is when he is conscious of a distinct vocation for certain kinds of artistic combinations which it takes delicate organs to appreciate, and when experience has shown him that this kind of combination receives scanty welcome at the hands of art's official censors. And this is Mr Whistler's case.[22]

Some critics found the light and color of the gallery too cold and clinical for their tastes, but the general impression was of a warm and pleasing environment for the display of pictures. The gallery "presents a pleasant artist's studio appearance" wrote one, "with its crockery and painted screens, its furniture in plain but rich-toned brown covers, and its ranges of etchings and sketches in plain wood frames."[23]

Henry Blackburn, who unfortunately did not carry out his promise to make a drawing of the gallery for the next issue of *Pictorial World,* provided the following account.

> The visitor is struck, on entering the Gallery, with a curious sense of harmony and fitness pervading it, and is more interested, perhaps, in the general effect than in

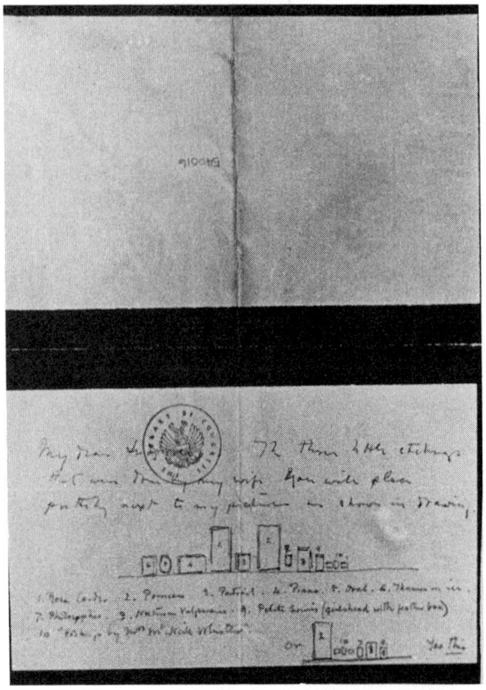

Fig. 3.3. Letter from Whistler to Albert Ludovici, with drawing showing the arrangement of his works for the first exhibition of the International Society of Sculptors, Painters and Gravers, 1898. Courtesy of the Library of Congress, Pennell Collection, Washington, D.C.

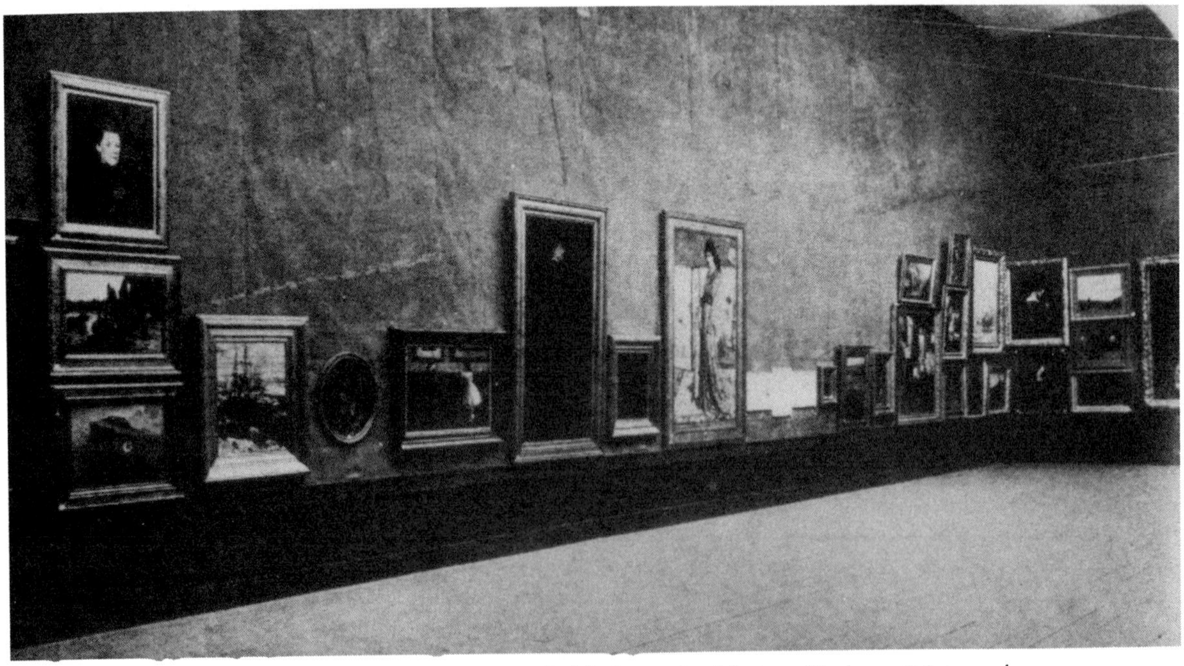

Fig. 3.4. Wall of the International Society of Sculptors, Painters and Gravers Exhibition, London, May 1898. Central group of works arranged by Whistler. From E. R. & J. Pennell, *The Whistler Journal*, 1921.

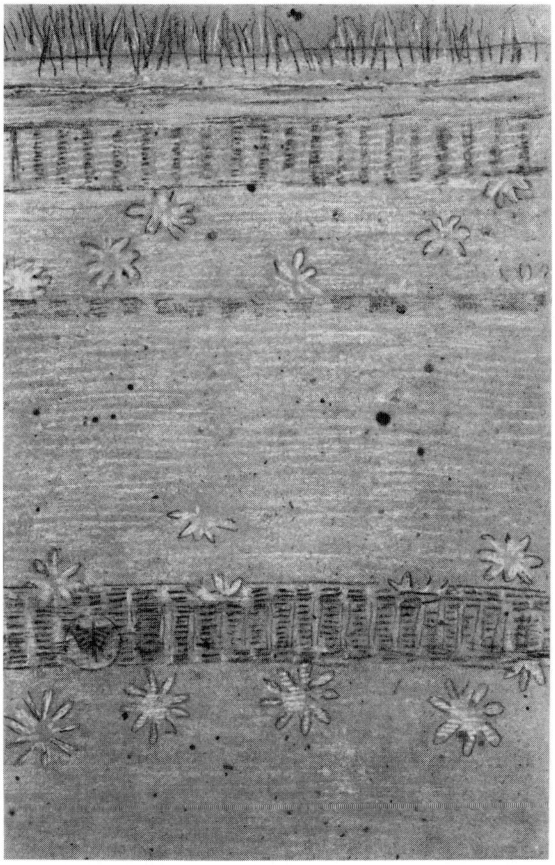

Fig. 3.5. James A. McN. Whistler, *Design for matting*, c. 1873. Pastel 11¼ × 7¼ in. By permission of the Fogg Art Museum.

> any one work. The Gallery and its contents are altogether in harmony—a "symphony in colour", carried out in every detail, even in the colour of the matted floor, the blue pots and flowering plants, and, above all, in the juxtaposition of the pictures. . . . If anyone wishes to realise what is meant by true feeling for colour and harmony—born of the Japanese—let him sit down here some morning, within a few yards of, but in the secure shelter from, the glare of the guardsman's scarlet tunic in the bay window of the club opposite, just out of hearing of Christie's hammer, and just out of sight of the conglomeration of a thousand pictures at the Royal Academy. A "symphony" is usually defined as a "harmony of sounds agreeable to the ear", here, at 48 Pall Mall, is a harmony of colour agreeable to the eye.[24]

The pleasant artist's studio appearance of 48 Pall Mall was not new in the field of "home improvements" in 1874. Whistler had already used distempered decoration rather than wallpaper as well as "quiet harmonies" of color for the interior of his own houses and for the dining room of Aubrey House, Campden Hill, the home of W. C. Alexander (who had commissioned Whistler to paint his two daughters). Whistler's decorative scheme was never carried through, although one of his designs for the dining room approximates to the effect created at 48 Pall Mall in 1874 (figs. 3.7, 3.8).

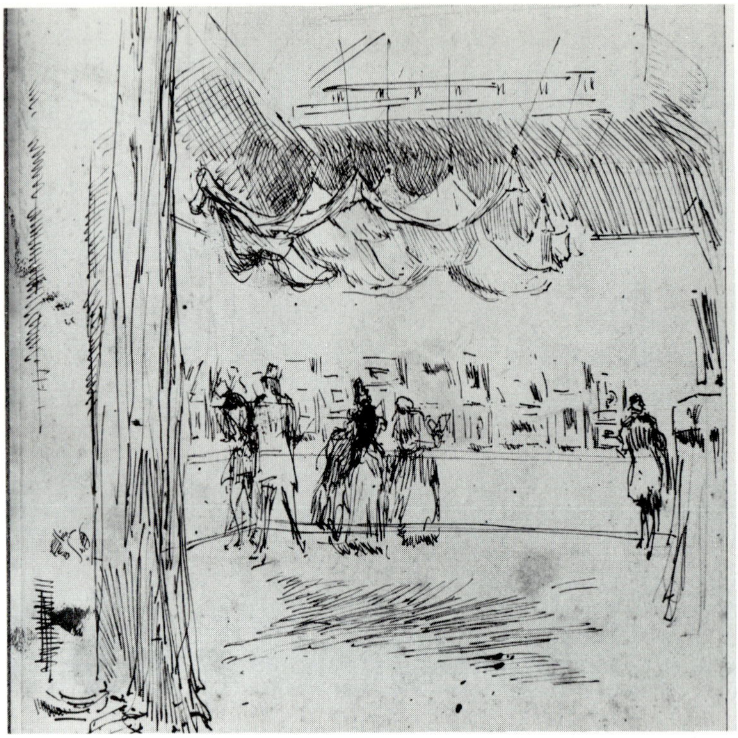

Fig. 3.6. James A. McN. Whistler, *Interior of the British Artists Exhibition*, 1887. Pen, 7⅞ × 6¼ in. © Ashmolean Museum, University of Oxford.

Well-spaced hanging and a consideration for the general ambience beyond the picture frame were clearly Whistler's priorities in 1874. Yet this was not the first time that a less cluttered display of pictures was exhibited in London outside the Royal Academy exhibitions. The exhibitions of the Society of French Artists, under the management of Charles Deschamps, at the Old German Gallery, 168 Bond Street, were noted for their uncluttered appearance and pleasing atmosphere. The galleries consisted of two rooms, one above the other, and had the appearance of Whistler's Pall Mall exhibition. "The pleasure which we feel on visiting this exhibition," wrote Frederick Stephens of the sixth exhibition, which opened on 21 April 1873, and included works by Degas, Manet, Monet, Pissarro, as well as Fantin-Latour's *Hommage à Delacroix*,

> is due to two circumstances, the high character of most of the pictures contained, and the sober aspect of the gallery, where the very frames and fittings have been considered with a view to a homogeneous effect. Nor is the small number of the paintings on view in any respect a disadvantage to the visitor or the contributor. We have protested many times against the injurious effects of the English practice of hanging as many pictures as the walls of our galleries will hold. Not only does such a mode of proceeding make the adoption of a low standard inevitable, but the visitor is wearied before he can gain even a faint idea of the more meritorious pictures in such crowded gatherings.[25]

Two letters written by Whistler to Deschamps in the winter of 1872–73, one in which he asks Deschamps to take his pictures from the Dudley Gallery and have them "hung in the Whistler gallery under your own good protection" and a second in

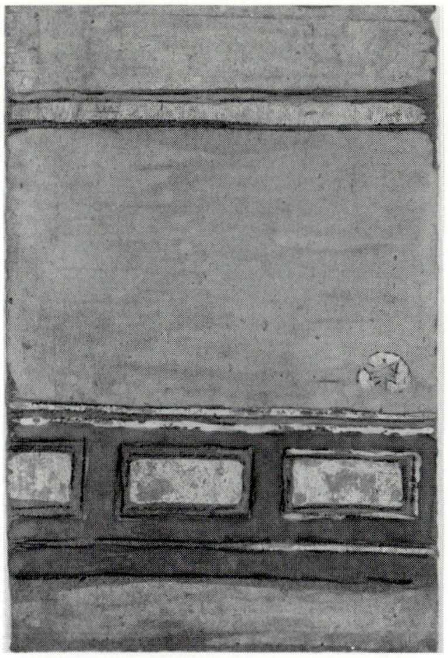

Fig. 3.7. James A. McN. Whistler, *Colour Scheme for the Decoration of Aubrey House*, c. 1873. Body color on brown paper, 6 × 4 in. Birnie Philip Bequest, University of Glasgow.

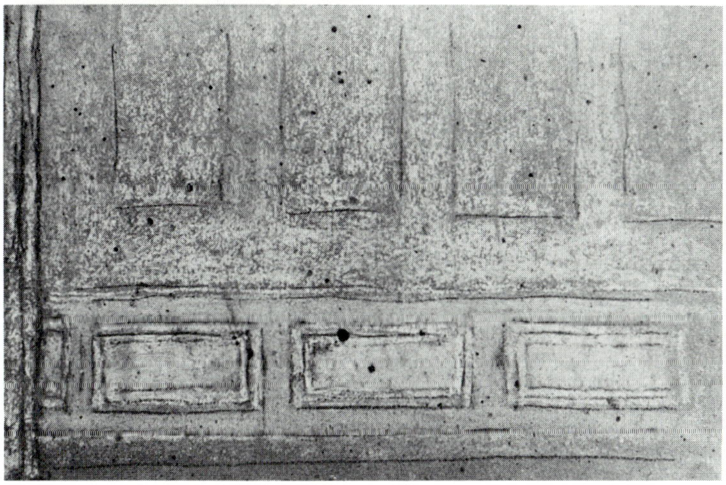

Fig. 3.8. James A. McN. Whistler, *Colour Scheme for the Decoration of Aubrey House*, c. 1873. Pastel. By permission of the Fogg Art Museum.

which he asks "whether my pictures from the Dudley are now safely hanging in your care upstairs in my gallery,"[26] are strongly suggestive of Whistler's hand in the interior design of the Society of French Artists exhibitions. Whistler's Pall Mall exhibition was also the occasion of his first brown-paper-covered catalogue (see fig. 3.9), coarse paper that Whistler used for pastel and charcoal drawings that he had first obtained from the French printer Auguste Delâtre. Deschamp's catalogues were of a similar design (see fig. 3.10).

> The very catalogue they sell you in Bond Street is a different thing from that which you have to buy elsewhere. It is nicely printed, and covered with stiff grey paper of a pretty tint; it is not too big for one hand, nor too small for two; and it

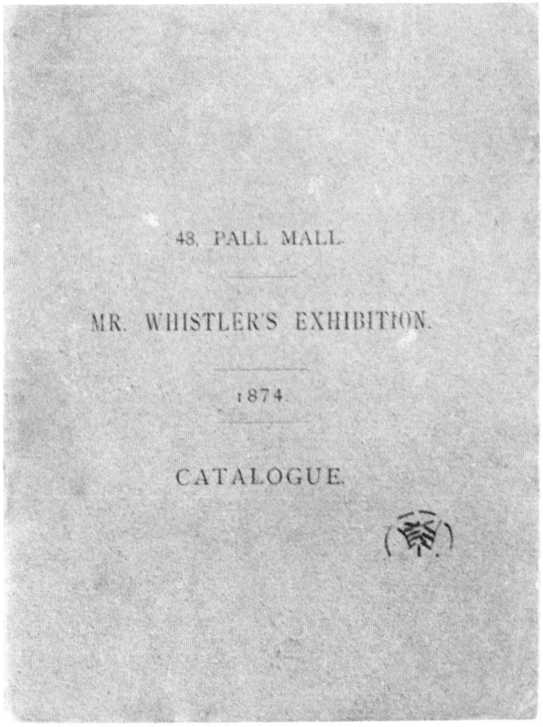

Fig. 3.9. Cover of catalogue for Whistler's Pall Mall exhibition 1874, designed by Whistler and signed in pen with a butterfly. Birnie Philip Bequest, University of Glasgow.

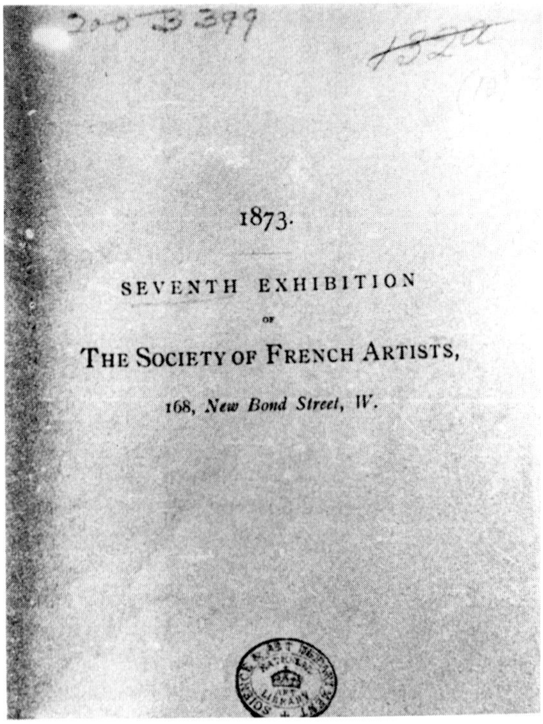

Fig. 3.10. Cover of catalogue for the seventh exhibition of the Society of French Artists, London, 1873. Victoria and Albert Museum Library, London.

has a margin in which you can write, the pages not having been, like the thing the Royal Academicians sell, cropped to the very bone.[27]

Because Whistler took such pains with the presentation of his exhibition, few critics took notice of individual works but confined themselves to describing the novel impression created by the gallery. However, the critic of *The Hour,* rashly writing in the mistaken belief that Whistler's full-length portraits which he favorably compared to Velázquez were not of recent date, earned one of the artist's first public rebuttals.

> This artist feeling, probably, that his works were not seen to advantage when placed in juxtaposition with those of an essentially different kind, has determined to have an exhibition of his own, where no discordant elements should distract the spectator's attention. ... With the exception of a complete set of his well-known etchings, half a dozen full-length portraits, and as many of those eccentric and apparently aimless exercises in colour with which he has of late perplexed the world, comprises the whole [*sic*]. Apart from the etchings, which we shall consider later, the motive in all these is essentially decorative. Mr Whistler has the finest sense of the quality of colour, and the power of producing the most exquisite combinations. Each of his pictures has a distinct and well-considered scheme of colour, and to this everything is made subordinate; in adapting the materials of his subject to his he does not hesitate to suppress any fact that may interfere with it, or to introduce any ingredient, however incongruous, that may aid in its manifestation. In his latest productions the most important elements of decorative art—beauty of form and harmony of line—have been entirely absent. The principle—if principle it can be called—on which the artist has lately worked, and which has caused him to ignore every element of art but one, is founded on fallacy. Colour, however pure and perfect in tone, when divorced from the forms with which it is associated in nature has no significance, and appeals only to the senses....
>
> The portraits are far more agreeable to contemplate. ... Among them is the full-length portrait of a young girl, which in execution and general treatment bears a strong resemblance to the works of Velasquez. The figure is admirably drawn, and natural and unaffected in action, and the colour delicate in its gradations and perfect in tone.... The large portrait of Thomas Carlyle is a later and less satisfactory work. The figure, which is seated and seen in profile, is well drawn and characteristic; but the head is loosely painted, and shows no very profound insight into character, while the tone is less fine and subtle than in the pictures already mentioned; it appears to be unfinished. An almost entire negation of colour is shown to be consistent with richness of tone in two portraits which hang on the opposite wall. Black, white, grey, and a small amount of flesh colour comprise the entire scale; the arrangement is very skilful, and the effect powerful....
>
> This exhibition causes one to form a high estimate of Mr Whistler's artistic knowledge and power; but it gives rise to the melancholy reflection that the best works are not of recent production, and that the latest are the least satisfactory.[28]

In order to forestall similar criticisms, particularly where they might concern the identification of Whistler's most recent work, Whistler wrote to *The Hour* on June 10th to explain why he chose to hold a one-man exhibition.

> Sir, I have read the intelligent remarks of your critic upon my pictures, and am happy to be able to remove, I think, the "melancholy" impression left upon his

mind by the supposition that "the best works are not of recent date". Permit me to reassure him, for the paintings he speaks of in glowing terms—notably "the full-length portrait of a young girl" which he overwhelms me by comparing to Velasquez, as well as two life-size portraits in black, "in which there is an almost entire negation of colour" (though I, who am, he says, a colourist, did not know it)—are my latest works, and but just completed.

May I still further correct a misconception? The etchings and dry-points in the gallery do not form a complete set. There are only fifty exhibited, making about half the number I have exhibited.

Again it was from no feeling that "my works were not seen to advantage when placed in juxtaposition with those of an essentially different kind", that I "determined to have an exhibition of my own, where discordant elements should distract the spectator's attention". It is true that occasionally it has been borne in upon my mind that those whose "works are of an essentially different kind" are unwilling to place mine in juxtaposition with their own.

My wish has been, though, to prove that the place in which works of art are shown may be made as free from "discordant elements which distract the spectator's attention" as the works themselves.

Marvelling greatly that the "principle" that has led me (in his eyes at least) to paint so that he speaks of me in the same breath with Velasquez, should be "founded on fallacy"—I remain, sir, your obedient servant,

June 10, 1874[29]

In the wake of the Ruskin libel trial ten years later, when he regularly sought critical confrontations, Whistler further elevated his modern art above that of the Spanish master by allowing his anecdotal riposte "Why Drag in Velázquez?" to pass into oral history. It swiftly became a part of the hagiography of the Whistler myth.[30] But in 1874 even *The Hour* had to concede Whistler's preeminence as an etcher, and his powers with the medium were rarely disputed by others. Whether or not Whistler's letter played any part in encouraging more favorable criticism is open to question, but subsequent reviews of the exhibition were better informed, and Whistler was praised equally for his portraits as well as his etchings. Comparisons with Velázquez were frequent. "His rare, though eccentric, genius will certainly raise his reputation as a portrait painter,"[31] wrote one. The exhibition, with its dominating full-length portraits, was obviously intended by Whistler to demonstrate his ability and potential as a fashionable portrait painter. The inclusion of three of the "Six Projects" also provided evidence of Whistler's capabilities as a decorative figure painter at a time when major commissions for London house interiors were being awarded to Morris, Burne-Jones, and other Pre-Raphaelite followers.[32]

From fellow artists too came approval. Rossetti was taken by Whistler to the exhibition and thought the portraits of his mother, Carlyle, and Cicely Alexander were "very fine works indeed in their own way"; but although he thought the portrait of Mrs. Leyland to be "a graceful design," he could not see "that it is at all a likeness."[33] On 9 September, Whistler's mother wrote of

> so many favourable notices in the leading London papers have been published about the Artist Whistler's Gallery at 48 Pall Mall. So he has at least acquired fame, tho not yet money in proportion to the expenses attendant upon it—But as he is unwearied in working and has orders more than enough, I trust his hopes

> may be realized and my prayers answer for him, for they are for more than he has yet aspired to.[34]

It was not until 1876, with Leyland's *Peacock Room,* that Whistler had the opportunity of a major decorative commission. Meanwhile, the exhibition produced no immediate commissions for portraits, although he still had in hand portraits of the Leyland family. On 22 June, Whistler sold the *Nocturne in Grey and Gold* (Y117) of Southampton Water from the exhibition as well as a *Nocturne in Grey and Silver-(Battersea)* (Y160) for 200 guineas to Alfred Chapman, the Lancashire managing director of the engineering firm Fawcett, Preston & Co. At the same time, he was finishing a nocturne of Valparaiso that was begun as a daylight picture in 1866 (Y76). It was completed and sold in 1875, a year when the subject of fireworks in a night sky was to particularly occupy him. The gallery at 48 Pall Mall seems to have stayed open to the public until the end of July 1874,[35] but Whistler's lease of the premises lasted until the end of the year, by which time the "expenses attendant upon it" mentioned by his mother were to be stretched even further. In September and the winter of 1874–75 Whistler conducted much of his business from Speke Hall, the Liverpool home of Leyland. He was also in Liverpool in October 1874 to see the exhibition of his etchings that his solicitor James Anderson Rose lent to the Liverpool Art Club,[36] an exhibition that later opened at the Hartley Institution, Southampton, and which was accompanied by the first published catalogue of Whistler's etchings compiled by Ralph Thomas.

Whistler seems to have conveniently forgotten about the last installment of rent due on 48 Pall Mall and the expiry of the lease at the end of the year. On 21 January 1875, Clifton Griffith wrote to remind Whistler that no one had come "to touch the gallery," to "be restored to the condition in which you found it." Clifton Griffith held Whistler responsible for rent until the work was completed and estimated that the cost of redecoration would come to "about £30."[37] He had found a new tenant, E. F. White, who sent Whistler a telegram on the twenty-second offering to relieve him "from all trouble" and to do the gallery up himself if Whistler would contribute £20. White told him that the maroon cloth Whistler had removed could not be replaced until the painting and stenciling was finished and repairs to the roof had been carried out; and that further, he warned, Griffith could claim rent from Whistler up to the day the repairs were completed, which in practice could never be finished by the beginning of February.[38] Whistler immediately wrote to Griffith claiming that his agreement with him had not "precluded me from painting it any colour I liked." Griffith's servant Mr. Lamb had told Whistler's decorator Frederick Fox "that the cloth was not worth rehanging and consequently it was not done." Whistler therefore took no steps to replace the fixtures before his term expired because Griffith had suggested "the incoming tenant might not require any change."[39] This had been a rash assumption a year before because now Whistler was "wrong to paint out the decorations" or "alter the gallery" without his permission. Griffith's immediate reply on the 23rd, "as the state in which you have left it is a bar to my letting" and already in the autumn had lost him "one good tenant." "As a gentleman" he expected Whistler to do what was right "without pressure." After accommodating him with regard to the payment of rent, he expected "a like sentiment of courtisies [*sic*] and good feeling," and unless Whistler arranged matters satisfactorily, he would at once instruct his solicitors to take proceedings.[40] Whistler felt that the gravity and injustice of Griffith's charges warranted a considered reply and he drafted two letters.

Speke Hall

Dear Sir—I fail altogether to understand what you can mean by having through me lost a tenant in the autumn, when my possession of the Gallery extended to the 14th of January!—

Our relations as landlord & tenant are clearly laid down in the Agreement drawn up by your Agent and signed by me—this seems to me, though no business man, evident to the merest child—Otherwise the Agreement itself means nothing and is only a farce.—

Now any attempt on your part to obtain from me more than I am therein bound to perform, becomes to me simple extortion, and your appeal, to what you are pleased to call "courtisies" (*sic*), absurd and pitiable.—

Against this sort of thing, be assured, I should defend myself to the uttermost, notwithstanding my disadvantage when compared to your superior knowledge of business.—

Meanwhile I learn that my man Fox and his assistants went to the gallery yesterday to hang the cloth and were prevented from so doing—the Gallery itself being in the hands of other workmen—therefore I shall have nothing more to do with it—.

Yours truly

E. Clifton Griffiths Esq. [*sic*] JMcN. Whistler[41]

Speke Hall—near Liverpool
Jany. 24th 1874

Dear Sir—Your memory plays you, I fear, a treacherous trick, or you would not forget that my intention to redecorate the Gallery and paint it as I pleased was openly expressed to your Agent and known to yourself when I took it;—that you were continually present during the alterations;—that, in company with my friend Mr Morris [William, or the artist Phil Morris?] I met you myself in the Gallery while the work was proceeding; (with Fox and his paint pots all about the place;?)—and that you never made the faintest objection whatever, nor in any way allowed me to suppose that I was at all running the risk with which you now threaten me!

On the contrary conversed pleasantly, after your manner, about the matter and took the pains to point out where you thought one of my new panels was, according to your fresh eye, a little out of the square, and might be bettered—"that you were not sure whether you appreciated the new colors, but would wait until the whole was complete. . . . "—

In the face of these facts I am afraid your Solicitor would have but a mild opinion of your "case"—

However far be it from me to offer advice—

Meanwhile I refer you, for all answer, to my letter of the 22nd—, only adding that if Fox and his men are opposed in putting up the cloth, as I gather, from Mr. White's letter to me, they have been, the delay is of your making, and I will not be at the expense of their lost time—

Yours truly

E. Clifton Griffiths Esq. [*sic*] JAMcN. Whistler-[42]

Whistler's pleas left Griffith unmoved, and Griffith telegrammed him informing him if the decorations were not paid he would take legal action which on January 29th he did, by entering a Writ in the Court of Exchequer of Pleas claiming "£68. 17s in respect of rent, repairs, and dilapidations."[43] Severely disadvantaged by being at such a distance from London, Whistler sent a telegram to his brother Dr. Willie Whistler, also a client of Rose, asking him to take all the papers relating to the Flemish Gallery round to Rose immediately. Willie was ill in bed with influenza, but Whistler's mother was on hand to help.[44] Immediately after the writ had been issued against him, Whistler shot off a check to Griffith for £48 15s. 0d., the balance of rent due, but withheld £20 2s. 0d. for the "repairs, alterations and dilapidations." "I want to fight Griffith—and I know you can beat him," he wrote to Rose.[45] Rose immediately went into action on behalf of his client. He took evidence from Walter Slater, a Chelsea carpenter acting on instructions from Whistler, who had been sent to the Gallery with the decorator Frederick Fox to rehang the cloth. He had found workmen already there with tressels and boards ready to redecorate the gallery. Fox asked Lamb, Griffith's servant, to fetch Griffith, "but he could not or he would not come." Then White, the new tenant, arrived and said to Fox, "Well you can't do it now." White "complained about the color on the walls & he never saw such a color before in a Gallery & that he had written to Mr Whistler to contribute £20 towards the redecoration of the Gallery which he himself would have sent if he had been in Mr Whistler's place & he asked Mr Fox to see Mr. Whistler and if he had any influence in the matter to persuade him to send a cheque even if it was not to the amount of £20—he did not say who he was to send the cheque to."[46]

The redecoration of the gallery at 48 Pall Mall began on January twenty-fifth and was finished by February sixth. It met White's requirements and presumably Clifton Griffith's tastes. The brown distemper Fox had painted on the ceiling was washed off, and the ceiling was stained with oil color, prepared, and distempered gray. The white painted skylight was once more obscured, and its surrounding woodwork rubbed down and painted in three shades. The pink gray distempered walls were washed and cleaned and stopped with parian plaster and calico. Eighteen feet of molding were erected between the end wall and the ceiling with prepared wood, and the cross battens were painted green to match green paper that was hung on the upper parts of the walls and between the battens. The staircase—Fox had painted it white—was painted with two coats of brown lake, and the old maroon cloth was sewn and once more tacked to the dado. The small back room—Whistler had it painted primrose—was cleaned, the woodwork painted with two coats of green, and the walls were papered to match. The work was labor intensive compared with the two months "on and off" that Frederick Fox had worked the previous year. Three tradesmen-decorators each worked 50 to 56 hours for two weeks at 10½ pence an hour. One assistant or apprentice worked for nine days at 4 shillings a day; and one laborer worked for fourteen hours at 6 pence an hour. A woman cleaned and sewed the cloth for 40 hours at 5 pence an hour. The labor cost amounted to £17 1s. 5d., while the total cost of £29 17s. 3d. was made up by materials, including paint, paper, and scaffolding.[47]

Meanwhile Rose planned a visit to the North Western Hotel, Liverpool, to see his client on February 16th, but Whistler missed him and left an invitation from Mrs. Leyland for him to stay at Speke Hall. "Meanwhile that ass Griffiths has sent an acknowledgement of the cheque of £48 15s., so surely he cannot sue me on the writ of £68 17s. ... putting all the rest out of the question—I hope you are going to roast him—Tell Ralph Thomas with my kindest thanks that I have received a copy of the Catalogue [of Whistler's etchings] he sent me."[48] Notwithstanding the check for £48 Whistler had sent, two days later the specific counts of Griffith's claim had grown to £100. It was wholly due to Rose's professional skills that the plaintiff's proceedings were severely delayed in the following weeks. On February 26th the court ordered Whistler a week's time to plead and gave a further five days on March 5th. A stay of proceedings was issued yet again on the 10th and 15th, and on the 17th and 23rd of March the court twice ordered "a further and better account in writing" of Griffith's demands. Not only had Rose negotiated these delays, but he also finally reduced Griffith's claims to £29 17s. 3d., which represented the cost of redecorating 48 Pall Mall to White's and Griffith's specifications.[49]

Clearly Griffith's demands had been excessive, a view endorsed by the judgment of the court when the case finally came to trial on April 5th with Mr. Warburton Pyke as Whistler's counsel. The plaintiff withdrew any further prosecution and accepted the sum paid into court in satisfaction of the cause of the action, asking only for costs. The action cost Griffith £5 15s. 1d. and the loss of an original scheme of decoration by Whistler. The action cost Whistler £6 11s. 8d. and the loss of an exhibition gallery.[50]

The rent of £315 for the Pall Mall Gallery represented a colossal investment by Whistler. The rent of his thirteen-room house, 2 Lindsey Row, Chelsea, was still only £80 a year in 1874.[51] This was the difference between the village of Chelsea—only recently joined to the rest of London by the Embankment—and the center of London within walking distance of the Royal Academy and the dealers' galleries, where the real business of the Victorian art world was conducted. The gallery at 48 Pall Mall no doubt served as a studio and centrally located venue for Whistler's patrons and friends after July when his exhibition closed. As such, it became an extension of the artist's studio and home and a complement to the more intimate setting of Chelsea where Whistler held his "breakfasts." Visiting the artist's studio cum home was, of course, a widely practiced and traditional social custom. Whistler's independent venture in 1874, together with the Kensington homes of Leighton, Watts, and others, must have crossed the mind of Sir Coutts Lindsay when in 1877 he planned a deluxe and much enlarged emporium for the sort of art, including Whistler's, which had already taxed the hospitality and hanging space available at the Royal Academy. In the same year Whistler was to build the White House in Tite Street, Chelsea, initially at a total cost of £1910,[52] where he combined a modern residence with a spacious studio commensurate with his ambitions as a fashionable artist and portrait painter, a career that was temporarily halted in 1878 by the Ruskin's libel suit and Whistler's subsequent bankruptcy.

APPENDIX

Mr. Whistler's Exhibition, London, Flemish Gallery, 48 Pall Mall, 1874. Catalogue (8pp.) annotated by Whistler with prices in the Birnie Philip Bequest, Glasgow University (fig. 3.1).

Oil Paintings

1. Portrait, "Arrangement in Black."
2. Portrait, "Symphony in Flesh Colour and Pink."

3. Portrait, "Arrangement in Black, No. 2."
4. "Arrangement in Grey and Black, Portrait of the Painter's Mother."
5. Portrait, "Harmony in Grey and Green."
6. Portrait of Thomas Carlyle, "Arrangement in Grey and Black, No. 2."
7. "Harmony in Grey and Peach Colour."
8. Harmony in Grey, No. 100 gs
9. Blue Waves.
10. Nocturne in Grey and Gold. 250 gs

Sketches for Large Paintings

11. Symphony in Blue and Pink.
12. Variations in Blue and Green.
13. Symphony in White and Red.

Screen—Blue and Silver

Etchings and Dry Points

1. Dry Point, "The Storm."
2. Dry Point, "The Forge."
3. Etching, "Old Chelsea Wharf." 4 gs
4. Etching, Portrait, "Delâtre, the Printer."
5. Etching, "Saverne—night."
6. Dry Point, Portrait. Very few proofs 6 gs
7. Etching, "Fumette."
8. Etching, "La Vielle aux loquecs [*sic*]."
9. Etching, "Limehouse."
10. Etching, "Black Lion Wharf." One proof only 10 gs
11. Etching, "Old Westminster Bridge."
12. Etching, "Billingsgate."
13. Etching, "Tyzack, Whitely, & Co." One proof only 10 gs
14. Etching, "Thames Police."
15. Etching, "Rotherhithe."
16. Etching, "Thames Tunnel Pier."
17. Etching, "Battersea Dawn."
18. Etching, "The Limeburner's Yard."
19. Etching, "Old Hungerford Bridge."
20. Etching, "Thames Warehouses."
21. Etching, "Portrait of Mons. Becquet, sculptor," known also as "The Violinist."
22. Dry Point, Portrait.
23. Etching, "La Mère Girard."
24. Dry Point, Portrait.
25. Dry Point, Portrait. 3 gs
26. Etching, "Saverne."
27. Dry Point, Portrait.
28. Etching, "Café des Pieds Monilles."
29. Etching, Portrait.
30. Dry Point, Portrait.

31.	Etching, Portrait.	
32.	Dry Point, Portrait.	
33.	Dry Point, Portrait.	5 gs
34.	Etching, Portrait, "Mons. Drouet, sculptor."	
35.	Dry Point, Portrait.	5 gs
36.	Dry Point, Portrait.	
37.	Etching, Portrait.	5gs
38.	Dry Point, Portrait (known as "The Wood Engraver").	
39.	Dry Point, Figure resting. Very few proofs	5 gs
40.	Etching, "La Marchande de Moutarde."	
41.	Etching, "Liverdun."	
42.	Dry Point, "Fumette."	
43.	Etching, "Long Shore Men."	
44.	Etching, "Le Parasol."	
45.	Etching, "Old Greenwich Pensioner."	
46.	Etching, "Interieur de Chiffonier."	
47.	Etching, "La Ratameuse."	
48.	Dry Point, "The Miser."	
49.	Etching, "The Old Farm."	
50.	Dry Point, Portrait.	10 gs

Drawings

1.	Head, Portrait.	
2.	Head, Portrait.	
3.	Design for Child's Costume.	
4.	Design for Screen.	20 gs
5.	Portrait with Fan. (Design).	5 gs
6.	Resting Figure.	
7.	Design for Portrait.	
8.	Head.	3 gs
9.	Portrait.	
10.	Portrait.	5
11.	"The Dress Maker."	7 gs
12.	Seated Figure.	10 gs
13.	Crouching Figure for Large Picture.	10 gs
14.	Portrait.	3
15.	Design for Mozaic.	10
16.	Design "Variations in Violet and Blue."	25 gs
17.	Design Figure for Bridge Picture.	5
18.	Design Figure for Bridge Picture.	5
19.	Design for Dress.	
20.	Figure for Bridge Picture.	10 gs
21.	Kittens.	2 gs
22.	Head, Portrait.	
23.	Design for Picture, "Variations in Yellow and Brown."	18
24.	Snow Piece.	
25.	Portrait.	
26.	Sunset.	

27. Portrait.	
28. Portrait. "Tatting."	10 gs
29. Design for Dress.	
30. Design for Dress.	
31. Standing Figure.	
32. Sketch of Carlyle.	10 gs
33. Sketch Portrait.	3
34. Portrait.	
35. "A Grey Note."	20
36. "Old Battersea Bridge."	5

NOTES

1. Elizabeth Gilmore Holt, *The Art of All Nations: 1850–1873, The Emerging Role of Exhibitions and Critics* (Princeton University Press. New Jersey: 1982).

2. "Fine-Art Gossip," *Athenaeum* (5 December 1868): 758.

3. E. R. and J. Pennell, *The Life of James McNeill Whistler,* 2 vols. (J. B. Lippincott Company & William Heinemann, Philadelphia & London: 1908), 1:153.

4. "Fine-Art Gossip," *Athenaeum* (22 November 1873): 666. Vol. 1, Whistler's press cuttings, Birnie Philip Bequest, University of Glasgow (GUL).

5. Jeremy Maas, *Gambart, Prince of the Victorian Art World* (Barrie & Jenkins, London, 1975), 241.

6. For further references to Whistler's paintings cited here see Andrew McLaren Young, Margaret MacDonald, and Robin Spencer, with the assistance of Hamish Miles, *The Paintings of James McNeill Whistler,* 2 vols. (Yale University Press. New Haven and London, 1980). All text references to illustrations in this catalogue are preceded by the letter Y (for Young).

7. Ibid., 1:84.

8. Fantin-Latour's reaction to Whistler and the Impressionists is discussed by the author in "Whistler, Manet and the Tradition of the *Avant garde,*" *Studies in the History of Art,* 19 (1987).47–64.

9. Oswald Doughty and J. R. Wahl, eds., *Letters of Dante Gabriel Rossetti,* 3 vols. (Clarendon Press, Oxford, 1967), 3:1287.

10. Pennell Collection of Whistler MSS, Library of Congress (LC).

11. Memorandum of agreement between E. Clifton Griffith and J. A. McNeill Whistler, 2 pp., 19 January 1874 (LC).

12. 48 Pall Mall is listed in *Kelly's Post Office London Street Directory* (1866) as "Gallery of Fine Arts." In 1867 "E. Clifton Griffith" is named as being at that address, and in 1868 his address is also given as "31 The Cedars, Putney SW." In 1871 the premises are listed as "Life Association of Scotland—Griffith, E. C." In 1873 Griffith is described as local secretary of the "Life Association of Scotland (branch of)." In 1874 Griffith's name appears with two others. In 1875 "Whistler, James McNeill, artist" appears with four other names.

13. *Art Journal* (February 1872): 62.

14. Draft of the Affidavit of Fox in the handwriting of James Anderson Rose, 4 pp., 1875 (LC).

15. Pennell, *The Life of James McNeill Whistler,* 1:179.

16. *Illustrated Review* (17 June 1874): 391 (GUL).

17. A copy of the catalogue, annotated by Whistler, is in GUL. See Appendix.

18. Whistler's own collection of press cuttings (GUL) includes the following reviews. Henry Blackburn, "A 'Symphony' in Pall Mall," *Pictorial World* (13 June 1874); Anon., "Mr. Whistler's Pictures,"

The Hour (9 June 1874); *The Tribune* (byline dated 13 June 1874); *Illustrated Review* (17 June 1874), 391; *Evening Standard* (24 June 1874); *Manchester Examiner & Times* (8 June 1874); *Builder* (5 July 1874); "Exhibition of Mr Whistler's Paintings and Drawings," *Globe* (n.d.); "Mr Whistler's Paintings and Drawings," *Art Journal* (June 1874): 230; and four unidentified reviews. See Robert H. Getscher and Paul G. Marks, *James McNeill Whistler and John Singer Sargent, Two Annotated Bibliographies* (Garland Publishing Inc. New York and London, 1986), 275–77.

19. This is specifically recorded in the *Illustrated Review* (GUL). The etching could have been one of three interiors by Whistler: *The Forge* K68 (cat. 2), *Longshoremen* K45 (cat. 43), or *The Miser* K69 (cat. 48).

20. *Manchester Examiner & Times* 8 June, 1874 (GUL).

21. Francis L. Fennell Jr., ed., *The Rossetti-Leyland Letters; The Correspondence of an Artist and his Patron* (Athens, Ohio: Ohio University Press, 1978), Letter 57, 47–48.

22. Sidney Colvin, "Exhibition of Mr Whistler's Pictures," *The Academy* 5 (13 June 1874): 672–73.

23. *Builder* (GUL).

24. Blackburn, "A 'Symphony' in Pall Mall," *Pictorial World* (13 June 1874) (GUL).

25. Frederick Stephens, "Exhibition at the Society of French Artists," *Athenaeum* (26 April 1873): 540.

26. Whistler to Charles Deschamps, from Speke Hall, near Liverpool, n.d. [Dec.?] 1872 (LC).

27. Frederick Stephens, "Exhibition at the Society of French Artists."

28. *The Hour* 9 June, 1874 (GUL).

29. Whistler reprinted his letter under " 'Confidences' with an Editor" in J. M. Whistler, *The Gentle Art of Making Enemies* (London: William Heinemann Ltd., 1892), 47–48.

30. The "Why drag in Velázquez?" story first appeared in the *Suffolk Chronicle* (26 July 1884). It was reprinted elsewhere, with variations, and published in Sheridan Ford, *The Gentle Art of Making Enemies* (Paris, 1890), 246, 250. The volume was suppressed by Whistler who omitted the story in his own edition of *The Gentle Art.* See Robert H. Getscher and Paul G. Marks, *James McNeill Whistler and John Singer Sargent, Two Annotated Bibliographies,* 258–59.

31. Unidentified review (GUL).

32. Such as that by William Morris and Burne-Jones in 1872 for the Hon. George Howard at No. 1 Palace Green. Bill Waters, "Painter and Patron, The Palace Green Murals," *Apollo* 102 (November 1975): 338–41.

33. Doughty and Wahl, 3:1307.

34. Anna McNeill Whistler to Mary Emma Eastwick, Wednesday 9th, [September 1874] (LC).

35. By which time the advertisements for the gallery, published in the *Athenaeum,* cease.

36. "Fine-Art Gossip," *Athenaeum* (24 October 1874): 550.

37. E. Clifton Griffith to Whistler, 21 January 1875 (LC).

38. E. F. White to Whistler, 22 January 1875 (LC).

39. Whistler to E. Clifton Griffith, 22 January 1875 (LC).

40. E. Clifton Griffith to Whistler, 23 January 1875 (LC).

41. Whistler to E. Clifton Griffith, n.d. [24 January 1875] (LC).

42. Whistler to E. Clifton Griffith, 24 January 1875 (LC).

43. E. Clifton Griffith to Whistler (telegram), 25 January 1875 (LC); Writ of the Court of Exchequer to appear within eight days, Westminster 29 January 1875 (LC).

44. Anna McNeill Whistler to James Anderson Rose, 6, 8 February 1875 (LC).

45. Whistler to James Anderson Rose, 7 February 1875 (LC).

46. Draft of the Affidavit of Slater regarding the rehanging of covering of the walls at the gallery, in the handwriting of Rose, 2 pp., 19 March 1875 (LC).

47. "In the Exchequer of Pleas between Edward Clifton Griffith and James A. MacNeill Whistler. Further and better particulars of the Plaintiff's claim delivered pursuant to the Order of Master Butler dated the 17th day of March 1875," 3 pp. (LC).

48. Whistler to James Anderson Rose, 16 February 1875 (LC).

49. "Orders of the Court" dated 26 February, 5, 6, 10, 17, 19 & 24 March 1875; "particulars of the claim," 2 pp., 15 March 1875; "further and better particulars of the claim," 3 pp., 23 March 1875 (LC).

50. Brief of the case for the defendant, rough draft, with opinions and points to plead, inscribed "Mr. Warburton Pike, 1 gna," dated 31 March 1875; Replication, 5 April 1875; part of Whistler's Bill of Costs, 3 pp., April 1875; Bill of Costs, 5 pp., 7 April 1875 (LC).

51. Agreement between Whistler and Mr. Robert Booth Latter of Bromley, Kent, for the lease of 2 Lindsey Row, Chelsea, December 1866 (LC). In 1870 Whistler attempted to rent Merton Villa, Fulham, at a rent of "less than £130." Anna McNeill Whistler to James Anderson Rose, 28 July 1870 (LC). In her letter Whistler's mother states, "Jemie says all the Studios now being built when he had hoped to have one, are totally wrong, he must therefore have one & soon as possible, built according to his own views."

52. Contract between Whistler and his builder, B. Nightingale, 5 November 1877 (LC).

4

S. BING in AMERICA

GABRIEL P. WEISBERG

S. Bing's prominence as a major proponent of the art nouveau movement at the close of the nineteenth century is now well established.[1] His business, located at the corner of 22 rue de Provence and 19 rue Chauchat in Paris, was the center of numerous exhibitions and artistic gatherings that brought together an international audience of artists and designers. In addition, his pavilion at the Paris Exposition Universelle of 1900 became a showplace for work designed and executed by craftsmen working directly under Bing's sponsorship with the clear intention of creating an international style.[2] Bing's impact is well-known, but his methods for achieving such successes have been largely undocumented. An active entrepreneur involved in commercial enterprises, Bing made a fortune through the dissemination of art objects (not always of the highest aesthetic quality) that pandered to the fashionable craze for all things Japanese that was sweeping Europe.[3] Therefore, in order to understand how Bing operated, it is necessary to reconstruct, in part, the world of entrepreneurial activity out of which he emerged;[4] a picture of his modus operandi will demonstrate how closely art and commercial activity were intertwined during the latter part of the century.

Bing's activities in the United States lie at the center of this study since it was with this country—and with the so-called captains of artistic industry—that Bing found himself in open competition. From this relationship, Bing learned a great deal and was able to increase his capital, as he found untapped markets for the sale and distribution of Japanese objects in America—markets that were not as discerning or as concerned about primary quality as those in Europe. An understanding of Bing's dealings in America helps elucidate his mastery of capitalistic as well as artistic manipulation.

The EARLIEST METHODS

Bing's first contact with the United States occurred long before he showed any interest in sponsoring American craftsmen in Europe. According to documents housed at the Metropolitan Museum of Art (New York), on 2 October 1882, Bing wrote to the director of the institution (L. P. di Cesnola) to offer a gift of a Chinese porcelain vase to the budding oriental collections.[5] This offer was not an unusual gesture, as it was a common practice among art dealers to open new relations with a prospective client by giving such an object. While Bing's motives were, in part, decidedly commercial, they also showed Bing's disinterested obsession with the creation of collections in institutions that could eventually bring oriental art to a broader public. In the case of the newly opened Metropolitan Museum, he wrote, "I have intended to make some contribution to the collection of the Museum ... matching with interest the efforts of your liberal citizens to establish a museum of art."[6] He added that the piece had been sent as an addition to the Avery Collection which, he said, "I believe is deficient in pieces of this character."[7]

This correspondence marks Bing as an inveterate museum watcher who knew when to cultivate a new area as a means of expanding the market. Since Bing had extensive dealings with the Metropolitan Museum of Art later on, this early exchange was prophetic of things to come. Once associated with an institution, Bing never relented in his contacts; he would continually send information to officials with the hope of making additional sales. Often Bing would send emissaries from his Paris office to a museum to work on business matters; for example, he announces in a letter to the Metropolitan on 13 March 1896, that his nephew Enrique Baer would soon arrive to work out other business matters involving the sale of some Japanese art objects.[8]

Bing often used business associates as emissaries on his behalf during his promotion of Oriental art. When art nouveau objects entered the Metropolitan Museum of Art in 1926, they too came to the New York institution through a dealer in Oriental art, René Haase, who had succeeded Bing in business.[9] In a sense, then, Bing's influence on the American art scene and on the art market came directly through his promotion of all types of Oriental art objects and only indirectly through his advocacy of design reformers in the United States.

Bing promoted Oriental art in the United States avidly. His activity in sales (especially through large auctions in New York and Philadelphia) enabled him to sell innumerable items to a voracious American clientele, who were attracted by the glamour associated with his name, especially since he brought objects from France directly to the United States. Bing's association with collectors brought the dealer into intimate contact not only with those who had money to spend on the newest craze but also with artists and some serious connoisseurs who wanted to develop collections of value. Bing's contacts with wealthy patrons often led him to museums, since these individuals were frequently on the boards of such institutions and were instrumental in seeing that collections and special exhibitions were cultivated. The latter involvement often led to shows under Bing's sponsorship, which gained large followings through reviews in newspapers and journals. Thus, Bing cultivated a taste for Oriental art—specifically the art of Japan—on new shores and emerged as the central figure in American Japanism just as he had established himself in Europe.

The SALESROOM as EFFECTIVE TOOL

Despite the widespread general belief that Bing's ties with the United States are largely linked to his treatise *La Culture Artistique en Amérique*, Bing's other side often appeared elsewhere at an early date. The first Oriental art sale was held in April 1887 (fig. 4.1) at Moore's Art Galleries at 290 Fifth Avenue in New York. The preliminary viewing of the objects that were to be sold, however, took place in an unusual location, "the

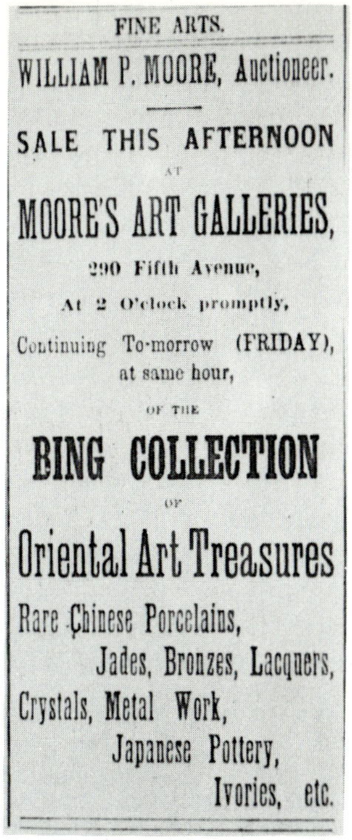

Fig. 4.1. Cover of the auction catalogue for Moore's Art Galleries, New York, April 1887.

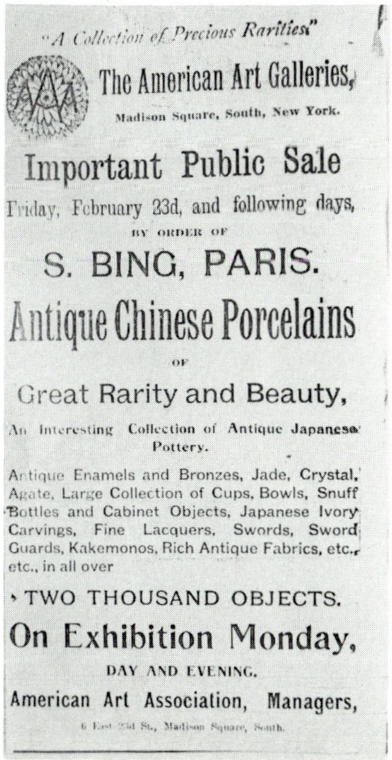

Fig. 4.2. Advertisement for Oriental sale, New York, 1894.

rooms of S. Bing, 220 Fifth Avenue on April 25th," revealing that by this date Bing had his own address in the largest United States metropolis.[10] It also demonstrates that he was willing to work in tandem with an American auctioneer in order to dispose of excess stock from France.[11] Several advertisements announcing the public sale appeared in the daily press including one in *The New York Commercial Advertiser* (on April 23) and another in *The Evening Post* (April 21). Both the official catalogue for the sale and the printed flyer noted that the sale included "some rare and antique porcelains, superb bronzes, exquisite lacquers, remarkable jades, crystals and hard stones."[12] Bing was clearly selling all types of "orientalia," but the quality of these objects is less apparent.

Despite the hyperbole in the advertisement, the material that Bing was selling was probably largely Oriental "stuff." Bing may have shipped these objects to the United States because he recognized that the country was ripe for them: Americans did not have a discerning background, and there were few who could spot the difference between pieces of extreme rarity and those of lesser significance. In France, Bing had followed the same commercial path in the early 1880s, during the promotion of contemporary Japanese art objects (those made concurrently in the Far East), which found a ready clientele with a limited means.[13] A similar entrepreneurial vision led him to recognize that these types of objects could be sold in America at public auction.

The 1887 sale proved so important that it was reviewed in *The New York Times* and *The Art Amateur.* The latter provided a good example of the taste and enthusiasm in the general arena, as the reviewer noted that

> the Bing auction sale at Moore's afforded golden opportunities for embryonic collectors of Japanese bronzes and Chinese and Japanese porcelains. The first two days the goods were almost given away.[14]

The quantity of available objects may have overwhelmed Americans at first, making it difficult for them to respond to what was being offered. It is also apparent that while some Americans did not want to pay high prices for all the objects, some pieces, presumably those of more aesthetic significance, were being held in reserve for later in the sale. Still, the reviewer notes that the attendance at the sale was small and that the auctioneer was unequal to the occasion. He ends by noting that "the advantage of selling an excellent lot of Oriental art goods, with the guarantee of a house like Bing, was wholly thrown away."[15] Bing had a lot of work to do in order to coax an American audience to appreciate the value of Oriental art.

It is not known whether Bing had anticipated a small turnout for the auction, but he did not despair, since his willingness to experiment had prompted the sale. Bing was helping establish a beachhead for the public in a new country, and it was generally accepted that this would take some time. If we keep in mind that Bing was not sacrificing objects of great aesthetic value, then his shrewdness appears more cunning. Bing was starting his audience at a low level, while planning to work them up toward better quality pieces; in addition, he hoped to establish a broad foundation for *Japonisme* by having objects available to a large public. These aspects are worth remembering in a study of the second public sale in April 1888.

This second sale took place in Philadelphia. Cognizant of the developing interest in Oriental art there following the success of the Centennial exhibition of 1876, Bing held his auction at the Davis and Harvey Art Galleries on Chestnut Street.[16] Once again the public sale included Chinese and Japanese porcelains, faiences, potteries, bronzes, enamels, ivories, lacquers, carvings, silk, embroideries, and some furniture. All of the objects were to be sold directly under the sponsorship of Bing's firm, which was still at 220 Fifth Avenue in New York. In holding this new sale, presumably with a fresh stock that had been sent from Paris, Bing continued to establish his American network while he was beginning to launch the highly successful, and visible, *Le Japon Artistique*. He believed that he needed a series of cities actively committed to the collection and understanding of Japanese art if his American campaign was to be successful. Philadelphia, therefore, assumed as much significance in his overall plans as New York.

A third public auction, even larger than the two previous sales, took place in New York in 1888. It began on November 21st and ended on November 27th, after 1334 objects had been sold to a wide variety of clients.[17] This time the sale actually took place in Bing's own showrooms under the general supervision of the Fifth Avenue auction rooms.[18] This first sale in Bing's own quarters demonstrates that he was doing exceedingly well, and he could invite prospective clients to his own showrooms.

By 1888, in the official records for businesses in the city, Bing was listed as a New York City antique dealer.[19] Unlike his similar listing in Paris, however, Bing is noted as working with a partner—John Getz. While it was not completely unusual to find Bing's name associated with others (he even used this technique in Paris on several occasions), it is apparent that after a few years Getz assumed more and more importance in the relationship, eventually even overshadowing Bing in the United States. It suggests that Getz was counted on to solve any dilemmas in the new market area, as Bing rarely was able to come to the United States on his own. In fact, because of this association, one reviewer of the early exhibitions in which Bing and Getz were involved considered that the latter was Bing's resident partner in America.[20]

Getz assumed increasing importance in the public salesroom side of Bing's American business. He helped coordinate the early Oriental art sales by preparing the catalogues (often writing the entries) and identifying the origin and age of a number of the pieces that were to be sold. At the same time, Getz maintained another interest: he was a significant interior decorator who had close ties with some of the more popular firms in the east. Since he had worked with the Herter brothers, important designers of early Japanese style furniture, Getz was well-versed in ways to incorporate Oriental art objects into the American home. He may also have been instrumental in promoting, in his own right, a taste for things Oriental by incorporating lacquers and ceramics into American room interiors as part of a changing aesthetic climate. Such a two-pronged interest, representing the two practical poles of Bing's personality, helped meld both men together. They were both eager to work together to spread the taste for orientalia in America if it could generate a successful commercial income.

It is unclear where the pair met, although it is possible that Getz had met Bing in Paris in 1886. Getz was abroad then, visiting several European cities, and would have had ample time to visit Bing's emporium in Paris. Although the passenger list of the returning vessel to the United States (November 1886) does not list his profession, he certainly went abroad on some type of business venture to increase his contacts with dealers.[21] Bing recognized Getz as someone who could help him increase the American side of his business as well as someone who wanted to see Japanese design principles in objects crafted in the United States. (Getz was also a collector of Japanese prints.)

Getz remained intimately associated with Bing's gallery in New York through 1891, the date when Bing most likely ceased his operation on Fifth Avenue[22]—

a move which might have had something to do with Bing's desire to sell only objects of the best quality. Getz, however, still remained in contact with Bing in other ways through the 1890s and helped organize the exhibition of modern books that Bing initiated in his art nouveau shop in Paris in 1896. At the time, Getz gathered the American books at his own New York gallery (391 Fifth Avenue) prior to their being shipped abroad.

Getz was actively involved with Bing in the American salesrooms, but the Paris dealer was also highly capable of seizing the initiative. He wanted to see his business expand; therefore he originated sales at the American Art Galleries in New York to further cement his position as the dean of the Oriental art dealers. His strategy was demonstrated in February 1894, when Bing was in America, and another sale of Chinese and Japanese art objects was held in New York.[23] Getz played only a minor role, helping to compile the catalogue for the sale, since Bing was now working with a new company and a new auctioneer, Thomas Kirby. Like Bing's previous sales in America, this one was thoroughly advertised in the press (fig. 4.2). *The Evening Post, The Sun,* and *The New York Tribune,* for example, ran previews, providing a good amount of presale publicity. The previewer for *The Post* noted that "perhaps never, certainly not this winter, has there been shown here a collection so rich in antique Japanese pottery. Of this there are over 300 pieces, most of which, it is safe to say, will appeal alike to artist and collector ... there is something personal about each piece of this ware of which so much less is here known than of porcelains."[24] For the previewer in *The Sun,* "any aggregation of objects bearing his approval is sure to be well recommended."[25] He commented that Bing had set a high standard for himself. However, this favorable response was countered by another reviewer who found the effort so diversified that the overall impact remained commercial. Bing was trying to raise the quality of the objects he was selling on the American market by 1894, but some observers still saw his entire American effort in a decidedly mundane light.

BING'S AMERICAN CLIENTS

It is difficult to know how successful the different sales actually were or how much money Bing realized from them. But he held an impressive sale in New York in 1894 (as the catalogue cover adapted from a print by Hokusai indicates) (fig. 4.3) while he was visiting America to raise capital for his new enterprise—art nouveau—in the decorative arts.[26] But the significance of the success or failure of these sales pales beside another important issue, one as pivotal for the future of Japanese art collections in the country as it was for the type of dealer Bing had become: the question of the quality and authenticity of the pieces that he was selling. If we believe most of the reviewers assessing the sales, it appears that Bing and Cie. was selling only works of the highest aesthetic quality and the most authentic provenance. However, when one examines some of the American collections that Bing helped develop (albeit they were formed in a different manner), a slightly different picture emerges. Here, one realizes that what Bing and other Oriental art dealers sold must have been a decidedly "mixed bag." While this does not mean that reviewers were only writing propaganda about the sales they visited, it does suggest that the understanding of Japanese, and to a lesser extent Chinese, art on the part of critics and collectors was still in its infancy. While the resulting collections

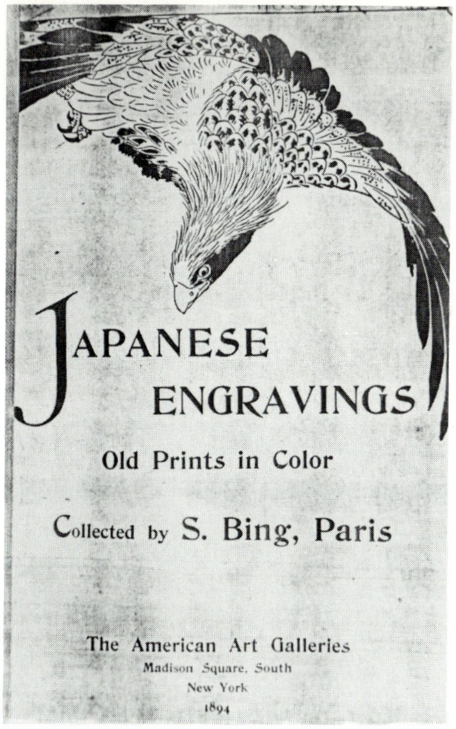

Fig. 4.3. Cover for 1894 Japanese print exhibition, New York. Courtesy of the New York Public Library.

do not suggest that Bing and others were willfully deceiving their clients, it does indicate that much had to be learned about the significance of individual pieces before they could be accepted as coming from a specific period or from a definite location in Japan.

One such collection exemplifying these issues is the Freer Collection in Washington, D.C. Bing openly assisted Charles Lang Freer in purchasing Japanese art—the second way in which the dealer worked. Their relationship got fully underway when the American entrepreneur asked Bing to help obtain pieces from the Goncourt sale in Paris in 1897.[27] The relationship between the men continued until Bing's death in 1905, but some of the pieces that Bing sold Freer have not turned out to be what they had been originally presented. Since Bing's personal collection of Japanese art work, which he kept housed in his private quarters on the rue Vézelay, was visited by extremely knowledgeable collectors from the United States, including E. S. Morse, who commented on the superb quality of Bing's Japanese pottery pieces, one suspects that Bing was not without a venal side, which was accentuated when he sold pieces to American collectors who lacked the necessary degree of sophistication to build a towering collection. This possibility is reinforced by the fact that Bing's own collection (sold in 1906) revealed that he had been a most discerning collector for himself. Bing may have followed two policies in working with private American collectors: first, he did not always sell pieces of the highest aesthetic quality and, second, he left it up to the collectors to choose the piece(s) they wanted. Thus, he could make a living through the contemporary market, while retaining the best pieces for himself in order to demonstrate his own level of significant connoisseurship.

The ties with Freer demonstrate that Bing was anxious to expand his business connections with wealthy American magnates. Some of these figures undoubtedly visited Bing's shops in Paris, negotiated with Bing's agents who came to America, and bought pieces from the sales that Bing organized in the United States. However, these sales also helped propagate Japanese art on even a more popular level.

The TRAVELING EXHIBITION

Bing also introduced Japanese art to the United States through traveling exhibitions with objects drawn from his own stock. This method had proven extremely effective in Europe, and Bing moved quickly to implement the same means in the United States. The most important of these itinerant exhibitions took place in March 1894, at the American Art Galleries, while Bing was also in the country. The show and its accompanying catalogue, titled *Japanese Engraving. Old Prints in Color. Collected by S. Bing, Paris,* represented Bing's increasing efforts to bring Japanese printmaking to an American audience (similar to the way he had done it in Paris with major exhibitions).[28] Two hundred and ninety pieces by some of the leading ukiyo-e printmakers ranging in date from 1608 until 1850 were included in the exhibition. Since the introduction to the catalogue had been prepared by Bing himself, it promised much for the American audience, giving the impression that one of the major sponsors and connoisseurs of Japanese art had decided to reach out to a popular American audience with the display of first-rate prints.

The exhibit did not go unnoticed. One critic reviewing the show for the magazine *The Critic* noted that "the exhibition of prints should be of great interest to all who care about the possibilities of color-printing, for no more artistic work has ever been done . . . than that produced by the popular school of Japanese art."[29] After the New York showing, Bing tried to have the prints exhibited in Philadelphia at the Pennsylvania Academy of Fine Arts. Since this institution was having its own show of Japanese objects and had asked Bing to contribute, the dealer thought that it would be ideal to have his prints included. While Bing did send some textiles to Philadelphia, it proved too late to show his Japanese prints. Thus, Bing lost a splendid opportunity to increase the awareness of his Japanese prints, although, true to his entrepreneurial ingenuity, he soon found another venue. He sent several hundred examples to the Boston Museum of Fine Arts in April 1894, when his friend Ernest Fenollosa was the curator in charge of Oriental art.[30] Bing's Japanese textiles eventually landed in the Metropolitan Museum of Art in New York.

None of these methods would have been quite as successful in reaching a public audience if it had not been for Bing's commercial promotion of *Japonisme* in America. Through the sale and distribution of *Artistic Japan* with its lavish reproductions and elaborate color plates, Bing stimulated trade, as individuals learned about Japan in a popular publication. The magazine was extensively reviewed in the United States, indicating that it was taken seriously as an educational tool and served as a commercial vehicle to let people know what was on the trade market. It also cleverly reinforced Bing's position in the United States, effectively promoting his name and firm.

Thus, by the mid-1890s, Bing had become a foremost promoter for all things Japanese—both good and bad. His methods had proven extremely successful in bringing him contacts; yet Bing was still eager to expand ties with individual collectors and with museums. Despite all of this interest in developing a market for *Japonisme* in America, however, Bing had another significant area of concern there.

BING and AMERICAN DECORATIVE ART

Bing's keen interest in the United States also grew from his broad study of American art—especially the decorative arts—and the impact that the American renaissance in this area had on his own perceptions of what an art dealer could do in his adopted country. When Bing decided to reenter the field of decorative design (he had first become involved while working with his father and other firms in the 1860s), conditions in Europe and the United States were ripe for change.[31] In fact, innovations had already taken place that helped convince Bing to move away from being seen solely as a dealer in Oriental art rather than as a promoter able to pursue his own passions for decorative design. Bing was certainly aware that France had lost its long-standing lead in the field of the decorative arts, a fact clearly evident at the 1893 Chicago World's Fair. Reports published after the fair by French art critics commented on advances made by European and American competitors admonished their countrymen to reform their methods of artistic production. A report written by Victor Champier (the editor of *Art et Décoration*) after the Chicago Fair, for example, was quoted in the French press: "It is certain that we have much to do if on the occasion of our next Exposition Universelle of 1900 we don't wish to see ourselves outdistanced on more than one point. French industrialists beware!"[32]

This anguished concern about the lost supremacy of French luxury products culminated in the organization of a national conference on the decorative arts in Paris during May 1894. This conference focused on increased competition from abroad (especially the United States) and tried to find solutions. Since Bing wanted to change the field of decorative design, he had probably remained allied to some craftsmen since the 1860s, while keenly following the situation. He had already returned from the United States when the conference took place; therefore he was personally aware of what had already been accomplished by American craftsmen, especially by Louis Comfort Tiffany.

Since records of Tiffany's firm have disappeared, Bing's relationship with him is difficult to document,[33] but they may have known each other since Bing first saw Tiffany's successful exhibition of stained glass windows at the Paris Exposition Universelle of 1889. Since Tiffany came to Paris then, it is likely (given Tiffany's penchant for Oriental art) that the American designer would have visited Bing's galleries. The two would have had much in common. Thus it is likely that when Bing came to America in 1894 he would have visited Tiffany's workshop and gotten a close look at the American's innovations; Bing may have gathered ideas to bring to France to help modernize the design world.[34]

Thus, Bing had several reasons to visit America in the late winter and early spring of 1894.[35] From February 12th until April 7th when he returned to France, Bing attended to business in conjunction with his sale of Japanese art, but, more im-

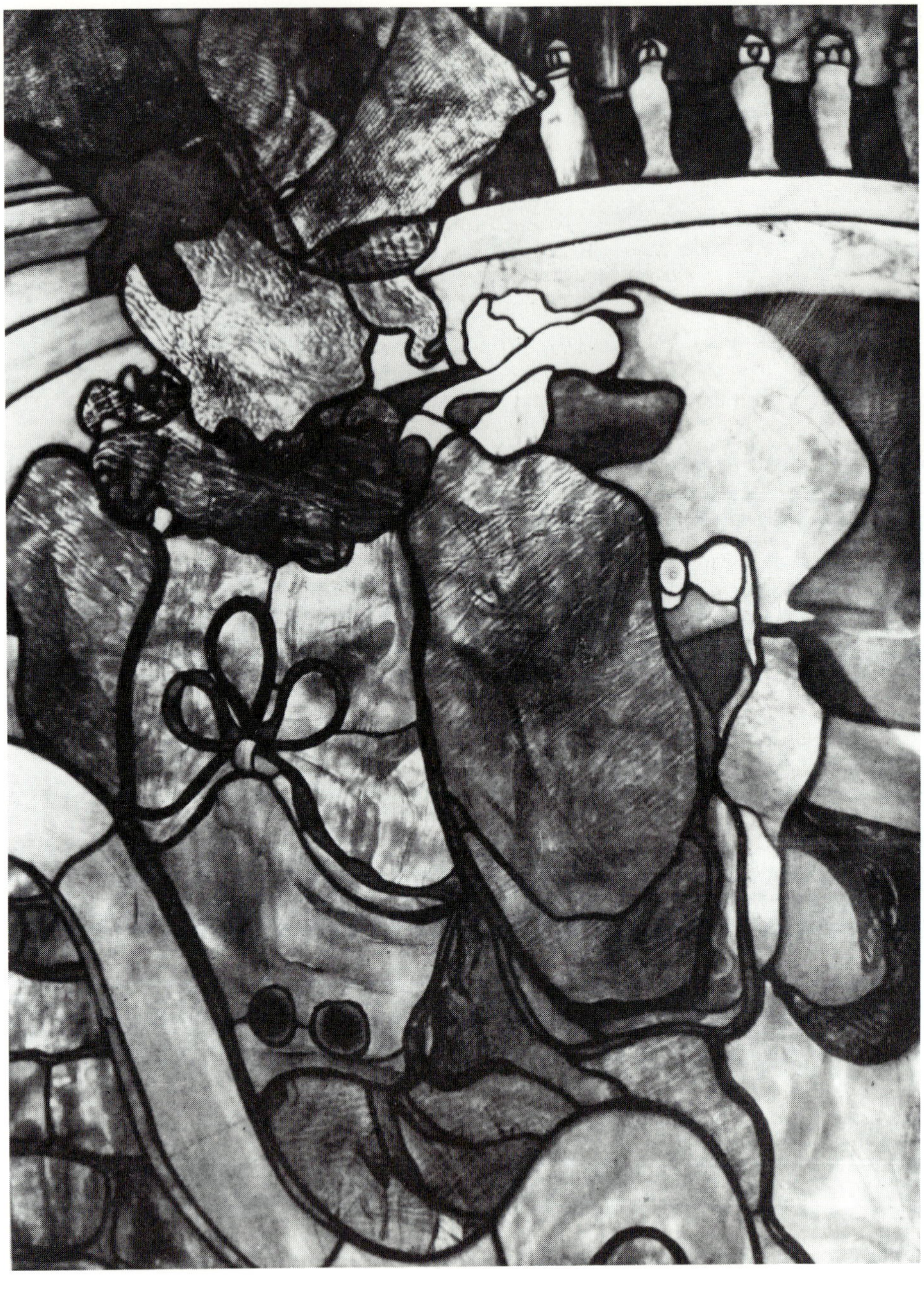

Fig. 4.4. Henri Toulouse-Lautrec, *Papa Chrysanthème,* stained glass window, 1894. Musée d'Orsay, Paris.

portantly, he found the time to study American art and the methods of American craftsmen.[36] He was determined to discover new perspectives and gain needed encouragement for his own renewed commitment to decorative design.

Bing met numerous craftsmen such as Tiffany, Samuel Coleman, and John Lafarge. Tiffany was the only one to become prominently featured in Bing's own

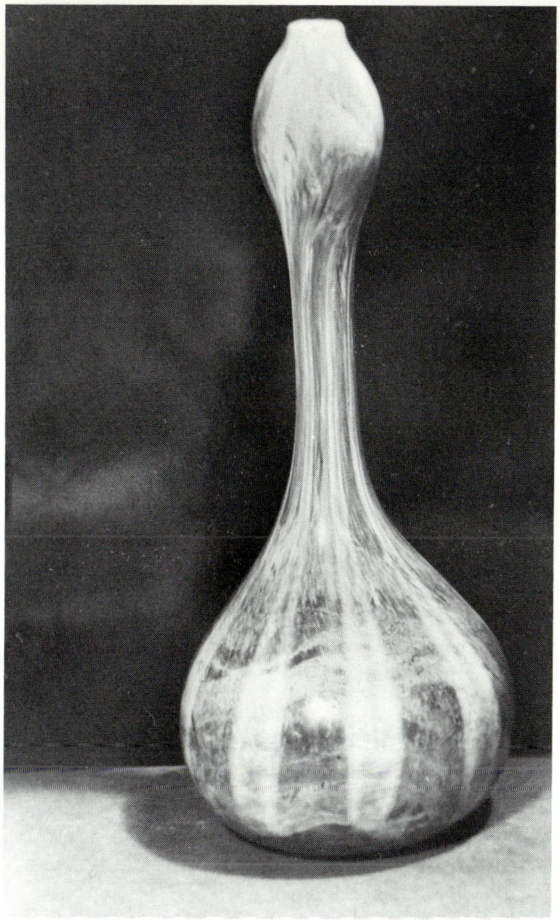

Fig. 4.5. Louis C. Tiffany, *Vase,* favrile glass, after 1895. Österreichische Museum für angewandte Kunst, Vienna.

business activities, but discussions with the others convinced the French dealer to seek craftsmen in cities throughout the United States. Still, Tiffany's methods and modern techniques most appealed to Bing. A visit to Tiffany's Brooklyn studios convinced Bing that a joint collaboration could be established in which Bing's ateliers would emerge according to Tiffany's model and Bing's own personal experience. Immediately after returning to France, Bing acted on his ties with Tiffany by soliciting from young French artists (the Nabis) sketches for stained glass windows that would be produced by Tiffany in America.

Bing's commitment to the Nabis is chronicled in a series of letters from him to members of the group who were going to do the project. Since the windows were to use the methods established by Tiffany, they signaled to Bing and his French colleagues that a new start in stained glass could be encouraged by working closely with America. When the completed windows were exhibited, first at the Salon of the Société Nationale des Beaux-Arts and later at Bing's first Salon of Art Nouveau in December 1895 (fig. 4.4), they attracted considerable reaction from visitors to the exhibitions and from the press. The critic for the *Revue Franco-Américaine,* an important journal that stressed relations between the countries, also believed them to be a series of "superb stained glass windows executed in New York. . . . The prestigious art of stained glass triumphs at the Champs de Mars."[37]

Most significant about these windows is the fact that during his trip to America Bing had the foresight to discuss this venture with Tiffany. Even with no previous training in stained-glass, Bing was confident that Tiffany was the figure to work with on this venture; therefore, upon returning to France, he acted to bring the young artists and Tiffany together. In this way, Bing pushed ever closer to the lead position as champion of the avant-garde in decorative art. As the project for the windows matured, Bing also became the primary sponsor for Tiffany favrile glass in Europe and organized exhibitions of Tiffany glass in Europe beginning in 1897 (fig. 4.5). Thus, in another way, Bing had the foresight to arrange a business relationship that permitted him to promote Tiffany throughout Europe solely through Bing's own company, L'Art Nouveau. By 1898, following Tiffany's major success at the Dresden International Exhibition, Bing organized further shows for the American; he also wrote articles on Tiffany pieces, further cementing the ties that he had established earlier.[38]

Aside from Tiffany, Bing singled out other American firms for the establishment of business relationships. Among these were the ceramic firms of Grueby and Company based in Boston, whom Bing undoubtedly visited in conjunction with his trip there to promote Japanese prints in 1894, and Rookwood and Company in Cincinnati, Ohio. Neither firm exhibited works at the first Salon of Art Nouveau, but many European museums bought Grueby and Rookwood pieces from Bing's shop once the dealer had negotiated with the American firms to be their agent in Europe.[39] The decorative arts museum in Nurnberg, Germany, for example, has several (figs. 4.6 and 4.7) exquisite Rookwood vases purchased from Bing in 1900 at the Paris World's Fair. Bing always maintained this keen interest in American craftsmen and firms, enabling them to sell wares to a large European audience. After 1895, he offered American sculptors and painters an opportunity to show their work in private exhibitions at L'Art Nouveau. Bing's close business ties with American craftsmen, and specifically with industrial firms that shaped his vision, demonstrated that he transported American ingenuity to France via examples of creative work that demonstrated a unified approach and by imitation of American methods in his own ateliers.

Bing's investigation of the contemporary American art scene also had another purpose, a less personal one than we have presented but one which would ultimately benefit the French nation. Bing also wanted to prepare a report on the state of artistic culture in America. When this was finally published in December 1895, it reached many of the leading designers throughout the world, including Henri van de Velde in Belgium, who had the slender volume carefully bound in leather. This pamphlet, published at the time of the opening of the first Salon of Art Nouveau, is a valuable document. Although it seems strange that Bing waited over a year before publishing the report, it is likely that he did not have the time to complete it during active preparations for the changeover of his business. Once the report was published, it went further than assessing the decorative arts. It provided a good, if conventional, survey of American art at the time.

La Culture Artistique en Amérique is divided into four sections: painting, sculpture, architecture, and the industrial arts. Bing found fault in the first sections,

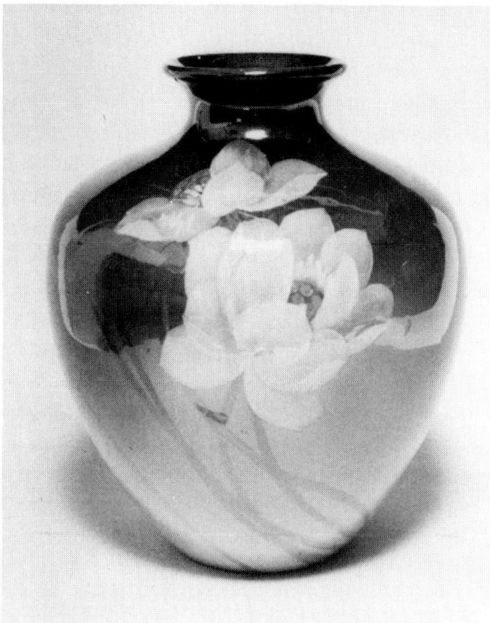

Fig. 4.6. Rookwood and Company, *Vase,* faience, c. 1900. Gewerbemuseum der L.G.A., Nuremberg.

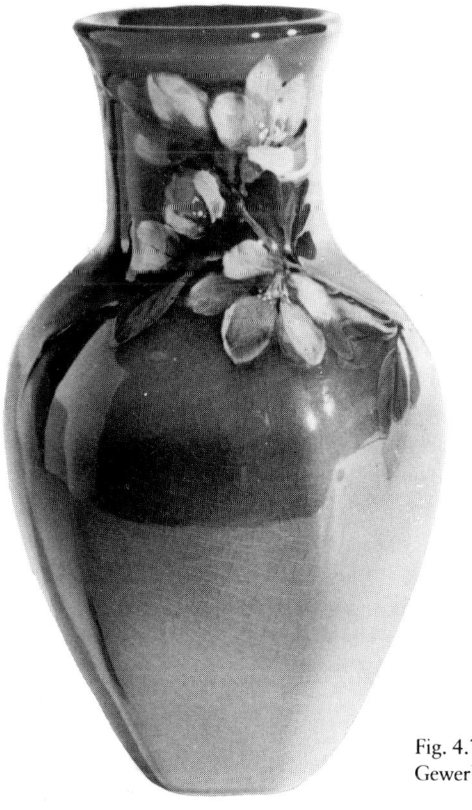

Fig. 4.7. Rookwood and Company, *Vase,* faience, c. 1900. Gewerbemuseum der L.G.A., Nuremberg.

believing that American art had not found a new ideal but was still subject to intense French influences. He stressed, however, that in light of the nation's level of energy and thrust toward the future, it was still "capable of forging a new art in her own image."[40] Sculpture did not impress him any more than painting; he thought that there were too many formal statues in the country. An American reviewer for *The Evening Post* (21 March 1896) took exception with Bing's opinion in these areas, commenting that "one might be tempted to believe, at first, that the report might have been written without crossing the Atlantic, for the only American painters the author seems to know well are those who have taken up permanent residence abroad." About the sculpture sections, the commentator notes that "if M. Bing knows little about American painting, he knows and cares less about our sculpture."[41] He continues in this vein, stressing that Bing's attitude could be explained by the other areas examined in the report.

> It is when Mr. Bing begins to deal with architecture that he reveals the reason for this attitude. He is one of those who came to the consideration of American art with a fixed notion that a new people should produce something entirely new, and that all art which resembles what has been done in other countries is therefore negligible. In our architecture he finds this new thing, and the cold critic of our painting and sculpture becomes the enthusiastic admirer of those high buildings which we, in our ignorance of what we have done best . . . are trying to suppress by act of legislature.[42]

While the critic for *The Evening Post* was astute in the evaluation of Bing's position on painting and sculpture, he may not have known that the Frenchman had little time for a full investigation of the arts of America during his short visit to the country. At the same time, the reviewer failed to understand the significance of what Bing wrote about architecture and the industrial arts. He only gives passing recognition to Bing for having enthusiastically endorsed stained glass, noting that this may have been "influenced by Bing's commercial relations with a well-known firm of manufacturers."[43] Seen in retrospect, this was a penetrating jibe, based on a correct assessment of Bing's commercial interests.

Given Bing's support of architecture in *La Culture Artistique* and his subsequent enthusiasm for the industrial arts, both areas should be carefully examined. In the realm of architecture—an area limited by Bing's ability to actually see buildings in the various cities that he visited—Bing believed that no nation had "displayed more overwhelming vigour" than had America. He thought that what made American architecture new and exciting was American architects' ability to adopt what they had learned in Europe to their own environment. One of the primary models of this facility was H. H. Richardson, whom Bing thought conveyed an understanding of the need for architecture to be responsive to modern life. Bing believed that conditions in America were ideal for a new architecture, since commercial and public buildings—which could handle increasing numbers of people—demonstrated the importance of this area to the spirit of the nation.

Bing wrote about commercial buildings, transportation centers, hotels, and specific architects who exemplified the new horizons. His stay in New York and his awareness of buildings in Chicago, Cincinnati, Albany, and Pittsburgh led him to champion Louis Sullivan in addition to Richardson. But at the same time as he examined such large structures, Bing praised the vitality of the American home with its new interior. Here, practicality had been wedded to art in order to allow the new home builder—or owner—the opportunity to use the new techniques provided by achievements in interior design. In addition, the impact of Japan had led some American designers and architects toward the realization that space and taste without pretentious details were needed.

Bing's keen understanding that interior design was burgeoning led to his recognition that the industrial arts could play a central role in home decoration. For a long time, France had been learning about American inroads in this field, including the ability to use industry to create new art objects, and Bing's evaluation was extremely timely and valuable to many, including the director of the Beaux-Arts, Henri Roujon, who had been helpful in [illegible] to the United States.

Bing's [illegible] trenchant for the French, and he developed his case carefully, noting [illegible] and wealth of the United States was not initially reflected in a new [illegible] decorative idiom. For a long period, America had relied on European imports, since the country had not fully mastered an independent ability to produce luxury items. [illegible] had primarily occurred with small objects, rather than furniture. The craftsman most responsible for the later shift was Edward C. Moore, who was among the first "to comprehend the real value of the art treasures just emerging from the Orient."[44] Using the United States as a model, Bing contrasted the situation in France. While America had forged ahead, he believed, France had stagnated under the weight of dead period styles and poor training of craftsmen in state institutions.

As Bing develops his lengthy essay in *La Culture Artistique* it becomes apparent to him that the American support of democracy, with its abiding belief in the equality of all areas of art, was responsible for freeing the decorative arts from being perceived as a base craft unworthy of consideration as high art. This significant message became a guiding and animating force for craftsmen in 1895 who were trying to establish a new style on equal footing with older areas such as painting and sculpture. Thus, the propagandistic force of Bing's message should not be underestimated. Since he was writing from the standpoint of a private entrepreneur, Bing increased awareness of the industrial arts while encouraging a renewal of energy in France to match what he had witnessed in America.

Bing's observation of the Tiffany ateliers and his desire to reestablish himself as a *chef d'atelier* led him to observe that all aspects of such a system could be welded together, producing an impression of harmony both in the objects and in the way the artisans worked with one another. Comradeship was encouraged; within the production of luxury items, Bing sought solidarity. To him, Tiffany provided the ultimate example of what could be achieved: a vast factory, a central workshop, and an army of craftsmen all working in relevant media. Bing was deeply impressed by American ingenuity, and he conveys this message in his writings. By 1900, the formation of his own ateliers helped him create a harmonious style for himself in all areas of the crafts.

Bing also found American design unpretentious, commenting that "the natural flow of lines, dictated by function" was "a thousand times more attractive than any artificial attempt"; and he asks whether it is "their continuing contact with Japanese art which has made Americans turn so enthusiastically toward nature?"[45] Since it was to Bing's advantage to see Japanese art as the force that had animated American design, he isolated these aspects of American decorative design that he hoped would revolutionize the French system.

CONCLUSION

In a sense then, Bing's trip to America and the subsequent publication of his report as *La Culture Artistique* became a symbolic mission. It was known in creative circles in France that Bing had gone to the United States to increase his commercial markets so that he would have more money and hence, freedom to find answers to what he hoped to do in the decorative arts in his own country. The trip emphasizes Bing's ingenuity as an entrepreneur, while making it abundantly apparent that Japan and the industrial reform movement in the arts were united in his mind. Bing could not see one without the other, and his American sojourn unmistakingly underscores this fact.

While Bing's trip to America in 1894 can be seen as the height of his interest in the United States, it was not the end of the relationship. Bing continued to work with wealthy American clients until his death in 1905. He sold numerous Japanese art objects and found some clients who were seriously interested in his form of art nouveau. As a businessman and entrepreneur, Bing never closed a door behind him. His ambitions and his hopes reveal America's centrality in forcing him to remain modern and energetic in a burgeoning new age that blended the commercial and the artistic to forge new paths.

NOTES

1. For further reference see Gabriel P. Weisberg, "L'Art Nouveau Bing," *Arts in Virginia Bulletin* 20 (Fall 1979): 1–15; Idem, "S. Bing's Craftsmen Workshops: A Location and Importance Revealed," *Source* 3 (Fall 1983): 42–48. Bing was the subject of a large-scale exhibition prepared by the author under the aegis of the Smithsonian Institution during 1986–87. This exhibition, "The Paris Style 1900: Art Nouveau Bing," sets Bing's contribution to the decorative style of 1900 into proper perspective.

2. Weisberg, "S. Bing's Craftsmen Workshops," 42–48. This article documents ways in which Bing worked with individual craftsmen on his own premises with the belief that his objects would forcefully contribute to an international decorative style.

3. The *Japonisme* movement was largely stimulated by Bing's promotion of art objects he had obtained in the Far East. Bing held a number of early sales to help spread this phenomenon; in the mid 1870s, he sold an extensive collection of Japanese art objects to the Victoria and Albert Museum, London. For reference to this sale, see *The Academy* (20 November 1875): 539. Throughout the 1870s and 1880s, Bing's Parisian shops (he often had several outlets) attracted numerous artists and collectors eager to acquire Japanese art works. Bing's trip to the Far East (and his well-established ties with the Orient) demonstrated that he could sell both ancient objects of high aesthetic quality and examples of a contemporary mode created for the Western trade. By 1888, Bing's promotion of the Far East reached a pinnacle with his sponsorship and publication of *Artistic Japan,* a monthly periodical prepared in three languages with glossy reproductions to assure distribution of the periodical to those who were wealthy and who might want to purchase expensive items. In this way, through his ability to merchandise a taste, Bing became a focal point for an entire movement.

4. The question of entrepreneurial patronage and class distinctions developed by those men who built collections or championed individual figures has not been dealt with in the literature of nineteenth-century art. The one article of significance is Albert Boime, "Entrepreneurial Patronage in Nineteenth Century France," in *Enterprise and Entrepreneurs in Nineteenth and Twentieth Century France* (Baltimore and London: The Johns Hopkins University Press, 1976), 137–207.

5. Letter of S. Bing to L. P. di Cesnola, 2 October 1882. Metropolitan Museum of Art, New York. Archives. Office of the Secretary, Correspondence files, 1870–1950. Whether Bing actually came to the United States at this time has not been determined, although he must have had prior contact with either the

director of the museum or the institution itself before he made his donation. Contact with Bing, however, could have been established solely in Paris. Bing's shops were recognized meccas for those interested in Far Eastern art, and the presence of a member of the museum staff at Bing's underscores this aspect.

6. Ibid.

7. Ibid.

8. Letter from S. Bing to the Metropolitan Museum, 13 March 1896. Metropolitan Museum of Art, New York. Archives. Office of the Secretary, Correspondence files, 1870–1950.

9. The exact nature of the business relationship between René Haase and Bing is difficult to establish with certainty. Bing may have worked with members of the Haase family at an early date when he was manufacturing porcelain. René Haase did take over the Bing Oriental business after the death of S. Bing's son, Marcel, in 1921, and hence, would have had access and title to whatever remained of the art nouveau stock still in the possession of Marcel Bing when he died. For this reason, in the mid-1920s, the Metropolitan Museum of Art found itself negotiating with Haase for art nouveau pieces manufactured by Bing. For further reference, see the notation of 6 October 1926, of an approval to purchase furniture, ceramics, and glass from R. Haase for $2,000, in the Metropolitan Museum of Art Archives. The money was drawn from the Edward C. Moore fund for the purchase of modern decorative art. Haase supplemented the purchase with other objects made for Bing as gifts to the Metropolitan.

10. See *Moore's Art Galleries, 290 Fifth Avenue, The Collection of S. Bing of Paris. Chinese Porcelains, Jades, Bronzes, Japanese Pottery, Crystals, Lacquers, Metal Work, Ivories, etc.* Exhibition at 220 Fifth Avenue, Sale at Moore's Galleries, New York, April 26–29, 1887, 1–60. A detailed examination of the official business records and address listings in New York for this period has revealed no documentation on Bing's presence in the city. It could be that Bing was subletting rooms from another dealer (as was often the case) or that he had a partner who was helping him establish himself in America. Hence the official records, if they have survived, could be under the name of Bing's associate in the United States.

11. The relationship with Moore's Auction Galleries is curious. This firm was well established as an auction house, and Bing may have been working with them to dispose of items as well as to establish his credentials in America. The availability of a large stock suggests that Bing could not dispose of everything on the Parisian art market. It also implies that the French dealer saw America as a logical area for some of his secondary goods. Thus, statements in the catalogue that many of the objects were "rare," "exquisite," or "remarkable" were nothing more than promotional hype—a convenient business ploy—to help Bing sell pieces to a new clientele.

12. A similar tone was found in the advertisement for *The Evening Post* (21 April 1887), 3. For further review of the sale see "Bric-à-Brac, The Bing 'opening,' " *The Art Amateur* 17 (November 1887): 124–25.

13. Tribunal de Commerce, Paris. "Dépot des Statuts de la Société en commandite par actions S. Bing et Cie.," July 1, 1884. This firm expressed the goal of selling contemporary Japanese art that was being imported to meet the current taste. Thus, by 1887, Bing may have been liquidating one aspect of his stock, especially the more mundane items, in order to assume the mantle of dean of tastemakers for serious Japanese art.

14. Montezuma, "My Notebook," *The Art Amateur* 17 (June 1887): 3.

15. Ibid. As was the case with early sales, objects of quality were sold amid a massive number of secondary examples.

16. For further reference, see *Catalogue of Rare and Valuable Art Objects comprising Chinese and Japanese Porcelains, Faiences . . . including many Specimens for Collectors and Amateurs to be sold by auction under the direction of the firm of S. Bing, 220 Fifth Avenue,* New York, at Davis and Harvey's Art Galleries, no. 1212 Chestnut Street, April 16–20, 1888. The catalogue was compiled by John Getz.

17. *Catalogue of Bronzes and other Works of Art comprising Antique Chinese and Japanese Porcelains . . . to be sold by auction under the direction of the firm of S. Bing at their art rooms, nos. 220 and 222 Fifth Avenue,* New York, Nov. 21, 1888.

18. Ibid.

19. *Throws's New York City Directory* 101 (New York, 1887–1888), 155. See entries for "S. Bing antiques, 220 Fifth Avenue," and "Bing and Getz, antiques, 220 Fifth Avenue." By 1889, Bing had changed his reference in this volume to "S. Bing (firm of) importers, 220 Fifth Avenue" (p. 157). A search of the New York City rent records under the general address numbers for this date has yielded no accurate reference to Bing, despite his being listed in the official directory.

20. In *Throw's* (1888), Bing and Getz were linked at 220 Fifth Avenue. See also Montezuma, "My Notebook," *The Art Amateur* 17 (June 1887): 3, citing Getz as Bing's "resident partner."

21. Passenger lists of vessels arriving in New York, 1820–1897. *La Normandie,* November 23, 1886. National Archives, Washington, D.C. Getz's destination was listed as New York.

22. *Throw's New York Directory* (1892), 108 and 467. There is no reference to Bing after this particular date. Getz was, however, listed as a publisher whose offices were found at 304 Fifth Avenue.

23. See *Catalogue of Antique Chinese and Japanese Porcelains, Pottery, Enamels . . . to be sold at Public Sale by order of S. Bing, Paris,* on Friday, February 23d . . . at The American Art Galleries, Madison Square South, New York, 1894.

24. *The Evening Post,* 20 February 1894, 8.

25. "Fine Oriental Pottery, Mr. S. Bing's Collection of Chinese and Japanese Porcelains, Enamels and Bronzes," *The Sun,* 20 February 1894, p. 3.

26. It is not clear how Bing fully financed the renovations for the first Salon of Art Nouveau in December 1895, other than by tapping his own financial reserves. However, if the American sale of Japanese objects had really been lucrative and pieces that Bing had in stock for a long period were sold at high prices, then Bing would have had the capital with which to work without depleting his reserves. Judging from his careful planning, the American sales would seem a very useful way in which he partially financed art nouveau.

27. For reference to Bing and Freer see the papers in the Freer Gallery of Art documenting their ties. Further reference to Freer's activities with Bing (and others) is found in Helen Tomlinson, "Charles Lang Freer: Pioneer Collector of Oriental Art," Ph.D. diss., Case Western Reserve University, 1979.

28. *Japanese Engravings, Old Prints in Color Collected by S. Bing, Paris,* The American Art Galleries, Madison Square South, New York, 1894.

29. "Art Notes," *The Critic* (17 March 1894).

30. "The Fine Arts," *Boston Herald,* 8 April 1894, p. 13. The reviewer called Bing's collection "magnificent," noting that it illustrated the history of art until current times.

31. For reference to Bing's earlier involvement with the manufacturing of ceramics see Gabriel P. Weisberg, "A Note on S. Bing's Early Years in France, 1854–1876," *Arts Magazine* 57 (January 1983): 84–85.

32. Une Mission en Amerique (Enclosure no. 2 with Dispatch no. 22). Consular Dispatches from Paris, 1790–1906, T 1–27. January 2, 1890–December 29, 1893. National Archives, Washington, D.C.

33. The location of records or documents that would demonstrate the closeness of the Bing-Tiffany relationship is continuing. From those documents that do exist (often partially reconstituted from materials in the archives of European museums), Bing and Tiffany were associated in numerous business and exhibition matters.

34. It is likely that Bing stayed with Tiffany when he was in New York in 1894. For further reference see Robert Koch, *Louis Comfort Tiffany, Rebel in Glass* (New York: Crown Publishers, 1964).

35. Passenger List, New York, February 12, 1894–March 16, 1894. Mic. M 237, R 623, no. 172. National Archives, Washington, D.C. Bing arrived on *La Champagne* as a first-class passenger, listing his occupation as an art critic.

36. See *Courrier des États Unis,* 7 April 1894. Bing left for France on *La Bourgogne.*

37. "Home," *La Revue Franco-Américaine* 1 (June 1895): 95.

38. S. Bing, "Die Kunstgläser von Louis C. Tiffany," *Kunst und Kunsthandwerk* (1898): 105–11.

39. Similar to documentation of ties with Tiffany, the papers of agreement between Grueby or Rookwood and Bing remain unlocated.

40. S. Bing, *Artistic Culture in America,* ed. Robert Koch (Boston: M.I.T. Press, 1970).

41. "Literature: Books on Art, *La Culture Artistique en Amérique,* par S. Bing, Paris: 22 rue de Provence, New York: Drysen and Pfeiffer, 1896," *The Evening Post,* 21 March 1896, p. 16.

42. Ibid.

43. Ibid.

44. S. Bing, *Artistic Culture,* 121.

45. Ibid.

II

The Importance of Exhibitions in the Promotion of Art and Artists

5

HOKUSAI and the FRENCH DIPLOMATS

Some Remarks on the Collection of Baron de Chassiron

GENEVIÈVE LACAMBRE

ELIZABETH HOLT has made a number of stimulating contributions to the study of the artistic relations between Japan and the West in the 1850s and 1860s, most notably by drawing attention to the presence of Japanese objets d'art at the New York Universal Exposition in 1853.[1] The advent of *Japonisme* in general has been the subject of numerous publications in the last few years.[2] These in turn have inspired the remarks that follow regarding the arrival in France of some early Japanese illustrated albums, especially those acquired in Yeddo (Tokyo) by the Baron de Chassiron[3] now in the collections of the Musée d'Orbigny-Bernon in La Rochelle.[4] Chassiron obtained them on October 6, 1858, just three days before the signing of the Franco-Japanese treaty by Baron Gros on October 9.

Before going into a detailed discussion of these early precursors of French *Japonisme,* it might be helpful first to recall an apocryphal anecdote recounted in 1905 by Léonce Bénédite, who claimed to have heard it from the etcher Félix Bracquemond. At Delâtre's, a printer's shop to which Bracquemond had brought his engraving, *Les Canards l'ont bien passée,* the etcher had seen a small book, oddly bound in red paper, which "because of its supple and springy material had been used as packing for some porcelains sent back by some French people settled in Japan." The volume was the *Manga* of Hokusai. The etcher was not able to acquire it at the time, but "a year or eighteen months later he came upon it again in the hands of the engraver Lavieille, the brother of the painter." Bracquemond obtained it through a trade and never parted with it.[5] Bénédite says this happened in 1856, the date that Philippe Burty and Henri Béraldi proposed for Bracquemond's engraving. Jean-Paul Bouillon, however, has pointed out that the copyright for the engraving was in fact 1859,[6] and art historians, myself included, have also questioned the correctness of the 1856 date on other grounds.[7]

Japan was not entirely unknown before the Franco-Japanese treaty, which established commercial relations beginning 15 August 1859, was signed, a treaty that had resulted from earlier difficulties the French had encountered in dealing with the Japanese. But when it comes to earlier examples of relations between them, the destruction of Admiral Cécille's Japanese souvenirs at Brest during the last war can only be deplored. Cécille had reached the Ryukyu Islands in 1846 and anchored at the port of Nagasaki. Recent investigation, however, has turned up an abundance of other in-

Translated by Yvonne M. L. Weisberg.

dications of Japanese material in France quite early on—for example, by 1843 the Cabinet des Estampes of the Bibliothèque Royale in Paris had volume six of Hokusai's *Manga,*[8] and many Parisian libraries owned several works by Baron von Siebold. They became even more numerous after 1853,[9] when the American Commodore Perry finally forced the Japanese to open their ports. It is precisely in that year that 125 copies of the *Catalogue librorum et manuscriptorum japonicorum a Ph. Fr. de Siebold collectorum, annexa enumeratione illorum, qui in museo regio Hagano servantur* were printed by the author in Leiden.[10] In it, item 531 is the *Book of Insects* by Utamaro in its 1799 edition; and beginning with item 547, eleven works in twenty-three volumes by Hokusai, including one edition in ten volumes of the *Manga,* are listed. But this material remained remote from French artists. It was not until 1861 that the French—including the Jacquemarts and the Goncourts[11]—began to visit the Siebold Collection. On 14 September 1861, on a trip through Holland, the Goncourts stopped in Leiden, were attracted by an Indian god, Ganesha, and reported that at the Musée Siebold "the ink sketches of the Japanese artists . . . have the spirit and the picturesque touch of a sepia by Fragonard."[12] Several months earlier, on 8 June 1861, they had mentioned in the *Journal* the already well-established shop at 36 rue Vivienne called A la Porte Chinoise, which sold tea and, now that trade between France and Japan had been made possible, also began to trade in lacquers from Japan. "The other day," wrote Goncourt, "I bought some Japanese designs at the Porte Chinoise printed on paper that resembles cloth, with the softness and elasticity of wool. I have never before seen anything so wonderful, so whimsical and so poetic as this art." He compared them to works of Dürer and to the "naiveté of the Primitives." In sum he found Japanese art to be "a wonderful art, natural and varied as a flower, fascinating as a magic looking-glass."[13]

The pivotal year is still 1861, however. In 1878 Ernest Chesneau wrote that it was in 1862 that a painter, "browsing around a merchant's shop among curiosities from the Far East . . . discovered in a recent shipment from Le Havre some single leaves painted or printed in color, some albums of sketches enhanced with flat tints."[14] But it is not impossible that he purchased these prints and albums a few months earlier, as Goncourt had done as well as the engraver Lavieille's before Lavieille had traded it to Bracquemond. What remains, however, is to determine precisely when the most important and the most reliable episode in Bracquemond's testimony—namely his discovery of the "small Japanese album" at the printer Delâtre's, which was so crucial in the history of *Japonisme*—took place. Delâtre could not have given the book to him since it was not his to give. Martin Eidelberg has quite rightly connected its presence there to the publication by Delâtre of a work by Adalbert de Beaumont and Eugène V. Collinot called *Recueil de dessins pour l'art et l'industrie.*[15] In it, plate 110, which shows various individuals—acrobats, archers, and artisans—reproduced from pages in the first volume of the *Manga,* carries the notation, "Japanese sketch, from the collection of Baron Gros." This suggests that the *Manga* volumes, or at least volumes one, two, and six, as well as other works by Hokusai that Adalbert de Beaumont used (he seems to have signed all the plates identified by Martin Eidelberg as inspired by the Japanese,[16] namely, the *Cent vues de Mont Fuji, Ga-ka,* and *Rin-Ga*), were borrowed from Baron Gros who, after signing the treaty with Japan, returned to Paris, where he arrived on June 6, 1859. In a letter from Yeddo (Tokyo) dated 6 October 1858, to Count Walewski, then minister of foreign affairs, Baron Gros tells us that "on September 26 (Sunday), I landed at Yeddo. . . . I have already been able to procure books, maps, and other objects, and some curious documents that Lord Elgin did not have."[17]

Little is known about Adalbert de Beaumont. He was probably a member of the aristocratic family of senators and state counselors Gustave Vapereau lists in the *Dictionnaire des contemporains*, and it was quite possibly through family connections that he was able to see the albums brought back by Baron Gros and use them as models.[18] In doing so, however, he did not always remain faithful to the style of the Japanese prototypes. Beaumont transformed them in part through the medium—shifting from colored woodcuts to back-and-white etchings—and in part through combining designs of differing origin, but mainly through using horizontal lines to suggest horizons or water at the feet of figures and animals, which gave any artist using his designs a Westernized version of the original Japanese models. Fascicules of Beaumont's work that provided the first Japanese designs had begun to appear in 1861 and not in 1859 as Martin Eidelberg, basing his argument on the title page, claims. The title page does in fact read, "Collection of designs for art and industry engraved by Adalbert de Beaumont, Paris, 1859. Depot gl- Avenue de Saxe, 9. M^ON^ Collinot et Cie, Imp. d'A. Delâtre 171 r. St. Jacques," but the copy of this album in the Cabinet des Estampes at the Bibliothèque Nationale bears the seals of the copyright[19] and provides important details about the date. Plates 1–18 were, as the title page says, deposited in December 1859, but the rest were deposited later: plates 19–24 on March 6, 1860; plates 26–54 on August 4, 1861; plates 55–88 on April 3, 1862; and plates 89–126 on May 8, 1863. The remainder were deposited at various times up to 1873, when the printer was no longer Delâtre but the venerable house of Lemercier.

The work had 247 plates in all, but only those printed by Delâtre are of interest here. Japanese designs appear in the issues registered at the copyright registry of the Seine on August 4, 1861, which contained eleven designs on six plates (31, 35, 40, 47, 50, 52). Two were from volumes one and two of the *Manga*. In 1862, seven Japanese designs were contained on four plates (57, 60, 61, 68), and in 1863 eleven designs on seven plates (97, 99, 102, 107, 110, 119, 120). After 1863 Lemercier printed another eighteen plates containing Japanese motifs. The Japanese works identified by Martin Eidelberg as inspiring Adalbert de Beaumont are the *Rin-Ga*, which the artist used as early as 1861, and the *Ga Ka* and *Views of Mount Fuji* which he used in 1863. By this time the engraver had some notion of the models he was using, for he wrote at the bottom of plate 107, "The design was taken from a cheap little Japanese children's book."

We can assume that Beaumont already had in his possession a fairly large number of Japanese albums. We can also assume that even if he gives what is probably an incorrect title, "Decoration from a panel in old Japan lacquer," to the *Pheasant on a Branch* that Martin Eidelberg identifies as an illustration from *Rin-Ga* by Hokusai,[20] there is no doubt that he could have seen Japanese lacquer in Baron Gros's collection.

The facsimiles used by Baron Charles de Chassiron (a member of the mission sent to the Far East that Baron Gros headed) to illustrate his book, *Notes sur le Japon, la Chine, et l'Inde 1858–1859, 1860,* published in Paris in the last days of 1861 (the dedication reads, "A mon père, Paris 1er decembre, 1861"), just a few months after Beaumont's, are quite a different story. Aside from a few missing pieces, the books, lacquer objects, netsukes, and other mementos brought back by Chassiron, can still be found in the collection he willed to the city of La Rochelle. The account of his trip, his will, and the collection itself were originally in the Museum of Natural History and are now in the Musée d'Orbigny-Bernon. The documents are of prime importance and should be thoroughly studied[21] for the information they can add to our knowledge of the first examples of Japanese art and crafts brought back to France by early visitors to

Japan, especially those allowed to enter Yeddo (Tokyo). Most visitors were restricted to foreign settlements along the coast because the 1858 treaty stipulated that foreigners could not reside in either Edo or Yeddo (Tokyo) before January 1, 1862, or in Osaka before January 1, 1863.[22]

The inventory of the Chassiron collection, established in Paris on 25 August 1871,[23] tells us more about the man than any reference book. It informs us that Charles Gustave Martin, Baron de Chassiron, was born on 5 December 1818; that he was descended from a baron of the Empire; that he had been an attaché first at the French embassy in Tunisia in 1848, then in Japan from 1858 to 1860; that he died in Tarbes on 20 June 1871; and that he had been a state counselor, a general counselor for the Charente Inférieure and a mayor of the commune of Nuaillé near La Rochelle where his chateau, called Beauregard, was located. It is there that he prepared his will dated 13 December 1869, and its codicils dated 21 August 1870, and 18 January 1871. His widow was the Princess Caroline Letizia Murat, who lived in Paris but was staying in Stuttgart when the inventory was made. The collection was housed in Paris at 9 rue de Douai, the Far Eastern objects in a "little red room" decorated with two trophies of Oriental arms and a vitrine that contained as many souvenirs of China—especially costumes—as objects and books from Japan. However, if one compares this inventory, drawn up after his death and often imprecise as to origin, with that made by the museum at La Rochelle as an exact record of the entire ethnographic collection from the Far East that was transferred in 1936 from the Museum Lafaille (Museum of Natural History), we discover that an estimated 391 of a total of about 658 objects were in fact brought back from Japan by Baron de Chassiron. Not all remain in the collection, however, and not all are of equal interest.

Among the pieces on the earlier inventory that can be securely paired up with items on the museum list are two swords, "one long and one short," purchased in Yeddo on 5 October 1856, with the governor's authorization.[24] It is more difficult to identify the "seven Chinese and Japanese walking sticks"; only six are in the inventory of the museum.[25] Two lacquer writing boxes (figs 5.1 and 5.2) described as "Chinese" in the first inventory are actually Japanese pieces from the Edo period.[26] Of the "two small lacquer cabinets," one of which contained a silver-covered copper case, which are identified as "lacquer inlaid tea cabinets,"[27] one is in fact a black paint box inlaid with silver and gold, and the other is a picnic box richly decorated with polychrome irises on a red background. Several other lacquer objects—chalices, trays, and bottles—and porcelain bottles cased in wicker, were purchased, if one is to believe the testimony of Baron de Chassiron and the Marquis de Moges,[28] at the port of Shimoda, their first stop in Japan. They were not, however, purchased at just any curio shop in the course of a stroll but must have been found at a bazaar the government kept for foreigners, because after his visit, Chassiron, having first noted that the Japanese were "great artists, great workers," remarks that "the officers of the governor also doubled as cashiers at the bazaars."[29] Two fans (fig. 5.3) were also probably acquired during this first layover at Shimoda. Both are covered with notes and sketches made on the spot. Chassiron writes in his diary, "I almost forgot to say that before we all sat down at the table, the governor handed each of us a simple, undecorated fan with a bamboo mount. The paper, made from white nettles, was thick and remarkably strong. Mine became instantly useful during the meal; when no one was looking I used it to take notes which I then filled in later on in the evening."[30]

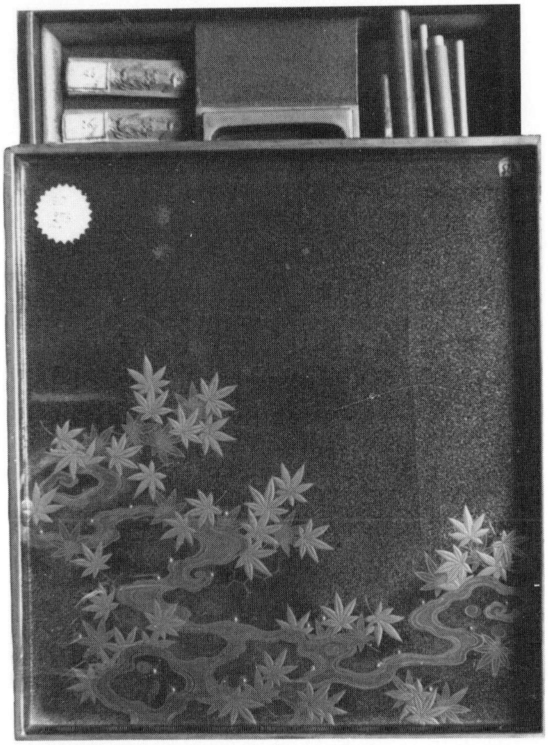

Fig. 5.1. Lacquer writing box, interior. La Rochelle, Musée d'Orbigny-Bernon.

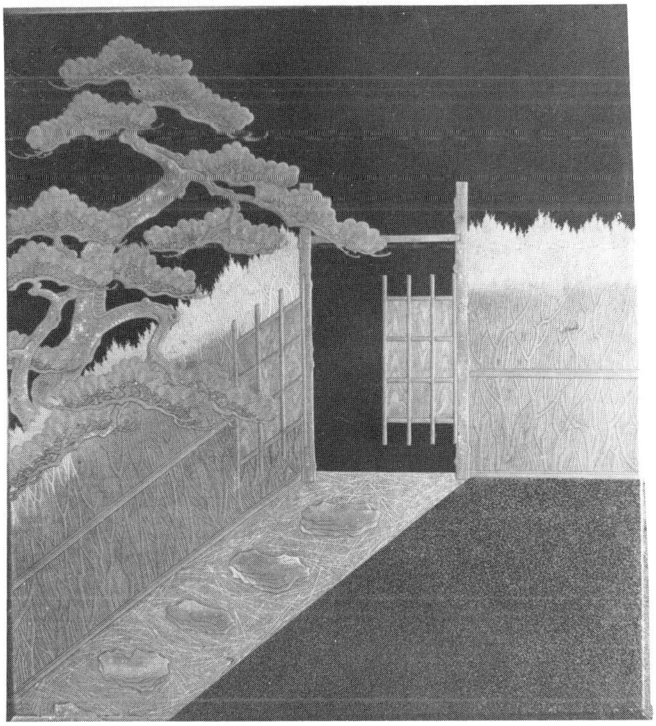

Fig. 5.2. Lacquer writing box, exterior. La Rochelle, Musée d'Orbigny-Bernon.

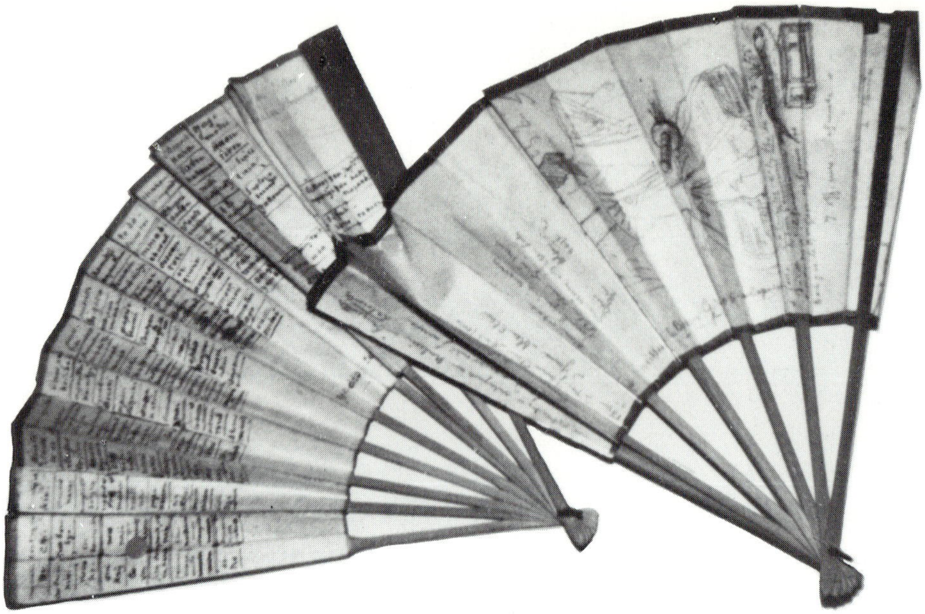

Fig. 5.3. Fans obtained at Shimoda by Baron de Chassiron.
Musée d'Orbigny-Bernon.

After this layover arranged for foreigners, the possibilities for exploring the shops of Yeddo brought some real aesthetic revelations. The mission arrived there on September 19. On October 3, Baron de Chassiron wrote, "I continued my pursuit of old ivories and old wood sculptures, which incidentally the Dutch are as fond of as we are. My best finds in this genre all come from pawnshops."[31] The inventory made after his death gives a long list of netsukes in ivory and wood which he acquired, but there are only eight left, four of ivory and four of painted wood.[32] An article on the collection that appeared in 1874 in *Le Magasin Pittoresque* (fig. 5.4) reproduces three of them, two of which still remain and one, *A Wild Sow Resting,* is now lost. It was "executed in a marvelous and absolutely realistic way"[33] and must be the *Wild Sow Resting on Branches* listed in the inventory made after the baron's death.

Among the ivories still in the collection, two carry the signature of Minkoku[34] (figs. 5.5 and 5.6) and are described as "a washerwoman and her child" and "a Japanese lady and her child in traditional dress" (in fact, the latter portrays an actor dressed in a costume worn by the nobility). The second one has a sticker attached to its back that probably carries the name of the dealer. A similar sticker is found on the back of a third netsuke described in the inventory as "an old masked woman and her child," which also in fact is again an actor and is in a similar style. The fourth, with an unidentified signature, is described as an "old man with a gourd" and is actually one of the gods of good fortune. The four wooden netsukes, made of boxwood decorated with a still fresh polychrome highlighted in gold, also represent gods of good fortune. We can recognize the *Old Man Carrying a Gourd* and the Chinese general from the legend of Shoki, who appears in the collection again in a larger version, a statuette 11 centimeters high but in similar style; it, however, appears to be unsigned.[35] The four netsukes are

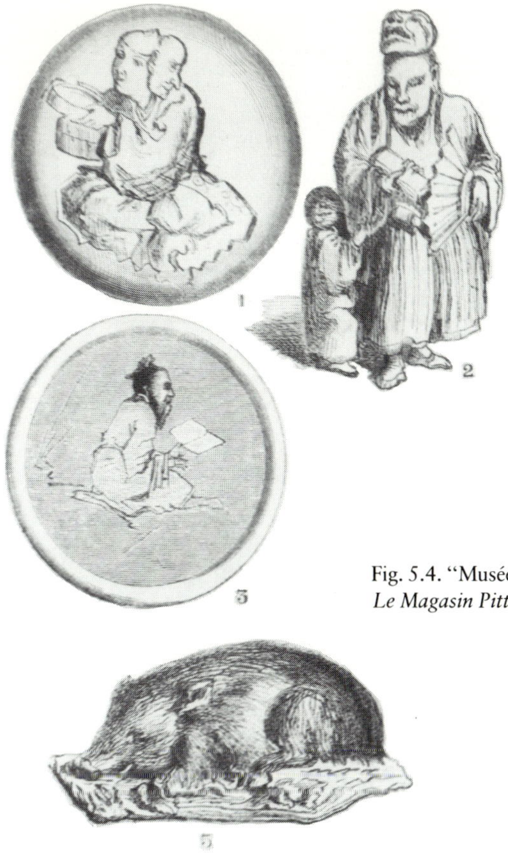

Fig. 5.4. "Musée de la Rochelle—curiosités japonaises," from *Le Magasin Pittoresque,* 1874 (detail).

signed by the artist Shuzan (fig. 5.7), and all are typical of the style of Nagamachi Shuzan, an artist of the Osaka school at the beginning of the nineteenth century.[36] It is not surprising that the Baron de Chassiron—even if he thought he was buying ancient pieces—actually purchased objects of relatively recent and sometimes even modern production, as without doubt the lacquers acquired at Shimoda were.

The problems of dating objects from the Edo period make it difficult to know if the "three lacquered or sculpted wood pagodas containing idols" are from the beginning of the nineteenth century or are older (fig. 5.8) and comparable to the seventeenth-century miniature sanctuary found in the British Museum.[37]

The part of the collection that is most fascinating—because it offers the rare opportunity of comparing reproductions that appeared in 1861 with their originals—comprises the remainder of the "fifty-one Japanese printed and colored albums" listed in the first inventory. Twenty-eight are left, of which one is a work in six volumes on morality *(Fugaku ...).* There are several gaps: volume one of Hokusai's *Manga,* several pages of which were reproduced in 1861, has disappeared. Some of the missing albums are possibly among those listed in the museum's 1936 inventory as being of Chinese origin—their titles are translated into Russian on the cover—and their provenance was unclear in the absence of the characteristic sticker of the Chassiron collection. One small thick volume with a light-blue cover has the following inscription on the back: "Baron de Chassiron, Yedo, octobre 1858," demonstrating conclusively that it

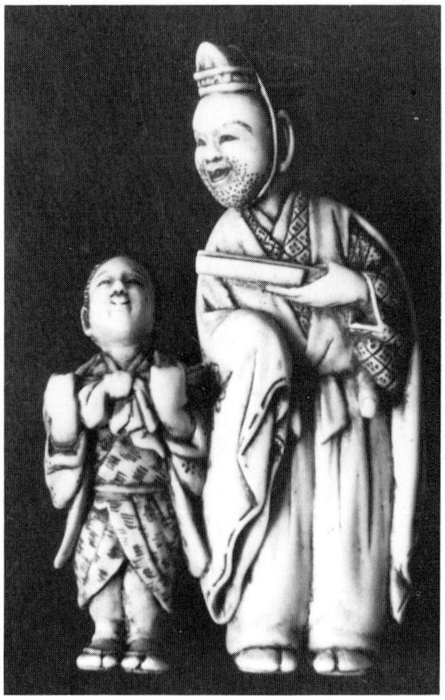

Fig. 5.5. Netsuke signed "Minkoku." La Rochelle, Musée d'Orbigny-Bernon.

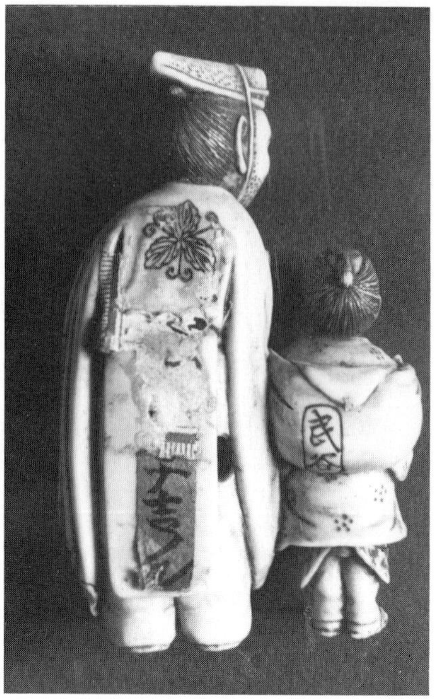

Fig. 5.6. Netsuke, detail of the signature. La Rochelle, Musée d'Orbigny-Bernon.

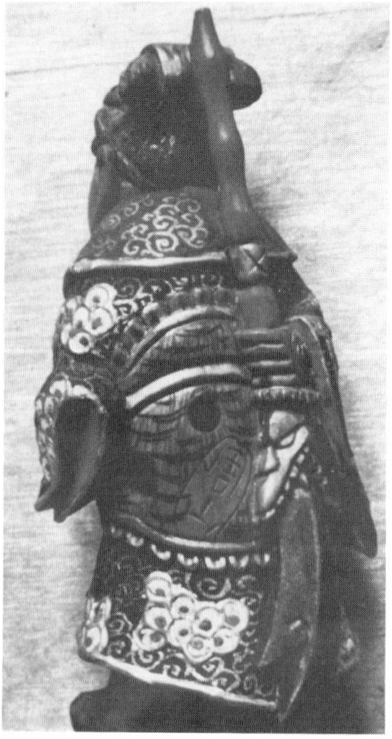

Fig. 5.7. Netsuke signed "Shuzan," detail. La Rochelle, Musée d'Orbigny-Bernon.

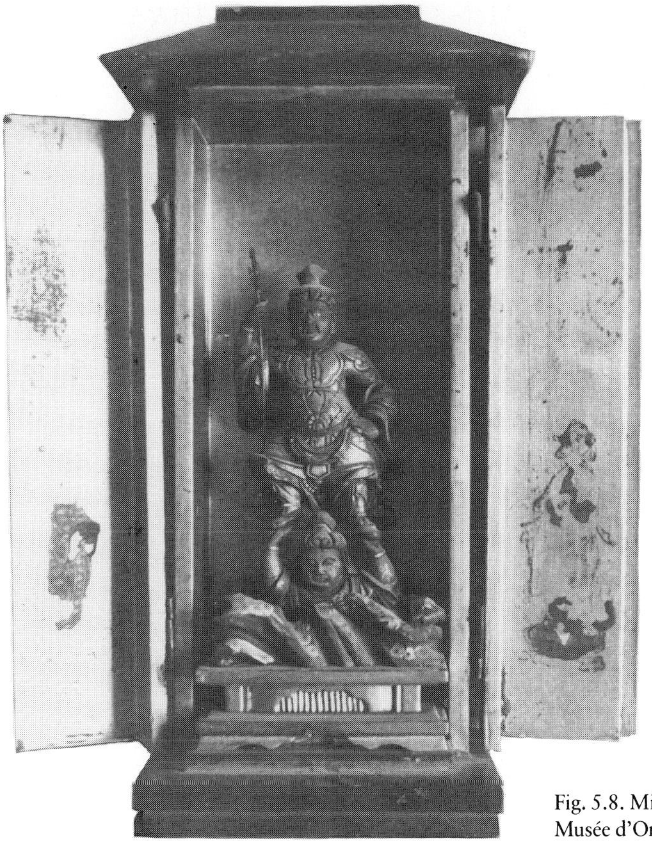

Fig. 5.8. Miniature sanctuary, lacquered wood with gold. La Rochelle, Musée d'Orbigny-Bernon.

was actually purchased on the first French mission to Japan. Titled *Haya Biki Moncho*, it is a volume of symbols or arms printed in black and white.[38] Quite possibly it belongs among the objects Chassiron bought on 6 October 1858, an event he also recounts in his book.

> Today I went alone to the city where I bought the objects on which, next to the old ivories, I place the greatest value. I extorted—and I am using the word quite literally and almost fought with one of the Japanese officers in the process—from the stalls of a curio shop a bundle of colored prints, engravings, and maps . . . the authorities have given instructions of the utmost severity regarding foreigners so far as maps are concerned, because it is feared that foreigners might obtain information dangerous to national security.

The map of Yeddo purchased that morning is reproduced in the book of 1861.[39] Chassiron continues:

> I have also been able—thanks to the ease which came with the use of an official escort—to build a rather complete collection of works from the sciences, the arts, and professions of Japan. I even gathered volumes of caricatures. Those small volumes, printed or engraved on wood—I do not yet know how—with the

> utmost care are intended for the education of the people. They are very cheap; each sells for 25 or 30 centimes in our money, and consequently they are within the reach of everyone.[40]

The difficulties the French experienced in securing books in Japan in 1858 are also mentioned in the accounts of Laurence Oliphant, member of an English mission who was in Japan between 1857 and 1859 and recounted his experiences in a book published in 1860. "It is evident," he writes, "that the government has given the order not to sell books to foreigners," but he adds that he "has made a good catch." Even though he was only able to carry away part of a map, "we were able to acquire a considerable number of illustrated books ... besides books which only contain engravings, there are illustrated novels with wood engravings printed on the same page with the printed text."[41]

The collections at La Rochelle include books from both categories. Eleven large-format (about 22.5 cm by 15.5 cm) and two in medium format (18 cm by 22 cm) are fully illustrated. Eight of small format (about 17.5 cm by 11.5 cm) contain both text and pictures; the illustrations are in black and white, but the covers are in color. One of them[42] has a cover signed by Toyokuni (probably Toyokuni II whose dates are 1777–1835); the text is illustrated by Kunitsuma (1805–1868). Kunitsuma also illustrated the second volume.[43] The Edo artist Yoshitora,[44] a student of Kunyoshi, is also represented. Later famous for his representations of foreigners stationed in Yokohama, he began as a modest illustrator of books. Another, dated 1853, is signed Kunimasa.[45]

Among the volumes that only have pictures are two in small format. One, a book of morals, is dated the Year of the Serpent of Ansei (i.e., 1858) and is the work of Kunyoshi (1797–1861).[46] Among the large-format volumes are volumes six and seven of Hokusai's *Manga,*[47] the third volume of the *Hundred Views of Mount Fuji*[48] also by Hokusai, volumes two and four of the *Banshoku Zuko* illustrated by Katsushika Taito (again Hokusai),[49] and finally the first volume of *Hokusai Gafu,*[50] of which one double page illustration representing eleven blind people crossing a river (fig. 5.9) is reproduced in Chassiron's book published in 1861.[51] Others are the *Shoshin Gafu,* published in 1858;[52] the *Koso Gafu,* a book of illustrations by Shoso-Koji first published in 1832 and reissued in 1852;[53] and the fourth volume of the *Shinji Andon.*[54] The last, a work in five volumes which appeared between 1829 and 1847, is a collection of satirical poems *(senryu)* illustrated by Oishi Shinko or Motora (1794–1833) and is particularly important because it identifies a hitherto unknown reproduction in the book by Chassiron.[55] The page represents a "false painter" painting an ex-voto or *yema* with two chopsticks; its ironical subject is an upside-down horse, and a "false doctor," actually a barber, taking care of a patient (figs. 5.10 and 5.11). The gray, blue, and surprisingly bright orange of the original are considerably toned down in the facsimile, where the orange becomes a pink that is somewhat stronger than that used in the reproductions of the *Manga* by Hokusai.

What can we conclude from this rapid survey of the Japanese books in the La Rochelle collection?[56] It is clear that Chassiron regarded them as remarkable documents of Japanese life. He used some of them for illustrations in his 1861 book, confidently selecting from the greatest of them, Hokusai, thirteen illustrations for his natural history of Japan: eight scenes of rural and peasant life from the first volume of the *Manga,* two from the *Hundred Views of Mount Fuji,* and finally one caricature from the first volume of the *Manga,* one from his *Gafu,* and one from the *Shinji Andon.*

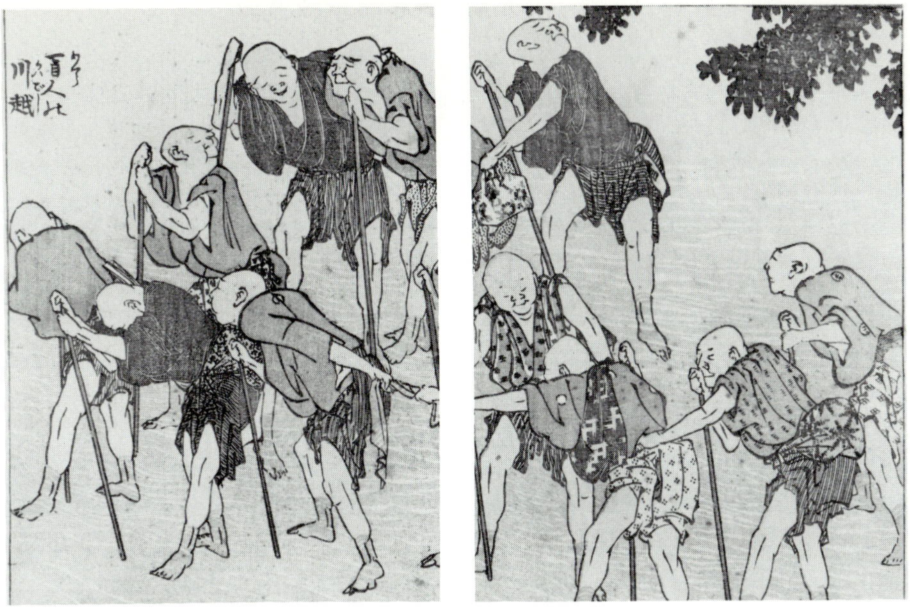

Fig. 5.9. Page for *Hokusai Gafu* reproduced in facsimile in Chassiron's 1861 book. La Rochelle, Musée d'Orbigny-Bernon.

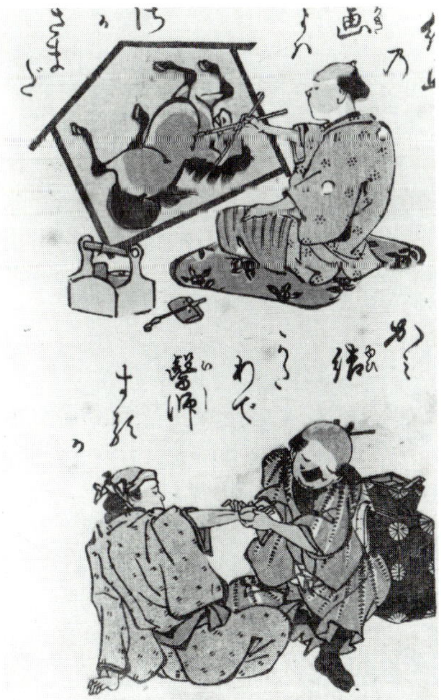

Fig. 5.10. Page from the *Shinji Andon* reproduced in facsimile in Chassiron's 1861 book. La Rochelle, Musée d'Orbigny-Bernon.

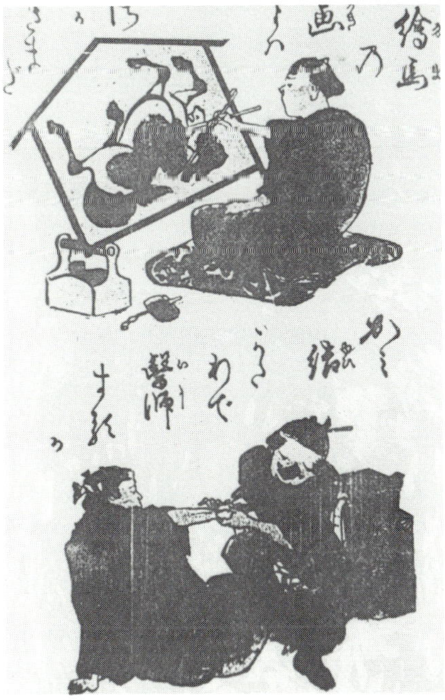

Fig. 5.11. Page from the *Shinji Andon* reproduced in facsimile in Chassiron's 1861 book. La Rochelle, Musée d'Orbigny-Bernon.

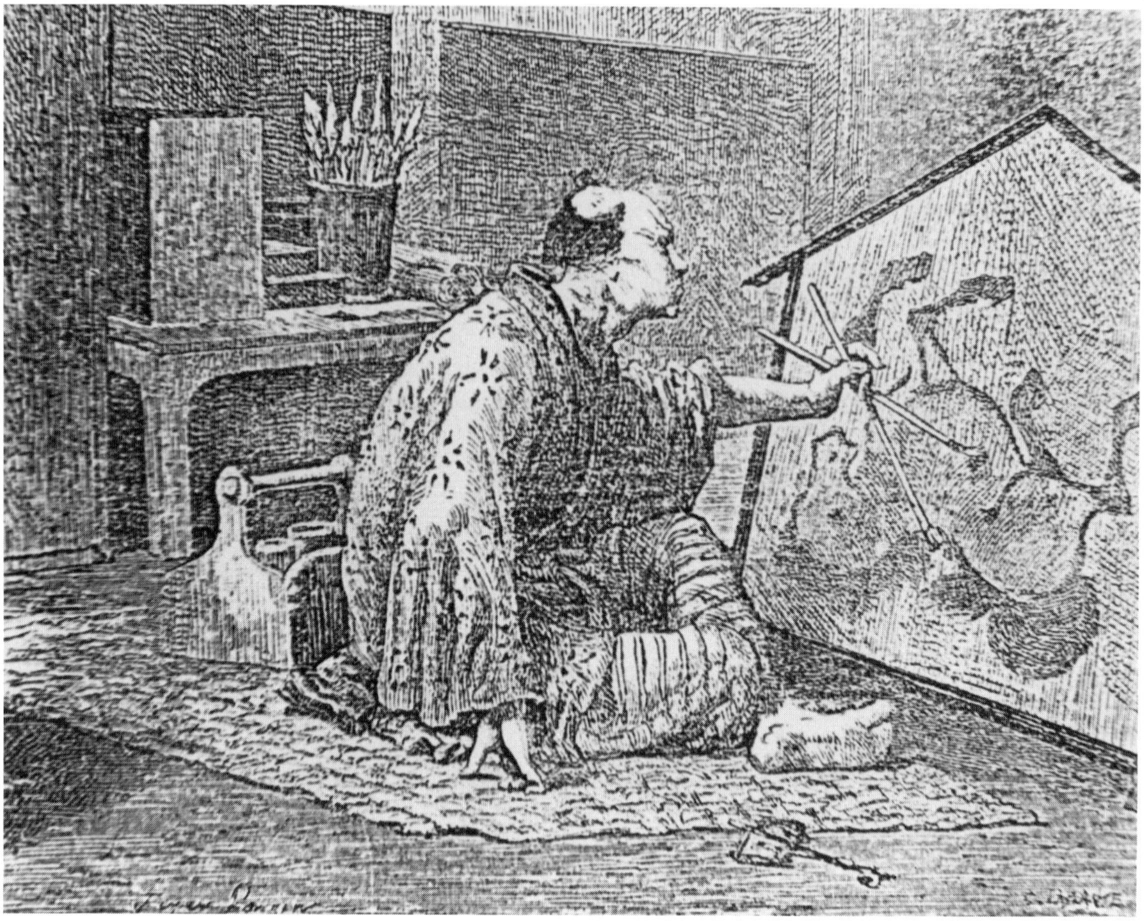

Fig. 5.12. "Artist painting a yema, drawing by Feyen-Perrin after an original Japanese sketch," from *Le Tour du Monde,* 1867.

The importance of Hokusai and the seminal role played by the *Manga* among Western artists is well-known. Hiroshige played a similar part, although there are no examples of his work at La Rochelle. Nor should the importance of the *Shinji Andon* be underestimated. Chassiron was not the only one to bring back a copy with him. Sir Rutherford Alcock took from it several illustrations for his *Capital of the Tycoon: A Narrative of a Three Years' Residence in Japan,*[57] though he must have picked it up later than Chassiron, since he did not reach Japan until 26 June 1859.[58] Further evidence for the spread of the *Shinji Andon,* or at least the reproductions from it that appear in Chassiron's 1861 book, is the reproduction of the "false painter"—this time inverted so that the painter becomes left-handed (fig. 5.12)—by François-Nicholas-Augustin Feyen-Perrin. He used it as an illustration for the account of Aimé Humbert's trip to Japan, which appeared as a serial in *Le Tour du Monde.*[59] It turns up again in *Le Japon Illustré,* a book published by Hachette in 1870. Feyen-Perrin, a naturalistic artist, does not really appreciate the quick graphic style of the Japanese work and tries to Westernize the figure by placing it in a room. However, for this *Japanese artist painting a "yema"* he very seriously draws the improbable upside-down horse, and the satire on incompetence is destroyed completely.

Although there is little documentation to tell us how well-known the Chassiron collection was, we can at least suggest that quite a number of people were acquainted with it and that the worlds of the diplomat and the artist were not as widely separated as one might at first suppose. Chassiron's wife was a member of the Murat family and related to Princess Mathilde, who in turn knew the Goncourts and at least once (on 16 August 1862) received them at Saint-Gratien[60] (the Goncourts even mention in their *Journals* under 20 July 1868,[61] some unflattering remark the princess made about Caroline de Chassiron). Certainly these early volumes brought back by members of English and French diplomatic missions, in spite of the measures the Japanese took to prevent it, were regarded as irreplaceable evidence on the life and attitudes of the Japanese. They were also recognized as revelations of a remarkable art. It is certainly unlikely that the Baron de Chassiron used them to pack porcelain!

NOTES

1. See Elizabeth Gilmore Holt, *The Art of All Nations, 1850–1873* (New York: Anchor Books, 1981), 360–77, and "The Documentation for the Contribution of Three Mid-Nineteenth Century Exhibitions to the Popularization of Japanese Art," in *Art, the Ape of Nature: Studies in Honor of H. W. Janson* (New York: Harry M. Abrams; and Englewood Cliffs, N.J.: Prentice-Hall, Inc., 1981): 639–50.

2. See, for example, Toshio Watanabe, "The Western Image of Japanese Art in the Late Edo Period," *Modern Asian Studies* 18, no. 4 (October 1984): 667–84.

3. Baron Charles de Chassiron, *Notes sur le Japon, la Chine, et l'Inde 1858–1859, 1860,* Paris: E. Dentu and Ch. Reinwald, 1861), 114–15.

4. I saw them in a collection of mementos brought back from the Far East by various travelers on the top floor of the Musée d'Orbigny-Bernon, where they were reorganized about fifteen years ago by Lise Carrier, then curator of the La Rochelle Museums. Thanks to Annie Dagout, of the Musée d'Orbigny-Bernon, and Alain Parent, curator of the Musée de Nouveau Monde at La Rochelle and acting curator for the other city museums, I was able to study them in 1984. Both were also generous with their help in the preparation of this article.

5. Léonce Bénédite, "Félix Bracquemond, l'animalier," *Art et Décoration* 17 (February 1905): 39–40.

6. Jean-Paul Bouillon, "Remarques sur le Japonisme de Bracquemond," in *Japonisme in Art. An International Symposium* (Tokyo: The Committee for the Year 2001 and Kodansha International, Ltd., 1980), 97.

7. See Watanabe, 670, n. 9.

8. Gisèle Lambert, "Le Fonds japonais ancien du Cabinet des Estampes de la Bibliothèque Nationale," *Nouvelles de l'Estampe* (January-February 1984): 15.

9. The library of the Musée d'Histoire Naturelle in Paris owns a folio edition in six volumes (call no. 23846) of the *Nippon Archiv zur Beschreibung von Japan;* the title page bears the date "Leiden 1852" except for the first volume which is dated 1832. In 1843 the administration of the Bibliothèque Royale considered placing an order for the book with the agent Roret; it did not assemble the parts it had already received until 1853. See the letter of Gustave d'Eichthal, dated 12 July 1853, found in volume one (call no. fol. O^2o/213). See also Phylis Floyd, "Documentary Evidence of the Availability of Japanese Imagery in Europe in Nineteenth-Century Collections," *The Art Bulletin* 68 (March 1986): 105–41.

10. The copy at the Bibliothèque Nationale (Réserve X621) was purchased from the book dealer Duprat for 24 francs on 27 August 1853.

11. See Deborah Johnson, "Japanese Prints in Europe before 1840," *The Burlington Magazine* 124 (951) (June 1982): 343–48.

12. Edmond and Jules de Goncourt, *Journal* (Paris: Edition Ricatte, 1956) 1: 962.

13. Ibid, 931.

14. Ernest Chesneau, "Exposition Universelle—Le Japon à Paris," *Gazette des Beaux-Arts* 18 (November 1878): 386–87.

15. Martin Eidelberg, "Bracquemond, Delâtre and the Discovery of Japanese Prints," *The Burlington Magazine* 123, no. 937 (April 1981) 221–27. Adalbert de Beaumont et Eugène V. Collinot, *Ornements du Japon. Recueil de dessins pour l'art et l'industrie* (Introduction par Fr. Favre) (Paris: Canson, 1859). See also Gabriel P. Weisberg, et al., *Japonisme. Japanese Influence on French Art 1854–1910* (The Cleveland Museum of Art, the Rutgers University Art Gallery, and the Walters Art Gallery, 1975–76), 142.

16. Eidelberg, 227, pl. 47–59.

17. Archives des Affaires Etrangères. Courrier diplomatique. C. P. Chine, vol. 26. Lord Elgin, the English envoy, had just signed an Anglo-Japanese treaty that then served as a model for the Franco-Japanese one. See Marquis de Moges (a member of the French expedition), "Voyage en Chine et au Japon, 1857–1858," *Le Tour du Monde* 20 (1860): 161.

18. For a Chinese motif (pl. 116 in Beaumont and Collinot) Adalbert de Beaumont cites Montigny's collection. Montigny had been consul general in China. Did they belong to the same circles?

19. The author is grateful to Mr. Claude Bouret, curator at the Cabinet des Estampes of the Bibliothèque Nationale, for having given the author the opportunity to consult the registers of the inventory for the Copyright Registry of the Seine.

20. Eidelberg, fig. 55 (pl. 68 of Beaumont and Collinot, Recueil).

21. Jacques de Caso, "1861: Hokusai rue Jacob," *The Burlington Magazine* 111, no. 798 (September 1969): 562–65, notes the book by Chassiron but thinks the collection is lost. See also Watanabe, 672, n. 15.

22. On the Franco-Japanese treaty of 1858, see Li Jin-Mueng, "Les Relations économiques et financières entre la France et le Japon de 1859 à 1914," Thèse de Doctorat de 3ème cycle (unpublished), Paris-Sorbonne, May 1977.

23. See Archives of the Musée d'Orbigny-Bernon, La Rochelle. This collection was willed to La Rochelle in 1871.

24. Chassiron, 110. He had acquired four swords, of which only two appear in the bequest.

25. *Inventaire du Musée d'Orbigny-Bernon, section Extrême-Orient* (Museum inventory numbers hereafter preceded by *EO*), 295.

26. *EO* 276, "three small ornamental dressing cases for men of letters. One of them is empty. China, Chassiron Collection."

27. *EO* 230.

28. Chassiron, 51, and Marquis de Moges, *Le Tour du Monde*, 162. Both noted, "In a huge shed the Japanese authorities had . . . collected together items produced by the country that could arouse the curiosity of foreigners. Japanese lacquer in many different forms and large displays of inkstands, boxes, trunks, and tables of all sizes and colors could be seen there."

29. Chassiron, 52.

30. *EO* 146.

31. Chassiron, 107.

32. *EO* 29: "Collection of netsukes (carved toggles attached to strings in ivory and painted or unpainted wood)." With no indication of number.

33. See "Musée de La Rochelle. Curiosités japonaises," *Magasin Pittoresque* 42 (1874): 372, pl. 1, no. 5. Number 2 on this plate is the *Masked Actor and Child* mentioned below; on page 373, pl. II, no. 11 reproduces the *Old Man Carrying a Gourd*, also mentioned below.

34. Pieces signed "Minkoku" are in the collections of the British Museum. See Richard Barker and Lawrence Smith, *Netsuke. The Miniature Sculpture of Japan* (London: British Museum Publi-

cations, 1976), nos. 99 to 100. They come from the collection of Sir Augustus Wollaston Franks (F. 692, F. 1253, and F. 438). The ivory *manju* signed in the same manner as those of La Rochelle are from the nineteenth century. The identical signature is, in fact, cited by Gonse in *L'Art Japonais,* new edition (Paris: 1926), 183. This applies both to the netsukes and to wood sculpture. See the bouquet-holder from the Louis Gonse collection which is reproduced on p. 195 and is engraved by Henri Guérard. Gonse dates it in the eighteenth century.

35. *EO* 267.

36. On this author, see Raymond Bushell, *Collectors' Netsukes* (New York-Tokyo: Weatherhill, 1971), 19 and figs. 6–7, and Joe Earle, *An Introduction to Netsuke* (London: The Museum Warminster: Compton, 1980), pl. 73.

37. Cf. Lawrence Smith and Victor Harris, *Japanese Decorative Arts from the 17th to the 19th Century* (London: British Museum Publications, 1982), 65, fig. 42.

38. *EO* 63. The dimensions are H. 8.7 cm by L. 12.7 cm by W. 2.2 cm.

39. Chassiron, 14: 114.

40. Ibid., 14: 115.

41. Laurence Oliphant, *La Chine et le Japon. Mission du Comte d'Elgin pendant les années 1857, 1858 et 1859,* trans. M. Guizot (Paris, 1860), 2:156–7, appeared in France without illustrations, but the English edition of 1859 reproduced works by Toyokuni, Hiroshige, and Hokusai. There is also a French edition dated 1875, which is illustrated. Oliphant mentions (p. 157) the purchase in Yeddo of two or three volumes in Chinese characters.

42. *EO* 62/20.

43. *EO* 62/27.

44. *EO* 62/21 and *EO* 62/22.

45. *EO* 62/23.

46. *EO* 62/15.

47. *EO* 62/12 (vol. 6) and *EO* 62/7 (vol. 7).

48. *EO* 62/13.

49. *EO* 62/17 (vol. 2) and *EO* 62/18 (vol. 4). According to the general inventory of the books published in Japan, the *Kokusho so mokuroku,* the first three volumes were published in 1835 and the last two in 1850.

50. *EO* 62/9.

51. Thirteenth and last facsimile of illustration. Certain details found in the blue background have been eliminated in the reproduction, but the overall design and color is quite faithful.

52. *EO* 62/16.

53. *EO* 62/11.

54. *EO* 62/19. Volume 1 of the same work is in the Stockholm Royal Library: J. S. Edgren, *Catalogue of the Hordenskiold Collection of Japanese Books in the Royal Library* (Stockholm, 1980), no. 878.

55. Facsimile illustration 12; see de Caso, 565.

56. I would like to thank my colleagues and friends Akiko Mabuchi, Akiya Takahashi, Shuji Takashina, and Suzanne Esmein who helped me identify many of the Japanese books through photographs from La Rochelle.

57. The first edition of the *Capital of the Tycoon* appeared in London and New York in 1863. In that edition, as well as the two-volume edition that came out in New York in 1877 (with different pagination), the illustration in vol. 1, ch. 5, p. 267, entitled *Mode of Protecting Land from Birds,* comes from vol. 4 of the *Shinji Andon.* From the same work also are *Manuring Process,* 1:265; *Clothing Merchants,* 2:254; and *Lanternmaker,* 2:264. There could be others.

58. See Haga Toru, "The Diplomatic Background of Japonisme: The Case of Sir Rutherford Alcock," in *Japonisme in Art: An International Symposium,* 27.

59. *Le Tour du Monde* 16 (1867): 372.

60. Goncourt, *Journal* (1956), 1:1111–12.

61. Ibid., 2:441–42.

6

RODIN and HIS AMERICAN COLLECTORS

RUTH BUTLER

A GREETING

I wish to send . . . greetings to all my friends in America, and to express my profound gratitude for their sympathetic appreciation of my art; it has been a great encouragement to me.

I sincerely admire your young country, which possesses a veritable thirst for the beautiful, and which will in time grasp and comprehend all that is greatest in art.

De grand coeur,
Auguste Rodin, 1911[1]

RODIN FREQUENTLY felt himself an outsider in France. The first time he ever exhibited his sculpture was in a foreign country—in Belgium. And ever after he sought patrons and courted critics from many nations.

The United States, the youngest industrialized nation in the world, found that, among all the arts, sculpture was the most difficult to understand. Until the 1870s Americans did not really collect sculpture. It was only then that William T. Walters and W.W. Corcoran started to amass their bronze Jean Antoine Louis Baryes by the dozens.

So how was it that this Rodin—controversial in France in the 1880s, an aggravating presence but one of great aura in the 1890s, lionized by the world in 1900, only to be rejected in the twentieth century by an art world moving on to abstraction—how was it that he became America's darling? He was the first living artist to be honored by having his own gallery at the Metropolitan Museum of Art; the gallery was the first public collection of his work anywhere. The Metropolitan staff was hard at work creating it when Rodin wrote his lovely epistle to America. Rodin has been unique in this country in having a monument, in the form of *The Thinker,* on prominent display in ten different American cities. He has his own museum in Philadelphia, just as he does in Paris; there are major collections of his works on both coasts of the United States, including a new sculpture garden at Stanford University.[2]

America and Rodin first took each other into account at the Philadelphia Centennial, where Rodin exhibited not as a Frenchman but as a Belgian, for in 1876 Rodin was living in Brussels. He shipped eight works across the Atlantic, more than any other sculptor from Belgium. He assigned them titles such as *The Rose, Loving*

Thoughts, *Large Grapes*, and *Field Flowers*. It is doubtful that any of these works remained in America; if they did, they probably sit quietly as decorative additions to Victorian parlors or are even stowed away in attics, unrecognized as early works by a renowned artist.

The fine arts were not the strong point of America's Centennial.

> The art galleries in the Centennial exhibition are not models of good arrangement, nor can the collections be said to be altogether well selected and representative. Nowhere, indeed, in the whole exhibition is hasty and inexperienced management more apparent, or the commercial spirit more obtrusive, than in the art department.[3]

The Italians dominated the Centennial art galleries, especially because they sent more than three hundred sculptures, a display that represented a tour de force of marble cutting; the English artists were considered the best, and the French disappointing. Henry James was in France during Centennial summer; his brother William wrote him from Philadelphia:

> France has nothing good to show.... Not that there were any very good American works, but there was nothing vile, such as every foreign school gives you in its degenerate pupils... without a grain of inward decency.[4]

The majority of Americans who went to Philadelphia in 1876 saw an art show for the first time in their lives. And it was difficult for them to understand why there were so many nude figures in every possible attitude "without a spark of reason for their nudity."

Most of Rodin's entries at the Centennial would have been female heads, but during Centennial summer he himself was hard at work on his first great life-size nude, the one we know as the *Age of Bronze*. To be sure America was not ready for a nude from Rodin's hand and would not be until the next great world's fair, the Columbian Exposition in Chicago, and then just barely.

Rodin's works came to the attention of Americans in a true sense via London where he exhibited the *Head of St. John* and the *Man with a Broken Nose* in 1882. Boston journalist Arthur Warren saw them at the Royal Academy and the Grosvenor Gallery and he told the readers of the *Boston Transcript* that the *Head of St. John* was the finest thing at the Academy even though it was "only a reproduction" (it would be a while before the majority of Americans understood that a bronze cast was not necessarily a reproduction), and that *The Man with a Broken Nose* was "a head which may be said without exaggeration to approach the best art of Greece."[5]

More important was the role of another critic who took himself to Europe in these years—William C. Brownell, a man whom Edith Wharton considered the "most discerning literary critic of our day." Brownell is the first American whom we know to have sought out the controversial sculptor in his atelier at 182 rue de l'Université. Probably he did it at the urging of W. E. Henley. Brownell had spent time in London writing for the gifted editor of the *Magazine of Art*. Henley and Rodin were already the best of friends. In the spring of 1884 Brownell appeared at Rodin's door, and he then began to assemble material for an article on *le nouveau mouvement* in sculpture for *Century* magazine. In 1889 the article still had not appeared and an embarassed Brownell wrote from New York:

> You must think that I'm not very serious—I come to you, I ask innumerable explanations about your way of thinking and your work . . . I accept your hospitality, I borrow an enormous number of photographs, I shake your hand, I leave and for years you hear nothing.[6]

The article finally came out in *Century* in November 1890, and it was reprinted as a chapter in Brownell's *French Art*, a book that remained a standard reference in America for understanding French art well into the twentieth century.

Brownell's delay resulted in his being scooped by a man who surely had no intention of doing any such thing. In 1889 the New England sculptor Truman H. Bartlett published the most complete account of Rodin's art and life that had ever been written *in any language*.[7]

Bartlett discovered Paris on his way to Italy in the 1860s. Although he had planned on enhancing his knowledge of the sculptor's art in the traditional centers of Rome and Florence, he found that it was Paris, not Italy where there were "the greatest living sculptors and the best schools of art."[8] So he settled into a studio at Pont-Marly where he created works for the Paris salons of the 1870s and where he trained his son Paul to draw and to model. The latter effort was even more successful than the first; when Paul Bartlett turned fourteen he had his first work accepted at the Salon.

It was young Paul, not Truman, who first encountered Rodin. He had taken a studio on the Passages des Favorites right around the corner from the studio Rodin occupied on the rue de Vaugirard. Rodin must have been hugely impressed by this young man, just the age of his own son, a youth who vexed him by showing no talent in art. When the two older sculptors met they found they really got on. They talked a great deal. Truman took notes and began to shape their conversations into what was to become his famous series for the *American Architect and Building News*.

Out of these long hours of conversation came one of the richest descriptions of the sculptor and his work ever written, and for the first time Americans could read about this French artist:

> original, without limit, clear and penetrating; generative and dramatic in his conceptive vision, delicate in sentiment, and rapid and powerful in execution. These qualities, pushed into activity by an unsurpassed intensity, have enabled him to produce a new world of sculpture.[9]

If credit for bringing Rodin to the attention of the American public belongs to Bartlett and Brownell, recognition for the first purchases of works goes to that indefatigable buyer of bronzes from Baltimore, George A. Lucas. He met the sculptor in the fall of 1887. A few months later he bought his first Rodin, recording it in his diary on 12 January 1888: "At Rodins & bought statuette Bastien Lepage for 400fs."[10] In March he bought the *Bust of St. John the Baptist* for 1,200 francs; Lucas himself arranged to have it cast in bronze before sending it to Samuel P. Avery in New York.[11] A few years later, in 1893, Avery donated the bust to the Metropolitan Museum, making it the first Rodin to enter a public collection in America (fig. 6.1). This honor echoed

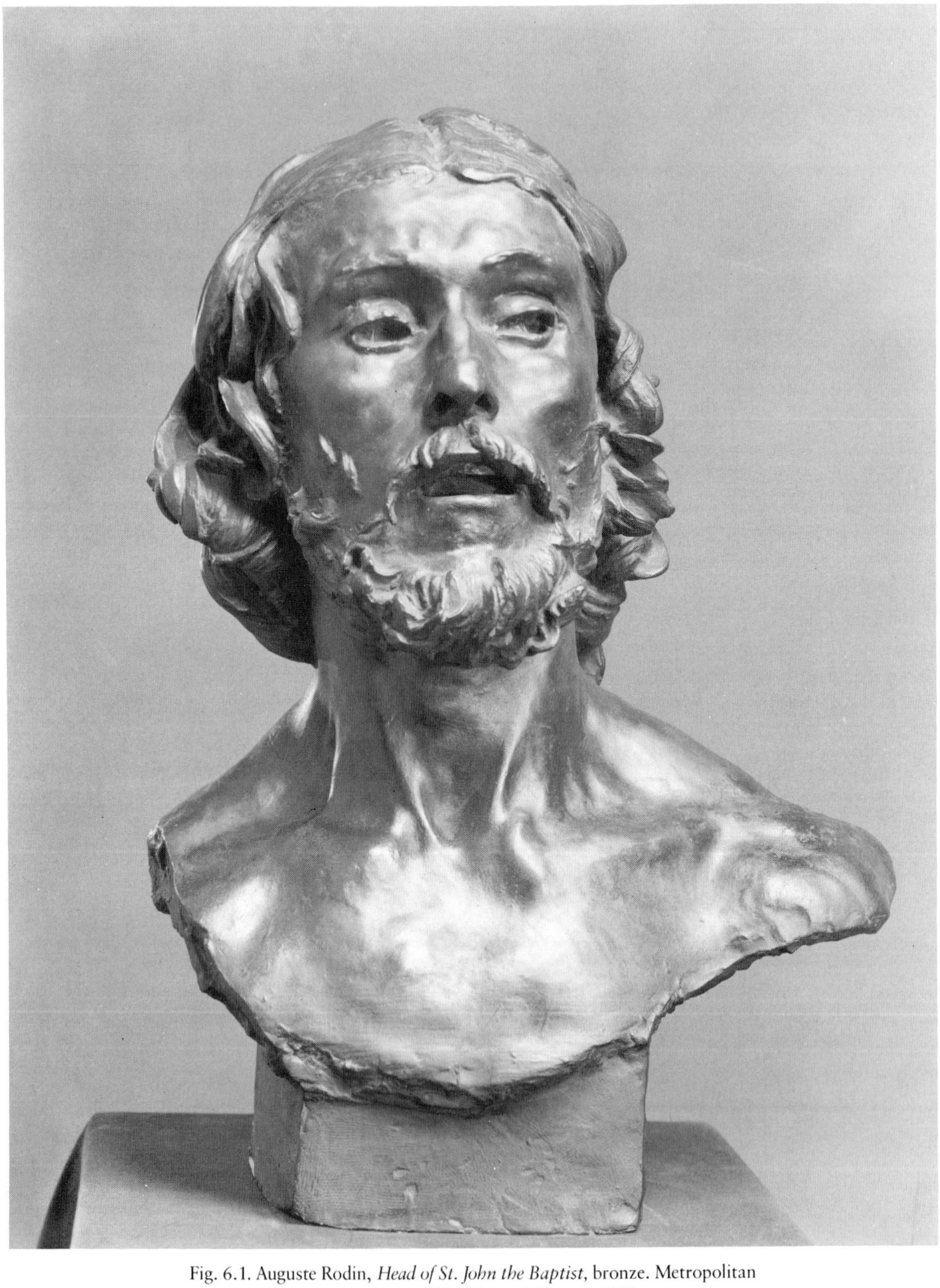

Fig. 6.1. Auguste Rodin, *Head of St. John the Baptist*, bronze. Metropolitan Museum of Art, gift of Samuel P. Avery, 1893.

the judgment of the French about its quality, for the *Bust of St. John* was the first work of Rodin's to receive an award at the Paris Salon. In 1889 Lucas considered two more Rodins—a small version of *Claude Lorrain* that he saw at Durand Ruel and the head of *St. George* that he priced at Rodin's studio—but in the end he did not buy.

From the early 1880s, one of Lucas' closest friends in Paris was Theodore Child. He became the third writer to celebrate Rodin's reputation on the other side of the Atlantic, publishing a long article in the *New York Sun* on 22 February 1891, and devoting a whole chapter to Rodin in *Art and Criticism* (1891) with the intention of bringing to Americans "the name of the most original, the most realistic, and at the same time the most literary of contemporary French sculptors."

The books by Child and Brownell were among the most important books on art to be published in America circa 1890. It is interesting to consider their dedication pages. *French Art* is dedicated "To Auguste Rodin," and *Art and Criticism* "To the Cultivated Women of North America." It was the winning combination, the one that provides the material for one of the most fascinating chapters in the story of how this provincial country, America, opened itself up to the possibility of "modern art." In the telling of this story no moment is more important than 1893, the World's Columbian Exposition, and no person than Sarah Tyson Hallowell.

Once Chicago had managed to wrest the fair from New York and Washington, the energy of the western city exploded. The American frontier had only closed in 1890; now Chicago was setting out to create on the shores of Lake Michigan the largest exhibition ever held. And she succeeded.[12] Henry Adams caught the spirit of the improbability of all this.

> That the Exposition should be a natural growth and product of the Northwest offered a step in evolution to startle Darwin; . . . the Beaux Arts artistically induced to pass the summer on the shore of Lake Michigan—could it be made to seem at home there? Was the American made to seem at home in it?[13]

No person felt more intensely about how the art exhibitions should look than Sarah Hallowell. She had been mounting art shows ever since she moved to Chicago and began building modern art collections in Chicago just as Lucas was building them in Baltimore and New York. It was widely rumored that she would become the director of fine arts for the fair, but she was edged out, mainly because of her sex. In 1891 Hallowell wrote to Bertha Palmer: "I know there is no person in this country of equal experience with my own . . . but with me as art director, much more would be expected than from a man—no shortcomings on my part would be tolerated. . . . "[14] In the end Miss Hallowell became an assistant to Halsey C. Ives, the commissioner of fine arts for the Exposition.

In the nineteenth century, world's fairs created the spirit of rivalry and competition between nations that we associate in the twentieth century with the Olympic Games. France set a new high standard in 1889; the Eiffel Tower still stands as a symbol of that triumph.

America learned much in Paris in 1889, and when the United States commissioners returned from France they sent a message to Congress that something was wrong with art in America. Their report particularly stressed the problems with sculpture.

> Our public statues . . . and other monuments erected to perpetuate the memory of distinguished men . . . and great events . . . constitute one of the most discouraging chapters in our national history. Of the many hundreds and possibly thousands of such works which exist on our soil, it is quite safe to assert that there are not more than twenty-five which, from an art standpoint, are fairly good.[15]

This is an extraordinary statement and the report had a tremendous impact on the Columbian Exposition. For the first time, sculpture was not ignored. Rather, as Elizabeth Holt has pointed out, "The entire exposition was a tremendous 'sculpture show.' "[16]

The United States commissioners who had been in Paris in 1889 did not neglect to report on "that wonderful artist, Auguste Rodin," who "unlocks the secrets hidden in the human form, and applies them to the noblest and grandest uses of art." They thought that his finest work was the *Burghers of Calais,* "a truly noble work, lofty in conception, and most impressively treated."[17]

They must have been pleased when the French government sent one of Rodin's *Burghers of Calais* to Chicago as part of the official French exhibition. It remained at the Art Institute when the fair was over (fig. 6.2). Rodin was also represented in the French section by his *Bust of Dalou.*

Official exhibits, however, were not the most exciting thing that happened in Chicago in the summer of 1893. The single most important event for the arts, the one that attracted everyone's attention, was the "Loan Collection of Foreign Masterpieces Owned in the United States." It was the centerpiece of Sarah Hallowell's efforts at the fair. In putting it together her competitive spirit swung into action: "I am of course eager to make the gallery of French pictures owned in America surpass what is sent from here," she wrote from Paris.[18] If American art was inferior to French art, at least the quality of American taste could be shown to best effect. The French admitted that the Loan Collection was the "veritable clou de l'Exposition,"[19] some complaining that the works, these "prisioners" in the American galleries, would never again return to Gallic shores.

The loan show was an exhibition of painting. With the exception of the great Barye collections in Baltimore and Washington, Americans did not collect sculpture, let alone contemporary sculpture. But Hallowell knew that if any sculptor should have been represented in the Loan Collection it was Rodin. Thus she urged Mrs. Palmer to buy. "I do hope you will conclude to order the Rodin marble. In all America, there is nothing of sculpture to equal this work of his which it would be so fine for you to own. . . . "[20] But she met with no success.[21]

Next we hear of urging from another quarter. From a letter that Hallowell wrote to Rodin in November 1892, it is clear that he had suggested the Columbian Exposition as the perfect setting for a Rodin exhibition! This idea, a one-man show at a universal exposition, was the scheme he carried out so grandly in Paris in 1900. He sent her his photograph. Miss Hallowell thanked him, assuring him that it was "beaucoup moins beau que l'original" and mentioning that she would just love to have the bronze portrait Mlle. Camille Claudel had made of him and that everyone—just everyone—thought a Rodin exhibition was a wonderful idea, but it was against the rules. "But I have another idea." The letter continues:

> I could show your works in my collection of French masterpieces owned by Americans. What would you be able to do for me? Could you send four or five works? I would put them in the catalogue as being in the collection of someone

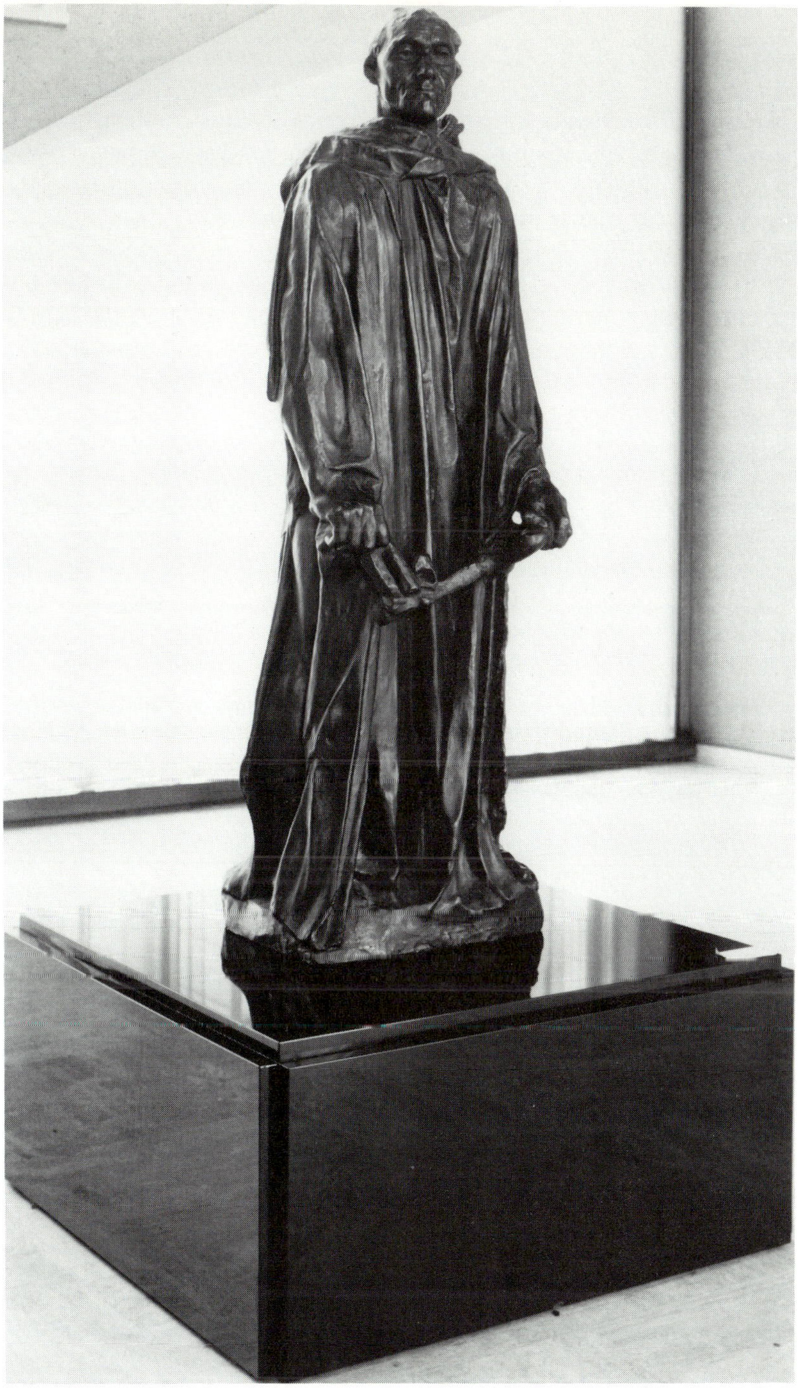

Fig. 6.2. Auguste Rodin, *The Burgher of Calais* (Jean d'Aire), 1889, plaster. © The Art Institute of Chicago, gift of A. M. H. Ellis, 1893.

whose name I would make up. I think this is legitimate because it is monstrous that so far none of your great works are in our country. What do you think? Let me know as soon as possible.[22]

Hallowell's fabrication has created a certain confusion about Rodin's participation in the Loan Exhibition. If we consult the big *Official Catalogue of the Exhibits at the World's Columbian Exposition* at the end of the section on art of the United States we find the private collectors. The last three works are:

2989 Auguste Rodin Francesca and Paolo (marble group)
2990 Auguste Rodin Francesca and Paolo (marble group)
From the "Gates of Hell" commissioned by the French Government for the Museum of Decorative Arts
2991 Auguste Rodin Andromeda (marble)
Lent by Mr. Henry Sargent, New York[23]

This is the catalogue copy that Hallowell invented.

If we look at the little catalogue that was published just for the Loan Collection we find what was really there:

123 Auguste Rodin Cupid and Psyche [fig. 6.3]
124 Auguste Rodin Sphinx (marble) [fig. 6.4]
125 Auguste Rodin Andromeda (marble)

No collector is mentioned.[24]

This confusion has not been made easier by the fact that one week after the show opened, the Rodins were no longer on view.

> When the loan exhibit of masterpieces owned in America was opened to the public three beautiful statuettes, the work of Auguste Rodin, were seen there. Yesterday they were no longer in place. Inquiry elicited the information that it had been decided not to exhibit them.
>
> ✤
>
> The subjects of the three marbles which Miss Hallowell of the Art Department of the Columbian Exposition secured with great difficulty for the loan exhibit are "Andromeda," "Cupid and Psyche," and "The Sphinx."[25]

The article in the *Chicago Tribune* described the works as "replicas of portions of a portal . . . for the Museum of Decorative Arts." Through the writings of Bartlett, Brownell, Child, and others, Americans had heard about *The Gates of Hell.* This should have been an enticing event for art lovers in Chicago in the summer of 1893. But since the works were not on view, although access could be gained with special permission, very few people actually saw the first works in America that gave some idea of Rodin's new approach to the human figure (figs. 6.3 and 6.4).

In the fall, the *Chicago Herald* ran a long and richly illustrated article under the headline, "Fought Against Fate, The Struggle of Sculptor Rodin." The author ended his piece with a discussion of the portal that "has aroused extraordinary fervor in artistic circles everywhere."

> Two illustrations of it are in the Fine Arts Building at Jackson Park. They are wonderfully beautiful, and executed with extraordinary delicacy. The room in which they are concealed is accessible to anyone who applies to a guard, and contem-

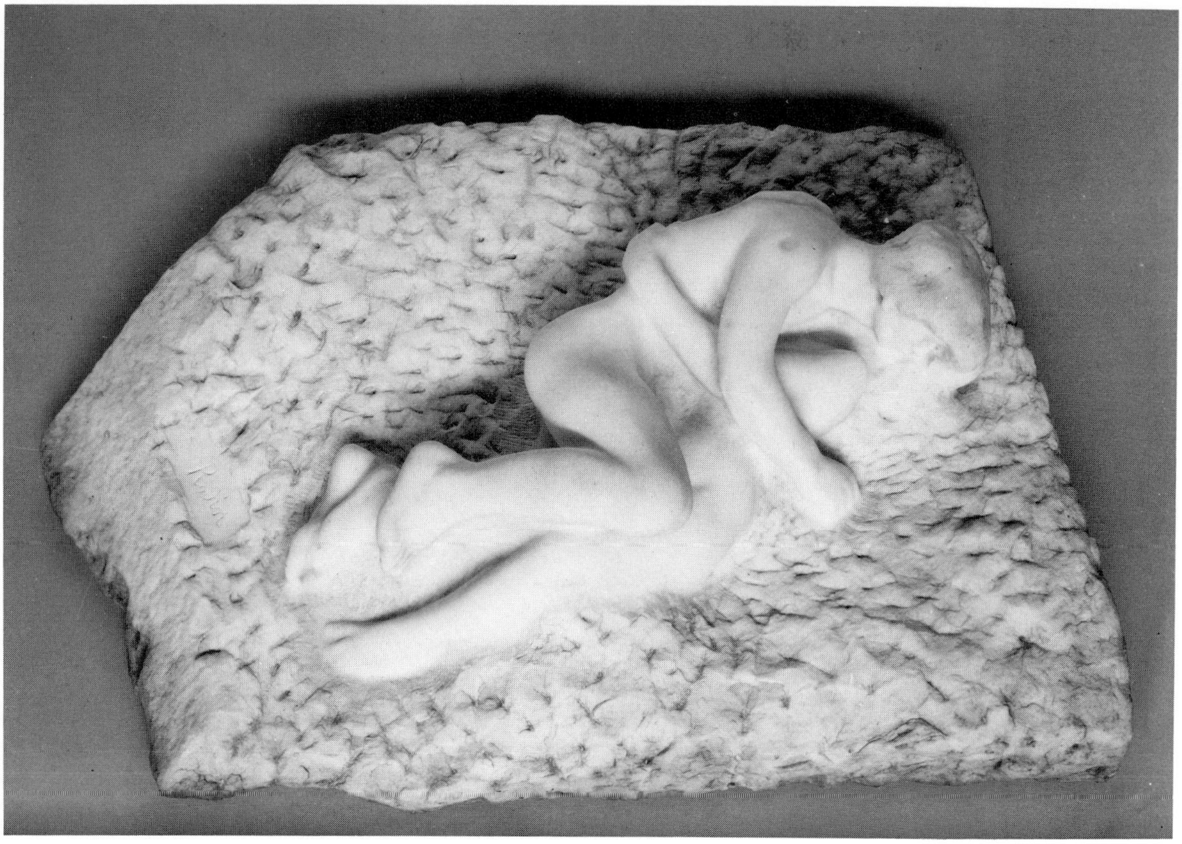

Fig. 6.3. Auguste Rodin, *Love and Psyche*, marble. Metropolitan Museum of Art, gift of Richard Anthony Strong and Alexander Milliken Stewart, 1938.

> plation of them justifies the care and reserve which have been exercised in their behalf. If such works were placed in the open of the sculpture corridors they would have been brutally defaced and ruined months ago.[26]

And he went on to describe *Paolo and Francesca* (à la Dante, not Rodin), so we know that even the critic had not seen the works that he was reviewing.

Rodin was the sculptor of carnal love and *volupté*. This imagery is at the very heart of *The Gates of Hell,* and it came to rest for a few moments on the shores of Lake Michigan in the summer of 1893, only to be speedily ushered out of view. If we consider the norms of taste and contemporary concepts of morality in America at the end of the nineteenth century this action should be viewed as correct.

In 1892, Will H. Low and Kenyon Cox were thinking about how to prepare the public for the great art exhibition about to take place when they published their article, "The Nude in Art." They pointed out that nudity in antiquity and the Renaissance was an artistic convention as it was now, but that it had been "better understood by the people than it is to-day because the people were more artistic than those of to-day, and better understood all matters of art." They built their pro-nude platform around the old truth and beauty formula.

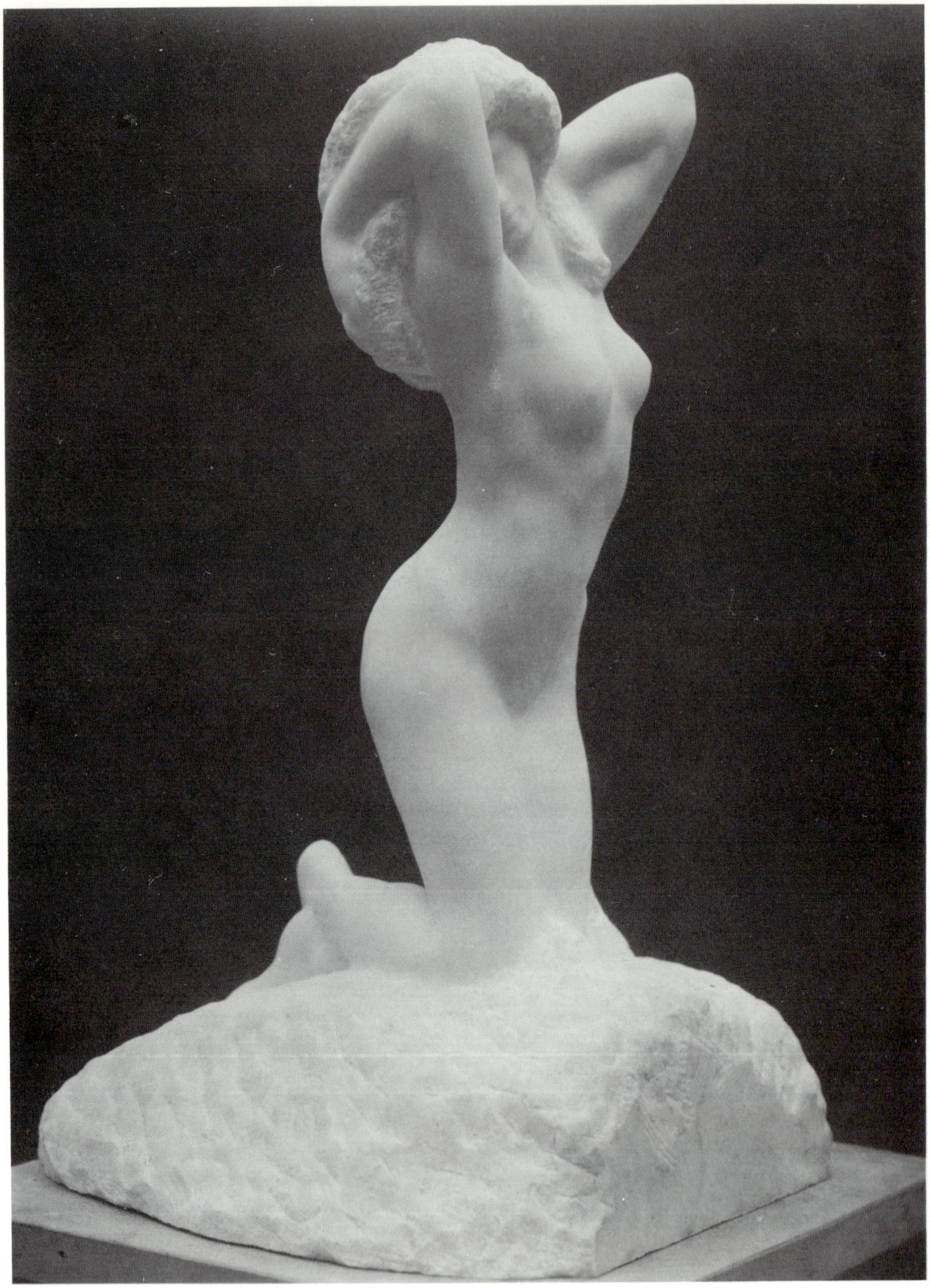

Fig. 6.4. Auguste Rodin, *The Sphinx*, marble. Whereabouts unknown.

> Surely, if art be the expression of man's delight in the beauty of nature, its highest and purest form is the expression of his delight in what is highest and most beautiful in nature, the human figure.[27]

Such thoughts never prepared anyone for a naked boy and girl lying in each other's arms on a bed of marble with nothing more to cover them than a mythological title.

Sarah Hallowell had promised Rodin she would sell the works in America, but she found no buyers; she begged off for reasons of financial crisis. The panic of 1893 was the worst the country had ever experienced, but it was the workers and the farmers who were deprived of income, not the rich. Americans could take Rodin's portrait heads and his *Burgher* in sackcloth, but not the turmoil contained in the nudes he created for *The Gates of Hell.*

Rodin was appreciative of all that Hallowell had done. To show her just how much it meant to him, he gave her a bronze version of the *Sphinx* in 1893. And in 1895 she wrote to him of her enchantment with "mon beau marbre, mon petit groupe en bronze et ma belle esquisse en terre." Sarah Hallowell now had the biggest collection of Rodins in America.

But in 1894 two more Rodins had arrived in Chicago at the Michigan Avenue home of Charles T. Yerkes. Yerkes, the "traction king" responsible for replacing horses with cables and thus giving Chicago five-hundred miles of new surface transportation with the ingenious downtown Loop as its centerpiece, frequently saw Hallowell in Paris. Surely it was her influence that was crucial to the purchase of the large marbles, *Cupid and Psyche* and *Orpheus and Eurydice* (figs. 6.5 and 6.6). How appropriate that the person who was the real life prototype for Theodore Dreiser's fictional character of Cowperwood, a man with an insatiable curiosity about eighteen-year-old girls whose motto was "I satisfy myself," was the first American to buy works by Rodin in this uninhibited new taste. Soon they were on view at the Art Institute, where Lorado Taft saw them.

> The limbs are of impossible proportions. And yet they seem to feel—do these little marble people. They are not puppets, nor even skillful actors, but real, loving, suffering humanity. You cannot help feeling with them.[28]

Hallowell may not have been able to sell Rodin's works out of the exhibition halls, but it was against the background of the Columbian Exposition, an occasion at which Europeans and Americans got to know each other in a new way, that Rodin's name came truly into view in America. The American Art Association purchased four of his works for a sale in New York in 1895;[29] others showed up in Boston in 1895 and 1896.[30] In Paris, Americans in ever greater numbers took to stopping by at 182 rue de l'Université where Rodin received on Saturdays. Henry Adams was there in the summer of 1895. Disappointed that he could find so little to buy in the shops, he decided as a last resort, to go "call on Rodin, and try to buy one of his small bronze figures. They are mostly so sensually suggestive that I shall have to lock them up when any girls are about, which is awkward, but Rodin is the only degenerated artist I know of, whose work is original." After the visit he wrote to Elizabeth Cameron again.

> I have passed an hour with Rodin in his studio looking at his marbles, and especially Venus and dead Adonis [fig. 6.7] which he is sending to some exhibition in Philadelphia, and which is quite too too utter and decadent, but like all his things

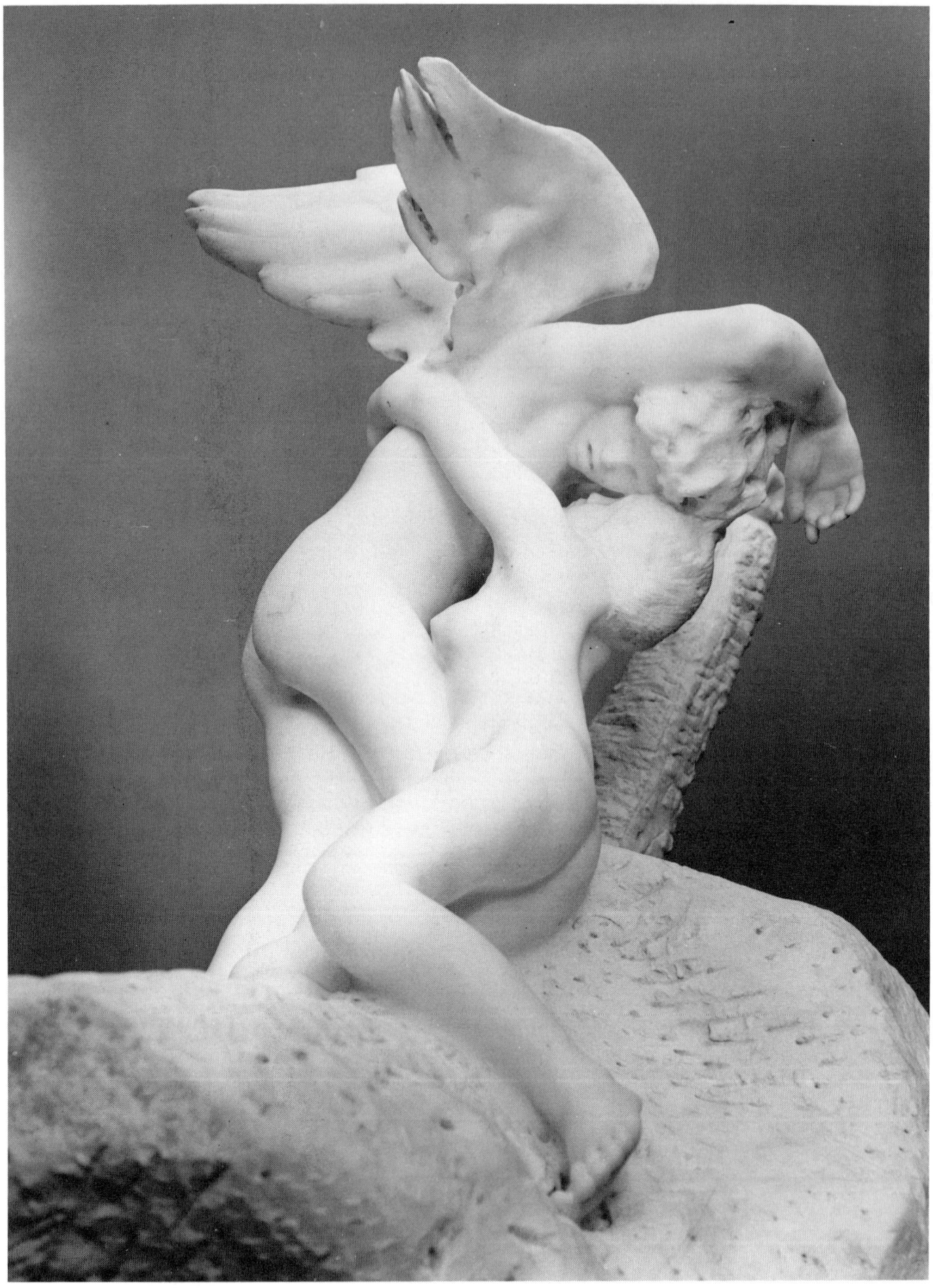

Fig. 6.5. Auguste Rodin, *Cupid and Psyche*, marble. Metropolitan Museum of Art, gift of Thomas F. Ryan, 1910.

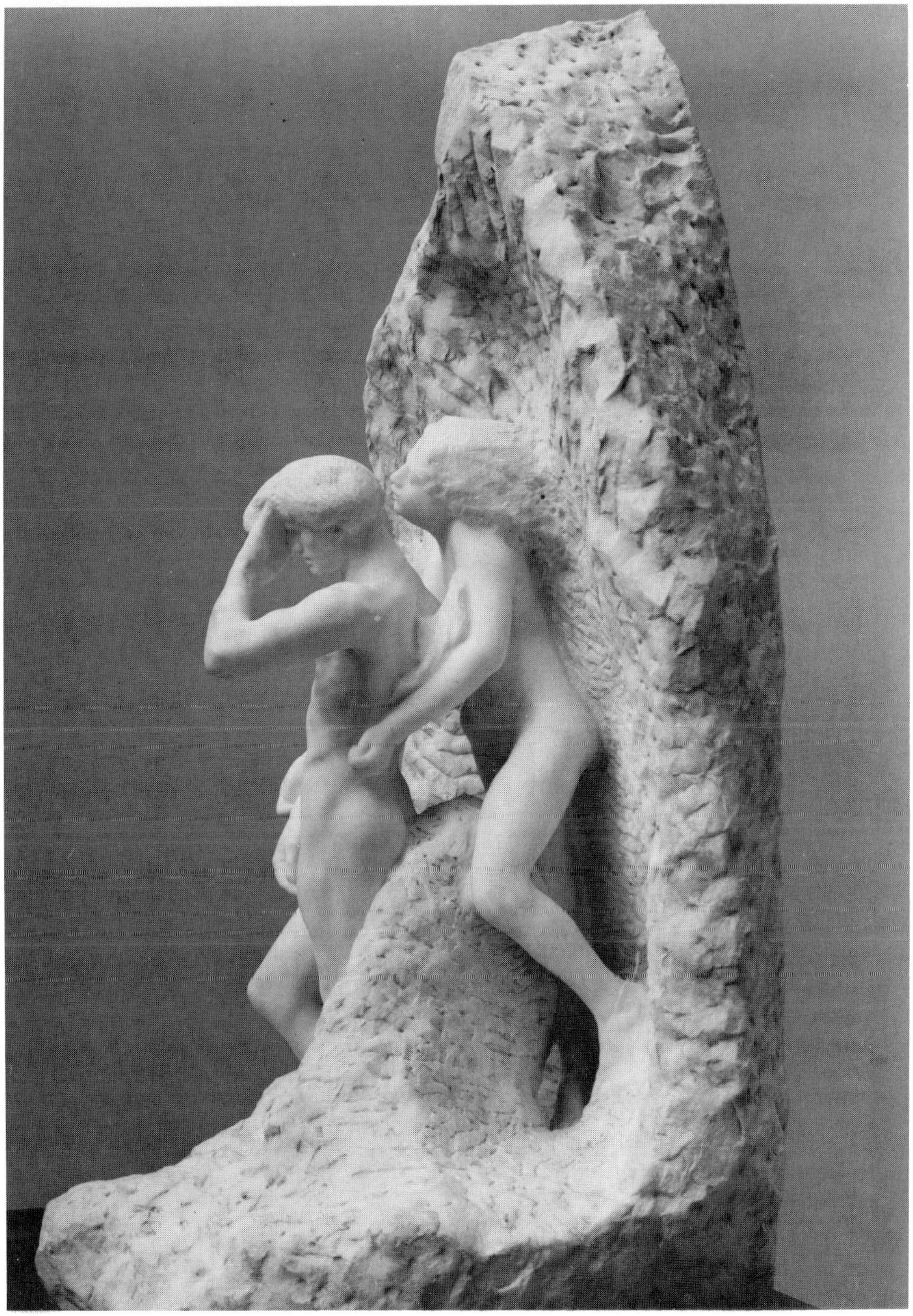

Fig. 6.6. Auguste Rodin, *Orpheus and Eurydice*, marble. Metropolitan Museum of Art, gift of Thomas F. Ryan, 1910.

> hardly made for *jeunes personnes* like me and my breakfast-table company. Why can we decadents never take the comfort and satisfaction of our decadence. Surely the meanest life on earth is that of an age that has not a standard left on any form of morality or art, except the British sovereign. I prefer Rodin's decadent sensualities, but I must not have them.[31]

Such exquisite anxieties and pungent misgivings overtook the American as he contemplated Rodin's coupled nudes. Could the sculptor have understood this in any way? Yet it was the strongest thing that drew them to him.

Venus and Adonis was shown in Philadelphia, but it, too, found no buyers and was returned to Paris. The first work by Rodin that was found acceptable in Philadelphia for public viewing was the *The Age of Bronze,* which arrived in 1898. When we think about Rodin's life in 1898, the year his *Balzac* was rejected by the Société des Gens de Lettres in Paris and created a furor known as the "Dreyfus Affair of the Art World," somehow the *Age of Bronze* of 1876 looks old-fashioned and tame. But not in Philadelphia, where only a few years earlier Thomas Eakins had been asked to resign as president of the Philadelphia Academy because of the importance he gave to studying the nude. He had posed male models in female life classes, and by so doing he had precipitated a crisis. Paul Bartlett wrote to Rodin on 7 January 1899, "Yesterday, I saw your plaster in Philadelphia . . . they are enchanted to have it." It was surely safer for those girls to work from a plaster than a real live man.[32]

By 1899, Charles T. Yerkes found himself politically blocked and socially ostracized in Chicago. So he sold out and moved to the house that he had built in New York at the corner of 68th Street and Fifth Avenue. And he took his marbles with him as well as the rest of his immense art collection.

As we consider American cultural history using the limited measure of Rodin sculptures, we should see this move of the Yerkes collection as appropriate. For the story of how America opened itself up to new art is not one that can be told in Philadelphia, in Boston, or in Chicago. It is a New York story, one that is part of the ferment of the early twentieth century when obsolete mores and styles came under attack in the new cosmopolis. New York was a place that made "291," Alfred Stieglitz's group that showed at the gallery at Fifth Avenue and 31st Street, possible. New York was the receptive climate in which Mabel Dodge could establish her salon at 23 Fifth Avenue in Greenwich Village, where thinkers, writers, and artists could meet and exchange views, where one could hear Mrs. Sanger describe her birth-control crusade or A. A. Brill explain the strange theories of Dr. Freud. It was a generation seeking salvation through art, believing the artist might take the place of god in his ability to create a new way of seeing and of being. Their radicalness was in the area of cultural choices and sexual behavior, not in politics. In erotic emotions and voluptuous fantasies they found a new kind of beauty, one that had been sorely lacking in America.

An individual who was of them, though not with them, was Chicago's own Mary Louise Fuller. By the end of the 1880s she had become Loie Fuller of New York vaudeville, and in 1892 she departed for Paris where she made her debut at the Folies-Bergère, becoming a success without precedent in that theater. When Stéphane Mallarmé saw her in 1893, it was "an enchantress, creating her own environment" who danced across the stage, colored lights from below illuminating the movements of her body under silken scarves.

Rodin was one of the many who fell under her spell, and she under his.

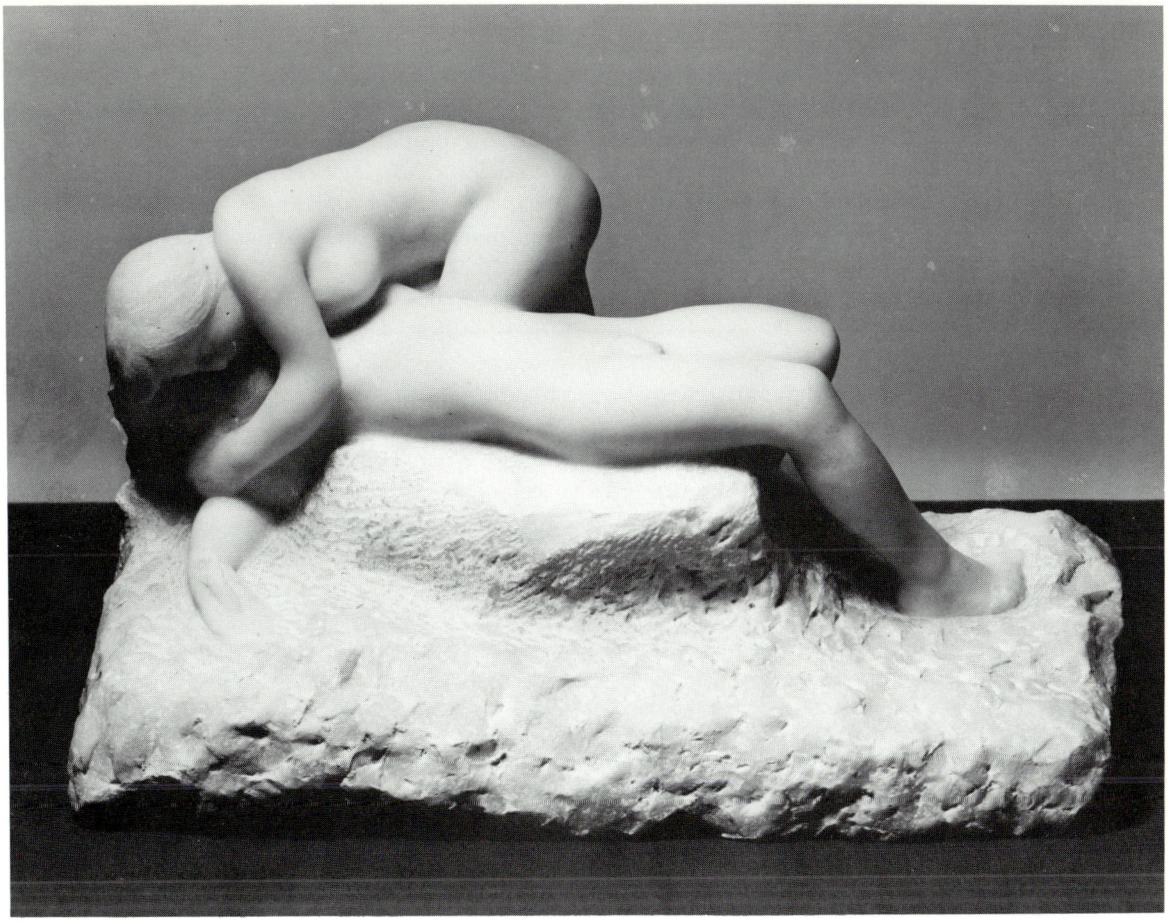

Fig. 6.7. Auguste Rodin, *Venus and Adonis*, marble.
The Walters Art Gallery, Baltimore.

They probably knew each other by 1896, but their real friendship dates from 1900, when they had pavilions facing each other at the Universal Exposition. Loie's pavilion was called a Museum of Dance. She not only danced there but had brought together a collection of sculptures and paintings of which she, Loie, was the subject. For the occasion of the 1900 exposition Rodin had put together a major retrospective of more than 150 sculptures, including *The Gates of Hell* and dozens of drawings, watercolors, and prints. It solidified his position as the most famous artist in the world.

Out of neighborly proximity at the exposition came a friendship, one that was not always easy, but one that resulted in the first real show of Rodin works in America. It took place at the National Arts Club on West 34th Street in Manhattan in May 1903. Though called "Miss Fuller's Collection," all the works were for sale. There were eighteen sculptures, eighteen drawings, and portraits of Rodin by Jean Paul Laurens, John Singer Sargent, and Camille Claudel. Here were versions of his most famous sculptures: *Adam, Eve, The Thinker,* heads of *Victor Hugo* and *Balzac, The Tower of Labor, The Hand of God,* and works in plaster that suggested something of what *The*

Gates were like. For New Yorkers it was powerful and unsettling. *The Times* reviewer found that "it excites and disquiets. But it makes one think and in the end compels one, however reluctantly, to acknowledge its power."[33]

A few months before the National Arts Club exhibition opened, the first issue of a new magazine, *Camera Work,* appeared. It featured a portrait of Rodin with his *Victor Hugo* in the background. This image, by a young photographer, Edward Steichen, was described as so powerful that it would end forever disputes over whether photography was an art or not. "A medium, so rich and so complete, one in which such a masterpiece can be achieved, the world can no longer ignore. The battle is won!"[34] In another article Charles H. Caffin described how privileged Steichen had been in working so closely with Rodin, that this opportunity had enabled him to come "under the inspiration of his grand and independent mentality," and that "these influences lit upon a young nature that has within it the capacity for corresponding qualities."[35]

When these articles were written, Steichen was living and working in a little studio on the top floor of 291 Fifth Avenue. It was the space that he and Alfred Stieglitz took as the setting for their famous exhibitions that would mean so much for modern art in America. For the first few years they showed only photography. When they discussed the idea of nonphotography shows they both agreed that they would start with Rodin drawings.

Steichen returned to Paris. Together he and Rodin selected the drawings, and an exhibition of fifty-eight works opened in January 1908.[36] It was well attended and widely reviewed. The Mexican artist, Marius de Zayas, whose work was also shown at 291 in 1908, recalled the Rodin show.

> Steichen must have seen in them all the elements needed to stir up things in New York. And they did. With this exhibition the Photo-Secession became the key which opened the doors of New York to modern art.
>
> The Rodin drawings exhibition started the ball rolling towards real modern art. Whether or not it was premeditated, this exhibition was a good beginning, an excellent "aperitif" for what New York had to swallow subsequently.[37]

Even when critics did not like the drawings at 291, where faces were "the merest twist of the pencil . . . gigantic female forms . . . sometimes one gets a bold line indicating a cheek, a breast, a thigh; sometimes a second line corrects the contour of a Gargantuan calf," you could feel the power of Rodin's work. This same critic evoked for his readers the scene from whence the images came.

> Imagine a Turkish bath, without steam, plus plaster and plaster casts . . . and a half dozen Adams and Eves walking, sitting and lying about . . . all striving to forget they are not clothed and are models hired by the day, and that some one is always watching them, ever on the alert to capture their lines, and curves, their unconscious poses and actions as they move.[38]

Charles de Kay enjoyed his racy recreation of Rodin's studio, presenting it in snide tones, but it was just the kind of thing that set the imaginations of the young rebels among the artists of 291 on fire. It only stimulated the flow of young people eager to pass through the great doors at 182 rue de l'Université. Agnes Ernst, a recent Barnard graduate connected to the Stieglitz group, met Rodin in the spring of 1909 through Eu-

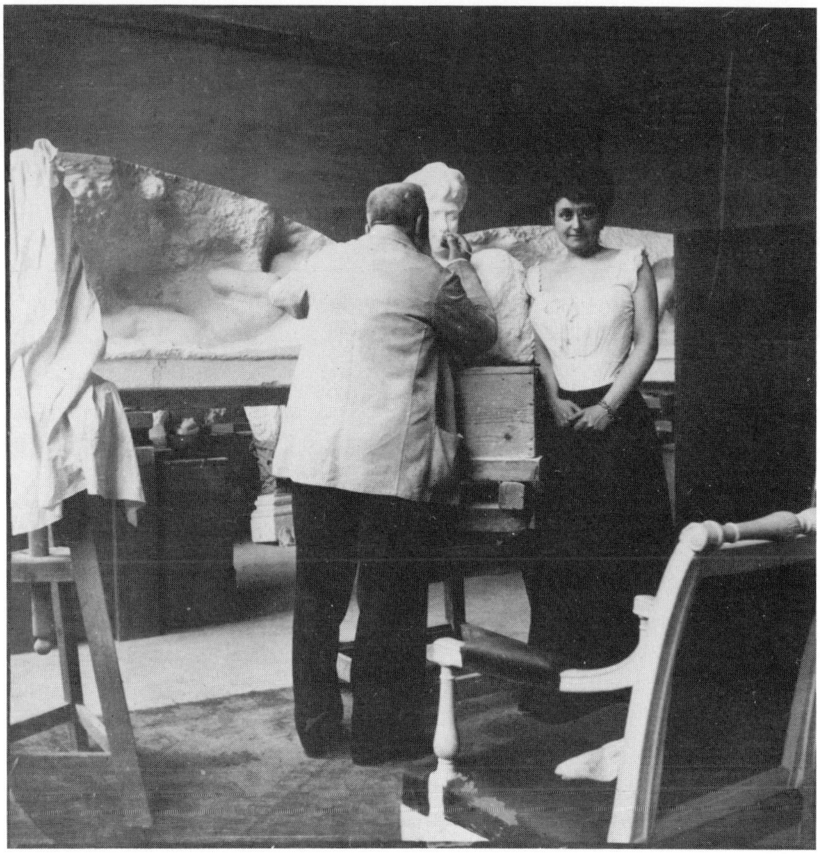

Fig. 6.8. Auguste Rodin at work on Kate Simpson's bust, 1902. Archives of the Musée Rodin.

gene Meyer, who would one day be her husband (as well as owner/publisher of the *Washington Post*). She remembered how:

> Rodin took me under his wing because he enjoyed my eagerness to learn. A curiously warm friendship sprang up between us which I had to defend now and then against his sensual attitude toward all women. Nothing I could say ever explained to him in convincing manner why I was unwilling to pose nude.[39]

Others stayed home and let the spirit of the man and his work exert its power over their will to create. In November 1908 the Metropolitan put Rodin's *Hand of God*, a recent gift, on exhibition. The work shows a gigantic hand rising from the marble block in order to let the forms of Adam and Eve tumble forth. The following year Cora Bennett Stephenson published her novel, *The Hand of God*, about the people of the Old Testament. Using the "sensual life of the Philistines" as background to the story of Samson and Delilah, she graphically depicted the "dances of sex and sun worship" of the ancient people. A nice new photograph of Rodin's *Hand of God* was the advertising image that appeared everywhere.

Rodin had another admirer in New York, one who stood at a certain distance from these adventurous downtown artists. She was Kate Simpson, the youngest daughter of New York banker and philanthropist, George I. Seney. She had married

John Woodruff Simpson in 1889, and by the end of the century, they had settled into 926 Fifth Avenue where they spent their winters. The rest of the year they traveled, and by 1901 their annual European trips included a stop at Rodin's.[40] This pattern came to an end only with the advent of the Great War. The visit of 1902 was particularly exciting; Rodin had begun Kate's portrait (fig. 6.8). The following spring, anticipating her return to Paris, Kate wrote: "Every day I remember you and your kindness; I am sure that my bust will show sensibilities that are so dignified and superior. In your heart I found both loftiness and tranquility."[41]

Rodin paid Kate a great compliment when he selected her bust as one of his two entries for the Salon of 1904. As he was hurrying to finish the work, he gave an interview to *The Craftsman*.

> "Almost invariably," he said, "there is intelligence in the faces of the women of this nation." "But," he added, casting a long look at the unfinished head which he turned toward me, "there is, furthermore, kindness of heart evidenced in the countenance of this model. That is what I shall attempt to express."[42]

By this time the Simpsons had begun to collect. In 1903 they had four Rodins: a *Thinker,* a *St. John,* a *Head of Balzac,* and a *Centauresse.* Every year more works arrived, including Kate's beautiful bust (fig. 6.9). In December 1906 Kate wrote to Rodin, "Each day I have a fresh impression of my beautiful marbles. You can not know what joy it gives me to possess them." She ends her letter by saying, "When you come to see me in April, I am sure that you will find these beauties well placed." It is the first time we hear of such a visit, but in 1908 it appeared in *The New York Times:* "Rodin Will Visit America This Winter." Rodin responded to the interviewer by saying:

> Yes, I expect to enjoy my visit to America for I hope to know its art better. I hear they have something fresh—Here, so long tempered by movements, isms—decadent—we must go back before we can make progress.[43]

Apparently Rodin was of the mind that he might have a better audience in New York than he did in Paris as Fauvism and Cubism began to make their way into the world of art.

There was another reason, however, for this wish to see America (one that was never fulfilled). Rodin had a new New Yorker in his life. She was Claire Coudert; she had married the Marquis de Choiseul in St. Patrick's Cathedral in 1891, a union that had been blessed by the Pope. The young society couple established themselves in Paris; by 1904 they had become acquainted with Rodin. Claire made the sculptor the goal of her life, and by 1907 she had achieved her heart's desire. She began to arrange his social life, pick out his clothes, think about how he should wear his hair; then she entered into his business affairs, fixing prices and deciding who should buy what. Since Rodin spoke no English, she moved into a particularly strong position when it came to American clients. And this intense little woman did not take kindly to rivals. Both Loie and Kate had to tread softly, although in order not to lose their friendship with Rodin, they tried their best to get along with her.

Even though La Duchesse, as she was called, had become all powerful, Kate Simpson still managed to play a role in Rodin's contacts with America. In 1909 she arranged for the genius of the American railroad system, H. L. Harriman, to meet with Rodin and to sit for his portrait. He died immediately after returning to New York.

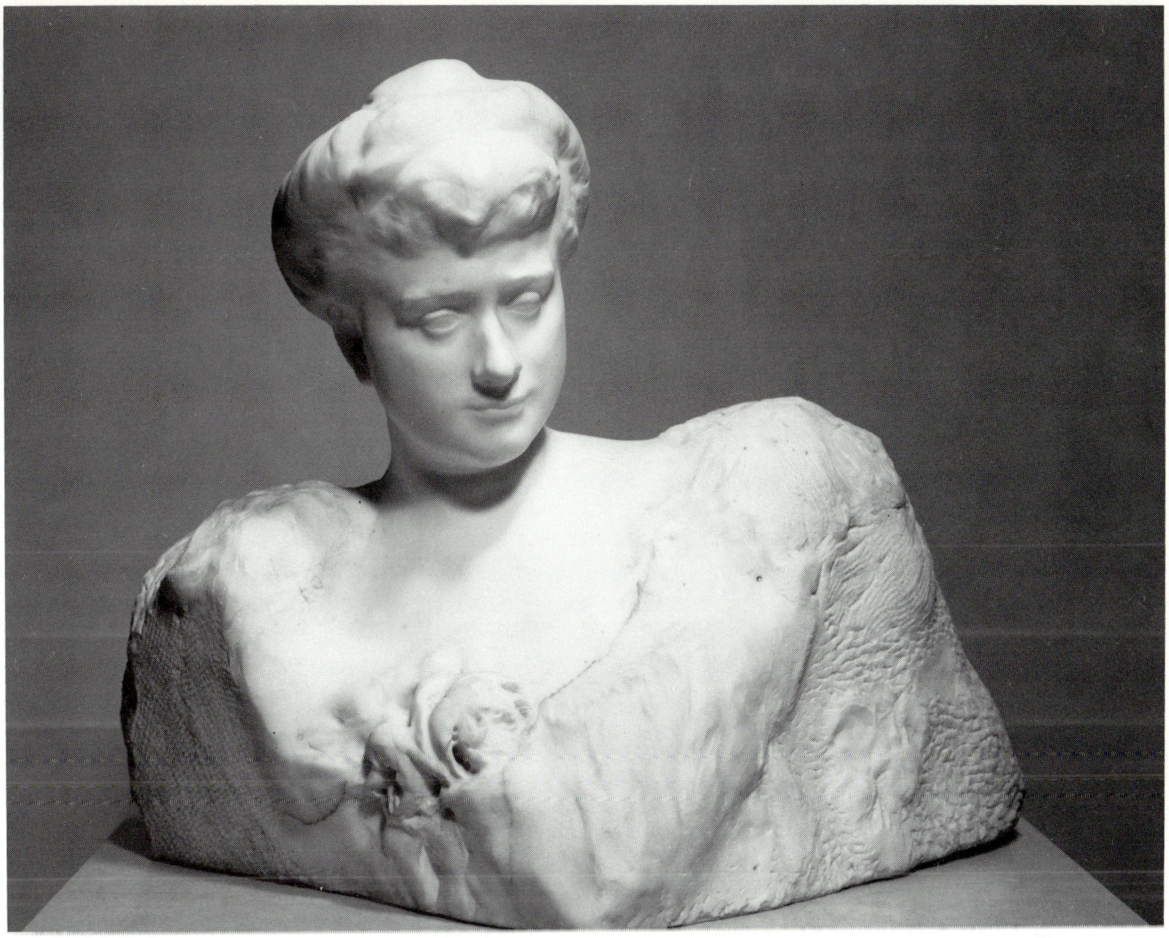

Fig. 6.9. Auguste Rodin, *Mrs. John W. Simpson*, marble. National Gallery of Art, Washington, gift of Mrs. John W. Simpson, 1942.

His daughter Mary wrote as soon as she was able, "The thing that gives me greatest consolation is to know that you have made Papa's portrait."[44] But her correspondence, too, went mainly to the Duchesse.

The bust was shipped in the fall of 1910 in the company of that of another New York millionaire, Thomas Fortune Ryan, a man with a drive similar to Harriman's as well as a comparable fortune. By 1910, when Ryan received his bust, he was in his sixties and was beginning to find that more and more he just wanted to retire to his sculpture garden at 858 Fifth Avenue. But Ryan, who had begun life as a penniless Irish orphan, felt that these pleasures should not be his alone. He had begun buying from Rodin in 1908 with the intention of donating the works to the Metropolitan. In 1910 he gave three marbles along with $25,000, indicating that the money was to be used for further Rodin purchases.[45]

In the summer of 1910, Daniel Chester French, America's most prominent living sculptor and chairman of the Metropolitan's Committee on Sculpture, set off with Edward Robinson, vice director of the museum, to visit Rodin's studio. They

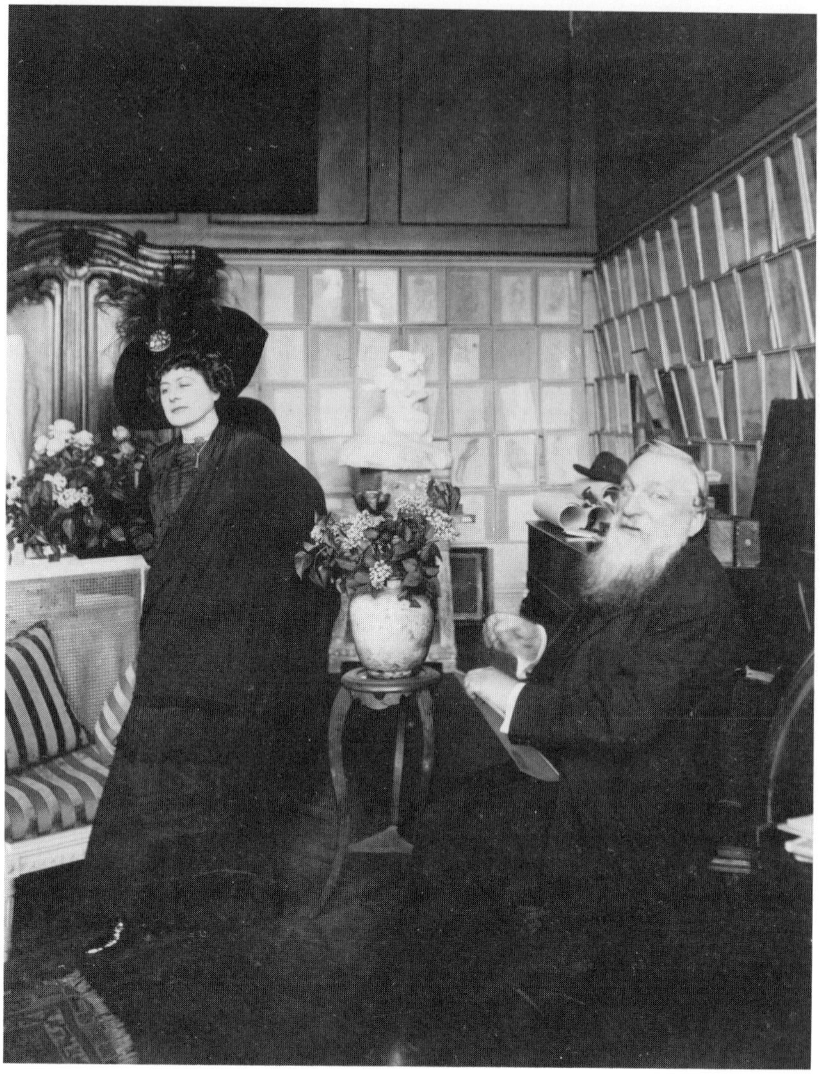

Fig. 6.10. Auguste Rodin and the Marquise de Choiseul at Hôtel Biron. Archives of the Musée Rodin.

went to review the recommendations made by the Metropolitan's European purchasing agent, John Marshall. He had drawn up a list of works in Rodin's studio in 1908, the ones he thought would be most suitable for the museum's collection. French took his wife and daughter along; they stayed at the Crillon and were frequently guests at Rodin's home in Meudon as well as at Hôtel Biron on the rue de Varenne, now his residence in the city where the Marquise de Choiseul acted as hostess. Mrs. French loved having lunch at this "wonderful palace," and she found Rodin "simple as a child . . . my daughter and I were flattered because he seemed quite as pleased at our liking his work as if our criticism had been really valuable."[46]

The crates began to arrive in New York in the fall. A gallery was selected. It would be the north corridor, just off the main hall. By spring of 1912 all was ready, and on May 1 a two-day celebration got under way. There was a banquet at the Waldorf in honor of the Lake Champlain tercentenary at which the French committee gave *La France,* a bronze bust by Rodin, to the American people: "This image we give to you as Champlain gave the best of his life to this land of yours." The next day the delegation, one of whom was the Marquis de Choiseul(!) (fig. 6.10), participated in the opening of the Rodin Gallery. There were forty sculptures, plus drawings and watercolors, the largest public collection of Rodin's work in the world. What was admired, and what we can admire again in the Meyer Galleries of the Metropolitan, was the diversity—marbles, bronzes, plasters, terra-cotta, large and small, finished and unfinished, early and late—a total view of the range of possibilities in Rodin's art was visible. As before, the favorites were the marbles, not only *The Hand of God* and the works from the Yerkes collection but also recent purchases such as the *Tempest, Madame X,* and *By the Sea.* Marble remained the chosen sculptural medium for Americans. Not only was it more expensive than bronze, but it also had a respectability inherited from the ancient past. Also they thought that marble was more "original," when actually it was just the reverse, for a bronze or a plaster is closer to the hand of the artist than a marble that has been pointed into existence by a practitioner. Rodin himself made a gift of a number of plaster sketches and fragments, as well as a bronze cast of the bust of Ryan, and a terra-cotta. With the exception of the Ryan bust, the works included in his gift would surely not have been selected by French and Robinson. They were too sketchy, too unfinished for their taste, but the presence of these small objects enlarged the picture and gave the possibility of understanding the process of sculpture as nothing else on view in America in 1912.

Rodin's place in American art history was embodied in the gallery at the Metropolitan in 1912; he was the artist who allowed people to know it was possible to have a sculpture that was neither monumental Beaux-Arts conservative nor naturalistic narrative genre. His work made it clear that the most daring distortions in the human figure and the most searching naturalism were not antithetical. Even more important, his work was frankly sexual; it was a powerful force that helped to break down the roadblock holding a portion of the creative energy of American artists in check.

For those enlightened enough to understand all this, it must have come as a shock to open the magazine section of the Sunday *Sun* on July 21st and read the headline: "Rodin, World Famous Sculptor, Lauds Greek Art. Great Master Insists That Student Who Loves Women Too Passionately Is Lost." There followed a strange interview full of agitation: "I have never made any erotic works." "... about the Futurists and others. They do not exist. All these new styles are fads." The interview ended with a profeminist statement: "The suffragettes are only trying to prove their value." This interview must be understood in the context of Rodin's personal life at this time, for it coincides with Rodin's breakup with Claire, an event covered on the front page of the *New York Times* in September.

> Paris society, recently back from fashionable resorts, talks of nothing but the quarrel alleged to have taken place between Auguste Rodin and a well-known Franco-American Duchesse, which, it is said, has caused the definite rupture of a friendship of such long standing that if you wanted to address yourself to Rodin you had to approach the Duchesse first.[47]

It does look like Rodin put off this dramatic change in his life until after the opening of the gallery. The Duchesse de Choiseul had been present at the visits from

American dignitaries and deeply involved in the decisions all along the way. Her husband (who long ago had given his blessing to the liaison) was a representative of France at the opening. It would not do to have made this move before May.

Kate Simpson, whose Fifth Avenue home had served as a private gallery for Rodin's work visited by scores of persons in the years preceding the opening of the Metropolitan gallery, suffered from bouts of jealousy and regret as she was forced into a secondary role during those years of preparation for the gallery. She wrote to Rodin in October that she knew he was alone at rue de Varenne.

> I have known you for a long time and I know that you will never be alone or sad as long as you are with your beautiful sculptures. On the contrary what you need is peace in order to bring your great work to completion. To my way of thinking there has been too much distraction in your life, too many people who have not let you have the tranquility you need to work. Fundamentally, you are of a simple nature; yet you are strong, you are a world unto yourself with your great thoughts and your great work.[48]

Rodin was almost 73 when this letter reached him. Few works would come from his hand during the five years that remained of his life. Friends and supporters closed around him, trying to keep other "adventurers" at bay, so that they might bring into being a great museum dedicated to his work.

Rodin did much for taste and for artistic freedom in America. In a way, America returned the favor. The adulation, the enthusiasm, the great love of Rodin on the part of his early collectors in the United States presented itself as both a challenge and an incentive for the French government, which in December 1916 voted to establish a Rodin museum at the Hôtel Biron in Paris.

NOTES

The author would like to thank the Florence J. Gould Foundation for a grant making possible the time for research on a biography of Rodin and writing of the present article.

1. *Art and Progress* 3 (December 1911): 409.

2. The B. G. Cantor Rodin Sculpture Garden at Stanford University was established in 1985.

3. *The American Architect and Building News* (1 July 1876).

4. Letter of 5 July 1876. Ralph Barton Perry, *The Thought and Character of William James* (Boston, 1935).

5. Arthur Warren, "Our London Letter," *Boston Transcript*, 20 May 1882.

6. Letter of 4 Feb. 1889. Archive, Musée Rodin.

7. "Auguste Rodin, Sculptor," *The American Architect and Building News*, nos. 682–703 (19 January–15 June 1889).

8. Truman Bartlett's notes found among the Paul Bartlett Papers, Library of Congress, Washington, D.C.

9. The Bartlett articles have been edited and republished by Albert E. Elsen, *Auguste Rodin, Readings on His Life and Work* (Englewood Cliffs, N.J.: Prentice-Hall, 1965), 105–106.

10. Lilian M. C. Randall, *The Diary of George A. Lucas: An American Art Agent in Paris, 1857–1909*, 2 vols. (Princeton, N.J.: Princeton University Press, 1979), 2:662.

11. Ibid., 2:666 and 1:98.

12. The Universal Exposition of 1889 in Paris occupied 72 acres as compared to Chicago's 686 acres.

13. Henry Adams, *The Education of Henry Adams* (Boston: Houghton Mifflin Co., 1916), 340.

14. The letter was written in January 1891. Found at the Chicago Historical Society and quoted in John D. Kysela, "Sarah Hallowell Brings 'Modern Art' to the Midwest," *Art Quarterly* 27 (1964): 155.

15. *Reports of the United States Commissioners to the Universal Exposition of 1889 at Paris* (Washington, D.C.: Government Printing Office, 1891), 2:4.

16. "American Collectors and French Critics of 19th-Century Sculpture," Symposium talk, Indianapolis Museum of Art, 1980.

17. *Report of the United States Commissioners*, 2:48–49.

18. Letter to Bertha Palmer, 9 July 1891, The Art Institute of Chicago. I should like to thank Susan Glover Godlewski for making this letter available to me.

19. Jacques Hermant, "L'Art à l'Exposition de Chicago," *Gazette des Beaux-Arts* (1 December 1893): 451.

20. Ibid.

21. In 1905 Hallowell finally managed to make arrangements for Mrs. Palmer to sit for a portrait by Rodin.

22. 15 November 1892, Musée Rodin. I should like to thank Mme. Hélène Pinet for helping me to get the material on Sarah Hallowell together. There are 121 Hallowell letters in the Musée Rodin, the first one dating from May 18, 1914.

23. I should like to thank Margaret Potter for her trek around to the Metropolitan Museum Library, the Frick Art Reference Library, the New York Public Library, and the New York Historical Society in search of Henry Sargent.

24. The works are cited by Georges Grappe as the ones that Rodin sent to the Columbian Exposition. Georges Grappe, *Catalogue du Musée Rodin, I-Hotel Biron* (Paris: Musée Rodin, 1944), 51, 56.

25. "Statuettes Withdrawn From View," *Chicago Tribune*, 17 May 1893.

26. *Chicago Herald*, 1 October 1893.

27. Will H. Low and Kenyon Cox, "The Nude in Art," *Scribner's Magazine* 12 (1892): 748.

28. Lorado Taft, "Auguste Rodin," *The Record*, 8 July 1895.

29. The sale took place on April 25 and 26 at Chickering Hall in Madison Square. The works were *Eve in Despair* (marble), *Bellona* (marble), *Milo* (bronze statuette), and *St. John* (bronze bust). *Catalogue of the Dissolution Sale of the Artistic Property Belonging to the American Art Association* (New York, 1985), 111–13.

30. *Boston Transcript*, 5 November 1895, and the *Worcester Spy*, 8 July 1896.

31. Letters of 29 August 1895 and 25 September 1895. Worthington Chauncey Ford, ed., *Letters of Henry Adams (1892–1918)* (Boston: Houghton Mifflin Co., 1938), 78, 87. The concrete result of the Adams-Rodin meeting was the purchase of five Rodins by Henry Lee Higgenson in 1902: *Ceres, Brother and Sister, Vulcan Creating Pandora, Flight of Love,* and *Death of Alcestis.*

32. This work remains to the present day in the Pennsylvania Academy of Fine Arts as a study work and not part of the regular collection.

33. *The New York Times*, 9 May 1903.

34. Sidney Allan, "A Visit to Steichen's Studio," *Camera Work* (January 1903): 28.

35. Charles H. Caffin, "Eduard J. Steichen's Work—An Appreciation," *Camera Work* (January 1903): 23.

36. The Rodin show took longer to assemble than anticipated. While Steichen was in Paris, Stieglitz hung drawings and watercolors by Pamela Coleman Smith, making this the first nonphotographic show at 291. William Innes Homer, *Alfred Stieglitz and the American Avant-Garde* (Boston: New York Graphic Society, 1977), 57–58.

37. Marius de Zayas, "How, When, and Why Modern Art Came to New York," Introduction and Notes by Francis M. Naumann, *Arts Magazine* (April 1980): 98.

38. Charles de Kay, "Memoranda of a Sculptor," *New York Evening Post*, 9 January 1908, p. 5.

39. Agnes E. (Ernst) Meyer, *Out of These Roots* (Boston: Little, Brown and Co., 1953), 84.

40. Among the photographs in the Simpson archival materials sold at Sotheby's 10 December 1982 (present whereabouts unknown) was one of Rodin's *Victor Hugo* by Steichen. Both Steichen and Rodin signed it with the date 1901. I interpret this as a document of the Simpsons, Steichen, and Rodin being together in 1901.

41. 3 April 1903, Musée Rodin.

42. *The Craftsman* (March 1904).

43. *The New York Times*, 4 October 1908.

44. Letter of January 1910, Musée Rodin.

45. Two of the marbles were the *Cupid and Psyche* and the *Orpheus and Eurydice*, which he had bought at the Yerkes sale on 10 January 1910. The third was *Pygmalion and Galatea*. See Clare Vincent, "Rodin at the Metropolitan Museum of Art," *The Metropolitan Museum of Art Bulletin* (Spring 1981), for a full description of the donation.

46. Mrs. Daniel Chester French, *Memoirs of a Sculptor's Wife* (Boston: Houghton Mifflin Co., 1928), 203.

47. *The New York Times*, 16 September 1912.

48. 16 October 1912, Musée Rodin.

7

NINETEENTH-CENTURY VISITORS to the FRANS HALS MUSEUM

PETRA TEN-DOESSCHATE CHU

THOUGH MUCH HAS BEEN WRITTEN about the nineteenth-century revival of Frans Hals and countless references have been made to the impact of his art on contemporary painting,[1] little has been done to link these phenomena with the establishment of the Frans Hals Museum in Haarlem, Holland.[2] Yet, the opening of this museum in July 1862 made accessible to the general public Hals's most ambitious and brilliant works, the civic guard and governors' portraits. These life-size group portraits of Haarlem burghers not only represented a unique and specifically Dutch type of painting,[3] which thus far had been associated primarily with Rembrandt and van der Helst, but also contained more portraits by the master than could be seen in the combined public collections in Europe at the time. Grouped together in the five civic-guard banquets and three governors' assemblies was a total of eighty-four figures. This was a staggering number considering that in 1862 the Louvre, then probably the most important museum in Western Europe, did not possess a single authentic Hals,[4] while the Rijksmuseum in the Trippenhuis in Amsterdam and the Mauritshuis in The Hague, the two major Dutch museums of the time, together owned a total of two portraits by the artist.[5]

In addition to increasing the number of works by Hals on public view, the opening of the Frans Hals Museum accomplished an important reversal of public opinion about the artist. Until then Hals had been commonly regarded as an irresponsible drunkard and dissipated bohemian, the counterpart of the jolly topers he so convincingly portrayed. This negative reputation, originated by the Dutch biographer Arnold Houbraken in the eighteenth century, had already begun to be challenged in the early nineteenth century by Dutch historians such as R. van Eynden and A. van der Willigen, as well as J. Immerzeel. These writers tried to prove that Hals, an officer in the Guild of St. Luke and a member of a civic guard company, must have been a respected citizen in Haarlem. They based their arguments both on archival documents and on the group portraits (then accessible by special request), which they felt could not have been painted by a drunkard. Notwithstanding their publications, Hals's negative reputation persisted, and it was not until the seventies and eighties, when the general public had become well-acquainted with the artist's group portraits in Haarlem (through visits to the museum, copies, or reproductive prints), that his name was gradually cleared.[6]

From the time of its establishment, the Frans Hals Museum became a magnet for artists, critics, and collectors who took advantage of the unique opportunity it offered to study the master's major works in his hometown. Their visits are well-documented in the visitors' registers of the museum, which have been preserved in their entirety[7] and list month by month and sometimes even day by day the names of those who came to the museum. It is the intent of this paper to reexamine the Hals revival in the light of these important documents, which provide information that may clarify both general and specific aspects of the artist's impact during the nineteenth century.

The presence of names of artists, critics, and collectors in the visitors' registers of the Frans Hals Museum is relatively scant during the sixties but rapidly increases during the next decade and culminates in the 1880s, after which it declines again. This trend is somewhat different from the general pattern of the nineteenth-century Dutch revival, which in many countries was well-established in the 1830s, culminated in the 1850s and 1860s, and waned in the 1870s.[8] In addition, the commonly held notion that the Dutch revival was associated primarily with the realist and proto-impressionist trends is contradicted by the registers, in which the signatures of François Bonvin, Henri Fantin-Latour, Louis Dubois, Edouard Manet, and Claude Monet are found side-by-side with those of academic painters such as Fernand Cormon, Paul Dubois, Jean-Léon Gérôme, Auguste Glaize, and Jules Lefebvre. However, the names that by far predominate are those of the naturalist painters—artists like Jules Breton, Jean-Charles Cazin, Pascal-Adolphe-Jean Dagnan-Bouveret, Virginie Demont-Breton, Léon Lhermitte, and Alfred Roll from France; Wilhelm Busch, Franz von Lenbach, and Max Liebermann from Germany; Mihály Munkácsy and Ilia Repin from eastern Europe; and William Merritt Chase, J. Alden Weir, and John Twachtman from the United States.

It would seem, then, from the registers that the revived interest in Hals not only outlasted the interest in other Dutch painters (with the possible exception of Rembrandt and Vermeer), but also that it was unique in touching avant-garde, conservative, and particularly *juste-milieu* groups of painters. The explanation for this phenomenon would seem to lie in the two different components of Hals's art that could appeal to nineteenth-century viewers: his subject matter and his technique. During the 1860s, the works of Hals were admired primarily for their typically bourgeois subject matter and their hearty, vigorous mood. The civic guard and governors' portraits were seen as heroic monuments to the middle class. During the 1870s and 1880s however, Hals's group portraits were admired less as celebrations of bourgeois life than for their masterful use of color and their dynamic, *alla-prima* facture. Hals's loose brushwork and verve made him a painter's painter whose craft appealed to artists of a wide range of artistic convictions.

A study of the reactions of the major critics who visited the Frans Hals Museum from 1862 to 1900 (for a full listing, see Appendix 1) clearly bears out the gradual change that Hals's reputation underwent during this period. Among the early visitors, the first who must be mentioned is the French critic and art historian Théophile Thoré, who contributed greatly to the reestablishment of Hals's reputation.[9] Thoré's alias signature, "W. Bürger," is found as early as 1863 (fig. 7.1) and again in 1866. Though his enthusiasm for Hals had been aroused initially at the epoch-making exhibition of old masters held in Manchester, England in 1857,[10] Thoré-Bürger's major and pioneering article on Hals, published in two installments in the *Gazette des Beaux-Arts* in 1868,[11] was not, indeed, could not have been written until after his visits to Haarlem. Thoré-Bürger was the prime representative of the first generation of Hals admirers who valued the master for his subject matter. He saw in Hals's work, and especially in the

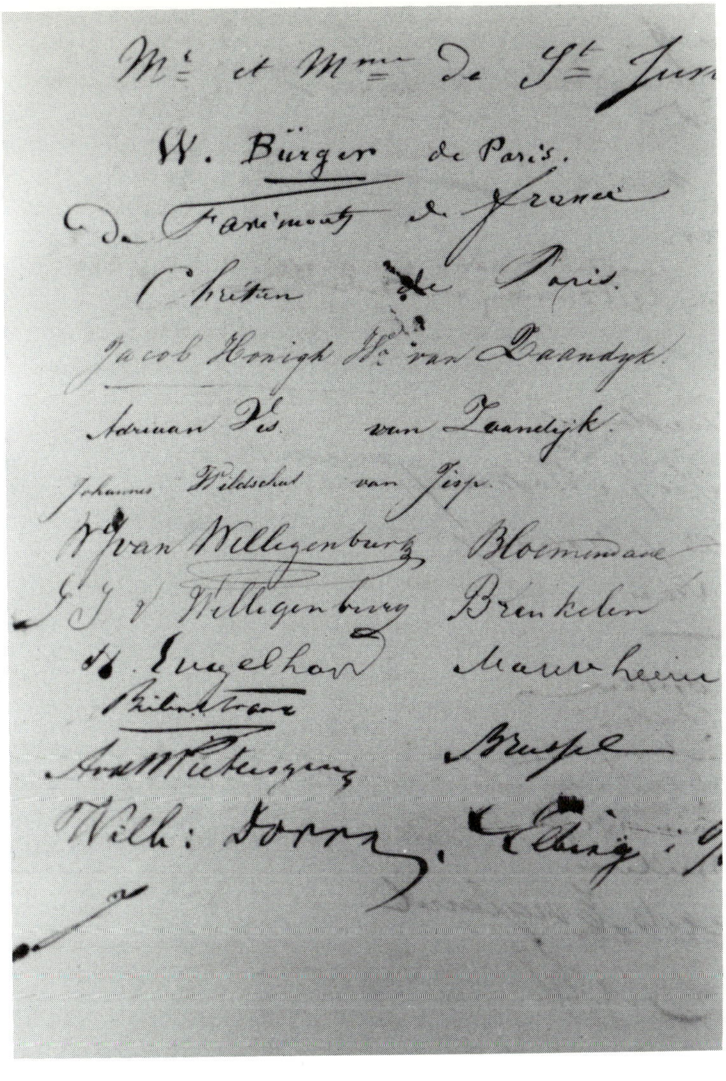

Fig. 7.1. Signature of W. Bürger (Théophile Thoré) in the visitors' registers of the Frans Hals Museum. Haarlem, Municipal Archives.

civic guard and governors' portraits, a clear affirmation of the bourgeois republican culture of seventeenth-century Holland that had initially attracted him to Dutch art. Writing in 1868, Thoré asked the rhetorical question, "Why should not those assemblies of Dutch citizen-soldiers be 'great art,' " and held them up as models to contemporary artists, encouraging them to paint similar gatherings of people of their own time: "an assembly of diplomats seated around a table . . . a professor surrounded by young people, a scene from the horse races, spectators leaving the Opéra, or a promenade on the Champs-Elysées."[12]

Signatures of other authors who contributed to the initial reevaluation of Hals also appear in the registers. As early as 1862 and again in 1864, 1873, and 1882, we find the name of Carel Vosmaer, the Dutch author-critic who wrote the introductory text to a folio volume of etchings by the German W. Unger after Hals's paintings, published in Leiden in 1873–74.[13] Conspicuously absent from the registers, however, is the name of Wilhelm von Bode, who defended his doctoral dissertation "Frans Hals und seine Schule" in 1870,[14] and, with M. J. Binder, published the first authorative oeuvre-catalogue of Hals's work in 1914.[15] From Bode's autobiography, *Mein Leben,*[16] we know that he visited the Frans Hals Museum in 1868 and possibly again during later trips to Holland in 1872 and the early 1880s. This should alert us that not all visitors signed the registers at all times, so that in no way they can be considered as a sine qua non for anyone's presence in the museum.

The French critic Zacharie Astruc, one of the first writers to emphasize the relationship between Hals and contemporary realist painting, signed the registers in 1875 and again in 1890.[17] To be sure, Astruc's visit to Haarlem, like Thoré's, can have done little more than heighten a long-entertained admiration for Hals's work. Had he not written, as early as 1866: "The reputation of this master will be due to a large extent to the modern school, which esteems him singularly and celebrates him as an inspirer. The truth is that he represents an approach that is healthy and invigorating, that he does not belie his vision, and that it is the moment par excellence to follow his sincere ways, if one wishes to strengthen and expand the domain of French art."[18]

Astruc's first visit to Haarlem almost exactly coincided with that of the painter-critic Eugène Fromentin, who in his well-known *Les Maîtres d'autrefois* likewise noted the connection between Hals and contemporary painting.[19] Whereas Astruc considered this relationship healthy and beneficial, however, Fromentin saw it in a less positive light.[20] Fromentin believed that the avant-garde of his time (Manet and the emerging Impressionists) took their cues not from the healthy and vigorous works of Hals's middle period but rather from the paintings of his old age,[21] notably *The Regents of the Old Men's Alms House* and *The Regentesses of the Old Men's Alms House*. To Fromentin, these were the works of a senile artist, a painter who was "three quarters dead," and he reproached his "young comrades" for consulting the work of an artist who was "no longer anything but a shadow of himself."[22]

Fromentin's attitude to Hals was, in general, ambiguous. He devoted an entire chapter of *Les Maîtres d'autrefois* to the Frans Hals Museum, which he singled out for the marvelous opportunity it presented "to embrace at a glance fifty years of the artist's labor, to be present at his researches, behold him in his successes, and judge him from his most important and best works."[23] In Fromentin's view, a visit to the Haarlem museum was crucial for the appreciation of the true artistic merit of Frans Hals. "Everywhere else," he wrote, "the idea that one forms of this brilliant master . . . is seductive, agreeable, clever, rather frivolous; but it is neither true nor equitable."[24] Yet in Haarlem, Fromentin found that Hals was "certainly one of the most clever and expert masters who has ever existed anywhere, even in Flanders in spite of Rubens and van Dyck, even in Spain in spite of Velásquez."[25] Although he exulted in Hals's workmanship, Fromentin regretted the lack of psychological and philosophical content in his work: "There is not much to divine behind the fine exterior execution of the Haarlem painter."[26] In this respect Fromentin sharply contrasted Hals with Rembrandt, behind whose exterior execution he found "a thousand things to discover."[27] In thus preferring Rembrandt over Hals, Fromentin gave evidence of his romantic roots. As Meyer Schapiro wrote in his perceptive introduction to the English edition of *Les Maîtres d'autrefois,* Fromentin was "a belated child of Romanticism who could no longer be content with an imagined world and yet could not accept the familiar reality as a matter for art."[28]

Fromentin's opinion of Hals as a "workman" rather than a "thinker" or a "mysterious painter"[29] was echoed in inflated form in the writings of the symbolist critic Joséphin Péladan, who visited Haarlem on 14 November 1892, when he signed the register as "Sâr Péladan, Grand Maître de la Rose + Croix."[30] Few modern bibliographies list his monograph on Hals,[31] which appeared in 1912 and consists largely of lengthy tirades against the ugly and ridiculous aspects of Hals's sitters. Yet, despite his negative attitude, Péladan had to admit that he felt strangely fascinated by the Haarlem group portraits, which he found at once repulsive and imposing: "I have never seen so many men [together] who were so mediocre, so boring, so nonexistent as these civic guard officers.... And nonetheless, they assert themselves, in spite of the boredom they embody, in spite of the irritation they produce by their complacent contentment."[32] This fascination was compelled by Hals's power of observation and above all his dynamic touch and "verve," which could lend spirited accent to the heaviest bourgeois.[33] To the symbolist Péladan, Hals represented both a "miracle and an abuse of artistic power."[34]

If we trace the *Rezeptionsgeschichte* of Hals from the middle of the nineteenth century to the fin de siècle, or from the realist through the symbolist period, the path it took can be clearly distinguished. The Hals of the sixties, his tarnished reputation only recently restored, was admired as the prototypical bourgeois painter and portrayer par excellence of middle-class life in republican Holland. The Hals of the seventies and eighties was the virtuoso technician whose talents matched or, in the eyes of some, even surpassed those of Velázquez, Rubens, or van Dyck. Finally, the Hals of the turn of the century was a painter of banal physicality whose only saving grace was his brilliant technique, or, to put it in the words of Odilon Redon, "The man who most masterfully has rendered animal life to the culminating point."[35]

Though the art critics and historians who visited the Frans Hals Museum in the nineteenth century were numerous, they were far outnumbered by artists, who flocked to the museum in the seventies and eighties as if heeding Fromentin's remark that "at Haarlem ... a painter in search of a fine strong lesson ought to give himself the pleasure of seeing Frans Hals."[36] Among the many hundreds of artists whose names are found in the visitors registers (for a complete listing, see Appendix 2), a few important painters will be singled out here and the specific impact of their visits on their work will be gauged. This, in turn, will lead to some general conclusions about the importance of Hals for the art of the second half of the nineteenth century.

One of the first artists to visit the museum from Belgium and France, Holland's southern neighbors, was the Belgian artist Louis Dubois, whose signature is found under 1866 and again under 1868. Dubois may have visited the museum on other, possibly earlier, occasions, because he is known to have made a number of full-scale copies after Hals's work. Of these, his copies after *The Regents of the Old Men's Alms House* and *The Regentesses of the Old Men's Alms House* (present whereabouts unknown) appear to have been best-known in the nineteenth century. According to a contemporary Flemish critic, they were so close to the originals that the members of the town council of Haarlem expressed the opinion that no one would notice were they to replace the genuine Hals paintings in their frames.[37] It is not known whether these copies or a copy of an earlier group-portrait by Hals inspired Fantin-Latour's *Homage to Eugène Delacroix* (fig. 7.2), exhibited at the Salon of 1864. Fantin's biographers maintain that this painting was originally planned as an allegorical composition but was

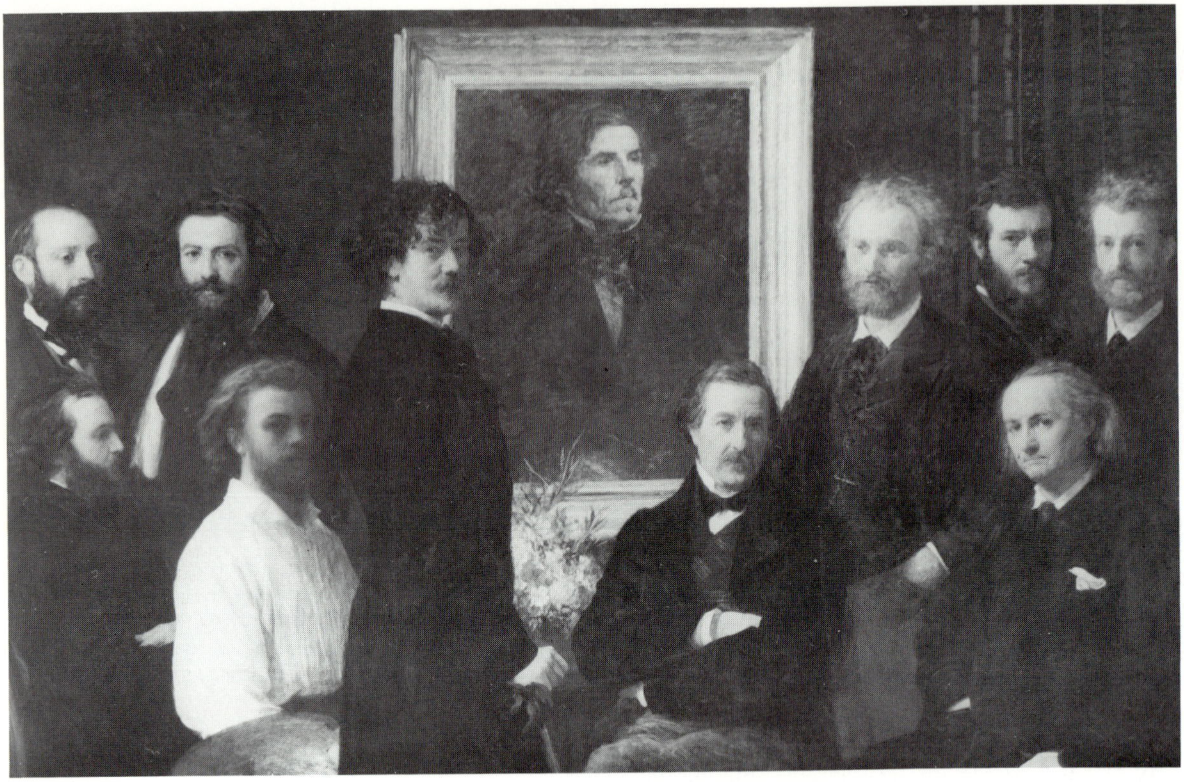

Fig. 7.2. Henri Fantin-Latour. *Homage to Eugène Delacroix*, 1864. Paris, Musée d'Orsay, Galerie du Jeu de Paume.

transformed into a characteristically realist group portrait once Fantin saw Dubois's copy after Hals.[38] The *Homage to Eugène Delacroix*, which predates Thoré's incitement to artists to paint groups of modern men in modern surroundings, clearly illustrates Hals's specific significance for the realists of the 1860s.

Fantin himself was not to visit the Frans Hals Museum until eleven years after he painted the *Homage to Eugène Delacroix* in 1875. By then, several French artists, mostly belonging to the realist school, had already preceded him. Although Gustave Courbet's only visit to Holland predated the opening of the Frans Hals Museum,[39] a number of his friends, including François Bonvin, Johan Barthold Jongkind, and Léopold Flameng, visited the museum in the course of the 1860s.

However, it was during and immediately after the Franco-Prussian War that the Dutch museums became favorite destinations for French artists, many of whom had taken refuge outside France. Antoine Vollon, for example, who had left Paris for St. Gilles, a suburb of Brussels, traveled to Holland in 1871 and visited the Frans Hals Museum in July of that year. He was to return to Haarlem in October of the following year, this time as a recipient of a grant from the new provisionary government of Versailles, which had commissioned him to copy *The Officers in the Company of St. George* for the Musée des Copies of Charles Blanc.[40] Another artist who went to Holland because of the Franco-Prussian War was Claude Monet, who had taken refuge in the small town

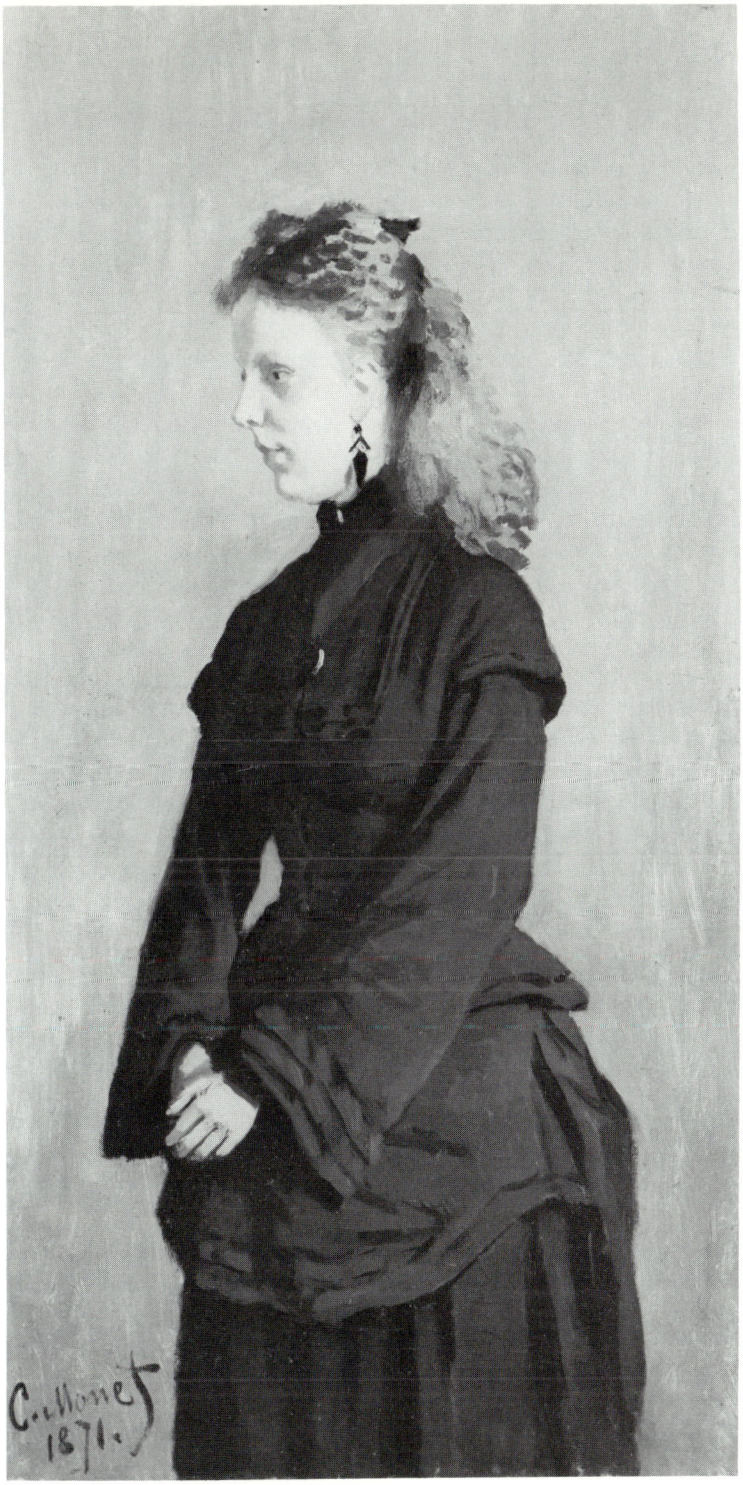

Fig. 7.3. Claude Monet, *Portrait of Guurtje van der Stadt,* 1871. Otterlo, Netherlands, Kröller-Müller Museum. (Photo: E. M. J. Heuker of Hoek)

of Zaandam, not far from Haarlem. His signature is found in the register under October 1871. A reflection of Monet's visit to the Frans Hals Museum may be found in his *Portrait of Guurtje van der Stadt* (fig. 7.3), which shows sober coloring and loose brushwork similar to that in Hals's later works (the matron in *The Regentesses of the Old Men's Alms House* comes to mind).

Monet's trip to Haarlem was closely followed by that of Edouard Manet, who visited the museum in June 1872 in the company of his brother-in-law, the Dutch-born sculptor Ferdinand Leenhoff. According to Antonin Proust, the boldness of Frans Hals made a deep impression on him.[41] The so-called *Le Bon Bock* of 1872 (fig. 7.4) is generally cited as the visible result of Manet's trip to Holland; in fact, when the work was exhibited at the Salon of 1873 it was immediately recognized as an attempt to paraphrase Hals. Indeed, when the critic Albert Wolff riled Manet for having put "water into his beer," referring to the old-master qualities of the picture, the painter Alfred Stevens retorted that it was "pure Haarlem beer."[42] Though the painting was a critical and public success, many of Manet's close friends considered it a step backward from his more experimental works of previous years; for example, *The Repose* of 1870, exhibited at the Salon of the same year, was felt to have a "spirit of modernity"[43] that *Le Bon Bock* lacked. That Manet, on the other hand, thought the example of Hals and modernity were not mutually exclusive, is revealed by his painting *The Railroad* (fig. 7.5). Exhibited at the Salon of 1874 but begun in the fall of 1872, immediately after Manet's return from Holland, this paradigm of modern painting in fact contains several elements that may well be derived from Hals. The way in which Victorine Meurend glances out of the picture, as if her attention has been momentarily attracted by the viewer, is very similar to a cliché pose used by Hals. The attitude of the head and also the gesture of the finger holding the page in the book in the Manet are found in Hals's Haarlem group portraits and single portraits in other collections as well. Moreover, though the background imparts a distinctly modern flavor to the picture, the figures are painted in a color scheme and technique that owe much to the Haarlem master. Other paintings of the early seventies by Manet may be related to Hals as well: the *Portrait of Berthe Morisot with a Bunch of Violets* (private collection) for example, and especially the *Portrait of Berthe Morisot with Hat, in Mourning* (private collection) recall Hals's late works both in the daubing brushwork and the predominantly black palette.

Fantin and Manet, the two leading artists in France to significantly feel the impact of Hals, respectively provided the realist and naturalist responses to Hals's challenge. Fantin was inspired foremost by Hals's subject matter, gatherings of contemporaries in contemporary dress and setting, while Manet drew upon the master's poses, palette, and technique.

When we move from a consideration of visitors from the French-speaking countries south of Holland to look at those from its German-speaking neighbors to the east, we are struck immediately by the predominance of artists from the Düsseldorf school in the register. Geography may have had much to do with this. Düsseldorf of all the major German art centers in the nineteenth century was closest to Holland. However, the German artists who were most impressed by their visits to the Frans Hals Museum came from other parts of Germany rather than from Düsseldorf. Wilhelm Busch, for example, who visited the museum in the fall of 1873, came from Wiedensahl near Hannover, though he had studied in Düsseldorf as well as in Antwerp, where his interest

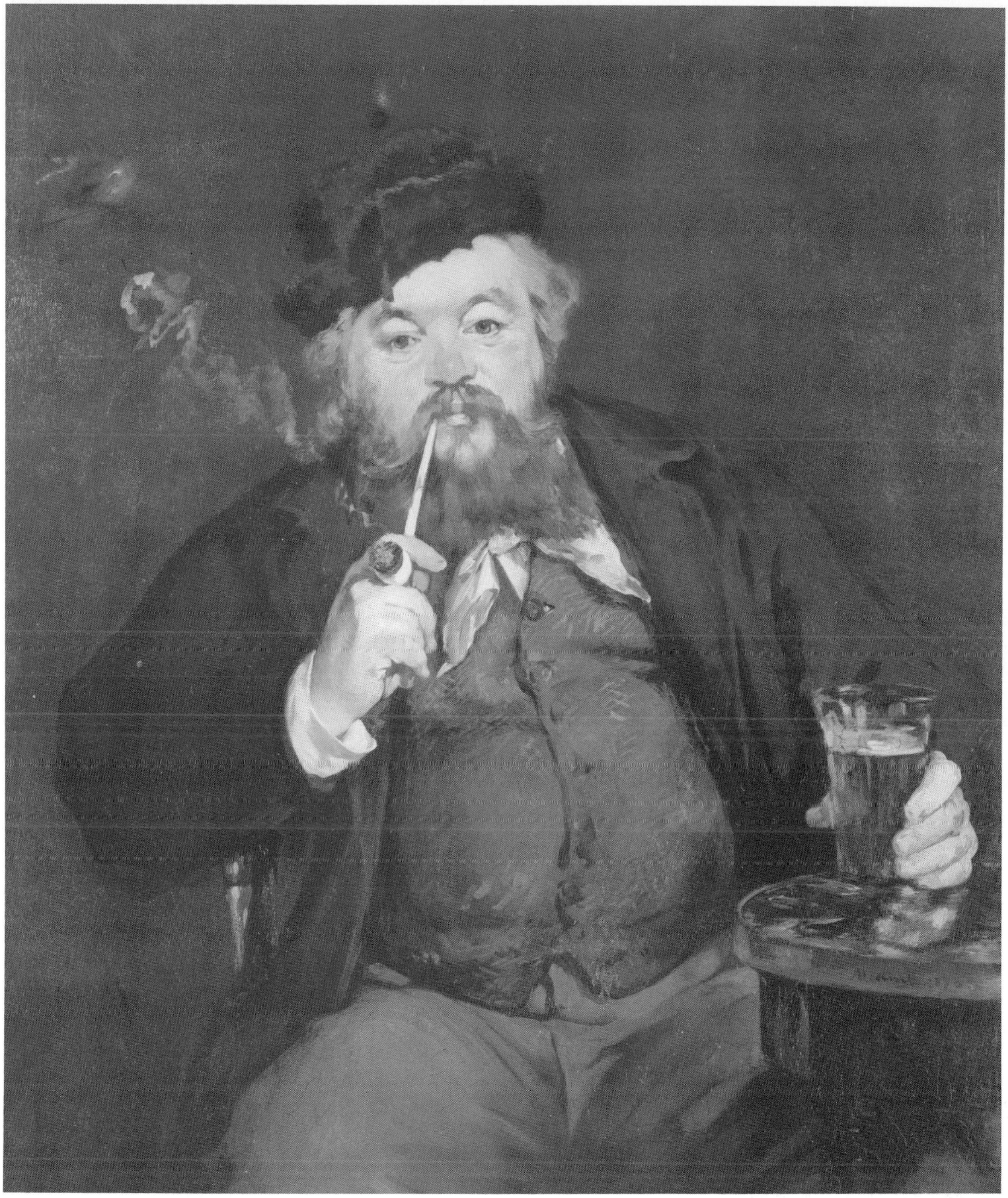

Fig. 7.4. Edouard Manet, *Le Bon Bock*, 1873. Philadelphia Museum of Art. Mr. and Mrs. Carroll S. Tyson, Jr. Collection.

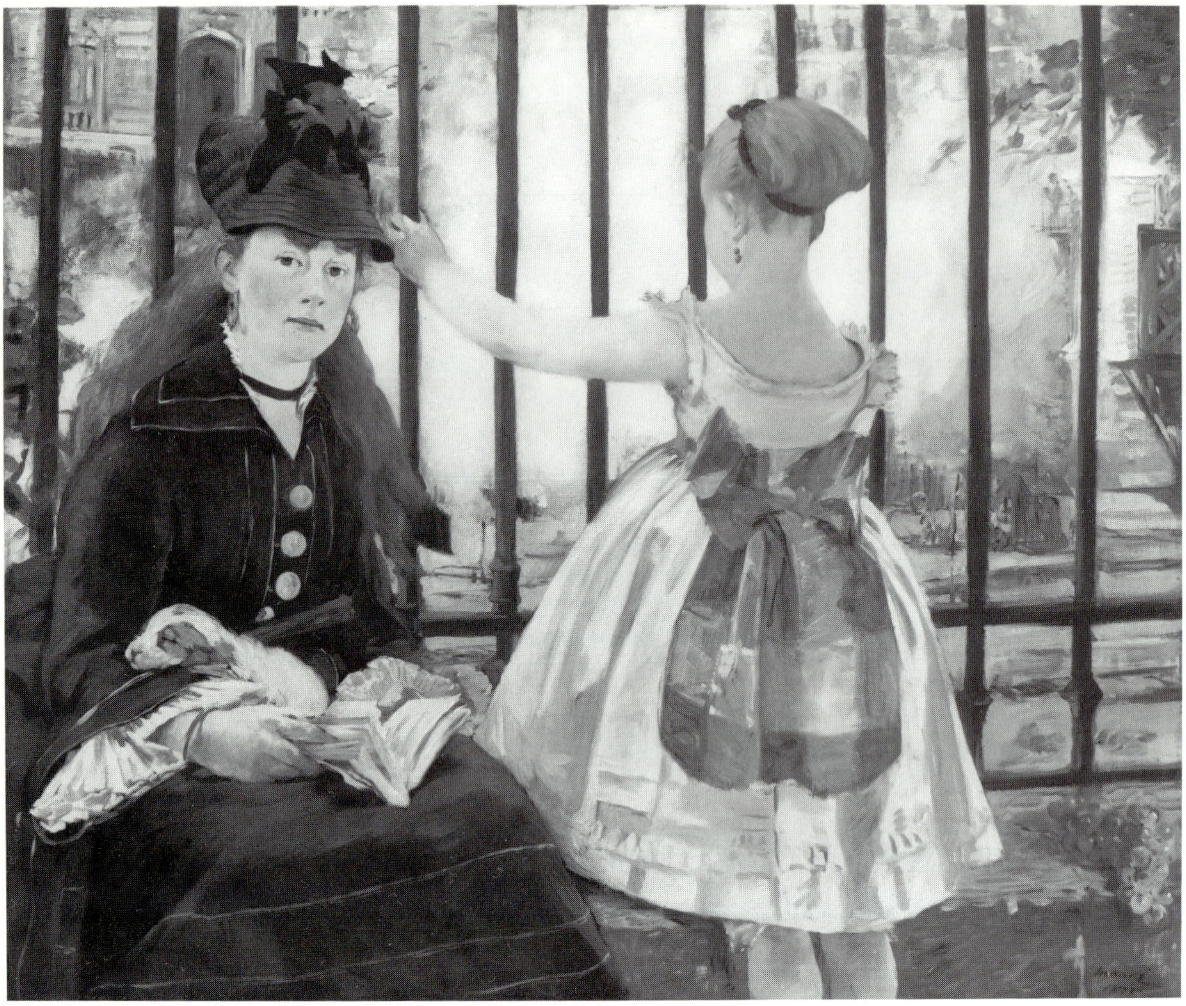

Fig. 7.5. Edouard Manet, *Gare Saint-Lazare,* 1873. Washington, National Gallery of Art. Gift of Horace Havemeyer in memory of his mother, Louisine W. Havemeyer, 1956.

in Dutch and Flemish painting may have been aroused. Known primarily as a satirical writer and illustrator of such German classics as *Max und Moritz* and *Die fromme Helene,* Busch was also a prolific painter, particularly of portraits and figure compositions.[44] That Busch's trip to Haarlem greatly impressed him is evidenced by a number of letters in which he reported his visit. In one of these, he wrote that his heart almost stopped beating when he saw Hals's large group portraits in Haarlem, which he found to be "forceful, unceremonious, and true."[45] In another letter he noted the "indestructible heartiness" of Hals, whom he referred to elsewhere as his "chosen favorite."[46] Hals's influence may be seen in a number of Busch's portraits and head studies of the early seventies, such as *Man in Seventeenth-Century Costume: Otto Busch* (Hannover, Wilhelm Busch Museum) and *The Merry Carouser* dated 1873 (fig. 7.6).

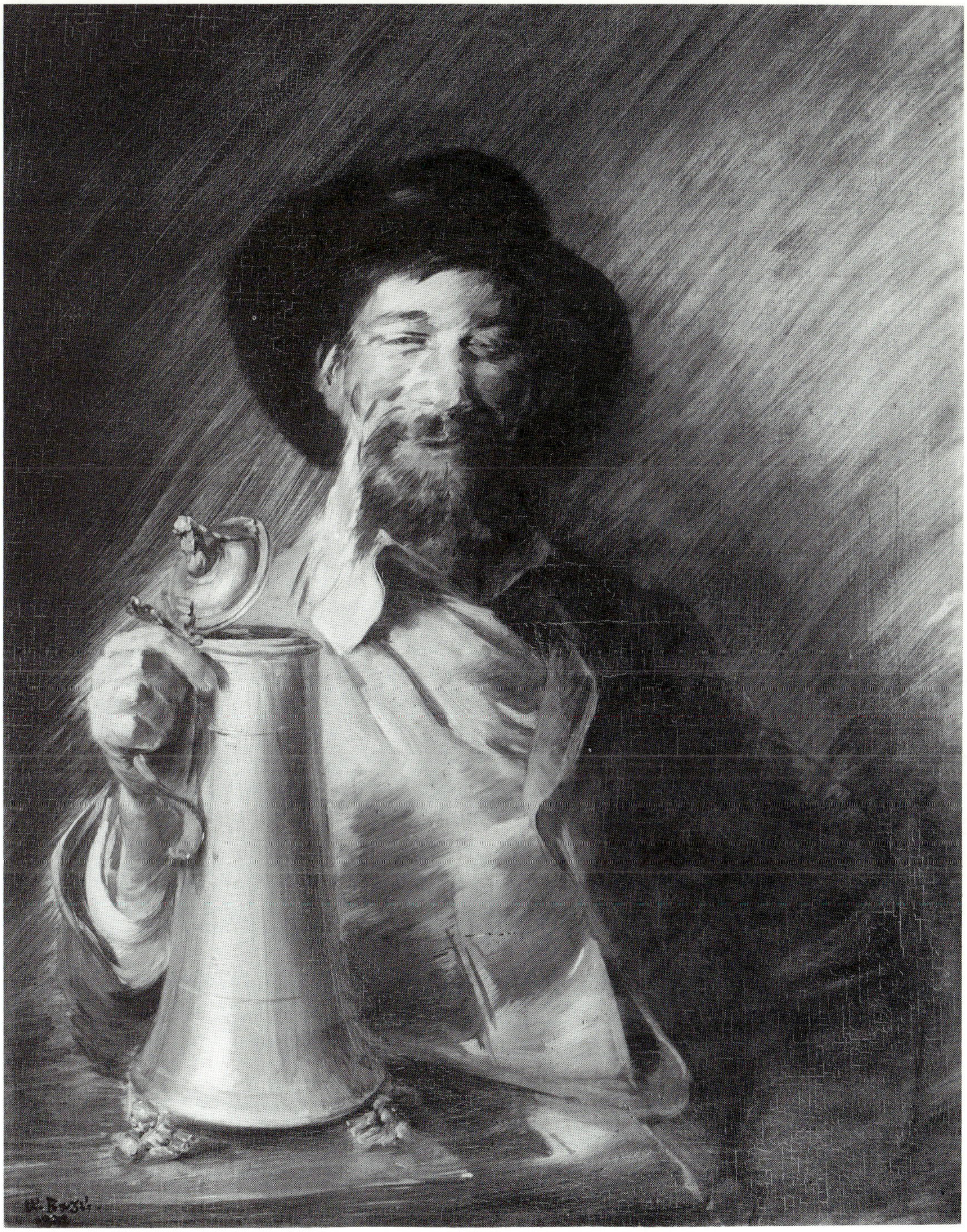

Fig. 7.6. Wilhelm Busch, *The Merry Carouser,* 1873.
Frankfurt, Städelsches Kunstinstitut.

Busch's close friend, the Munich painter Franz von Lenbach, is known to have traveled to Holland three times—in 1873, 1888, 1898[47]—but he signed the registers only on his first two visits. Lenbach, particularly during the later part of his life, was much taken by northern baroque painting and is reported to have been "as if intoxicated with Rembrandt, Rubens, and Frans Hals."[48] Though it is difficult to pinpoint specific examples of Hals's influence in Lenbach's work, the artist did much to popularize the Dutch master in Munich. An active member and one-time president of the artists' association Allotria, Lenbach played an important role in organizing Allotria's celebrated costume parties, which featured outfits derived from famous paintings by the masters of the past. One of the best-remembered of these was the Niederländerfest of 1881, at which Dutch group portraits were enacted in "living pictures," and at which Lenbach himself "wore a large millstone collar à la Franz Hals and a costume in style with it."[49]

More serious than Lenbach's involvement with Hals was that of the Berlin painter Max Liebermann. Liebermann, who made his first trip to Holland in 1872, returned there countless times throughout the course of his career. Though it is customary to stress Liebermann's interest in contemporary subject matter and scenery rather than museums in Holland, his admiration for Dutch seventeenth-century painting, notably that of Hals, should not be overlooked. During his first lengthy stay in Holland in 1879, Liebermann spent a good deal of time in Haarlem making copies after Hals's work, just as he had copied Hals's *La Bohémienne* earlier in Paris.[50] Max Friedländer, in his monograph on the artist, has analyzed the significance of Hals for Liebermann's work. "In Hals he found a temperament akin to his own. And this master became an example for him, gave him a yardstick like no other painter old or new."[51] At the same time, Friedländer warned against looking for specific Halsian elements in the artist's work. "Liebermann's originality has not been harmed by the intimate contact with this example; on the contrary, it brought him closer to nature and to himself. In his choice of themes and his mode of composing, he was not at all faithful to the great portraitist."[52] Today we might be more readily inclined to directly relate certain works by Liebermann, notably those of the seventies, to Hals. His multifigure paintings of women plucking geese or canning goods and of girls' schools and old-age homes are related to Hals in the way they stress both the uniformity and individuality in groups. Some of Liebermann's portraits are even closer to Hals's work; the *Portrait of Dr. Sachs* of 1878 (private collection) and the later group portrait of an *Assembly of Hamburg Professors* (fig. 7.7) are unthinkable without the master's example.

Liebermann's enthusiasm for Hals was shared by his good friend Miháli Munkácsy, whom he had first met in Dresden in 1872 and with whom he became closer while living in Paris from 1872 to 1878. Munkácsy visited the Frans Hals Museum in September 1872 (the same year as Liebermann) and again in 1888. Like Liebermann, he started his career by painting a number of large multifigure genre scenes, which are loosely related to Hals,[53] as are some of his early portraits, such as the *Portrait of the Pianist Grünfeld* of 1873 (private collection). Munkácsy was by no means the only eastern European artist to visit the Frans Hals Museum. Several Russian artists came to Haarlem, including the painter Ilya Repin. The latter was accompanied by Vladimir Vassiljevitch Stassov, an art critic and important spokesman for the Russian realist movement. Both Repin, in his autobiography, and Stassov, in his diary, make mention of this visit, which much impressed them, as Hals's group portraits apparently were

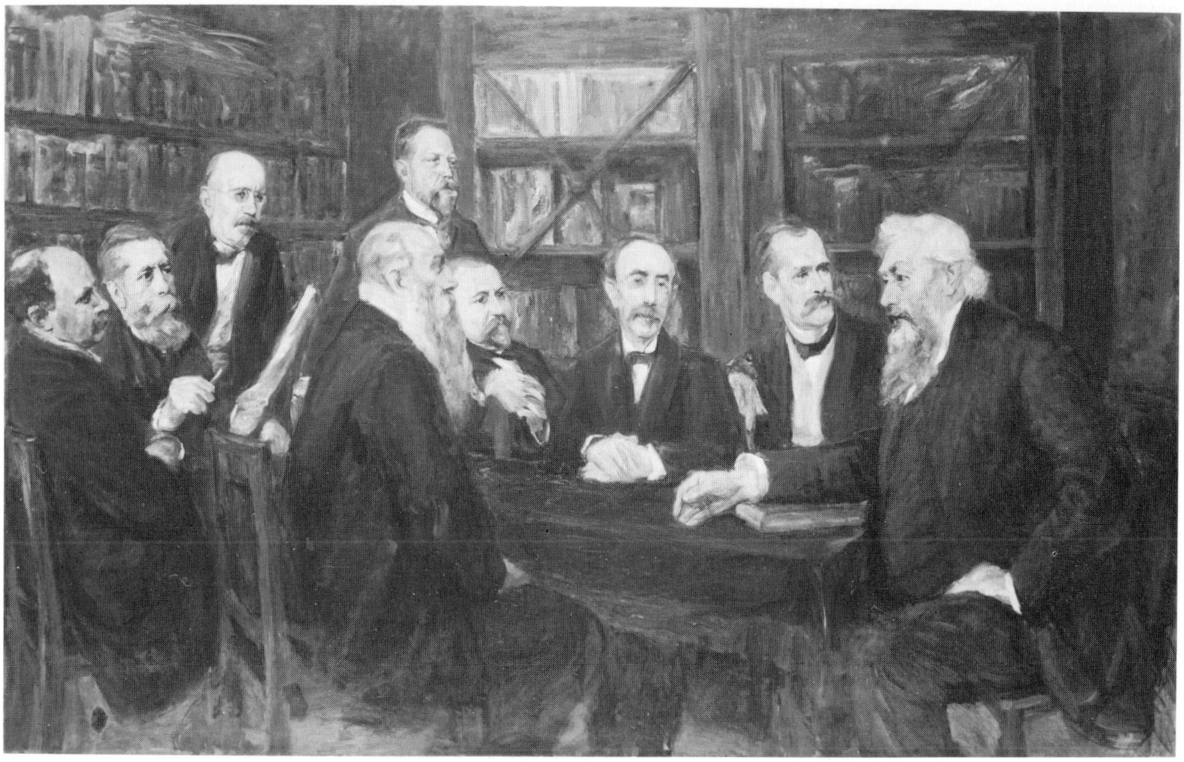

Fig. 7.7. Max Liebermann, *Assembly of Hamburg Professors,* 1906. Hamburg, Kunsthalle.

unknown in Russia (unlike those by Rembrandt, of which copies and reproductions were available). In his memoirs Repin calls the Frans Hals Museum "paradise," and Stassov's diary informs us that of all the Dutch and Flemish artists, Repin was most impressed with Hals.[54]

The admiration for Hals in American artistic circles was nurtured on both French and German soil. The American artists who came to the Frans Hals Museum were almost invariably those who studied in Paris, Munich, or Düsseldorf, where their interest in Hals was, if not initially aroused, certainly reinforced. Among the first American artists to visit the museum was Mary Cassatt, who came to Haarlem as early as 1873, when "she went for a jaunt to Holland."[55] Her name is not found in the register,[56] but a sketch copy she made after *The Officers and Sergeants of the St. Hadrian Civic Guard Company* has been preserved (fig. 7.8).[57] The immediate impact of Cassatt's acquaintance with Hals's works in Haarlem may be seen in the *Portrait of the Artist's Mother* (fig. 7.9), painted in Antwerp in 1873; here not only the figure's pose and facial expression but also the loose brushwork recall the figure of Adriana Bredenhof in *The Regentesses of the Old Men's Alms House.*

Less than two years after Cassatt's visit, in January 1875 J. Alden Weir came to Haarlem (he did not sign the register) and copied the same group portrait (fig. 7.10). In his letters from Haarlem he called Hals the "king of portrait painting" and a

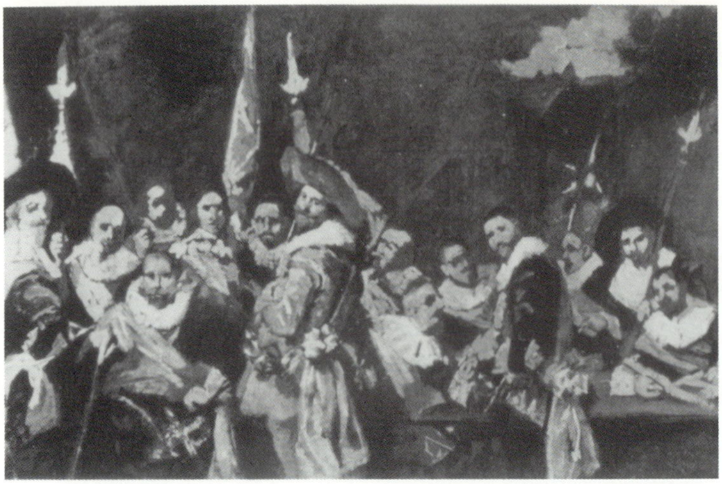

Fig. 7.8. Mary Cassatt, copy after Frans Hals, *The Officers and Sergeants of the St. Hadrian Civic Guard Company,* 1873. Private collection.

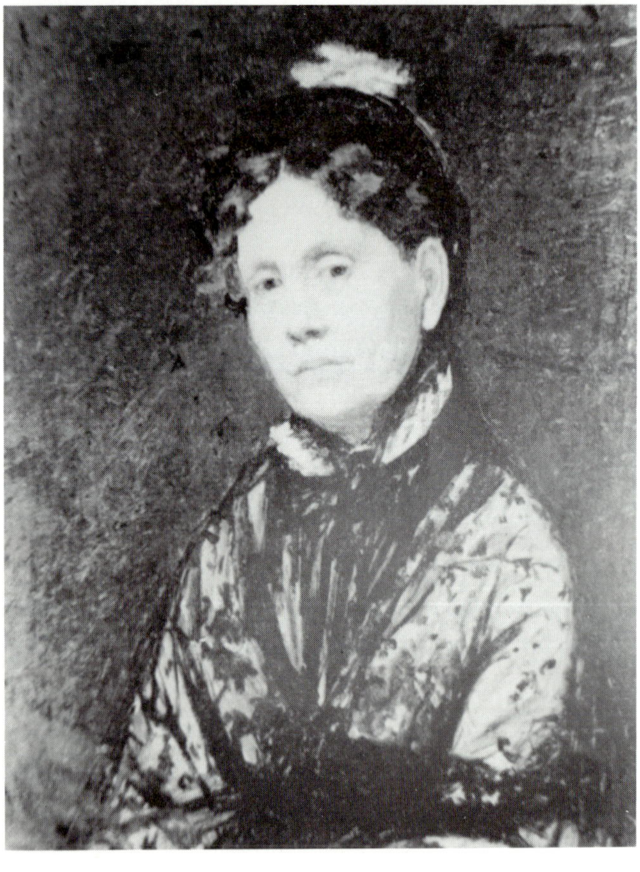

Fig. 7.9. Mary Cassatt, *Portrait of the Artist's Mother,* 1873. Private collection.

"wonderful man of genius . . . by the side of Titian, if not ahead of him, in portrait painting."[58] In her excellent Weir monograph of 1983, Doreen Bolger Burke states that the immediate result of the artist's trip was a plan, unfortunately never executed, for a group portrait of some of his fellow art students in Paris ("those of character and promise").[59] Had it been realized, the work might have resembled Fantin's Hals-inspired group portraits, such as the *Homage to Eugène Delacroix, An Atelier in the Batignolles,* or *A Table Corner.* Weir did carry out, upon his return to New York, another large multifigure painting titled *In the Park* (fig. 7.11). The painting, which was unfortunately cut up after it was exhibited, in its original form was a large canvas with six life-size figures closely grouped together in a narrow space and set against a landscape background. While compositionally akin to the left side of *The Officers and Sergeants of the St. Hadrian Civic Guard Company,* which Weir had copied, *In the Park* also calls to mind Hals's early genre scenes, and Burke points to the specific connection with *The Merrymakers at Shrovetide* in the Metropolitan Museum of Art, New York.[60]

Unlike Cassatt and Weir, William Merritt Chase became a Hals admirer in Munich. A student of A. von Piloty at the Munich Academy, Chase received a training in which the study of the old masters was strongly emphasized. His early identification with the Dutch masters, notably Hals, is evidenced by several photographs dating from his student days in which the artist is seen dressed up as a Dutch burgher. His particularly Hals-like pose in one photograph (fig. 7.12) may have been modeled after the servant in *The Banquet of the Officers of the St. George Civic Guard Company* of 1616. Chase first visited the Frans Hals Museum in 1878 and returned numerous times thereafter. He is known to have made several copies after Hals's group portraits or details thereof (see fig. 7.13).[61] Chase's admiration for Hals is reflected in some early works, such as the *Portrait of a Woman* (fig. 7.14) painted after his first trip to Haarlem, which in its strictly frontal pose of the figure and the asymmetrical placement of the hands calls to mind the portrait of Anna van Damme in *The Regentesses of the Old Men's Alms House.* However, Chase has not yet adopted Hals's loose brushwork, which manifests itself only in his work of the 1880s.

Of all the American artists who visited the Frans Hals Museum, Chase did most to spread the master's popularity in the United States. When he became a teacher at the Art Students League in New York in 1878, an anonymous reporter expressed the hope that the artist would "turn out many a Franz Hals from among the lively crowd of American disciples."[62] Chase did not disappoint the unknown writer. He encouraged his students to travel to Holland to study the master's work, and in 1903 he even took a summer class to Haarlem. This visit was so much appreciated by the town's inhabitants that Chase was presented with a medal, inscribed as follows: "Remembrance of the visit of William Chase, U.S.A. and his class to the Frans Hals Museum in Holland." In return Chase laid a wreath at the foot of the newly erected Hals monument in the presence of the mayor and the people of the town.[63]

After studying the importance of the Frans Hals Museum for foreign artists, a few words must be said about Hals's reputation at home. It is perhaps significant that, with the exception of Carel Vosmaer's introduction to the etchings by Unger after Hals, all major nineteenth-century texts on Hals were written by foreigners (Bode, Fromentin, Thoré, and Péladan). Indeed, it appears that while Hals was considered abroad to be the prototypically Dutch painter and Rembrandt "an exception" within the Dutch school of painting,[64] in Holland it was Rembrandt who was seen as the national

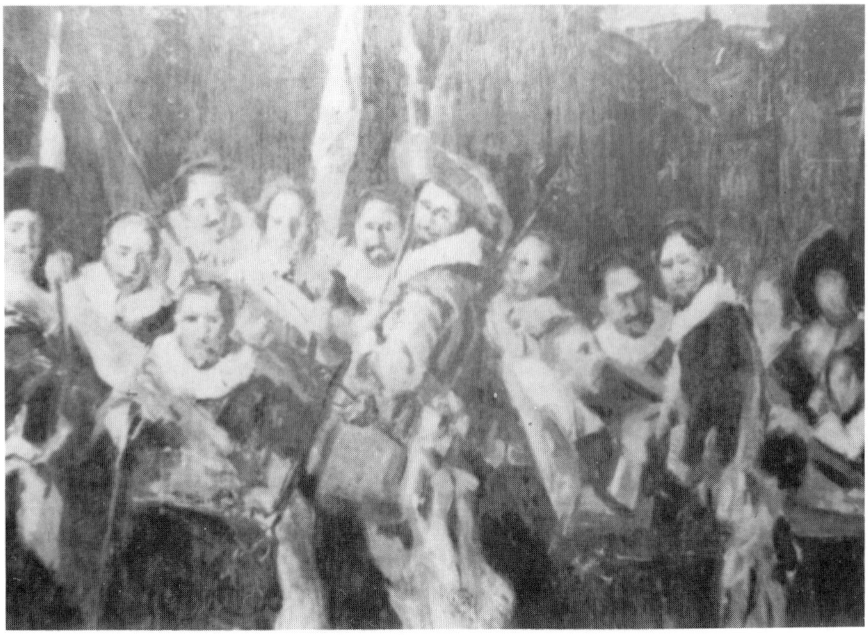

Fig. 7.10. J. Alden Weir, copy after Frans Hals, *The Officers and Sergeants of the St. Hadrian Civic Guard Company,* 1875. Private collection.

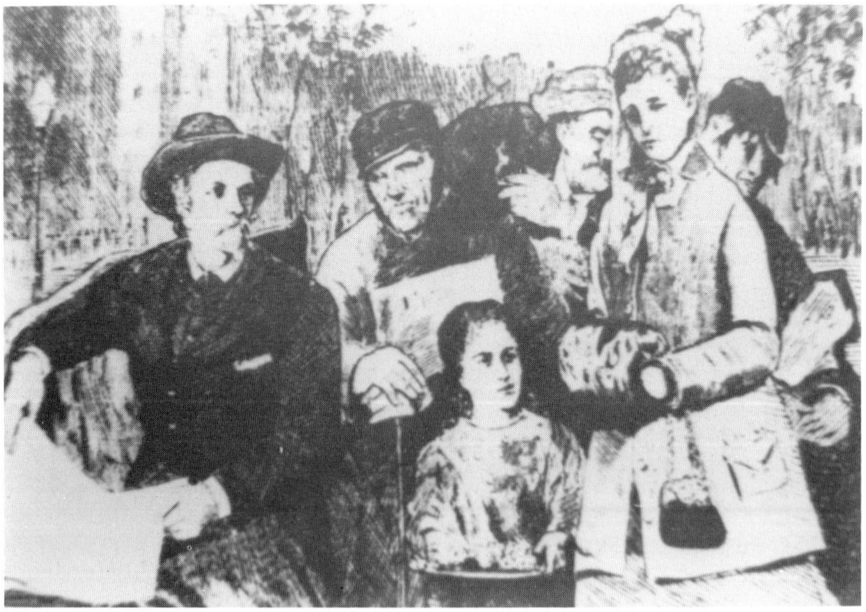

Fig. 7.11. Engraving after J. Alden Weir, *In the Park*, c. 1879. From *New York Daily Graphic*, 8 March 1879.

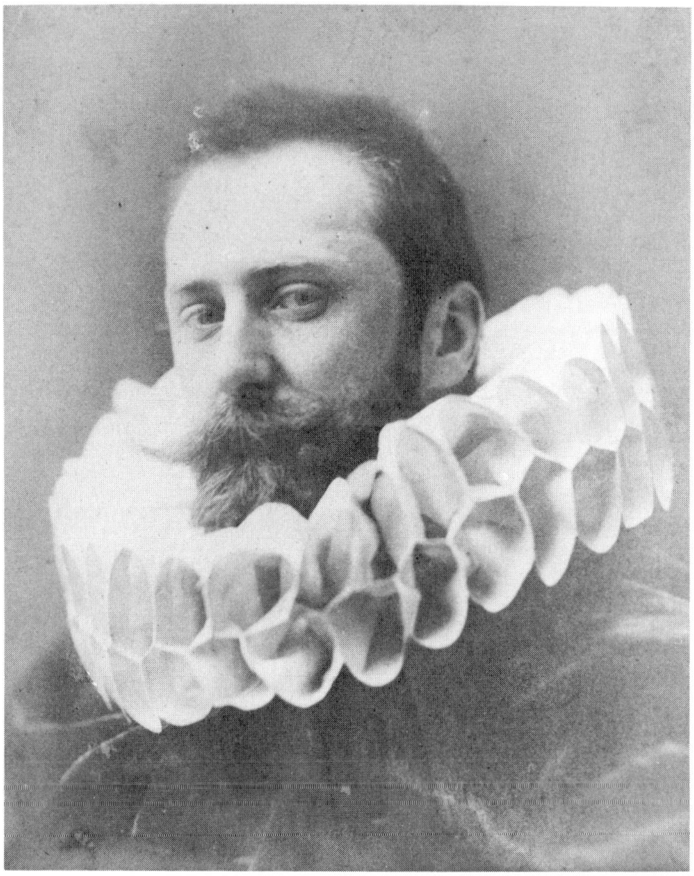

Fig. 7.12. Photograph of William Merritt Chase in seventeenth-century costume, Munich c. 1876. Southampton, New York, Parrish Art Museum, William Merritt Chase Archives.

artist. The unveiling of Rembrandt's statue (a twenty-three-foot high colossus) in 1852 was a major patriotic event, marked by grand festivities that lasted for several days.[65] No such honors were reserved for Hals, whose much smaller monument in Haarlem was not erected until 1900.[66] Though Dutch nineteenth-century artists visited the Frans Hals Museum diligently, his influence on them is difficult to evaluate. The main reason for this is that Dutch artists of the second part of the nineteenth century were primarily landscape painters and, as such, were less influenced by Hals than by Jacob von Ruisdael, Meindert Hobbema, or Willem van der Velde. Moreover, the few nineteenth-century Dutch artists who did paint the figure, such as Jozef Israels and later George Breitner and Vincent van Gogh, were primarily attracted to Rembrandt. This is clearly borne out in van Gogh's letters, which contain 111 references to Rembrandt and only 30 to Hals. To be sure, van Gogh appreciated Hals, whom he admired as "a colorist among colorists" equal to Veronese, Rubens, Delacroix, and Velázquez. But like Fromentin, he saw Hals as an artist "who always remains on earth," as opposed to Rembrandt whom he felt to be "so deeply mysterious that he says things for which there are no words in any language."[67]

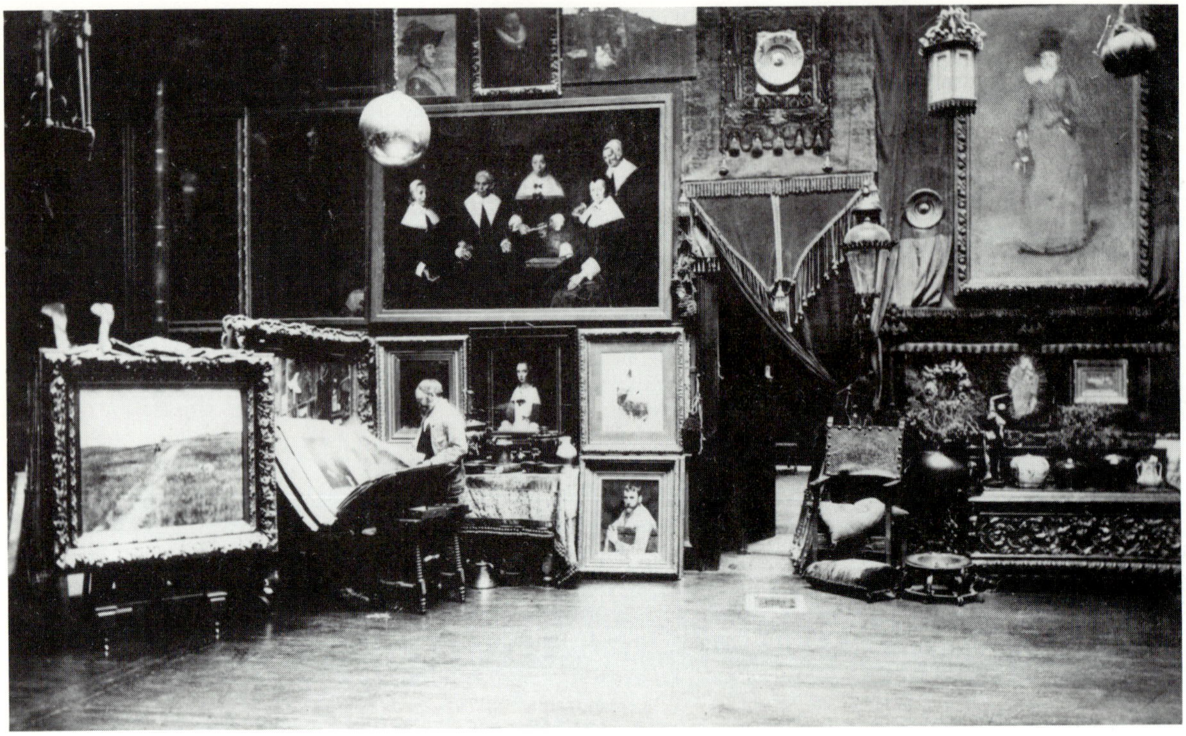

Fig. 7.13. Photograph of William Merritt Chase's Tenth-Street Studio. (The artist's copy after *The Regentesses of the Old Men's Alms House* is visible on the rear wall of the studio.) Southampton, New York, Parrish Art Museum, William Merritt Chase Archives.

In conclusion, it appears that the opening of the Frans Hals Museum in 1862 contributed significantly to the revival of interest in Frans Hals, which became an international artistic trend during the 1870s and 1880s that extended from Russia in the east to America in the west. Judging from the museum's registers, Hals's popularity in avant-garde artistic circles peaked in the early seventies—exactly when their interest in most other Dutch artists (Rembrandt excluded) began to wane—while among more conservative artists Hals's reputation as a great painter continued to thrive until the end of the century. The reason for this appears to be that Hals offered something that set him apart from the Dutch artists who had been admired during the previous decades (Bartholomeus van der Helst, Paulus Potter, Pieter de Hooch, or Frans van Mieris): namely a powerful vision and a bold virtuoso technique through which the artist could achieve both extravagant and subtle, sober effects as circumstance required.

For a short period in the late 1860s and early 1870s, Hals's paintings, with their bourgeois subjects and loose, free brushwork, offered to the avant-garde of the time an important signpost from realism to Impressionism; subsequently, during the late 1870s and 1880s, it presented to more conservative painters a viable alternative to Impressionism and Postimpressionism. To those who wished to leave realism behind but were not quite ready for the accentuated brushstroke and the "violettomania" of

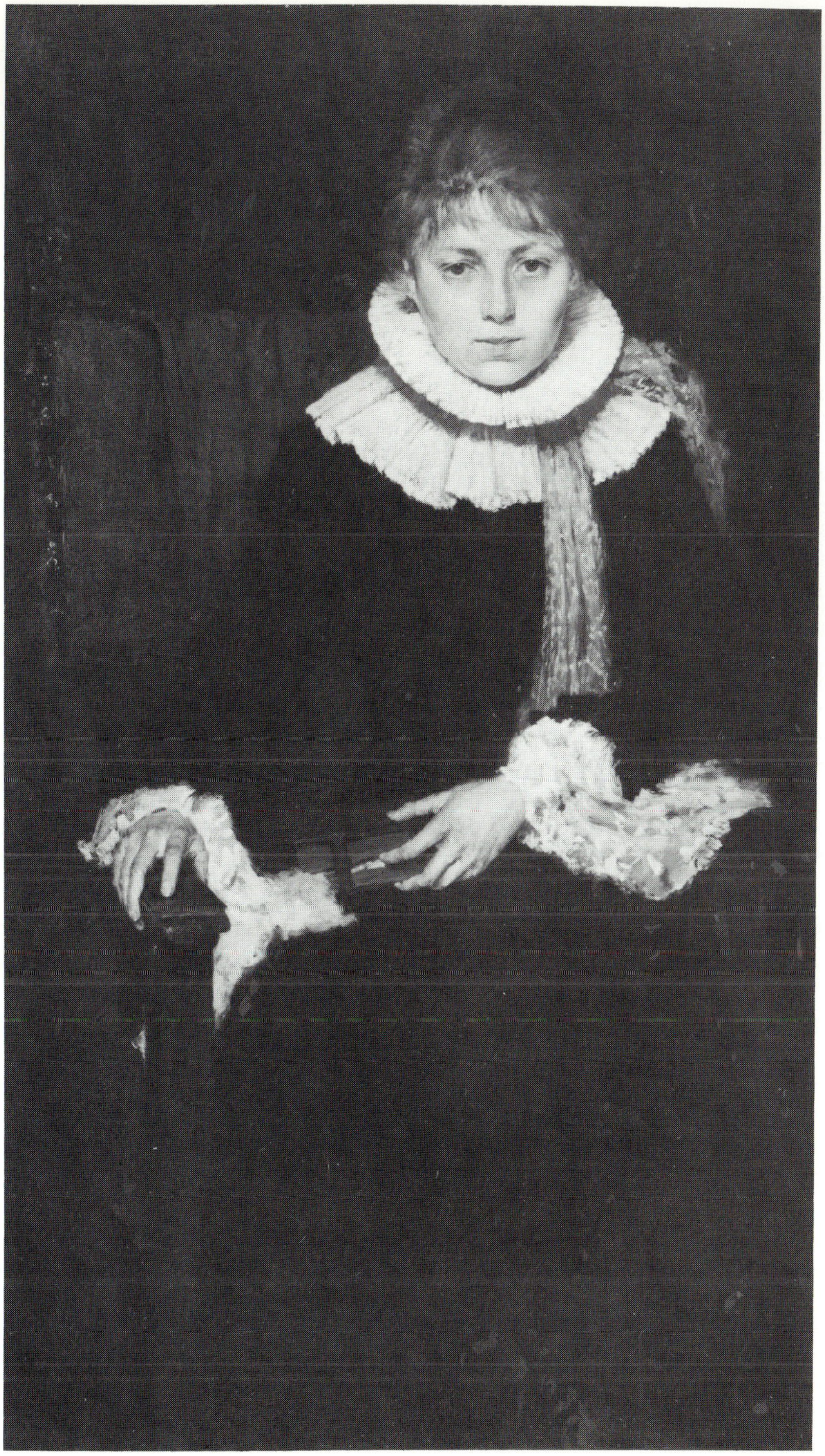

Fig. 7.14. William Merritt Chase, *Portrait of a Woman*, 1878. Courtesy of the Wadsworth Atheneum, Hartford, Connecticut.

Impressionism (or, later, for the dots of pointillism), Hals's painting furnished a free and loose facture without "anarchy," a lively palette without "madness," casual poses and animated gestures integrated in solid compositions, and the possibility of contemporaneity without the shock of the new—basically a middle-of-the-road formula that offered a guarantee of critical and public success.

APPENDIXES

Visitors to the Frans Hals Museum, 1862–1900

In perusing the voluminous visitors registers of the Frans Hals Museum, I culled from them the signatures of artists and art-related visitors with whom I was familiar as well as the names of those who qualified themselves as "artiste peintre," "Maler," "kunstschilder," "statuaire," "écrivain d'art," etc. No doubt, certain names of note have escaped me. Not only are the signatures often difficult to decipher, but also the mere quantity of names to be waded through will inevitably lead to omissions.

In the appendixes I have, whenever possible, provided the full names of the visitors, even when they signed only with their last names, or with last names and first initials. Life dates or, by default, major exhibition dates, if known, are added in parentheses. If a visitor is listed for the second time, dates are substituted by "v.s." Some names are crosslisted in both appendixes, in which cases parentheses will contain the indication, "see app. I," or "see app. II." Place names are those provided by the visitors themselves, unless they are in brackets. Material in quotation marks refers to notations made by the visitors in the registers. Parentheses contain my remarks.

APPENDIX 1
Art Critics, Historians, Dealers, and Collectors

1862		Carel Vosmaer (1826–1888), The Hague
1863		W. Bürger (pseud. of Théophile Thoré, 1807–1869), Paris
1864		Victor de Stuers (1843–1916), Maastricht (Netherlands)
		Hendrik Conscience (1812–1883), Courtrai (Belgium)
1868		Emile Montégut, Paris (with Adolphe Artz)
1869	Aug.	Jules Claretie (pseud. of Jules Arsène Arnaud, 1840–1913), Paris
	fall	Jan van Beers (1821–1888), Antwerp
1872		Samuel P. Avery (1822–1904), New York
		Henry Havard (1838–1921), Paris
1873	Aug.	Carel Vosmaer (v.s.)
	Aug.	Edmondo de Amicis (1846–1908), Florence
1873	fall	Roger Portalis (1841–1912), Paris
1874	spring	Roger Portalis (v.s.), Paris
1875	July	Eugène Fromentin (1826–1876), Paris
	Aug.	Zacharie Astruc (1833–1907), Paris
	Aug.	Hugo von Tschudi (1851–1911), Vienna
	Aug.	Vincent van Gogh (not the artist but probably the dealer)
	Sept.	Enrico Cernuschi (1821–1896) (with family)

1876	Sept.	Sully Prudhomme (1839–1907), Paris
	Sept.	Paul de St. Victor (1827–1881), Paris
	with	Charles Blanc (1803–1882), Paris
	with	Paul Chenavard (see Appendix 2)
1877	June	Oskar Berggruen, Vienna
1879	3/21	Th. van Gogh (probably Theo, Vincent's brother)
	7/7	Henry Havard (v.s.; with Maxime Lalanne)
	9/5	Marcellus Emants (1848–1923), The Hague
1880	4/20	Hendrik Conscience (v.s.), Brussels
	July	Carl Justi (1832–1912), Bonn
1881	Apr.	Jan Pieter Veth (1864–1925), Amsterdam
		Henry Thode (1857–1920), Berlin
1882	10/12	Carel Vosmaer (v.s.), The Hague
1883	5/7	Georges Lafenestre (1837–1919)
	May	Georges Ohnet (1848–1918), Paris (with Mrs. Ohnet)
	5/18	Vladimir Stassov (with Ilya Repin)
	June	Emilien Ernest Chesneau (1833–1890)
	July	Georges Lafenestre (v.s.), Paris
	July	Ch. Lauth, "directeur de Sèvres," Paris (with Mrs. Lauth)
	10/15	Abraham Bredius (1855–1946), Amsterdam
	Oct.	Mario Proth, Paris
1884	Sept.	Jules Destrée (b. 1863)
	Oct.	Georges Lafenestre (v.s.), Paris
1885	8/20	Barbet de Jouy (1812–1896)
1886	10/6	P. Haverkorn van Rijsewijk, Rotterdam (Director Museum Boymans)
	10/28	Camille Mauclair (1872–1944), Paris
1887	7/20	Abraham Bredius (v.s.), Amsterdam
1888	1/20	François Coppée (1842–1908), Paris
	7/30	Henri Hymans (1836–1912), "cons. Bibliothèque Royale, Bruxelles"
	with	Alfred Michiels (1813–1892), "collectionneur," Tirlemont
1889	4/9	T. van Gogh (v.s.), Paris
	5/3	Vincent van Gogh (v.s.), Amsterdam
	10/18	Charles Saunier (1815–1889), "rédacteur *Revue Art et critique*," Paris
1890	6/16	Emile Michel (1818–1909), Paris
	7/17	Paul Durand Ruel (1831–1921), Paris
	8/2	Zacharie Astruc (v.s.), Paris
	8/28	Roland F. Knoedler, New York
	8/28	V. van Gogh (v.s.), Amsterdam
1891	4/18	Royal Cortissoz (1896–1948), New York
	5/11	Cornelius Marinus van Gogh (dealer; with F. Leenhoff)
	5/15	Cornelius Marinus van Gogh (v.s.)
	5/23	Jan Six (1857–1926)
		Jules Destrée (v.s.), Charleroi (with Mrs. Marie Destrée)
	8/28	Georges Lafenestre (v.s.), Paris
1892	4/16	Siegfried Bing (1838–1905), Paris
	with	Marcel Bing, Paris
	May	Etienne Moreau-Nélaton (1859–1927), Paris
	9/16	Ulrich Thieme (1865–1922), Leipzich

	Sept.	Paul Eudel (1837–1911), Paris (with Mrs. Eudel)
	11/14	Sâr Péladan (1858–1918), "Grand Maître de la Rose + Croix"
1893	7/13	Cornelis Hofstede de Groot (1863–1930), The Hague
	8/1	Arsène Alexandre (b. 1859), Paris
	Oct.	Théodore Duret (1838–1927), Paris
1894	8/11	H. Galli, "Directeur de *L'Art Français*"
	8/16	Alfred Stieglitz (1864–1946; with Mrs. Stieglitz)
	Sept.	Max J. Friedländer (1867–1958)
1895	8/13	Georges Ohnet (v.s.), Paris
	with	Jean Richepin (1849–1926), Paris
	Oct.	Siegfried Weber (b. 1870), Heidelberg
1896	June	Octave Maus "Directeur de *La Libre Esthétique*"
	Aug.	Roland F. Knoedler (v.s.), New York
1897	7/30	Raymond Koechlin (1860–1931), Paris
	9/6	Georges Lafenestre (v.s.), Paris
	9/16	Pierre J. H. Cuypers (1872–1921), Amsterdam (architect, Rijksmuseum)
1898	4/2	Willem Vogelsang (1875–1954), Freiburg i/Br
	5/26	Georges Riat (1870–1905), Paris
1899	Sept.	Anatole France (1844–1924), Paris
	6/16	Bernhard Winter (b. 1871), Oldenburg
	6/18	Jan Apol (1874–1945), The Hague
	8/17	Max Liebermann (1847–1935), Berlin
	8/26	Fritz Werner (v.s.), Berlin, "Direktor der Kongl. Kunst-Academie"
	9/28	Hugo Vogel (1855–1934), Berlin
	9/30	Lizzy Ansingh (v.s.), Amsterdam
	11/16	Ferdinand Katona (b. 1864), Budapest
	Nov.	C. Franco de Amicis, Amsterdam, "peintre et écrivain"

APPENDIX 2
Artists

1862	7/28	Hendrick Frans Schaefels (1827–1904), Antwerp
	with	David Cot (sp.?), Antwerp
	Aug.	A. Hunck, Paris
	Sept.	Sebastian Buff (1829–1880), Switzerland
1863	Sept.	Jacobus Cornelis Gaal (1796–1866), Kampen (Neth.)
		Auguste-Clément Chrétien (b. 1835), Paris
		Johannes Bosboom (1817–1891)
1864	6/5	Franz Büchser (1828–1890), Solothurn (Switzerland) "Franz Büchser, Peintre artiste de Soleure, Suisse, auf seine Pilgrimsfahrt zum Altar der groszen Niederländischen Museen, den 5 Juni 1864, en complète admiration."
		Johann Philip Koelman (1818–1893), The Hague
	Aug.	Nicolaes J. W. de Roode (1814–1884), The Hague
		Jan Gerard Smits (1823–1910), The Hague
		Joseph Stallaert (1825–1903), Tournai (Belg.)
		Eduard Hübner (b. 1842), Düsseldorf
		Fritz Wedding, Düsseldorf

1865		Johannes Arnoldus Boland (1838–1922), Amsterdam
		Johannes Jacobus Mesker (1843–1890), The Hague
		Adine Pérignon Verdé-DeLisle (1805–1866), Paris
	with	Elisabeth Boulanger Cavé (b. 1809), Paris
		Peter Antoon Verlinde (1801–1877), Antwerp
		Adolphe Chappuis, Paris (Salon 1869)
1866		Johannes Hendrik Veldhuyzen (1831–1910), Amsterdam
		Louis Tuerlinckz (1820–1894), Brussels
		Thérèse Schwartze (1851–1918), Amsterdam
1867		Julius Jacobus van de Sande Bakhuysen (1835–1925), The Hague
		Cornelis Jan de Vogel (1824–1879), Dordrecht
		Alexander Friedrich ("Fritz") Werner (1827–1908), Berlin
		C. F. ("Frans") Lebret (1820–1909), Dordrecht
		Louis Dubois (1830–1880), Brussels
		Jean-Maxime Claude (1824–1904), Paris
		Jan van der Kaa (1813–1877), Rotterdam
		Hyppolite Moulin (1832–1884), Paris
	9/5	Salomon van Witsen (1833–1911), The Hague
		Pieter Oijens (1842–1894), Amsterdam
	with	David Oijens (1842–1902), Amsterdam
1868		François Bonvin (1817–1887), Paris
	Apr.	Cornelis Jan de Vogel (v.s.), Dordrecht
		Johan Albert Neuhuys (1844–1914), Utrecht
	with	Joseph Hendrick Neuhuys (1841–1899), Utrecht
	with	Bernardus Johannes Blommers (1845–1914), The Hague
	with	Joseph Jodocus Moerenhout (1801–1875)
	May	Norbert Schrödl (1842–1912), Vienna
		David Adolphe Constant Artz (1837–1890), Paris (with Emile Montégut)
		Albert Kappis (1836–1914), Düsseldorf
		Louis Dubois (v.s.)
	8/30	J. B. Jongkind (1819–1891), Paris
		Joseph-Michel Caillé (1836–1881; Paris)
		W. W. B. Jansen, Rossum (Netherlands)
1869		Adolphe Artz (v.s.), Paris
	with	John Dun (exh. at R.A. 1872–1884), Edinburgh
	6/7	Henri Rochussen (1812–1889), Rotterdam
	Aug.	Léopold Flameng (1831–1911)
		Jan Hendrik van de Laar (1807–1874), Rotterdam
	with	Anthonie Jacobus van Wijngaerdt (1808–1887), Haarlem
		Sientze van Houten (1834–1909), The Hague
	with	Alfred Jacques Verwee (1838–1895), Brussels
	with	Hendrik Willem Mesdag (1831–1915), The Hague
		Edmond de Schampheleer (1824–1899), Brussels
		Edouard Piechter, Paris
1870		Bernard Blommers (v.s.), The Hague
		Charles Théodore Sauvageot (1826–1883), Paris
		Ch. Paul Schauwaloff (Russia)
	with	P——A. Rogoluboff (Russia)
		Hendrik Willem Mesdag (v.s.), The Hague
	12/22	Salomon van Witsen (1833–1911), The Hague

1871 Edouard Detaille (1848–1912)
Ferdinand Roybet (1840–1920)
Paul C. L. Nanteuil Leboeuf (b. 1837), Paris
Emile-Auguste Carolus-Duran (1838–1917), Paris
July Antoine Vollon (1833–1900), Paris
with Jean-Marie Rollion (1846–1929), Paris
Charles-Léon Cardon (b. 1850), Brussels
Hendricus Franciscus Martinus ("Henri") Schelfhout (1839–1910)
Adolphe Mouilleron (1820–1881), Paris
Etienne Gautier (1842–1903), Paris
Sept. Charles Daubigny (1817–1878), Paris
with Karl Daubigny (1846–1886), Paris
Oct. Osbert Burr Loomis (b. 1813), New York
Oct. Claude Monet (1840–1926)
David Bles (1821–1899)
with Julius Jacobus van Sande Bakhuyzen (1835–1925)
with Elchanon Verveer (1826–1900)
with Gerke Henkes (b. 1844)
with Johan Gerard Smits (1823–1910)
Emile Boetzel (Salon 1880), Paris

1872 1/31 Salomon van Witsen (v.s.), The Hague
"Henri" Schelfhout (v.s.) (with Mrs. Schelfhout)
5/15 Fritz W. Sonderland (1836–1896), Düsseldorf
with Wm. Seelig, Düsseldorf
with Ernst Anders (b. 1845), Düsseldorf
with Fritz Beinke (1842–1907) Düsseldorf
with Hugo Crola (1841–1910), Düsseldorf
with F (?). W. Schade, Chicago
May Georges Jan Hendrik ("Geo") Poggenbeek (1853–1903), Amsterdam
6/26 Edouard Manet (1832–1883), Paris
with Ferdinand K. A. C. Leenhoff (1841–1914), Johannes Stortenbeker (b. 1821), The Hague
Ernest Journault (Salon 1864 ff.), Paris
with Léon Bonnat (1834–1923), Paris
Léon Glaize (1842–1932), Paris
with Frederik Hendrik Kaemerer (1839–1902), Paris
Georges Becker (b. 1845), Paris
with Louis-Joseph Devémy (1808–1874), Paris
Aug. Fernand Cormon (1845–1924)
Aug. Edmond van der Meulen (1841–1905), Brussels
Sept. Adolphe Artz (v.s.), Paris
with Auguste Glaize (1807–1893)
Sept. Mihāli Munkácsy (1844–1909), Paris
Oct. Paul Joseph Constantin Gabriel (1828–1903), Brussels
Antoine Vollon (1833–1900), Paris
with Robert Mols (1848–1903), Antwerp
Cornelis Jan de Vogel (v.s.), Dordrecht
J. Wolkenburg, Amsterdam

1873 Charles Storm van s Gravesande (1841–1924), Brussels
Aug. Moritz Daniel Oppenheim (1800–1882), Frankfurt
8/7 François Bonvin (v.s.), St. Germain (with Louis de Turenne)
Franz Seraph von Lenbach (1836–1904), Munich

	Aug.	Léopold Flameng (v.s.), Paris
	with	François Flameng (1856–1923), Paris
	fall	Wilhelm Busch (1832–1908), Frankfurt
		G. de Schampholz, Brussels
1874	3/20	Salomon van Witsen (1833–1911), The Hague
	with	Willem Karel Nakken (1835–1926), The Hague
	Mar.	Paul Milliet (1844–1920), Paris
	Apr.	Georges Duplessis (b. 1852), Paris
	Apr.	Jacobus Adrianus Maigret (1812–1893), Amsterdam
	with	Johannes Albertus Hesterman (1848–1916), Amsterdam
		Antoine-Gabriel Favard (1829–after 1877), Rome
	May	Jean-Léon Gérôme (1824–1904), Paris (with A. Goupil)
	June	Pierre Marie Beyle (1838–1902), Paris
	with	Alphonse E. F. Lecadre (1842–1875), Paris
	with	Henri Martin, Paris
	Sept.	Ernst Müller (1823–1875), Rome
	with	Willem Johannes Martens (1838–1895), Rome
	Sept.	Thomas Walter Wilson (b. 1851), London
	Oct.	Théodule Ribot (1823–1891), Colombes ("peintre d'histoire")
1875		Fritz Werner (1827–1908), Berlin
	with	Georg Oeder (1846–1931), Düsseldorf
	with	Henri de Braekeleer (1840–1888), Antwerp
		Axel Gillis Hafström (b. 1841), Sweden
	with	Frithjof Smith-Hald (1846–1903), Norway
	June	Ch. Drouet (1836–1908), Paris
		Pieter Stortenbeker (1828–1898), The Hague
	with	Emile Wauters (1846–1933), Brussels
		Felix Cogen (b. 1838), Brussels
	with	Louis Tytgadt (b. 1841)
		Eugène Fromentin (1820–1876), Paris
	July	Paul-Jean Clays (1819–1900), Brussels
	July	Alberto Vianelli (1841–1927), Paris
	Aug.	Edmond Marie Petitjean (1844–1925), Nancy
	Aug.	Johannes Stortenbeker (v.s.), The Hague
	Aug.	Henri Fantin-Latour (1836–1904), Paris
	with	Victoria Dubourg (b. 1840), Paris
	with	Edwin Edwards (1823–1879), London
	Aug.	Ludwig ("Ludovisi") Passini (1832–1903), Vienna
	Aug.	Emil Jacob Schindler (1842–1892), Vienna
	Sept.	Eugène van Gelder (b. 1856), Brussels
	Sept.	Jules Lefebvre (1836–1911), Paris
	with	Emile Vernier (1829–1887), Paris
	with	Jacques Lanquetin (d. 1889), Paris
		Georges de Dramard (1839–1900), Paris
		Geo Poggenbeek (v.s.)
1876		Geo Poggenbeek (v.s.)
		Adolphe Leleux (1812–1891), Paris
	with	Armand Leleux (1818–1885), Paris
	with	Emilie Leleux (1824–1885)
		Henri de Braekeleer (v.s.), Antwerp
	with	Franz Vinck (b. 1827), Antwerp
	with	Gustave Denzhuys (sp?), Ghent

	with	J. van Busbrouck (sp?), Ghent
		Ferdinand Carl Sierig (1839–1905), The Hague
	July	Eilif Peterssen (1852–1928), Christiania/Munich
	Aug.	Jean-Eugène Ducasse (b. c. 1817), Paris-Passy
		Hugh Carter (1837–1903) (with Sully Prudhomme and Georges Lafenestre)
		Paul Chenavard (1807–1895), Paris
	Nov.	Eugène van Gelder (v.s.), Brussels
	11/7	Charles Z. Landelle (1812–1908)
	Dec.	Pieter Jos. Menckens, Antwerp
1877		J. Valkenburg, Amsterdam
		Alfred Agache (1843–1915)
	May	Jacob Krauth (1833–1890), Mannheim
		Léon Philippet (1843–1902), Liège
	with	Alex(andre) Marcette (1853–1929), Liège
		Emile Claus (1849–1924), Vijve (Belgium)
		Karl (also Charles) V(u)illermet (1849–1918), Lausanne
	Aug.	Emile Michel (see Appendix 1)
	Aug.	Ernst Ferdinand ("Ernesto") Eichler (1850–1895), Rome
	Sept.	Paul Gabriel (v.s.), Brussels
		Auguste Bourotte (b. 1853), Brussels
	Nov./ Dec.	Jean-Jacques Henner (1829–1905), Paris
1878	3/13	Willem Roelofs (1822–1897)
	with	Pieter Oyens (v.s.)
	with	David Oyens (v.s.)
	7/17	Félix-Joseph Barrias (1822–1907)
	8/27	William Merritt Chase (1849–1916), America
	10/9	Hector Lemaire (b. 1846), Paris
1879	1/6	Philips Sadée (1837–1904)
	4/2	Charles Julien
	4/5	Alfred Roll (1846–1919)
	with	Paul Jacques Melon (Salon 1878), Paris
		Léon Couturier (1842–1935), Paris
	4/18	Paul Dubois (1829–1905), Paris, "Directeur de l'École des Beaux-Arts de Paris, membre de l'Institut."
	4/26	Carl Locher (1851–1915), Danmark
	with	Karl Madsen (1855–1938), Danmark
	7/7	Maxime Lalanne (1827–1886; with Henry Havard)
	8/12	Pieter Stortenbeker (v.s.)
	9/10	Pierre Loison (1816–1886), Paris (with Mrs. Loison)
	with	S. L. Adam (Salons 1883, 1892), Paris
	10/9	Philippe Zilcken (1857–1930), The Hague
1880	2/26	Adrien-Louis Demont (1851–1928)
	with	Virginie Demont-Breton (1859–1935)
	4/13	Alfred Roll (v.s.)
	with	Georges Bertrand (1849–1929)
	4/16	Achille Guédé (b. 1846), Paris
	5/17	John Everett Millais (1829–1896), London
	with	William Powell Frith (1819–1909)
	with	Andrew Gray (England)

	5/19	Jan Hendrik Weissenbruch (1824–1903)
	with	Pieter Stortenbeker (v.s.)
	with	Julius Jacobus van de Sande Bakhuysen (b. 1835)
	with	H. Rochussen (Henri, 1812–1889; or Hugo, b. 1821), Rotterdam
	6/9	Henri Stanislas Rouart (1833–1905), Paris
	6/27	Jules Breton (1827–1905), Courrières, "peintre, poète." (with Mrs. Breton)
	Sept.	Albert Martin (1827–1900), Leeuwarden (Netherlands)
1881	Apr.	Jan Pieter Veth (1864–1925), Amsterdam
		Pascal-Adolphe-Jean Dagnan-Bouveret (1852–1929), Paris
	with	Emile Wauters (1846–1933), Brussels
		Gustave Bettinger (Salon 1904), Paris
		Maurice Bompard (1857–1936)
	Aug.	Pierre-Nicholas Tourgueneff (1854–1912)
	Aug.	John Ferguson Weir (1841–1926), New Haven, Connecticut
	with	J. Alden Weir (1852–1919), New York City
	8/12	David Oyens (v.s.), Brussels
	with	Pieter Oyens (v.s.), Brussels
	Dec.	Ferdinand d'Huart (Exh. Brussels, 1910), Luxemburg
1882	July	Jean-Jacques Henner (v.s.), Paris
	Aug.	Albert-Pierre Dawant (1852–1927), Paris
	Sept.	Armand Berton (1854–1927), Paris
	with	Louis-Henry Devillez (b. 1855), Paris
	1/12	Henri Lefort (b. 1852), Paris
	with	James McNeill Whistler (1834–1903), London
	with	Matthew Robinson (Exh. 1856–1884), London
	with	George Francis ("Frank") Miles (1852–1891), London
1883	5/18	Ilia Repin (1844–1930) (with Vladimir Stassoff)
	July	A. A. Alleaume, France, "peintre verrier"
	July	Henri Harpignies (1819–1916)
	July	Charles Saunier (1815–1889), Paris (with Georges Lafenestre)
	July	Léon Bonnat (v.s.), Paris
	July	Emile Munck, Brussels
	Aug.	Theo van Rysselberghe (1826–1926), Brussels
	Sept.	Tsuyen (sp.?), Copenhagen
	Sept.	Alexis (sp.?) Perrignan de Frenoy, Brussels
	Oct.	Eberhard Stammel (1833–1906), Düsseldorf
	10/15	H. Rochussen (v.s.)
	Oct.	Hendrik Lodewijk Permeke, Antwerp
	Oct.	Hubert Bellis (1831–1902), Brussels
1884	June	William Merritt Chase (v.s.), New York
	with	Rosalie Gill (d. 1898), New York
	with	Sue-May Gill
	July	H. Hopkinson Smith (b. 1838), New York
	8/9	Geo Poggenbeek (v.s.)
	Aug.	Arthur Thevel (sp.?) Paris
	with	Pieter H. H. Tholen (1831–1913), Paris
	Sept.	H. Gobin, Paris
	Sept.	Hippolyte-Pierre Delanoy (1849–1899), Paris
	Sept.	Emile Bayard (1837–1891), Paris
	Oct.	Henri-Victor Devéria (1829–1897), Paris

1885	6/7	Paul Friedrich Meyerheim (1842–1915), Berlin
	6/11	John Henri Twachtman (1853–1902), Cincinnati, U.S.A.
	8/7	Jean Gigoux (1806–1894), Paris
	8/16	Theo van Rysselberghe (v.s.), Brussels
	with	H. Saeger, Brussels
	8/16	Jean-Joseph-Marie Carriès (1855–1894), Paris
	with	Frantz Charlet (1862–1928), Brussels
	8/16	Achille Varin, Paris
	8/17	William Merritt Chase (v.s.), New York
	8/21	Jean Mayné, Brussels (with Mrs. Mayné)
	with	Eugène van Gelder (v.s.), Brussels
	8/27	Emile Berchmans (b. 1867), Liège
	9/5	Walter Launt Palmer (1854–1932), America
	with	John Twachtman (v.s.), America
	with	William Meritt Chase (v.s.), America
	9/8	Edmund Harburger (1846–1906), Munich
	with	Wm. Harburger, Mainz
	9/11	Henri de Braekeleer (v.s.), Antwerp
	9/24	Tony Robert-Fleury (1839–1912), Paris
	11/2	Reinier E. J. Roeterink (1831–1913), Alkmaar
	with	C. J. van Kampenhorst, Haarlem
1886	Aug.	Jules Casiles, Paris
	8/31	Alfred-Henri Bramtot (1852–1894), Paris
	9/7	Georges Lufesne (sp.?), Paris
	with	Andrée Lufesne (sp.?), Paris
	9/27	Eugène H. E. Cuvillier (Salons 1887–1897)
	with	Henri Cross (1856–1910)
	10/2	Henri Cross (v.s.), Paris
	with	Eugène Cuvillier (v.s.), Paris
	11/26	Johannes Stortenbeker (v.s.), The Hague
	12/30	Geo Poggenbeek (v.s.), Amsterdam
1887	2/3	Philippe Zilcken (v.s.)
	4/16	Eugène Carrière (1849–1906)
	4/16	Jean-Baptiste-Georges Hébert (b. 1837), Paris
	5/16	Joseph Eysseric (1860–1932), Carpentras
	7/16	Heinrich Kühl, Munich
	8/3	E. Schalbroeck (1853–1935), Rotterdam
	8/16	Gerarda Hermina Marius (1854–1919), The Hague
	8/16	Rein (sp.?) Guérin, Paris
	8/16	Louis-Michel Eilshemius (1864–1942), New York
	9/7	Heinrich Rasch (1840–1913), Munich
	9/16	Hugo Vogel (1855–1934), Berlin
	9/19	Hermann Lasch (b. 1861), Düsseldorf
	with	Walter Peterson (b. 1862), Düsseldorf
	with	Edm. (sp.?) Matsen, Düsseldorf
	10/1	Charles Giroux (b. 1861), Paris
	12/23	Raoul Charles Verlet (1857–1923), Paris
1888	4/3	Omer Dierickx (b. 1862), Brussels
	with	Joseph Dierickx (b. 1865), Brussels
	with	Edouard Drugate (sp.?), Brussels
	with	Ad. Crespin (b. 1859), Brussels

	4/27	Jean Theodoor ("Jan") Toorop (1858–1928), Brussels
	5/3	Philips Sadée (v.s.), The Hague
	5/18	Louis-Auguste Girardot (b. 1858), Paris
	5/29	Walter B. Crane (1845–1915; with Mr. and Mrs. W. H. Crane, New York)
	6/2	Willem Adriaan van Konijnenburg (1868–1943), The Hague
	6/9	Afrund (sp.?), Munich
	6/11	Emile Wauters (1846–1933), Brussels
	6/15	Jose Salis y Camino (b. 1863), Irun (Spain)
	8/20	Franz von Lenbach (v.s.), Munich (with Mrs. von Lenbach)
	8/30	Ferdinand Leenhoff (v.s.), Paris
	9/7	Gustave Moreau (1826–1898), Paris
	with	Edmée Chéramy, Paris (with Mr. Chéramy)
	9/10	Hendrik Willem Mesdag (v.s.), The Hague
	9/12	Eugène Chigot (1860–1927), Paris
	with	Julien Dejardin (1857–1907), Valenciennes
	9/16	Mihály Munkácsy (v.s.)
	9/19	Mortimer Menpes (b. 1860), London [with R. M. Menpes]
	9/22	Jean-Joseph Weerts (1847–1927), Paris
	with	John Hughes (sculptor), Paris
	9/29	Georges Croegaert (b. 1848), Paris
	10/1	Alfred William Hunt (1830–1898), Paris
	10/22	Hendrik Antoon Pothast (1847–1924), Amsterdam
	10/27	Johan Thorn Prikker (1869–1932), The Hague
	11/7	Jean-Charles Cazin (1841–1901), Paris [with Mrs. Marie Cazin]
	with	Jean-Michel Cazin (1869–1917)
1889	1/24	Nils Gustav Wentzel (1859–1927), Kristiania
	with	Sverre Ihle, Kristiania
	with	Jo Visdal (1861–1923), Kristiania
	1/28	Max-Arthur Stremel (1859–1928)
	with	A. F. Seck (sp.?), Antwerp
	2/23	Johann Matthaus Keuffel (b. 1841), Frankfurt
	4/6	Charles Cottet (1863–1924), Paris
	4/6	Marcel Gauvaigne, Lille
	4/29	Alfred Boucher (1850–1934)
	5/6	J. van Lils, Antwerp
	5/20	Agnes Lunn (b. 1850), Denmark
	with	A. M. Brodersen (b. 1863), Billesholm (?)
	5/31	Pieter Oyens (v.s.), Amsterdam
	6/3	Anton G. A. van Rappard (1858–1892), Santpoort
	6/11	Henry Cumming, Russia
	6/25	E—— Cortin (sp.?), Berlin (and Mrs. Cortin)
	6/25	Adolphe Artz (v.s.), The Hague
	8/27	Anton G. A. van Rappard (v.s.)
1890	6/5	Jules du Jardin, Brussels
	6/12	Henri Fortuny (sp.?), Paris
	6/16	Emile Michel (see Appendix 1)
	6/16	Willem de Haas Hemken (b. 1831)
	6/25	Willem Albracht (b. 1861), Antwerp
	7/2	Herman Delgoufre, Brussels
	with	Rene Osyn (sp.?), Brussels
	7/10	A. Duverne (sculptor), Paris

	7/26	William Degouve de Nunques (1867–1935), Brussels
	7/26	Jean-Charles Cazin (v.s.)
	9/24	Paul Colin (1838–1916), Paris
	12/11	Nicolaes van de Waaij (b. 1855), Amsterdam
	with	Ernest Sigismund Witkamp (1854–1897), Amsterdam
1891	5/11	Ferdinand Leenhoff (v.s.) (with C. M. van Gogh)
	5/26	Jan Toorop (v.s.), London
	6/19	Léon Lhermitte (1844–1925)
	7/6	Marie Destrée, Charleroi (with Mr. Jules Destrée)
	8/28	Willem Roelofs (v.s.), The Hague
	10/10	Charles Vincent (1862–1918), Paris
	with	Paul Roussel (1867–1928), Paris
	with	Jules Breton (1827–1905), Paris ("membre de l'Institut de France")
	10/12	W. Wissing, Dresden
	10/15	Hedwig Nardi, Leiden
1892	5/4	Jacob Lömme, Norway
	with	Lili Lömme, Norway
	May	Etienne Moreau-Nélaton (see Appendix 1)
	8/3	Paul Poetzsch (b. 1858), Dresden
	8/13	Frans Lebret (1820–1909), Dordrecht
	9/28	Adolph Frederik Lange (1861–1938), The Hague
	Dec.	Willem Roelofs (v.s.)
1893	3/23	E. von Streter, Munich
	4/25	Evert Pieters (1856–1932), Antwerp
	5/26	Charles M. Webb (1830–1895), Düsseldorf
	6/5	Ludwig Noster (1859–1910), Berlin
	with	Adalbert Roessler, Berlin (1853–1929)
	8/15	Karel Otto (1830–1902), Amsterdam
	9/14	Arthur Stoughton, "élève de l'école des Beaux-Arts"
	9/16	Willem Johannes Martens (1830–1895), Berlin
	9/20	J. H. L. de Haan, Brussels
	9/22	Maria Elisabeth Georgina ("Lizzy") Ansingh (1875–1959), Amsterdam
	Oct.	Louis Mayer (b. 1869), Weimar
1894	5/15	Gustav Wendling (b. 1862), Düsseldorf
	6/25	V. Vallgren (b. 1855), Paris
	8/8	Jean Jules Antoine Lecomte de Noüy (1842–1923)
	Aug.	John Christen Johansen (b. 1876), Copenhagen
	6/16	Alfred Stieglitz (1864–1964) [with Mrs. Stieglitz]
	10/1	Kurt Wetzel
	10/2	Pierre Gusman (b. 1862), Paris
	10/11	Ernst Heckel, Munich
	10/12	J. (?) von Gutbier (sp.?), Dresden
	Nov.	Frans Smeers (1873–1960), Brussels
1895	9/17	Ernst L. Ostermayer (1868–1918), Stuttgart
	9/19	Gerard Portielje (b. 1856), Antwerp
	Oct.	Pieter Annanius ("Piet") van den Bergh (1865–1950), The Hague
1896	May	Roger Jourdain (1845–1918), Paris
	with	Jean-Louis Forain (1852–1931), Paris
	with	Pierre Tourgeneff (v.s.), Paris

	Aug.	Charles Guérin (1875–1939), Paris
	with	Marc Puys, Paris
	Aug.	Richard Pollak (b. 1867), Prague
	10/2	M. Bauer, Munich
1897	May	Evert Pieters (v.s.)
	6/7	Jean-Charles Cazin (v.s.), Paris
	6/7	Paul Peterich (b. 1864)
	with	Wilhelm Kumm (b. 1861)
	7/1	P. J. Th. ("Piet") Slager (1871–1938), den Bosch
	8/8	Eugène Dietz, Paris
	with	H. Palland (sp.?), Paris
	with	Edmé-Antony-Paul ("Tony") Noël (1845–1909), Paris
	8/12	Eugène Bénet (b. 1863), Paris
	with	Julia Brouilhony, Paris
	8/19	Théodore-Jacques Ralli (1852–1909), Paris
	8/24	Eugène Hantzlin (sculptor), Paris
	9/13	Peter Philippi (1866–1958), Düsseldorf
1898	May	Julien Perrey (b. 1871), Paris
	5/31	Joseph Stallaert (1825–1903)
	8/17	Ilse Conrat (b. 1880)
	9/21	Adolphe-Charles Marais (b. 1856), Paris
1899	May	Ernst Ramada, Vienna

NOTES

The writing of this chapter was made possible by a sabbatical leave granted to me by Seton Hall University. Many people have contributed to its genesis. It would like to thank, in particular, Jaap Temminck, archivist of Haarlem, and his staff for their friendly cooperation. For information and assistance of various kinds, I am indebted to Monique and Gerrit Berends, Doreen Bolger Burke, Lidy ten Doesschate, Carol Fuerstein, Anne van der Jagt, David Milgrome, Carol Forman Tabler, Yvonne and Gabriel Weisberg, and Julius Zsako.

1. The most comprehensive account of the Hals revival to date is Frances Suzman Jowell, "Thoré-Bürger and the Revival of Frans Hals," *Art Bulletin* 56 (March 1974): 101–17. On the influence of Hals on nineteenth-century painting, see, among others, Petra ten-Doesschate Chu, *French Realism and the Dutch Masters* (Utrecht: Haentjens Dekker & Gumbert, 1974), esp. ch. 5.

2. For a brief history of the museum, see Frans Hals Museum, *Frans Hals* (Haarlem, 1962), 9–12.

3. The uniqueness of the Dutch group portrait was first recognized by Alois Riegl in 1902. Cf. Alois Riegl, *Das holländische Gruppenporträt*, reprint ed., 2 vols. (Vienna, 1931).

4. The Louvre acquired its first authentic work by Hals, *La Bohémienne*, with the La Caze Collection in 1869.

5. *Marriage Portrait of Isaac Abrahamsz. Massa and Beatrix van der Laan* (then generally considered a self-portrait of the artist with his wife) and the *Merry Toper.* Both paintings were in the Rijksmuseum, which did not acquire any additional paintings by Hals until 1885. The Mauritshuis acquired its first paintings by Hals in 1880 (portraits of Jacob Pietersz, Olycan, and his wife Aletta Hanemans).

6. On Hals's reputation in the eighteenth and early nineteenth centuries, see Jowell, "Thoré-Bürger," 103–5.

7. Now in the Municipal Archives of Haarlem.

8. On the nineteenth-century interest in Dutch paintings, see Chu, *French Realism;* also Horst Gerson, *Ausbreitung und Nachwirkung der holländischen Malerei des 17. Jahrhunderts* (Haarlem: Erven Bohn, 1942); S. Heiland and H. Lüdecke, *Rembrandt und die Nachwelt* (Leipzig: Seemann Verlag, 1960); Stanley Meltzoff, "Nineteenth-Century Revivals," Master's thesis, Institute of Fine Arts, New York University, 1941; Henry Nichols Blake Clark, "The Impact of Seventeenth-Century Dutch and Flemish Genre Painting on American Genre Painting, 1800–1865." Ph.D. diss., University of Delaware, 1982; Lois Engelson, "The Influence of Dutch Landscape Painting on the American Landscape Tradition," Master's thesis, Columbia University, 1966; H. van der Tuin, *Les Vieux peintres des Pays-Bas et la critique en France de la première moitié du XIXe siècle* (Paris: Librairie Nizet, n.d.).

9. Jowell, "Thoré-Bürger," esp. 107–17.

10. Ibid., 107.

11. *Gazette des Beaux-Arts* 24 (1868): 219–30, 431–48.

12. Ibid., 436.

13. W. Unger, *Etsen naar Frans Hals,* with an introduction by C. Vosmaer (Leiden, 1873–74).

14. Published Leipzig: E. A. Seemann, 1871.

15. Wilhelm von Bode and M. J. Binder, *Frans Hals, sein Leben und seine Werke* (Berlin: Photographische Gesellschaft, 1914).

16. Wilhelm von Bode, *Mein Leben,* 2 vols. (Berlin: Hermann Reichendorf, 1930), passim.

17. Sharon Flescher, *Zacharie Astruc: Critic, Artist, and Japoniste* (New York and London: Garland, 1978), 73–74, mentions yet another trip to Holland in 1888.

18. Ibid., 299. My translation.

19. *Les Maîtres d'autrefois* was first published in installments in the *Revue des deux mondes.* I have used the English edition published by Schocken Books (New York, 1963) under the title *The Old Masters of Belgium and Holland* (introduction by Meyer Schapiro).

20. Fromentin, *The Old Masters,* 225.

21. Ibid., 234.

22. Ibid.

23. Ibid., 226.

24. Ibid., 224.

25. Ibid., 226.

26. Ibid., 233.

27. Ibid.

28. Ibid., xxxiv.

29. Ibid., 226.

30. Péladan's visit to Holland coincided with that of Paul Verlaine. For amusing details of the meetings of these artists, see Paul Verlaine, *Quinze jours en Hollande* (Utrecht and Brussels: Het Spectrum, n.d.), passim.

31. Joséphin Péladan, *Frans Hals* (Paris: Goupil, 1912).

32. Ibid., 13. My translation.

33. Ibid., 17.

34. Ibid., 14.

35. Odilon Redon, *A Soi-même* (Paris: H. Floury, 1922), 75.

36. Fromentin, *The Old Masters,* 224.

37. M. Véry, "A critique, critique et demi," *L'Artiste* 19 (August 1877): 261. Dubois was very proud of these copies and appealed to his friend Gustave Courbet for help in selling them for a good price in Paris. Cf. Louis Dubois to Gustave Courbet, Etterbeek, 15 May 1870, Courbet Papers, box 2, Bibliothèque Nationale, Paris (Cabinet des Estampes).

38. A. Jullien, *Fantin-Latour* (Paris: Lucien Laveur, 1909), 63 and Frank Gibson, *The Art of Fantin-Latour* (London, n.d. [1924]), 80.

39. Courbet visited Amsterdam and The Hague as early as 1846.

40. The whereabouts of this copy are not known. I am indebted to Carol Forman Tabler for providing information about Vollon's commission. On Charles Blanc's Musée des Copies, see Albert Boime, "Le Musée des copies," *Gazette des Beaux-Arts* 64 (1964): 237–47.

41. Antonin Proust, "The Art of Edouard Manet," *The Studio* 21, no. 94 (January 1901): 230.

42. Quoted in George Hamilton, *Manet and his Critics* (New Haven: Yale University Press, 1954), 167.

43. Adolphe Tabarant, *Manet et ses oeuvres* (Paris: Gallimard, 1947), 206.

44. For discussion of Busch as painter, see Hans Georg Gmelin, *Wilhelm Busch als Maler* (Berlin: Mann, 1980).

45. Friedrich Bohne, ed., *Wilhelm Busch, Sämtliche Briefe—Kommentierte Ausgabe in zwei Bänden* (Hannover, West Germany: Wilhelm Busch Gesellschaft, 1968), 1:115.

46. Ibid., 117, 133.

47. Sonja Mehl, *Franz von Lenbach in der Städtischen Galerie im Lenbachhaus München* (Munich: Prestel Verlag, 1980), 16, 29. Lenbach's first trip was in the company of Busch.

48. Ibid., 89.

49. Siegfried Wichmann, *Franz von Lenbach und seine Zeit* (Cologne: Dumont Schauberg, 1973), 84.

50. Max Friedländer, *Max Liebermann* (Berlin: Propyläen, n.d.), 48. According to Friedländer, Liebermann never copied any other artist's work. Asked why he liked to copy Hals's paintings, Liebermann is supposed to have answered: "It is not easy to say . . . but there is no one who has painted a head that way." Quoted in Gemeentemuseum den Haag, *Max Liebermann in Holland* (The Hague, 1980), 41. My translation from quotation in Dutch.

51. Friedlander, *Liebermann*, 46. My translation.

52. Ibid., 49. My translation.

53. Géza Perneczky, *Munkácsy* (Budapest: Corina Verlag, 1970), 17.

54. Ilja Repin, *Fernes und Nahes: Erinnerungen* (Berlin: Henschelverlag, 1970), 251, and Fan Parker and Stephen Jan Parker, *Russia on Canvas: Ilya Repin* (London and University Park, Pa.: Pennsylvania University Press, 1980), 72.

55. Mary Cassatt to Emily Sartain, Antwerp, 25 June (1873). Quoted in Nancy Mowll Mathews, *Cassatt and her Circle: Selected Letters* (New York: Abbeville Press, 1984), 121.

56. It appears that copyists in the Frans Hals Museum did not sign the visitors registers (cf. also Dubois, Vollon, Liebermann, Weir, and Chase). They may have entered their names in a list of copyists, but such a document has not been found.

57. Cassatt cherished this copy throughout her life and used to show it to young students. See Frederick A. Sweet, *Miss Mary Cassatt: Impressionist from Pennsylvania* (Norman, Okla.: University of Oklahoma Press, 1966), 27.

58. J. Alden Weir to Robert Walter Weir, 2 January 1875. Quoted in Dorothy Weir Young, *J. Alden Weir* (New Haven: Yale University Press, 1960), 62.

59. Doreen Bolger Burke, *J. Alden Weir: An American Impressionist* (Newark, Del.: University of Delaware Press, 1983), 96.

60. Ibid., 97–100.

61. Katherine Metcalf Roof, *The Life and Art of William Merritt Chase* (New York: Hacker Art Books, 1975), 328–29, mentions three copies, none of which I have been able to locate.

62. "The Art Students League," *The Art Amateur* 2 (January 1880): 24.

63. Roof, *Life and Art of Chase*, 213.

64. Fromentin, *The Old Masters*, 135.

65. See L. D. Couprie, "Rembrandt Was an Honourable Man: Dutch Celebrations in the Past," *Delta* 12 (Summer 1969): 89–95.

66. The statue, which is placed at the entrance to the Florapark in Haarlem, was a creation of Hendrik Adolphe ("Henri") Scholtz.

67. *The Complete Letters of Vincent van Gogh*, 3 vols. (Greenwich, Conn.: New York Graphic Society, 1959), 1:424, 417.

III

Documents as Sources for Revisionist Art History

8

A NEGLECTED COLLABORATION

Van de Velde, Lemmen, and the Diffusion of the Belgian Style

JANE BLOCK

TODAY THE NAME OF HENRI VAN DE VELDE evokes images of the indefatigable proselytizer of the "new style" at the turn of the century; of the creator of disparate architectural monuments such as his own home, Bloemenwerf, and the Werkbund Theatre at Cologne; and, perhaps, of the irascible old man presenting himself as the great father of the modern movement.[1] It does not bring to mind the name of van de Velde's friend and chief associate during the 1890s, Georges Lemmen.

This was not always the case. Contemporaries of van de Velde and Lemmen often linked the two as founders of the new Belgian revival. For example, in 1899 *l'Art Moderne* hailed van de Velde and Lemmen as the "initiateurs de la Renaissance," while the same year the *Zeitschrift für Bücherfreunde* joined their names with that of Théo van Rysselberghe as the leading creators of modern book design in Belgium.[2] By 1902 the *Jahrbuch der bildenden Kunst* could refer to the well-known "Lemmen–Van de Velde'sche Linie" without further explanation.[3] The following year *Dekorative Kunst* criticized Lemmen and van de Velde as creators of "Ornamentkunst," reflecting even at the decline of art nouveau the persistent linking of their names in the press.[4] So strongly were the two associated in the minds of contemporaries that thirty years later the first chronicler of the Belgian modern movement, Madeleine Octave Maus, vividly recalled their inseparability in the 1890s. Despite Lemmen's early death and van de Velde's separate career as an architect, Madame Maus quite naturally discussed one in terms of the other.

> Both valuable recruits for Les XX, these two young men were so different, yet their names were so frequently linked. . . . Distinguished by much intelligence and cultivation, both were adepts of Seurat's principles, both infatuated from its inception with the domain of everyday objects.[5]

Van de Velde and Lemmen's association in Belgium, France, and Germany during the 1890s has been slighted in modern scholarship, and the seminal influence of the precocious Lemmen on the emerging van de Velde all but ignored.[6] By tracing the careers and interaction of the two through published and unpublished sources, it is hoped that a more balanced view will emerge.

Henri van de Velde (1863–1957) and Georges Lemmen (1865–1916) came into close contact when they became members of the Belgian avant-garde exhibition society Les XX. As early as the fall of 1886, while still living in Antwerp, van de

Velde coveted membership in Les XX.[7] In 1887 he based his own group, l'Art Indépendent, on the Brussels model.[8] By 1886 Lemmen likewise hoped for election and in January 1887 was approvingly referred to in print as a "future Vingtiste."[9] Both men were finally elected in 1888; each exhibited paintings the following year. Immediately the two young artists came under the influence of Georges Seurat, whose work was first shown at Les XX in 1887. Along with van Rysselberghe and Willy Finch, Lemmen and van de Velde became the chief exponents of neoimpressionism outside of France.[10]

Responding to the emerging arts and crafts movement in England, Lemmen became increasingly absorbed in the decorative arts. His enthusiasm was soon shared by van de Velde. Lemmen's first book design, a cover for Georges Eekhoud's *La Nouvelle Carthage,* was created in the spring of 1889.[11] The following year he was commissioned to create Les XX's catalogue cover for the 1891 exhibition (fig. 8.1) and produced a design of historical importance. Drawing on the model of the *Hobby Horse* cover as well as the books of Walter Crane, Lemmen created one of the first designs in what was to be known as the art nouveau style. Drawn a year before Victor Horta's famous Tassel House was built, the cover's two-dimensional sun, symbolizing Belgium's creative rebirth, rises from the sea of undulating lines, while energized lettering explains the catalogue's content. The next year van de Velde turned to book illustration and produced the well-known cover to Max Elskamp's *Dominical* (fig. 8.2). To evoke waves and sun's rays by a striking simplicity of means, van de Velde drew from his friend's design to produce his own masterpiece.

As the two men explored the diversity of the decorative arts, their friendly rivalry became noticeable. After a visit from Lemmen, Max Elskamp playfully warned van de Velde that Lemmen was far advanced on a silk embroidery and a fire screen. Elskamp implies that van de Velde should hasten to create similar works and adds, "Vrai, tu n'as pas de chance."[12] Although Lemmen's two designs have disappeared, van de Velde's tapestry *La Veillée d'Anges,* drawn in 1892 and woven the following year, is among his most famous early arts and crafts objects.

This competitive aspect of their friendship did not diminish the warm ties between van de Velde and Lemmen. The intimate side of their relationship is revealed by the humorous congratulatory note Lemmen presented to van de Velde and his fiancée, Maria Sèthe, on the announcement of their wedding plans in 1893.[13] In the public arena, in 1894 Lemmen published a glowing review of van de Velde, declaring him the spokesman for the "art of tomorrow" and the "rejuvenation of art."[14] As if justifying their mutual attraction to the decorative arts, Lemmen quoted his friend's description of the artist's function: "To embellish all of life and to disseminate beauty everywhere."

Both artists realized that contemporary criticism was an ideal way to spread the gospel of the new art and early in their careers turned to writing about the Belgian style, often acknowledging its debt to England. Although van de Velde began writing reviews of local exhibitions in 1889, his first polemical article dealing with the arts and crafts movement, "Artistic Wallpapers," did not appear until 1893.[15] Meanwhile, in March 1891, Lemmen wrote a two-part essay on the decorative arts of Walter Crane, the "ouvrier d'art." Lemmen's attraction to Crane was as strong as van de Velde's was to John Ruskin and William Morris. He suggested that Crane be invited to exhibit at Les XX and in 1891 lent his personal copies of Crane's children's books for display.[16] Lemmen's subsequent writings remained firmly rooted in particular objects

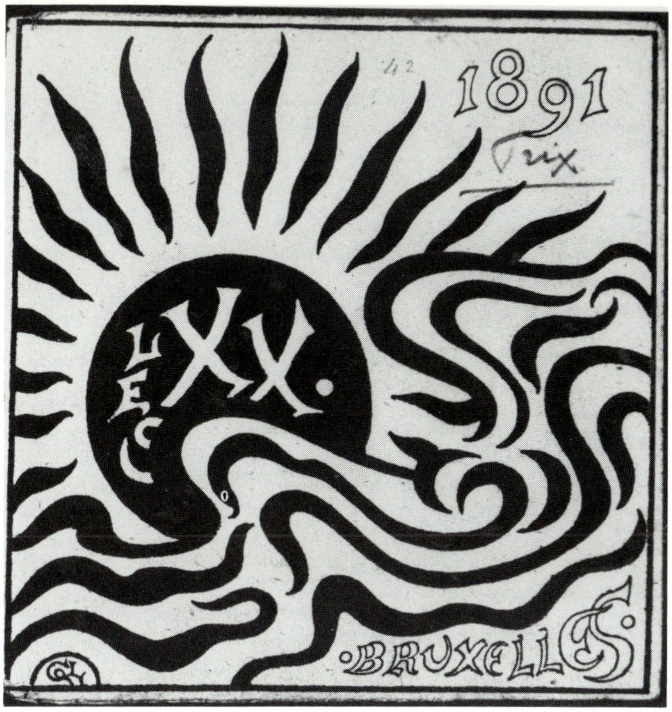

Fig. 8.1. Georges Lemmen. Cover for Les XX 1891 catalogue. © A. C. L. Bruxelles.

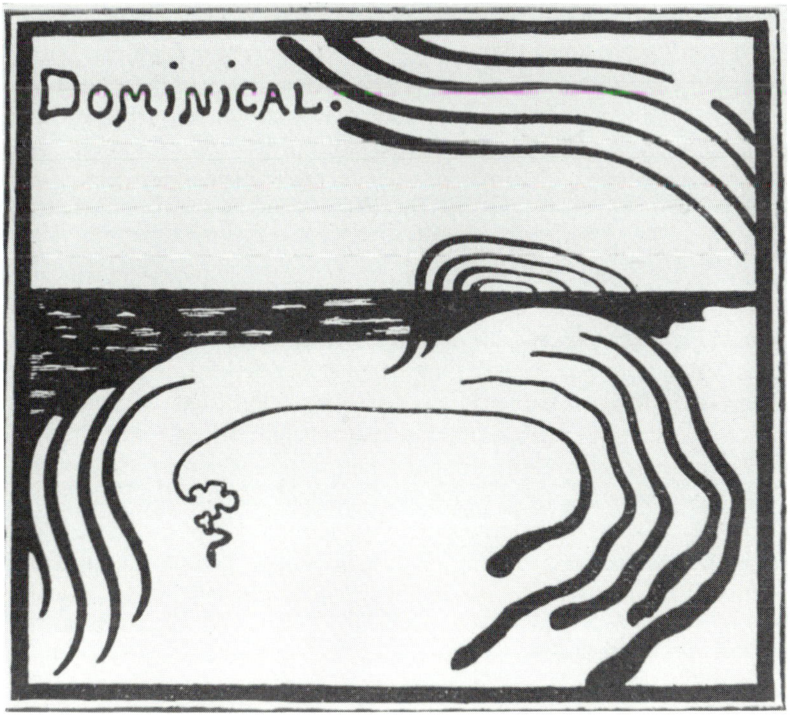

Fig. 8.2. Henri van de Velde. Cover for Max Elskamp's *Dominical*. Antwerp, J. E. Buschmann, 1892.

and styles to which he responded and are free of the messianic zeal found in van de Velde's *Le Déblaiement d'art* (1894) and *Aperçus en vue d'une synthèse d'art* (1895).[17]

Even after election to Les XX, van de Velde continued to organize groups in Antwerp patterned after it. In 1891 preparing the first exhibition of his new l'Association pour l'Art, van de Velde called upon his knowledgeable friend for assistance.[18] Lemmen secured on loan a group of Jules Chéret posters from a local collector and several works by Seurat from the symbolist poet Gustave Kahn.[19] Lemmen himself lent drawings, paintings, and books by Seurat, Constantin Guys, Ando Hiroshige, and Crane, and traveled to Antwerp to help hang the exhibition. A pleased Lemmen wrote to co-exhibitor and friend Jan Toorop: "It is truly the most artistic exhibition that we have in Belgium. No duds as with Les XX or at the Paris Independents—all the entries are interesting."[20]

As is so often the case, no subsequent personal appreciation of Lemmen's effort by van de Velde exists. Nevertheless, indirect examples of their reciprocal admiration abound. For instance, when van de Velde proposed to Lucien Pissarro the formation of a new Brussels review, he listed among his stable of "meilleurs dessinateurs" Georges Lemmen.[21] Likewise, when Lemmen attempted to organize a memorial album of prints in Seurat's memory, he wrote to Camille Pissarro soliciting his help and noting that van de Velde was among the important artists enlisted.[22]

The first project on which Lemmen's and van de Velde's artistic talents were combined in the same work was the new Flemish periodical *Van Nu en Straks*.[23] Van de Velde had been recruited by the editor Auguste Vermeylen to design the layout and provide ornamentation. In turn van de Velde enlisted Lemmen, as well as van Rysselberghe and such Vingtistes as James Ensor, Georges Minne, and Finch. Each artist created head- and tailpieces and occasional initial letters. For the first issue (April 1893), van de Velde designed a boldly abstract title page which continued the tradition of Lemmen's 1891 Les XX catalogue cover, but now at the expense of legibility. With a greater sense of how far a letter form could be stretched before losing its meaning, Lemmen began to develop in the mid 1890s a personal style of curvilinear ornament that could be combined effectively with his own lettering. After 1894, at the very time Lemmen began to work most closely with van de Velde, Théo van Rysselberghe replaced van de Velde as Lemmen's "friendly rival" and the artist whose lettering and decorative style can be most closely compared to Lemmen's.

Van de Velde and Lemmen's first architectural collaboration was also their first important opportunity to exhibit outside of Belgium. In mid 1895, Japanese art dealer Siegfried Bing asked van de Velde to design several rooms as part of his gallery remodeling at 22 rue de Provence, Paris.[24] Bing had met van de Velde in the spring of 1895 when he traveled to Brussels with his friend, art critic Julius Meier-Graefe. In the morning of their visit, the two transplanted Germans visited the year-old gallery, la Maison d'Art.[25] That afternoon, on the strength of an article by van de Velde, which Meier-Graefe had read with great interest, he and Bing paid a call on van de Velde in nearby Uccle.[26]

Van de Velde's claim that Bing's visit to la Maison d'Art encouraged him to found his Salon de l'Art Nouveau was shared by *l'Art Moderne*, which was quick to claim that Bing's refurbished shop was "a successor to the Maison d'Art in Brussels on the Toison d'Or."[27] Indeed, the similarity between the two galleries was striking. Both served as host to all the arts. Painting, sculpture, furniture, ceramics, glass, and books

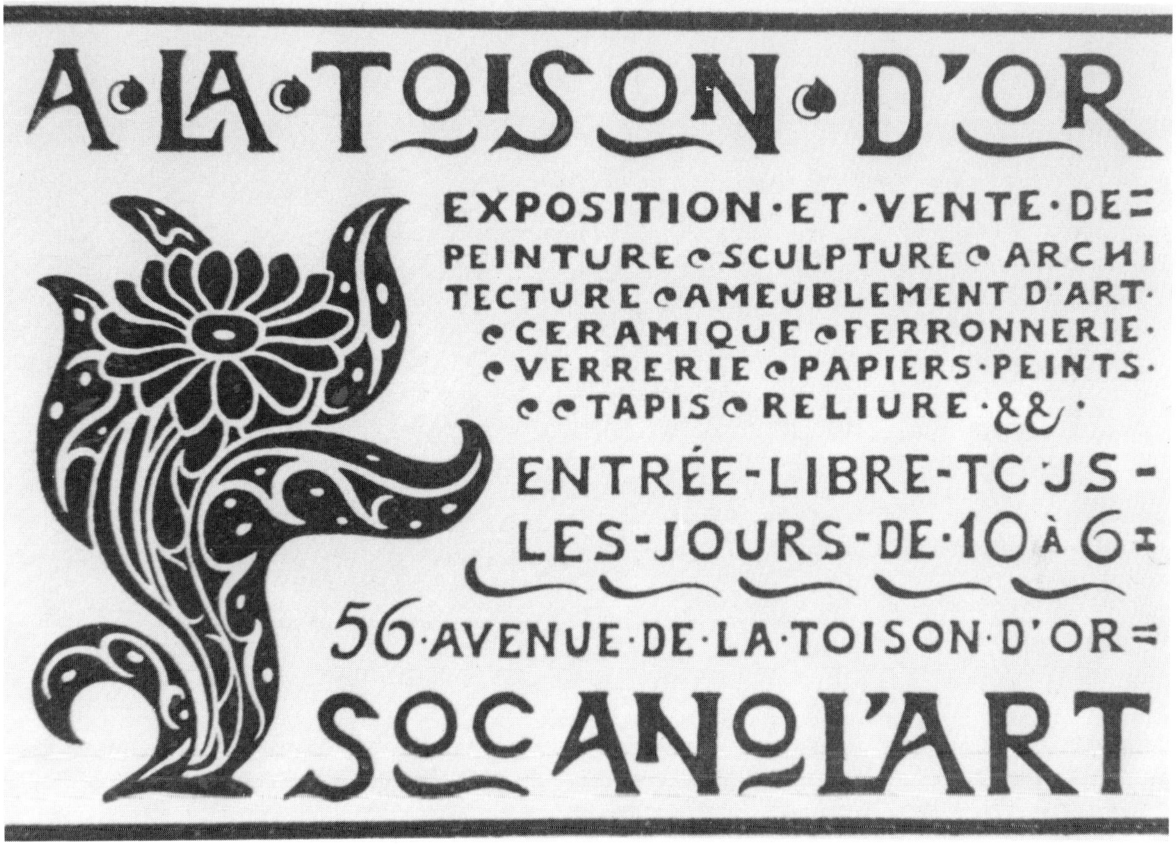

Fig. 8.3. Georges Lemmen. Poster for La Maison d'Art, "A la Toison d'Or," c. 1894–95. From *Decorative Kunst* 1 (1898): 110.

were displayed as integral parts of the total aesthetic environment. The Maison d'Art was self-consciously and deliberately elitist. In their "ivory kiosque" its members sought to unite a select group of aesthetes for "the diffusion, evolution and exaltation of art."[28] Unlike Bing's gallery, the Maison d'Art's raison d'être was not mercantile nor was it open to the public. Nevertheless, the clientele of each was probably much the same and the overall impression quite similar.

Lemmen was involved in several projects for the Maison d'Art. In 1894 he created the gallery's poster (fig. 8.3), which he decorated with a forceful, stylized sunflower bearing thick tentacle-like leaves. He also designed brochures and a mosaic in the form of an octopus. Although several artists designed for the Maison d'Art, van de Velde himself was not actively involved in the gallery.[29]

Shortly after his eventful trip, Bing acquired the services of Vingtistes van de Velde, Lemmen, and van Rysselberghe, and fellow Belgian Frank Brangwyn. In the absence of contracts, Bing's specific involvement in the meting out of projects is unclear. Whether van de Velde enlisted Lemmen after receiving Bing's commission, or whether Bing hired Lemmen directly is not known. It is telling that among the assignments that Lemmen was given were those he had fulfilled for the Maison d'Art: glass mosaics, an-

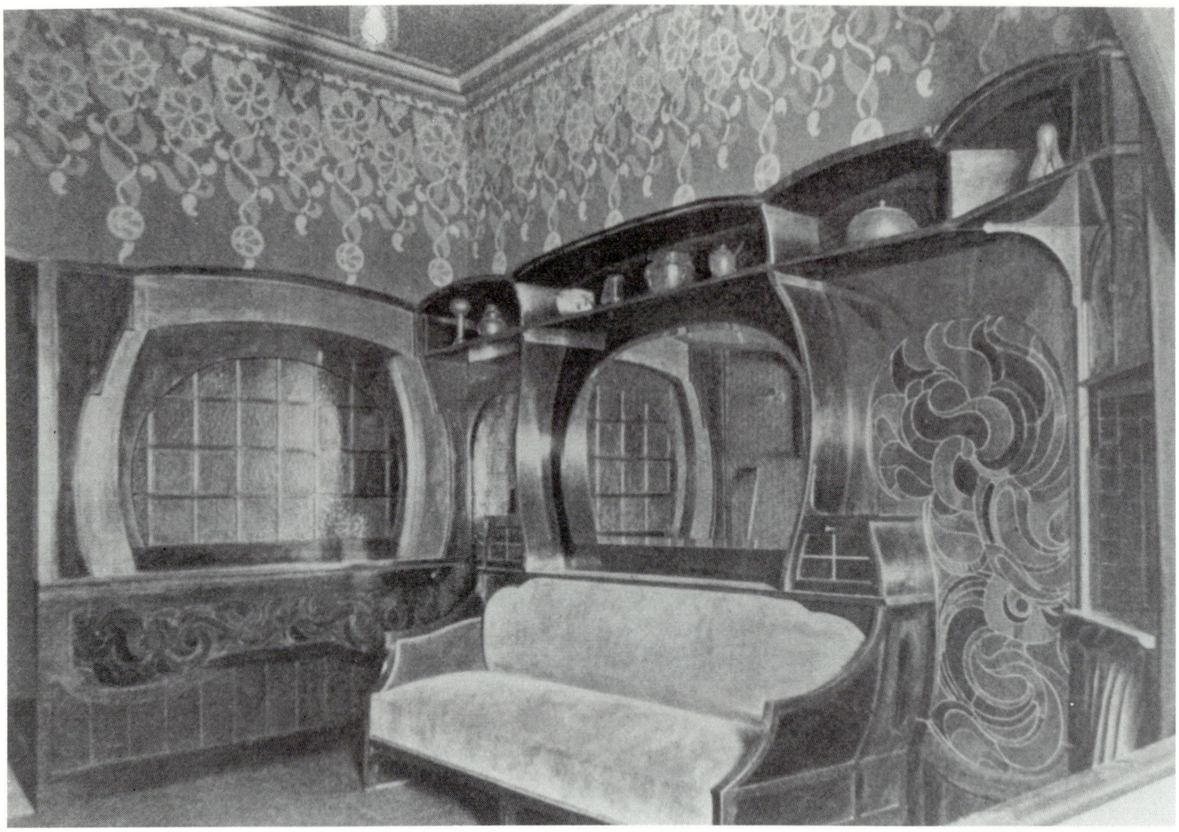

Fig. 8.4. Georges Lemmen and Henri van de Velde. Smoking Room for Siegfried Bing's Salon de l'Art Nouveau, Paris, 1895. From *l'Art Décoratif* 1 (October 1898): 19.

nouncements, and posters. Thus, it seems plausible that Bing hired Lemmen directly. Van de Velde in his turn was commissioned to design the architectural settings and furniture for three rooms. For one of these rooms, the "fumoir" (fig. 8.4), van de Velde worked closely with Lemmen to produce a remarkable synthesis of their two styles. To embellish van de Velde's austere omega arches, Lemmen added stained glass, glass mosaic, stencilled frieze, and a rug. Adjacent to van de Velde's benches, Lemmen inserted mosaics of asymmetrical, flame-like arabesques. Above the plate rail his stencilled frieze of swaying sunflowers makes a clear reference to the similar motif used on the Maison d'Art poster.[30] In addition to this joint creation, Lemmen was responsible for the gallery's graphic work. He produced the exterior poster that appeared next to Louis Bonnier's iron grillwork, the invitation to the gallery's reopening in December 1895, the manifesto announcing its aims, and the numerous advertisements that appeared in many of the new art magazines.[31] He also supplied endpapers for Bing and drew the dealer's personal stationery, executed in the fluid style whose name was taken from the gallery itself (fig. 8.5).[32]

Van de Velde's reputation was enhanced by his participation in the Dres-

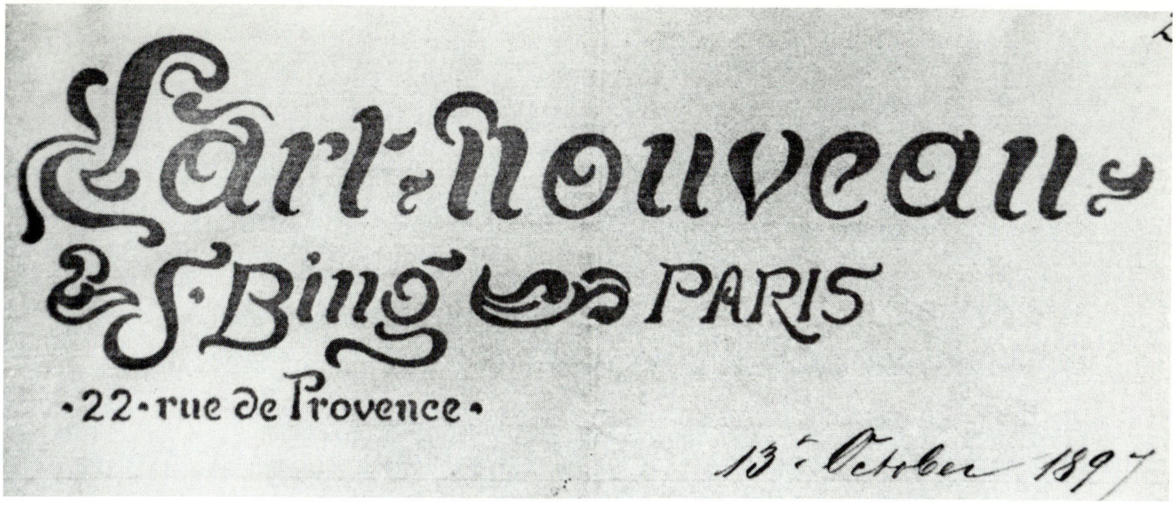

Fig. 8.5. Georges Lemmen. Stationery for Siegfried Bing's Salon de l'Art Nouveau, c. 1895. Kaiser Wilhelm Museum Archive, Krefeld. Photo Kruty.

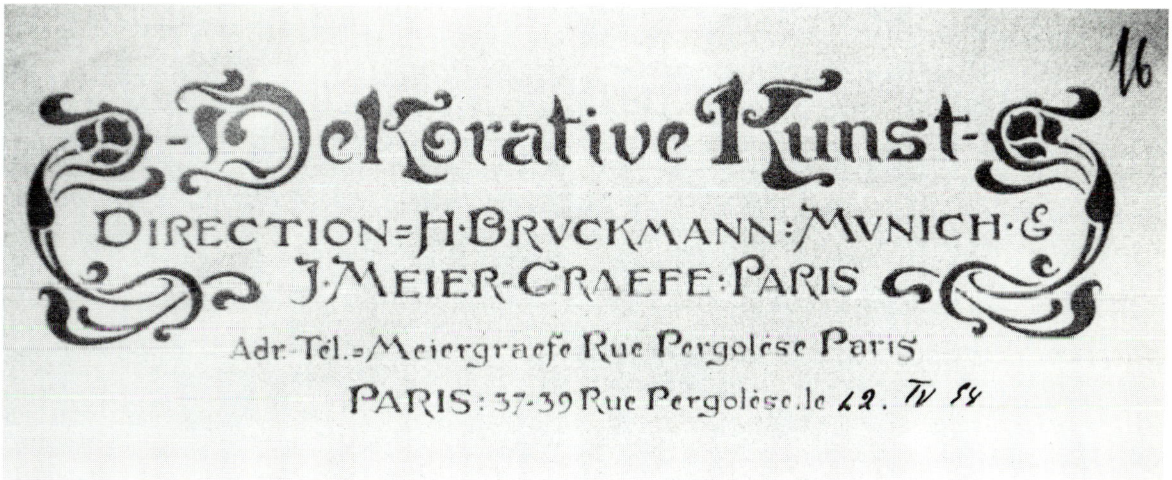

Fig. 8.6. Georges Lemmen. Stationery for Julius Meier-Graefe, c. 1897–98. Kaiser Wilhelm Museum Archive, Krefeld. Photo Kruty.

den International Exhibition of 1897. Under the banner of Bing's l'Art Nouveau, he exhibited the previously designed rooms for Bing's shop and a newly created lounge. As van de Velde reports, these rooms were greeted with great enthusiasm.

> Next morning awoke to find my name broadcast from end to end of Germany, and myself described as the man whose vigorous and completely untraditional conception of domestic decoration and design did not shrink from boldly severing the Gordian knot which for close on a century had kept the whole of Europe tied to servile imitations of past styles.[33]

This passage is characteristic of van de Velde's bombastic, florid style and his exaggerated sense of self-importance. Lemmen's name is conspicuously absent from this account.

The fame which came to van de Velde as a result of the Dresden exhibition was due in no small part to Meier-Graefe's influential acclaim.[34] When Meier-Graefe decided to contribute to the publishing boom with his own magazines, *Dekorative Kunst* in late 1897 and *l'Art Décoratif* in October 1898, he hired van de Velde to remodel his editorial office on rue Pergolèse in Paris. However, following Bing's lead, he commissioned posters and stationery (fig. 8.6) from Lemmen. Meier-Graefe's faith in the two Belgian artists was complete: the third issue of *Dekorative Kunst* included the first major article on Lemmen's decorative arts, reproducing his rugs, cushions, endpapers, and posters.[35] Similarly, the first issue of *l'Art Décoratif* was completely devoted to van de Velde and included wallpapers, bookbindings, and stained glass.[36] This article contained reproductions of the van de Velde/Lemmen smoking room for Bing and van de Velde's office for Meier-Graefe.[37] Above a doorway in the latter, Lemmen's poster for *Dekorative Kunst* is proudly hung next to Seurat's *Le Chahut*, which Meier-Graefe owned at this time. Meier-Graefe hired Lemmen as Belgian correspondent for *l'Art Décoratif* as well.[38]

A frequent visitor to Bing's gallery and personal friend of Meier-Graefe's was Count Harry Kessler. In 1898 van de Velde remodelled Kessler's Berlin apartment, but that same year Lemmen designed the young count's first major book, *Notizen über Mexico*, as well as Kessler's bookplate and bookplates for his circle of friends.[39] A series of Berlin commissions for van de Velde and Lemmen followed in rapid succession. In September 1898 the Keller & Reiner Gallery reopened in the salon created by van de Velde, and a month later van de Velde's art gallery for the publishers Bruno and Paul Cassirer was likewise ready for business.[40] Lemmen designed stationery and advertisements for both influential galleries. In Lemmen's Cassirer announcement (fig. 8.7), his hand drawn lettering has been purged of its florid arabesques and now has the consistency of movable type.

The repeated exposure of their oeuvre through Bing's gallery, journals, the yearly salons of La Libre Esthétique in Brussels, and the influential Dresden exhibition drew the attention of Friedrich Deneken, the progressive director of the Kaiser Wilhelm Museum in Krefeld. Determined to involve modern artists in the local textile industries, Deneken closely observed the various decorative arts movements. The first fruits of his work appeared shortly after the Kaiser Wilhelm Museum opened in 1897. Deneken mounted an exhibition of thirty new silk samples by Otto Eckmann, Willy von Beckerath, van de Velde, and Lemmen and wrote a preface to the catalogue about the "modern style in the textile arts."[41] By 1898 he was in constant correspondence with van de Velde, who came to visit the silk factories themselves and in August 1900 lectured on "Die künstlerische Hebung der Frauentracht" during the exhibition of artist-designed women's clothing at the museum.[42] Lemmen, too, was repeatedly invited and in 1898 showed fabrics and rugs at the exhibit "Künstlerischer Möbel und Geräte" along side works by Otto Eckmann and C. F. A. Voysey.[43]

Deneken relied on Meier-Graefe and Bing for advice and occasional samples from their galleries.[44] Although he often commissioned designs by mail, Deneken sometimes traveled to visit artists themselves. On 1 June 1898 he wrote to van de Velde of his intention to arrive in Brussels the following Friday "in order to explore all the

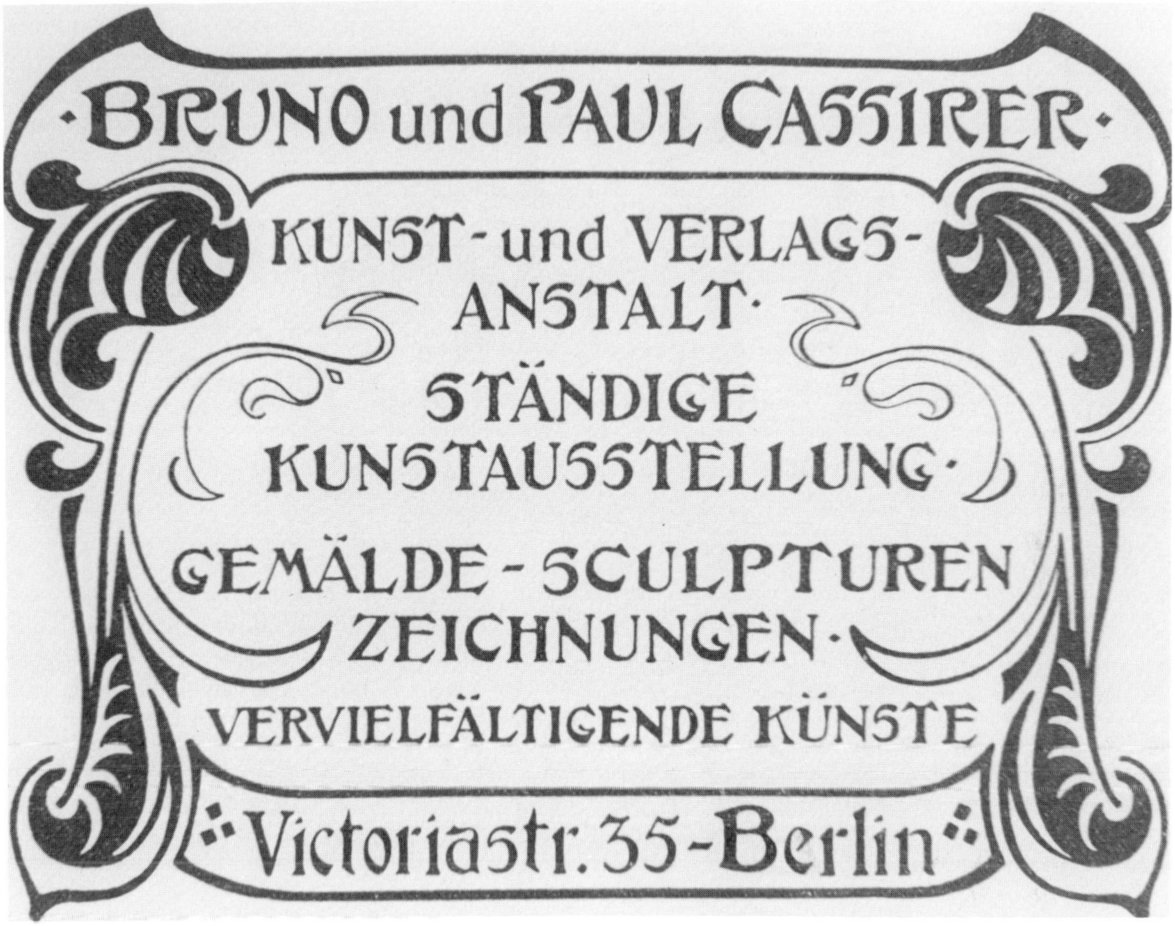

Fig. 8.7. Georges Lemmen. Announcement for Bruno and Paul Cassirer Gallery, 1898. From *l'Art Décoratif* 1 (1898): unpaginated advertisement.

shared interests of you and Herr Meier-Graefe."[45] He normally used van de Velde as an intermediary in dealing with Lemmen since, as he noted on 16 April 1898, "You are such good friends with Herr Lemmen."[46] The next year Deneken approached van de Velde with a local commission on the strength of the latter's supposed design for a magazine cover. Van de Velde declared that he, in fact, had not designed the cover and, neglecting to mention the name of the actual designer, Théo van Rysselberghe, instead recommended his associate as the man best qualified for the job.

> It wasn't I who created the cover for "Dekorative Kunst." I confess that at first glance the attribution is possible. . . . Yesterday I sent everything to my friend M. Lemmen, communicating to him your letter and explaining the impossibility in which I found myself of executing for you the masthead of a newspaper. . . . He promised to set to work today. He will send you directly his drawing and I am certain it will please you as much and more than one of mine.[47]

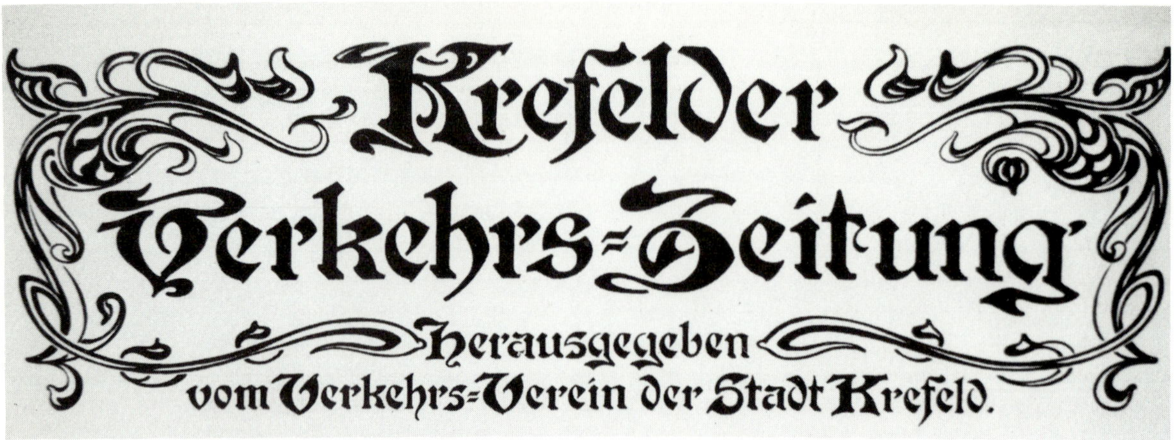

Fig. 8.8. Georges Lemmen. Drawing for masthead of the *Krefelder Verkehrszeitung*, c. 1899. Ink on paper, 175 × 497 cm. Kaiser Wilhelm Museum, Krefeld. Photo Kruty.

The banner which Lemmen created for the *Krefelder Verkehrszeitung* (fig. 8.8) continued in use for many years. For this weekly, to be printed in fraktur type, Lemmen provided a fusion of art nouveau with the traditional German lettering style. The original drawing was delivered to Deneken as promised by van de Velde and is still in the possession of the Kaiser Wilhelm Museum. It was exhibited in 1899 in Krefeld at an exhibition devoted to book arts, and in October 1899 the *Zeitschrift für Bücherfreunde* pronounced it "the only worthwhile artistic masthead of a German newspaper."[48]

At this time van de Velde and Lemmen continued to work on silk designs for Deneken. As van de Velde explained in the same note, ". . . We [he and Lemmen] are agreed to send you samples of various fabrics, but we still need three more weeks."[49] After 1900 van de Velde began working directly for the silk manufacturers Deuss and Oetker. On 21 January 1901, Deneken wrote to Lemmen in an attempt to connect him in a similar way to the firm of Mottau and Leendertz, dealers in velvet.

> Herr Van de Velde has already worked for a half year for one of the best-known silk factories. Now one of the leading velvet manufacturers also wishes to move in this direction. I am sending you separately several samples of pressed velvet for you to color.[50]

Unfortunately the designs Lemmen sent in April, after a fierce bout of influenza, did not please Herr Leendertz, and Lemmen's career in Krefeld came to an end.[51] Van de Velde remained in the service of Deuss and Oetker until after 1903.[52]

Encouraged by his reception especially in Germany, van de Velde formed his own company in Brussels, Arts d'Industrie et d'Ornamentation, in the fall of 1897 to manufacture his products. About the same time, Lemmen likewise decided to advertise his skills in the decorative arts and designed a letterhead with the same title (fig. 8.9). As van de Velde decorated his stationery with a "V" insignia, Lemmen adorned his own with a calligraphic "L."[53] Lemmen punningly referred to van de Velde's new trademark in a poster designed for a merchant of bottled water who coincidentally bore van de Velde's name.

Although van de Velde produced a sizable output of designs for posters, advertising, and bindings himself, in the commissions he shared with Lemmen he referred these to his partner, acknowledging Lemmen's growing reputation and ability in the separate world of typographic design.[54] Lemmen's interest in the creation of a modern lettering climaxed with another van de Velde collaboration, a deluxe edition of Friedrich Nietzsche's *Also Sprach Zarathustra* to be decorated by van de Velde, produced under the direction of Count Kessler, and published under the auspices of Nietzsche's literary executor, his sister Elizabeth Förster. In 1898 Lemmen was commissioned to design a new typeface for this monumental work. Though the book was not published until 1908, Lemmen and van de Velde each began working on their assignments in 1899.[55] The final product masterfully combines Lemmen's letters, derived from Roman faces but retaining several art nouveau idiosyncrasies, with van de Velde's later decorative style (fig. 8.10).

In September 1899 Meier-Graefe opened his own gallery for the display of contemporary decorative arts, La Maison Moderne.[56] He turned to van de Velde to redesign the existing facade and created a suitable interior with showcases and furnishings. As with the earlier series of galleries and Meier-Graefe's own office, Lemmen was assigned much of the graphic work.[57] He drew the advertising posters, stationery, and the lettering at the entrance. Although the monogram Lemmen created from "LMM," used with great frequency by Meier-Graefe, retains his characteristic art nouveau curves, the lettering he designed for van de Velde's severe exterior is more classic in form and reflects Lemmen's contemporary work on the *Zarathustra* typeface (fig. 8.11).[58]

Meier-Graefe's gallery came to supercede Bing's as the Parisian outlet for Lemmen's and van de Velde's work. By 1900 the two men had been replaced by a new set of primarily French artists at l'Art Nouveau, who created the rooms acclaimed at the Paris World's Fair and, two years later, in Turin.[59] Meier-Graefe, too, sent a range of products from the Maison Moderne to Turin, which included Lemmen's leather "Mappenwerke" and an embossed armchair.[60] In the nearby Belgian pavilion, van de Velde displayed furniture and bookbindings while his "collaboratore, G. Lemmen" showed rugs and drawings.[61]

In October 1900 van de Velde moved to Berlin to cultivate what he perceived to be richer ground. This move severed direct contact from his old friend, whose pleasure in traveling to France and England apparently did not extend to Germany.[62] Van de Velde, in his turn, was now less inclined to promote his Belgian associates. At the same time, Lemmen's independent dealings with *Die Insel* ended when the xenophobic editor Rudolph Schröder, who favored artists such as Heinrich Vogeler and E. R. Weiss, sought to purge the periodical of Belgian ornament.[63] Thus, when Lemmen stopped receiving commissions with van de Velde, his work for German clients ceased. The Germanization of van de Velde was made complete in 1902 when the Grand Duke of Saxe-Weimar appointed him his artistic advisor. Theoretical writings, such as *Die Renaissance in modernen Kunstgewerbe* (1901) and *Kunstgewerbliche Laienpredigten* (1902), continued to flow from van de Velde's pen, while his business and ability to sell his enthusiasm remained generally high. Lemmen, on the other hand, often felt the strain of limited finances and, in moments of despair, considered abandoning his artistic career.[64] His poverty, sickness, and family responsibilities prevented his move to Paris, as he now wished.

By 1903 the friendship between Lemmen and van de Velde had all but

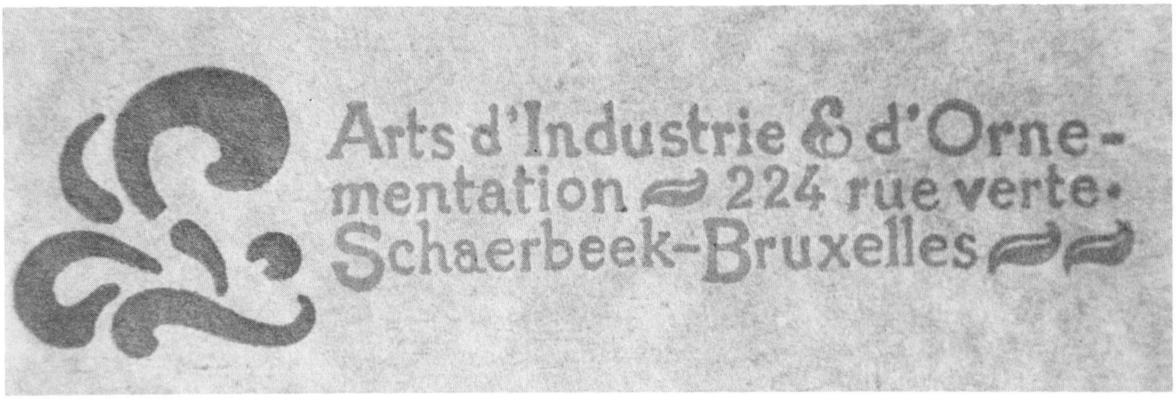

Fig. 8.9. Georges Lemmen. The artist's business stationery, c. 1897. Elisabeth Thevenin-Lemmen Collection, Toulon. Photo Kruty.

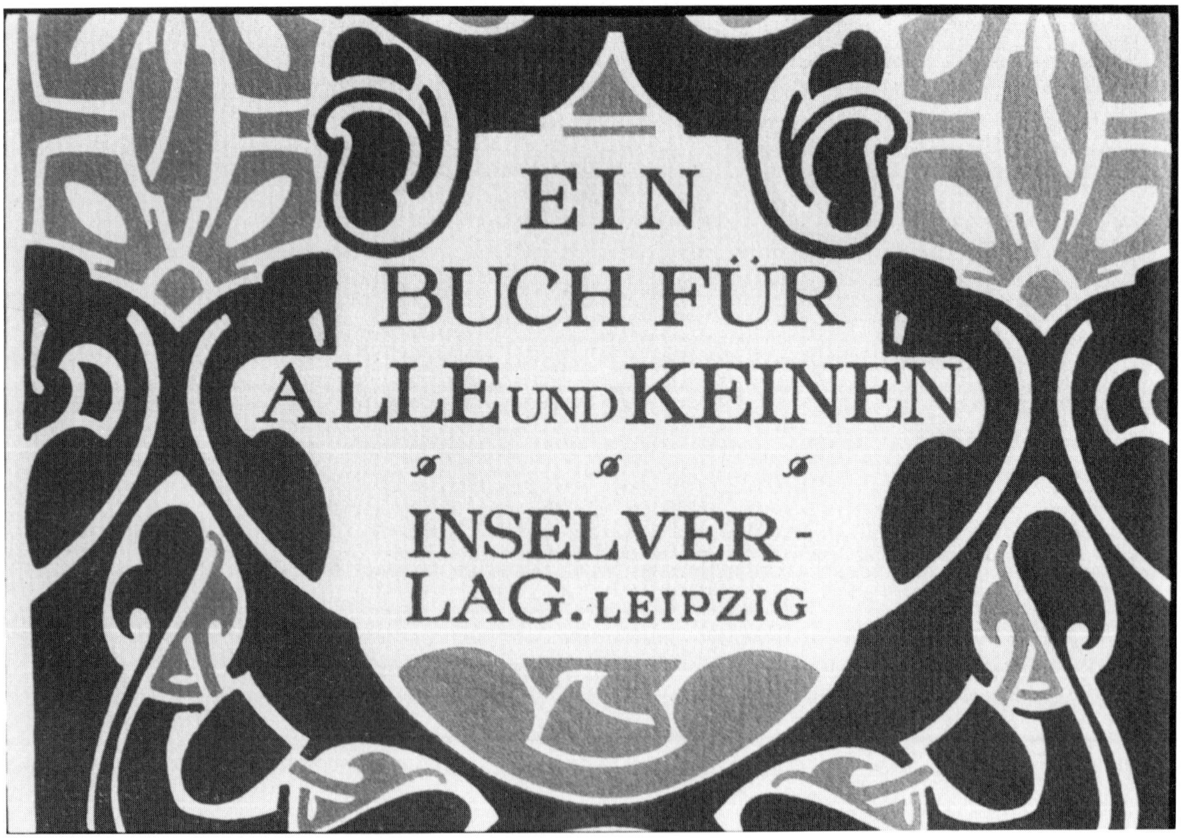

Fig. 8.10. Georges Lemmen and Henri van de Velde.
Title page for Friedrich Nietzsche's *Also Sprach Zarathustra*.
Leipzig: Insel Verlag. 1908. Princeton University Library. Photo Kruty.

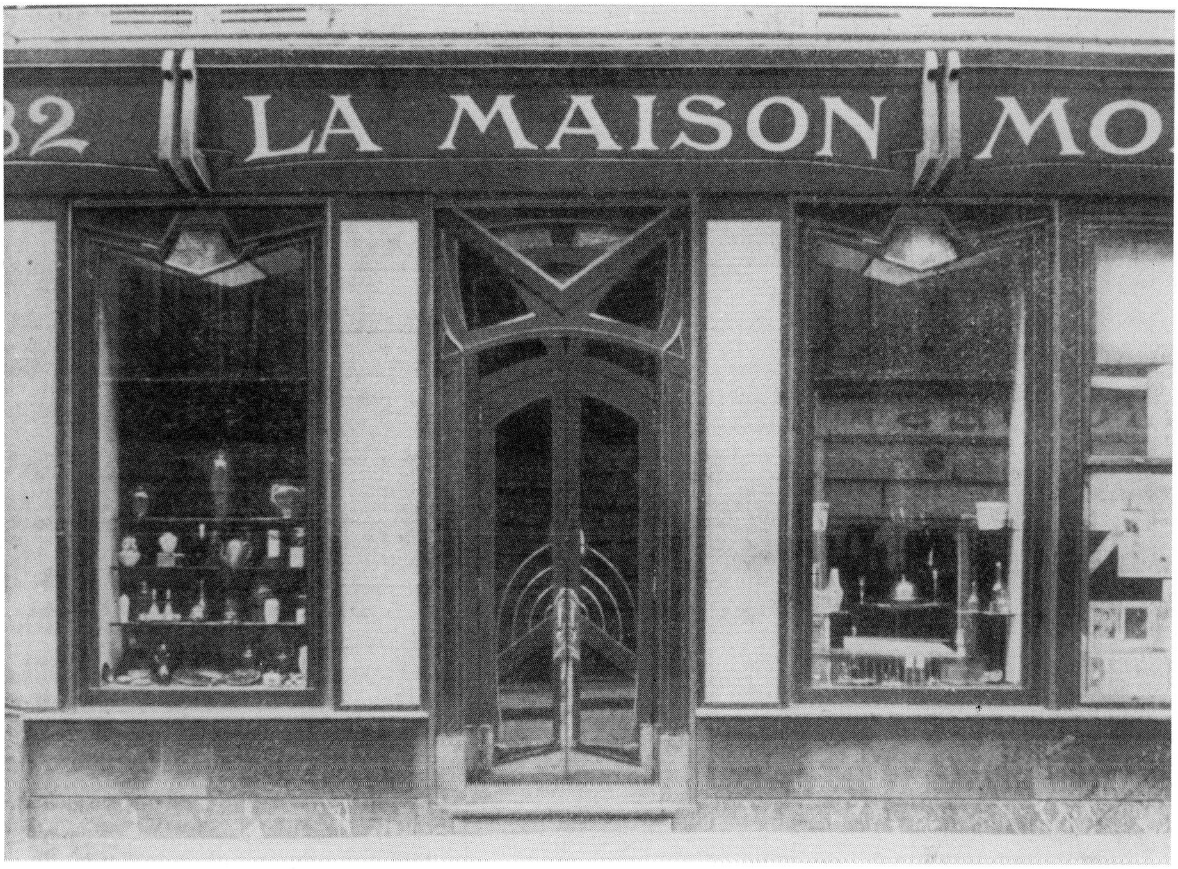

Fig. 8.11. Georges Lemmen and Henri van de Velde. Façade for Julius Meier-Graefe's La Maison Moderne, Paris, 1899. From *Deutsche Kunst und Dekoration* 7 (1900–1901): 99.

disappeared. Lemmen confessed to his friend Willy Finch his irritation at yet another complaining note from Maria van de Velde. The sycophantic Maria may have helped to widen the distance between van de Velde and Lemmen, but implicit in these remarks is a criticism of van de Velde as well.

> I just can't feel sorry for them. I really hate *cold* people, *utilitarianism,* and *big theories;* and I don't much care for grandiose ideas in tiny brains. "Our creations," "our house," "Henry's theories," . . . [65]

Thus ended more than a decade of close friendship and collaboration.

Brought together by their ardent interest in Les XX, Lemmen and van de Velde had shared their mutual discovery of the arts and crafts movement and played important roles in the creation of a new decorative style in Belgium which soon swept the continent. In 1895 their "friendly rivalry" turned into a partnership when they were invited to work together at Bing's Salon de l'Art Nouveau in Paris. What began as a marriage of convenience blossomed into a true romance in the next five years as the two went from commission to commission in France and Germany. After 1900 separate developments in their careers and a changing artistic climate in Belgium, France, and Germany effectively ended both the partnership and the friendship.

NOTES

The author would like to thank the following individuals for their assistance: Paul Kruty for his excellent counsel on typography and for reading and editing my manuscript; Jean Warmoes, Musée de la Littérature, Bibliothèque Royale, Brussels for access to the van de Velde papers; and Julian Heynen of the Kaiser Wilhelm Museum for help with the Krefeld documentation.

1. For the last point, see especially van de Velde's memoirs, *Geschichte meines Lebens*, ed. Hans Curjel (Munich: R. Piper & Co., 1962). Van de Velde's notes for this autobiography are housed in the Van de Velde Archive, Musée de la Littérature, Bibliothèque Royale, Brussels. Henry-Russell Hitchcock first rejected van de Velde's claim that he was the inventor of art nouveau. See H. R. Hitchcock's *Architecture: Nineteenth and Twentieth Centuries* (Harmondsworth, Middlesex: Penguin Books, 1958), 291.

2. "Petite Chronique," *l'Art Moderne* 19 (1 October 1899): 331; and Jean Loubier, "Die Kunst im Buchdruck," *Zeitschrift für Bücherfreunde* 2 (February 1899): 486.

3. "Die Kunst im Handwerk," *Jahrbuch der bildenden Kunst* 1 (1902): 57.

4. Karl Scheffler, "Eine Bilanz," *Dekorative Kunst* 6 (April 1903): 253.

5. Madeleine Octave Maus, *Trente années de lutte pour l'art* (Brussels: l'Oiseau Bleu, 1926; Brussels: Lebeer Hossmann, 1980), 85–86. The passage continues: "But we have seen through what paths the decorative arts led Van de Velde to his later career, while for Lemmen the creation of numerous models in the realm of applied arts never subverted his true calling as a painter." (All translations, unless otherwise indicated, are the author's.)

6. The one notable exception is Françoise Aubry, "G. Lemmen et les arts appliqués," in *G. Lemmen* (Brussels: Hortamuseum, 1980), 15–20.

7. In the fall of 1886 a friend of van de Velde's, the painter Adrien-Joseph Heymans, requested that Octave Maus, secretary of Les XX, visit van de Velde's atelier. Donation Albert Vanderlinden, 4733, Musées Royaux des Beaux-Arts de Belgique (hereafter cited as M.R.B.A.B.), Archives de l'art contemporain (hereafter cited as A.A.C.), Brussels. This suggestion was followed by Maus's emissary, Théo van Rysselberghe who reported on this visit to Maus. See M. J. Chartrain-Hebbelinck, "Les lettres de Van Rysselberghe à Octave Maus," *Bulletin des Musées Royaux des Beaux-Arts de Belgique* no. 1–2 (1966): 63–64.

8. For more information on Les XX and groups patterned after Les XX, see Jane Block, *Les XX and Belgian Avant-Gardism, 1868–1894* (Ann Arbor, Mich.: UMI Research Press, 1984).

9. "Petite Chronique," *La Wallonie* (15 January 1887): 69.

10. For additional information on the Belgian neoimpressionists see the following: Robert Herbert, *Neo-Impressionism* (New York: The Solomon R. Guggenheim Museum, 1968); Jean Sutter, *The Neo-Impressionists* (Greenwich, Conn.; New York Graphic Society, 1970); Ellen Lee, *The Aura of Neo-Impressionism: The W. J. Holliday Collection* (Indianapolis: Indiana University Press, 1983); *Exposition du Pointillisme* (Tokyo: Musée National d'art occidental, 1985).

11. Eekhoud's work was first published in 1888 by H. Kistemaeckers. On 20 April 1889, Lemmen wrote to Eekhoud asking permission to create a set of illustrations for the second edition that would capture the spirit of the work rather than literally transcribe passages. Lemmen to Eekhoud, 20 April 1889, Musée de la Littérature, Bibliothèque Royale, Brussels. Lemmen's illustration was, however, not used for Eekhoud's second edition, although Lemmen was sufficiently pleased with it to exhibit it repeatedly at Les XX in 1890, 1893, and at the Association pour l'Art in 1892.

12. This letter is cited in A. M. Hammacher's *Le monde de Henry van de Velde*, trans. Claudine Lemaire (Antwerp: Editions Fonds Mercator, 1967), 49–50. I wish to thank Roger Cardon, author of

the forthcoming catalogue raisonné of Lemmen's graphic oeuvre, for locating the original letter in the Archief en Museum voor het Vlaamse Cultuurleven, Antwerp, among the Elskamp-Van de Velde correspondence, E281 B. Contrary to Hammacher's statement that the letter is dated 1890, there is no written or postmarked date affixed to the letter. It seems more likely that the letter dates from 1891 when van de Velde was working on his initial project for the embroidery that was shown at Les XX in February–March 1892.

13. For a reproduction of this artistic document, see the exhibition catalogue *G. Lemmen* (Brussels: Hortamuseum, 1980), 17.

14. Georges Lemmen, "Chronique d'art: La Libre Esthétique," *Le Réveil* 4 (March 1894): 178.

15. "Artistic Wallpapers," *l'Art Moderne* 13 (18 June 1893): 193–95; and its sequel (25 June 1893): 202–204. For an extensive list and discussion of van de Velde's writings see Clemens L. Rességuier, *Die Schriften Henry Van de Veldes* (New York: The Delphic Press, 1955). This first article resulted from van de Velde's research for an upcoming course on applied arts to be taught at the Antwerp Academy. By this time he had not yet traveled to England. When he heard that his future wife, Maria Sèthe, would be visiting there, he asked her to visit the three firms of Morris, Jeffrey, and Essex for samples. (Henri van de Velde Archive, F.S.X. 784, Musée de la Littérature, Bibliothèque Royale, Brussels). Lemmen, by contrast journeyed to London at least twice in the early 1890s. Van de Velde later paid homage to William Morris not only by including him in his course on the applied arts but by lecturing in 1898 on "William Morris, Artisan et Socialist" at the Section d'art of the Maison du Peuple, the headquarters of the Parti Ouvrier Belge. This lecture was published under the same title in *l'Avenir Sociale* 3 (1898): 35–48, 65–67.

16. Lemmen wrote the article for the influential review and organ of Les XX, *l'Art Moderne*. See Georges Lemmen, "Walter Crane," *L'Art Moderne* (1 March 1891): 67–69 and its sequel (15 March 1891): 83–86. Lemmen followed this up four years later with a shorter piece on Crane: "Chronique d'art," *Le Réveil* 5 (February-March 1895): 154–55.

17. See for example Lemmen's articles in *l'Art Moderne*, "La Question des refusés," (23 March 1897): 164–65; "Exposition internationale à la Haye," (9 June 1901): 197–98; "Jakob Smits," (30 June 1901): 222–23; "Propos d'actualité," (6 March 1904): 73–75; "La Société des Peintres-Graveurs," (3 February 1907): 34–35.

18. This unofficial outpost of Les XX was bolstered with membership from Brussels. Boch, Toorop, Finch, George Minne, van Rysselberghe, and, of course, Lemmen and van de Velde exhibited there in 1892. Correspondence and documents for the Association pour l'Art is to be found at the Musée de la Littérature, Bibliothèque Royale, Brussels.

19. Kahn's name was suppressed (at his own request) as owner of the Seurats which were listed as *Les Poseuses*, *Embouchures de la Seine (Honfleur)* and drawings for *La Baignade* and *La Parade* (catalogue for the Association pour l'Art, 1892).

20. Lemmen to Toorop, Toorop Archive, May 1892, Koninklijke Bibliotheek, The Hague.

21. Van de Velde to Lucien Pissarro, 14 December 1894, Pissarro Archive, The Ashmolean Museum, Oxford.

22. Lemmen to Pissaro, 16 July 1891, Carton 86, dossier 1, liasse 7, Bibliothèque d'art et d'archéologie (Fondation Doucet), Paris. My thanks to Roger Cardon, Antwerp, for sharing this information with me.

23. Devoted to art and literature, *Van Nu en Straks* (1893–1901) sought to rival the French language reviews such as *l'Art Moderne* and *La Wallonie*. For further details see *Van Nu en Straks; Belle epoque en Vlaanderen* (Ghent: Centrum voor kunst en Cultuur, 1983). Lemmen considered some of the motifs used in *Van Nu en Straks* important enough to repeat in the French language periodical, *Le Réveil*.

24. For additional information on Bing see Samuel Bing, *Artistic America, Tiffany Glass, and Art Nouveau* (Cambridge, Mass.: M.I.T. Press, 1970); Robert Koch, "Art Nouveau Bing," *Gazette des Beaux-Arts*, 6th ser. 53 (March 1959): 179–90. Among the numerous articles by Gabriel P. Weisberg may be cited "Samuel Bing: Patron of Art Nouveau," *The Connoisseur*, 172 (October 1969): 119–25; 172 (December 1969): 294–99; 173 (January 1970): 61–68. Also see Weisberg, *Art Nouveau Bing* (New York, 1986), where Bing's name is established as Siegfried.

25. The account of van de Velde's first meeting with Bing is available in van de Velde's memoirs, *Geschichte meines Lebens*, 102–111. See also "Henry van de Velde: Extracts from his Memoirs: 1891–1901," ed. P. Morton Shand, *Architectural Review* 112 (September 1952): 151–53. An unpublished version

is available at the van de Velde archive, "Histoire de ma vie," farde 26, 12–13, Musée de la Littérature, Bibliothèque Royale, Brussels.

26. The essay "Déblaiement d'art," was issued in *La Société Nouvelle* (April 1894): 444–56 and published as a separate volume also in 1894 (Brussels: Mme Vve. Monnom). Meier-Graefe mentioned the Brussels enterprise in the periodical *Pan;* see "Notizen-Verschiedenes," *Pan* 1 (April-May 1895): 47.

27. Van de Velde, *Geschichte meines Lebens,* 104; and *l'Art Moderne* 16 (19 January 1896): 22. In addition to reviews in *l'Art Moderne,* the principal source of information on the Maison d'Art are the eight brochures published by Edmond Picard in 1895 under the heading *Maison d'Art, "A la Toison d'Or"* (Brussels: P. Weissenbruch). The Maison d'Art was founded on 7 March 1894 as the Société Anonyme l'Art by Octave Maus, Edmond Picard, Emile Verhaeren, and Charles Buls. By the end of 1894 its headquarters were 56 avenue de la Toison d'Or, home of Edmond Picard. Picard, a lawyer and co-founder of *l'Art Moderne,* ran the gallery with one of his three sons, William. The gallery was later enlarged and reopened 10 December 1895; see *l'Art Moderne* 16 (19 July 1896): 229 and F.(ernand) K.(hnopff), "Studio Talk," *Studio* 7 (February 1896): 50. Brochure 2 describes the Italianate-Flemish Renaissance *hôtel* with its exhibition, theatrical, concert, and lecture facilities.

28. The two quotations come from Brochure 1, "A la Toison d'or: Une Maison d'art à Bruxelles," 5, and Brochure 2, "Notice sur la Maison d'art," 7.

29. Posters for the Maison d'Art designed by Gisbert Combaz and Emile Berchmans may be found in the catalogue by Yoland Oostens-Wittamer, *L'Affiche Belge 1872–1914* (Brussels: Bibliothèque Royale, 1975).

30. Lemmen had in fact created a rug with a strikingly similar design. See his article, "Moderne Teppiche," *Dekorative Kunst* 1 (1898): 103. For a list of Lemmen's entries to the Salon de l'Art Nouveau see *Exhibitions of Art Nouveau* (New York: Garland Publishing Co., 1981).

31. These ads were reproduced in *l'Art Décoratif* 1 (October 1898). The poster, manifesto, invitation, and a late ad for Bing are reproduced in the exhibition catalogue *Japonismus und art nouveau: Europaïsche Graphik aus den Sammlungen des Museums für Kunst und Gewerbe Hambrug* (1981).

32. Lemmen writes to Kessler that Bing in 1897 had exhausted his stock of endpapers. Lemmen to Harry Kessler, 24 April 1898, Harry Kessler Papers, The Newberry Library, Chicago.

33. "Henry van de Velde: Extracts from his Memoirs: 1891–1901," 155.

34. Ibid.

35. O. G. Destrée, "Die Schmuckkünstler Belgiens: Georges Lemmen," *Dekorative Kunst* 1 (1898): 105–111. See also Lemmen's own article "Moderne Teppiche," *Dekorative Kunst* 1 (1898): 97–105.

36. *L'Art Décoratif* 1 (October 1898): 1–48. In addition, issue number 12 of *l'Art Décoratif* (September 1899) was devoted to the work of Lemmen, Finch, and van de Velde.

37. Ibid., *L'Art Décoratif,* Oct., 1898, 19, 25.

38. Georges Lemmen, "Bruxelles," *l'Art Décoratif* 1 (October 1898): 47.

39. Harry Graf Kessler, *Notizen über Mexico* (Berlin: F. Fontane & Co., 1898). The book has been reprinted without Lemmen's designs: Frankfurt-am-Main: Insel-Verlag, 1964. Lemmen's work for the *Notizen* was cited along with other important book designers at the fin-de-siècle in "Bucherschau: Modernen Buch-Schmuck in der Praxis," *Deutsche Kunst und Dekoration* 4 (April-September 1899): 384. For additional information on Kessler see his *Souvenirs d'un Européen,* trans. Blaise Briod, (Paris: Librairie Plon, 1936) and Alan Fern, "The Count and the Calligrapher," *Apollo* 79 (March 1964): 214–220.

40. Keller & Reiner Gallery was located at 122 Potsdamerstrasse, Berlin. It featured the decorative arts and showed works of Emile Gallé, Daumis Daum, Louis Majorelle, and Louis Comfort Tiffany. In addition, Lemmen showed his own works at the gallery. See "Die Wohnungsausstellung von Keller & Reiner in Berlin," *Die Kunst* 4 (1901): 211; "Petite Chronique," *l'Art Moderne* 21 (20 October 1901): 352; H.R., "Von Ausstellungen und Sammlungen," *Die Kunst für Alle* 17 (1 February 1902): 214. In fact Lemmen's rug (unidentified as such) is shown repeatedly in ads for the gallery's "Modernes Herrenzimmer." See *Dekorative Kunst* (1898) and *Die Kunst* 8 (November 1903). For a photograph of van de Velde's entrance hall see G. G., "Studio Talk," *The International Studio* 6 (February 1899): 286, and for a discussion of van de Velde's work see: "Sammlungen und Ausstellungen," *Die Kunstchronik,* neue folge, 10 (13 October 1898): 12–13. The Cassirer Gallery opened 1 October 1898 with an exhibition of the works of Edgar Degas, Con-

stantin Meunier, and Max Liebermann. See *l'Art Décoratif* (1 October 1898): 48. In 1901 Bruno and Paul Cassirer published van de Velde's *Die Renaissance in Modernen Kunstgewerbe.*

41. Gerda Breuer, "Deneken und die Krefelder Textilindustrie," in *Der westdeutsche Impuls: 1900–1914: Von der künstlerseide zur Industriefotografie* (Krefeld: Kaiser Wilhelm Museum, 1984), 91.

42. The lecture was published by Kramer & Baum of Krefeld in 1900. Maria van de Velde wrote the introduction to an album on women's clothing: *Album modernen nach Künstlerentwürfen ausgeführter Damenkleider* (Dusseldorf: Friedrich Wolfrum, 1898). For additional information on the Krefeld silk industry see Herbert Kisch, *Prussian Mercantilism and the Rise of the Krefeld Silk Industry: Variations Upon an Eighteenth-Century Theme,* Transaction of the American Philosophical Society, 58, no. 7 (Philadelphia, 1968); Hae-Bon Chung, "Das Krefelder Seidengewerbe in 19. Jahrhundert (1815–80)" (Ph.D. diss., Bonn, 1974).

43. Ausstellung Künstlerischer Möbel und Geräte (Krefeld: Kaiser Wilhelm Museum, 1898). Lemmen's entries are numbers 88–90. For additional information on the museum, see "Kaiser Wilhelm-Museum zu Crefeld," *Deutsche Kunst und Dekoration* 1 (January 1898): 140; "Studio Talk-Crefeld," *Studio* 13 (April 1898): 203–4.

44. Meier-Graefe to Deneken, 13 March 1899, #61, Kaiser Wilhelm Museum (hereafter cited as KWM), Krefeld. See also Bing correspondence in the KWM.

45. Deneken to van de Velde, 1 June 1898, #14, KWM, Krefeld.

46. Deneken to van de Velde, 16 April 1898, #11, KWM, Krefeld.

47. Van de Velde to Deneken, undated, #102, KWM, Krefeld.

48. Walter von zur Westen, "Der kunstlerische Buchumschag," *Zeitschrift für Bücherfreunde* (October 1899): 261. According to the City Archive in Krefeld, the Lemmen design was still being used as masthead in November 1903. Letter to author, 12 March 1984.

49. Van de Velde to Deneken, undated, #102, KWM, Krefeld.

50. Deneken to Lemmen, 21 January 1901, #62, KWM, Krefeld.

51. Deneken to Lemmen, 30 April 1901, #97, KWM, Krefeld. Lemmen wrote three replies to Deneken regarding the velvet designs: 24 January 1901, #65; 12 April 1901, #89; 20 April 1901, #94.

52. E., "Künstler-Seide von Deuss & Oetker in Krefeld," *Die Kunst* 8 (1903): 59–62.

53. For a reproduction of van de Velde's stationery see *Henry van de Velde, 1863–1957* (Brussels: Palais des Beaux-Arts, 1963), opposite p. 36. For Lemmen's poster for L. Vandevelde & Cie, see *G. Lemmen* (Brussels: Hortamuseum, 1980), 18.

54. Lemmen was included in Rudolf von Larisch's prestigious *Beispiele Kunstlerlischer Schrift* (Vienna: Anton Schroll and Co., 1900). Along with Lemmen's entry of artistic lettering were those of compatriot van Rysselberghe, his idol Walter Crane, and Otto Eckmann, Kolomon Moser, A. M. Mucha, Weiss among others.

55. Lemmen's execution of a new typeface which was cut and cast put him in the select group of other artist-typographers such as Eugène Grasset, Georges Auriol, Otto Eckmann, and Peter Behrens. For additional information on the genesis of the *Zarathustra* edition, the cult of Nietzsche and the collaboration of Lemmen, van de Velde, and Kessler, see the author's forthcoming *Pantheon* article, "The Insel Verlag Zarathustra: an Untold Tale of Art and Printing." For a synopsis of this, see Jane Block, "The Insel Verlag Edition of Nietzsche's Also Sprach Zarathustra," *The Princeton University Library Chronicle* 46 (Spring 1985): 321–23.

56. For more information on Meier-Graefe, see Kenworth Moffett, *Meier-Graefe as art critic,* Studien zur Kunst des neunzehnten Jahrhunderts, vol. 19 (Munich: Prestel Verlag, 1973). For more on La Maison Moderne see *Documents sur l'Art Industriel au Vingtième Siècle* (Paris: La Maison Moderne, 1901); "Exposition à la Maison Moderne," *Revue Blanche* 21 (1900–1901): 620–22; Julius Meier-Graefe, "La Maison Moderne," *Die Zukunft* 38 (January 1902): 279–84; Max Osborn, "La Maison Moderne in Paris," *Deutsche Kunst und Dekoration* 7 (November 1900): 99–103.

57. Other posters were designed for La Maison Moderne by Maurice Biais and Manuel Orazi.

58. The "LMM" monogram was skillfully used by Lemmen in the endpapers to Meier-Graefe's *Documents sur l'Art Industriel au Vingtième Siècle* and in a poster for his shop; see *G. Lemmen*

(Brussels: Hortamuseum, 1980), 22. Meier-Graefe closely followed the development of the *Zarathustra* typeface. In 1904 he lamented its failure to yet appear in *Entwicklungsgeschichte der modernen Kunst*, vol. 2, (Stuttgart: Jul. Hoffman, 1904), 666, n. 1.

59. Martin Eidelberg sees this as a conscious decision on Bing's part. See M. Eidelberg, *E. Colonna* (Dayton, Ohio: The Institute, 1983): 40.

60. "Die Sektion Frankreich," *Dekorative Kunst* 12 (September 1902); 460; and "Die Französischen Gewerbe Künste auf der Turiner Ausstellung," *Deutsche Kunst und Dekoration* 11 (January, 1903): 171.

61. Vittoria Pica, "La sezione Belga," *L'Arte decorativa all' Esposizione di Torino del 1902* (Bergamo: Istituto Italiano d'arti grafiche, 1903): 34. See also, Georg Fuchs, "Die Belgische abteilung auf der Turiner Ausstellung," *Deutsche Kunst und Dekoration* 11 (October 1902–March 1903): 147–160.

62. Lemmen may, in fact, have traveled to Leipzig in 1901 to supervise the proofs for his *Zarathustra* typography, but evidence is not conclusive. Lemmen to Toorop, 23 June 1901, Koninklijke Bibliotheek. The Hague.

63. Schröder expressed dissatisfaction with Lemmen's work upon seeing the proofs which arrived during his absence and saw that "eine Unmenge schauderhaften 'Buchschmuckes' von der Hand eines Herrn Lemmen aus Brüssel nicht nur eingetroffen war, sondern schon—nach der unleidlichen Manier jener Tage in diversen Verkleinerungen und Vergrösserungen gegossen—auf Probeblättern vorlag." See Klaus Schöffling, *Die ersten Jahre des Insel Verlags, 1899–1902* (Frankfurt-am-Main: Insel Verlag, 1981), 13.

64. Lemmen to Finch, 21 June 1902, 21809/1; 6 April 1907, 21809/16; 1 October 1907, 21809/20, M.R.B.A.B., A.A.C., Brussels.

65. Lemmen to Finch, 26 March 1903, 21809/8, M.R.B.A.B., A.A.C., Brussels.

9

ART and MUSIC at the SALONS de la ROSE + CROIX, 1892–1897

LAURINDA S. DIXON

"WE ALL KNOW in our own day, in the winters of 1892 and 1893, what nonsense there was in Paris over a revival of interest in this apparently vanished sect. ... Besides the picture exhibition, lecture courses were given—dull, of course; and plays also," wrote Alice Morse Earle in her popular and entertaining book of 1902, *Sun-Dials and Roses of Yesterday.*[1] Mrs. Earle was certain that the outrageous occurrences in fin-de-siècle Paris would never be forgotten—ridiculed, perhaps, but not forgotten. Reading her words three quarters of a century later, however, our memories strain to identify the subject of her derision—art nouveau? Postimpressionism? neoimpressionism? Not likely. These movements have been rescued only recently from the obscurity of the avant-garde and probably would not have been recognized by Alice Earle. The object of Mrs. Earle's discontent was Rosicrucianism, an old sect briefly revived in the late nineteenth century as a mystical order of artists and intellectuals led by their "Sâr," Joséphin Péladan.[2] The French Rose + Croix was concerned with restoring spiritualism and idealism to the arts by means of annual shows that reflected the group's philosophy. These salons, held between 1892 and 1897, were among the most curious events in the history of art.[3]

ROSICRUCIANISM in the CONTEXT of the LATE NINETEENTH CENTURY

Péladan's sect took its name from seventeenth-century Rosicrucianism, an occult movement which provided an aura of obscurity and ritual to which fin-de-siècle mystics were strongly attracted.[4] Members of the mythic sect claimed to possess superhuman, if not supernatural, powers. They held the secret of the "philosopher's stone," which gave them immortality, eternal wisdom, and the power to foretell the future. Seventeenth-century Rosicrucianism owed its emblems and symbols to alchemy, an ancient philosophy which had ceased to function as a legitimate science but remained powerful as a philosophy.[5] Nineteenth-century Rosicrucians further abstracted and occultized the old images and allegories, obscuring any vestige of utilitarianism by an overlay of philosophical, psychological abstractions, rooted in the turbulent social and intellectual climate of the time. They found inspiration in the libraries and archives of Paris, which were rich in holdings of ancient texts illustrated in the bizarre and esoteric visual language of a long lost, arcane science.[6]

The late nineteenth century was ripe for the Rosicrucian rebellion against the materialism of the industrial age, the unrelenting realism of the camera, and all other destroyers of spiritual idealism. The public was barraged with occultist periodicals[7] and mystical novels, while seances, ouija boards, and automatic writing were the parlor games of the fashionable elite. The artistic salons of the Rose + Croix catered to the same public tastes and were tremendously popular, drawing as many as 15,000 curious viewers in a single day.[8] The list of 231 invited participants was international in scope, including artists from France, Belgium, Switzerland, and Spain.[9] The works of Gustave Moreau, the English Pre-Raphaelites, and Puvis de Chavannes were exhibited as models for emulation, though the cautious Puvis protested strongly against this involuntary mentorship.[10] At the first salon of 1892, a large Manet hung in the foyer of the Gallerie Durand Ruel, where it was heckled and otherwise reviled as having been "painted with the elbow."[11] As a realist work, it represented all that the Rose + Croix preached against.

Joséphin Péladan's avowed intention was to ruin realism. He called for men of superior intellect to restore the "ideal," with tradition as its base and beauty as its means. The prescribed vehicles, listed in the Rosicrucian Manifesto of 1892, were subjects drawn from "the Catholic Ideal and mysticism . . . legend, myth, allegory, the dream, the paraphrase of great poetry, and finally all lyricism." History painting, genre, portraits (except those of the Sâr Péladan and the "super human" Wagner), landscapes, animals, still life, and "all humorous things" were banned.[12] In true monastic fashion, women were excluded from participation. Exceptions were made, however, for those humble female servants who wished to donate money to the order.[13] Initiates were hailed as priests, kings, and magi and summoned by the question, "Artists—do you believe in the Pantheon and St. Ouen, in Leonardo and in the Nike of Samothrace, in Beethoven and Parsifal? You will be admitted to the Rose + Croix."[14]

With the mention of the works of Beethoven and Wagner *(Parsifal)*, the Rosicrucian Manifesto linked musical and artistic philosophies in the common pursuit of a spiritual ideology. Péladan, echoing the symbolist poets of his day, believed that music possessed the incantory power to reveal the unconscious and the occult.[15] Accordingly, the catalogues of the salons de la Rose + Croix indicate that concerts were part of the exhibitions and that artistic contemplation was accompanied by sound. At first glance, these musical programs give the impression of variety and balanced eclecticism, featuring works by both early and contemporary composers (figs. 9.1 and 9.2). Indeed, it is difficult for a modern music lover to compare the musical "incantations" of Mme. Corrylange Moogenboom with the music of Mozart, Wagner, and Satie based upon anything other than variety and contrast. In the context of the Rose + Croix, however, music augmented the sense of sight and was therefore considered indispensable to the spiritual contemplation of art. In fact, the music and art of the salons de la Rose + Croix were specifically and intimately related by means of shared values and mutual ideals.

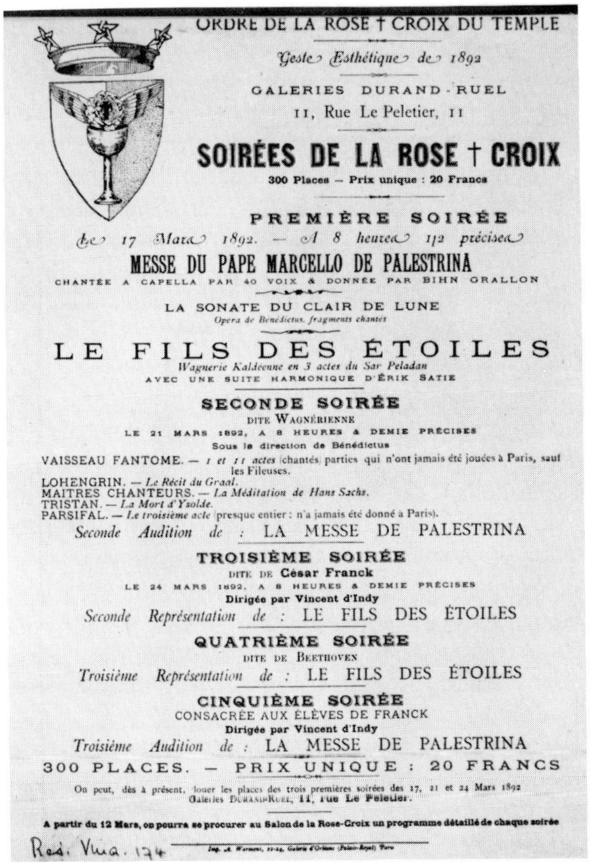

ORDRE DE LA ROSE † CROIX DU TEMPLE

Geste Esthétique de 1892

GALERIES DURAND-RUEL

11, Rue Le Peletier, 11

SOIRÉES DE LA ROSE † CROIX

300 Places — Prix unique : 20 Francs

PREMIÈRE SOIRÉE

Le 17 Mars 1892. — A 8 heures 1/2 précises

MESSE DU PAPE MARCELLO DE PALESTRINA

CHANTÉE A CAPELLA PAR 40 VOIX & DONNÉE PAR BIHN GRALLON

LA SONATE DU CLAIR DE LUNE

Opera de Benédictus, fragments chantés

LE FILS DES ÉTOILES

Wagnerie Kaldéenne en 3 actes du Sar Peladan

AVEC UNE SUITE HARMONIQUE D'ÉRIK SATIE

SECONDE SOIRÉE

DITE WAGNÉRIENNE

LE 21 MARS 1892, A 8 HEURES & DEMIE PRÉCISES

Sous la direction de Bénédictus

VAISSEAU FANTOME. — *I et II actes* (chantés) parties qui n'ont jamais été jouées à Paris, sauf les Fileuses.

LOHENGRIN. — *Le Récit du Graal.*

MAITRES CHANTEURS. — *La Méditation de Hans Sachs.*

TRISTAN. — *La Mort d'Ysolde.*

PARSIFAL. — *Le troisième acte* (presque entier : n'a jamais été donné à Paris).

Seconde Audition de : LA MESSE DE PALESTRINA

TROISIÈME SOIRÉE

DITE DE César Franck

LE 24 MARS 1892, A 8 HEURES & DEMIE PRÉCISES

Dirigée par Vincent d'Indy

Seconde Représentation de : LE FILS DES ÉTOILES

QUATRIÈME SOIRÉE

DITE DE BEETHOVEN

Troisième Représentation de : LE FILS DES ÉTOILES

CINQUIÈME SOIRÉE

CONSACRÉE AUX ÉLÈVES DE FRANCK

Dirigée par Vincent d'Indy

Troisième Audition de : LA MESSE DE PALESTRINA

300 PLACES. — PRIX UNIQUE : 20 FRANCS

On peut, dès à présent, louer les places des trois premières soirées des 17, 21 et 24 Mars 1892 Galeries DURAND-RUEL, 11, rue Le Peletier.

A partir du 12 Mars, on pourra se procurer au Salon de la Rose-Croix un programme détaillé de chaque soirée

Res. Vma. 174

Fig. 9.1. Concert advertisement, *Ordre de la Rose + Croix du Temple, Geste Esthétique*, 1892. Courtesy of the Library of Congress, Washington, D.C.

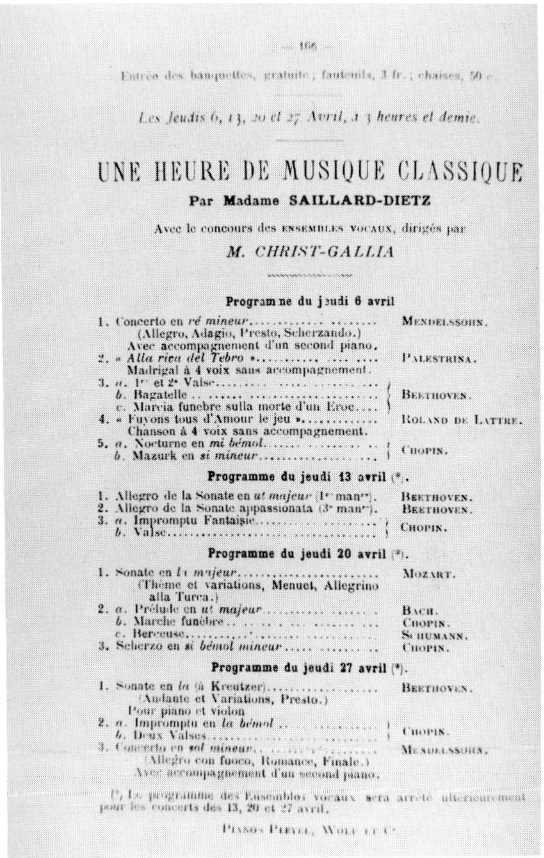

— 166 —

Entrée des banquettes, gratuite ; fauteuils, 3 fr. ; chaises, 50 c.

Les Jeudis 6, 13, 20 et 27 Avril, à 3 heures et demie.

UNE HEURE DE MUSIQUE CLASSIQUE

Par Madame SAILLARD-DIETZ

Avec le concours des ENSEMBLES VOCAUX, dirigés par

M. CHRIST-GALLIA

Programme du jeudi 6 avril

1. Concerto en *ré mineur*........ MENDELSSOHN.
   (Allegro, Adagio, Presto, Scherzando.)
   Avec accompagnement d'un second piano.
2. « *Alla riva del Tebro* »........ PALESTRINA.
   Madrigal à 4 voix sans accompagnement.
3. *a*. 1re et 2e Valse........ / *b*. Bagatelle........ / c. Marcia funebre sulla morte d'un Eroe.... } BEETHOVEN.
4. « Fuyons tous d'Amour le jeu »........ ROLAND DE LATTRE.
   Chanson à 4 voix sans accompagnement.
5. *a*. Nocturne en *mi bémol*........ / *b*. Mazurk en *si mineur*........ } CHOPIN.

Programme du jeudi 13 avril (*).

1. Allegro de la Sonate en *ut majeur* (1re manre). BEETHOVEN.
2. Allegro de la Sonate appassionata (3e manre). BEETHOVEN.
3. *a*. Impromptu Fantaisie........ / *b*. Valse........ } CHOPIN.

Programme du jeudi 20 avril (*).

1. Sonate en *la majeur*........ MOZART.
   (Thème et variations, Menuet, Allegrino alla Turca.)
2. *a*. Prélude en *ut majeur*........ BACH.
   b. Marche funèbre........ CHOPIN.
   c. Berceuse........ SCHUMANN.
3. Scherzo en *si bémol mineur*........ CHOPIN.

Programme du jeudi 27 avril (*).

1. Sonate en *la* (à Kreutzer)........ BEETHOVEN.
   (Andante et Variations, Presto.)
   Pour piano et violon
2. *a*. Impromptu en *la bémol*........ / *b*. Deux Valses........ } CHOPIN.
3. Concerto en *sol mineur*........ MENDELSSOHN.
   (Allegro con fuoco, Romance, Finale.)
   Avec accompagnement d'un second piano.

(*) Le programme des Ensembles vocaux sera arrêté ultérieurement pour les concerts des 13, 20 et 27 avril.

PIANOS PLEYEL, WOLF ET Cie.

Fig. 9.2. Concert advertisement, Ordre Laïque de la Rose + Croix du Temple et du Graal, Second Geste Esthétique, *Catalogue Officiel Illustré du Salon*, p. 166.

The WAGNERIAN SYNTHESIS

It is not surprising, then, that the guiding star of the French Rose + Croix movement was not a venerable artist, as one would expect, but the composer-philosopher Richard Wagner. In fact, the initial manifesto of the French Rose + Croix movement was drawn up in a flurry of inspiration after a performance of Wagner's *Lohengrin*.[16] Thereafter, Wagner's name was reverently intoned as a spiritual beacon to members of the order, appearing on the programs of every salon. The grand opening of the first exhibition in 1892 was heralded by a "Solemn Mass of the Holy Ghost," during which selections from Wagner's *Parsifal* were played. Four days later, a musical soirée dedicated to Wagner featured selections from *Tristan und Isolde, Meistersinger, Lohengrin,* and *Parsifal*.[17] The following year featured lectures at the piano by one "Benedictus" on the subject of *Parsifal,* with commentary by Péladan.[18] The years of the salons de la Rose + Croix marked a high point in Péladan's fascination with Wagner, evidenced by his scene-by-scene analysis of the Wagner music dramas published in 1895.[19]

The works of art exhibited at the salons reflected the musical presence of Wagner, paying homage to the story lines of certain music dramas. In addition to the inevitable portraits of Wagner, images of Lohengrin and Parsifal appeared as role models for modern Rosicrucians. In the Wagnerian mythology, these two knights were legendary guardians of the Holy Grail—pure, wise, and constantly tempted by female wiles to which they remained stoicly impervious. The "grail," once an alchemical symbol for the universal elixir, symbolized the Rosicrucian "ideal."[20] The allegorical search for the grail became the artist's search for the ideal, while Woman, particularly *Parsifal*'s Kundry and *Lohengrin*'s Elizabeth, represented the opposing lure of the real world. Amfortas, *Parsifal*'s Grand Master of the Grail, was also a popular subject. In fact, Bernard Du Pasquier's *Study for an Amfortas* exhibited in 1892 was actually a thinly disguised portrait of the Sâr Péladan. As "Grand Master," his official capacity in the hierarchy of the Rose + Croix corresponded to that of Amfortas in *Parsifal*.[21]

The Wagnerian presence at the salons de la Rose + Croix embraced far more than subject matter. The exhibitions were part of a veritable cult derived from the composer's music and writings.[22] Among the ideas shared by the Rose + Croix and Wagnerian philosophy were the concept of a union of the arts; the symbol; ambiguity; ambivalence toward women; the notion of ancient racial pride accompanied by fascination with a long lost, "glorious" past; social and intellectual reform; religious fervor; and, above all, the glorification of the role of the artist in society. In fact, Wagner's oft-stated philosophies read like a paraphrase of the Rosicrucian Manifesto.[23] One might well ask what attracted the delicate, decadent Rosicrucian aesthetic to the storm and stress of the Wagnerian music drama?

French symbolists were strongly drawn to the concept of the unification of the arts embodied in the Wagnerian *Gesamtkunstwerk*.[24] Wagner wrote his own libretti and supervised scenery design, but he was first of all a musician, and he emphasized the role of music above art and poetry in his artistic synthesis. It was his belief that the earliest forms of speech were musical; therefore, music was closest to the first pure universal mode of communication. Wagner believed that sound was capable of bypassing the veneer of acquired human culture, reaching the emotions directly. He justified this theory by citing a lofty example—ancient Greek declamatory verse—which he believed to have been sung rather than spoken.[25]

The Rosicrucians shared with Wagner the belief in a lost universal language. They, however, believed that the most direct route to the subconscious, the "soul," was through visual images, which are not dependent upon notes as intermediary vehicles of interpretation. In Péladan's theory of synesthesia, the written word evoked images in the imagination, while music produced a volatile impression that aided in the contemplation of these images. Music, language, and art mingled in each human soul, "sounding the keys of an interior clavier."[26] Like the symbolist poets, Péladan drew correspondences between the colors and moods evoked by Wagner's music, designating, for example, *Lohengrin* as grey-blue and *Tristan* as purple.[27] However, the musical notation necessary to Wagner's craft, was believed to put distance between art and thought. Because the visual arts require neither notes nor alphabets, Péladan raised art above music, declaring, "The painter alone employs the forms and colors of reality heard by all men."[28]

The symbol was important to both the Wagnerian *Gesamtkunstwerk* and the art of the Rose + Croix. Wagner's musical symbols, which he called *leitmotifs*, were equivalent in every sense to the visual symbols employed by fin-de-siècle artists. In the music of Wagner, the leitmotif is heard when its corresponding meaning is alluded to either directly or indirectly in the narrative. It accompanies its representation throughout the music drama, often cropping up independently to remind the listener of his, her, or its existence—sometimes inverted, augmented, ornamented, or interwoven with other leitmotifs to suit the scene or mood in which it appears.[29] Likewise, the emblematic swans, lilies, and sphinxes in symbolist paintings evoke a psychological context, which differs according to the unique state of each viewer's soul. Like the leitmotifs of Wagner, visual symbols remember, comment, reveal, and prophesy, adding an overlay of mystery and ambiguity to the basic form.

The symbol, because it appeals to the imagination rather than to reality, is by nature ambiguous. Wagner used musical symbolism to evoke vague sensations rather than concrete substance, declaring, "To make my intentions too obvious would get in the way of a genuine understanding."[30] He achieved musical vagueness by obscuring the borders between major and minor and consonance and dissonance. Wagner's continuous veil of sound, which lacks cadencial resolutions and traditional harmonic stability, suggests a perpetual stream of consciousness.

Péladan celebrated Wagner's ambiguity, noting that the indefinite character of music allows it to appeal differently to each soul. He called upon art to strive toward a similar vagueness, asking, "What do Beethoven and Leonardo say?" and answering, "What each person has in his own soul."[31] Péladan considered Leonardo's *Mona Lisa* to be the ultimate example of musical vagueness transmuted into visual enigma. He claimed that it was Leonardo's expertise as a musician that enabled him to evoke such mystery in his painting.[32] The *Mona Lisa*'s mysterious smile invited speculation as to whether she was "a madam or a madonna?" Confirming the Sâr's obsession with ambiguity, the salons of the Rose + Croix abounded with titles such as *Sphinx, La Vague, Enigmatique,* and *Mysteriosa,* which sometimes displayed *Mona Lisa*'s inscrutable smile. In double homage to Wagner and Leonardo, the preface to the catalogue of the third exhibition was titled "Leit motiv de la Joconde."[33]

The ultimate Rosicrucian ambiguity was achieved by blurring the distinction between the sexes.[34] Androgyne begged the ultimate question—is it male or female? The answer could only be "both and neither." The hermaphrodite of the Rose + Croix developed directly from one of the most important and oft-illustrated allegories of ancient alchemical philosophy. In a single image, it personified alchemists' successful "marriage" of ingredients with opposing characteristics (such as wet and cold with hot and dry) into a unified, undifferentiated whole. Typical of most early alchemical allegories, the androgyne also carried a philosophical meaning—the union of spirit (the male principle) and flesh (the female principle) achieved only by devout struggle and self-denial.[35] The unimpeachable hermaphrodite therefore represented both the fruit of the "chemical marriage" of opposites and the triumph of mind over matter. Wagner also celebrated the unity of androgyny. He recognized that the ideal hermaphroditic state could only be achieved by struggle, maintaining, "A human being is both man and woman, it is only when the two are united that the real human being exists."[36]

Delville's *Symbolization of the Flesh and Spirit* (fig. 9.3), shown at the second Rosicrucian salon, is an expressive illustration of Wagner's belief that sexual conflict exists at the core of each human psyche. This striking work depicts two figures engaged in a struggle. The voluptuous female, mired in what appear to be thorns and

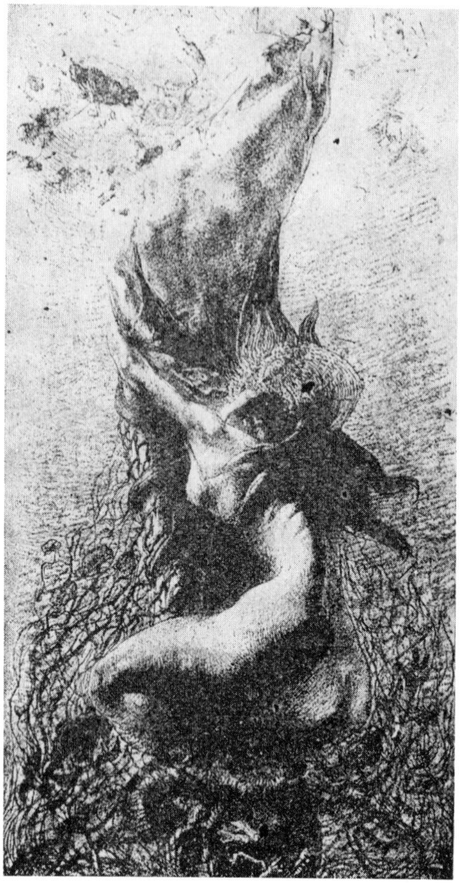

Fig. 9.3. Jean Delville, *Symbolisation de la chair et de l'Esprit*, 1893. *Catalogue Officiel Illustré du Salon*, No. 54.

vegetation, attempts to forcibly restrain her male companion from his upward ascent toward the realm of the spirit. Péladan chronicled a similar struggle in his series of novels, *La Décadence Latine*, which featured androgynous beings triumphing over adversity and temptation.[37] Consequently, paintings titled *Androgyne* by Armand Point and Alexandre Séon appeared at the salons, while Fernand Khnopff's contributions displayed that distinctive enigmatic face whose feminine sensitivity belies its masculine contours (fig. 9.4).[38]

If androgyne personified a state of unified grace, dominance of the female principle boded disaster. Women were positively represented by Wagner and the Rose + Croix only in capacities subservient to men or as embodiments of abstract ideals.[39] Wagner's Brunhilde personified the role of woman as nurturing muse. In this capacity, she and her Walkyrie sisters appeared along side numerous female saints and holy women at the Rose + Croix exhibitions. Brunhilde's opposite, Kundry, represented another favorite Rosicrucian leitmotif, the malevolent femme fatale. As an earth spirit bent on destroying the high resolve of the grail knights, Kundry represented instinct and emotion—threats to the Rosicrucian ideal. Her evil nature was confirmed by the *Kundry* exhibited at the fourth Salon of 1894 (painted by "Walter, from Saint-

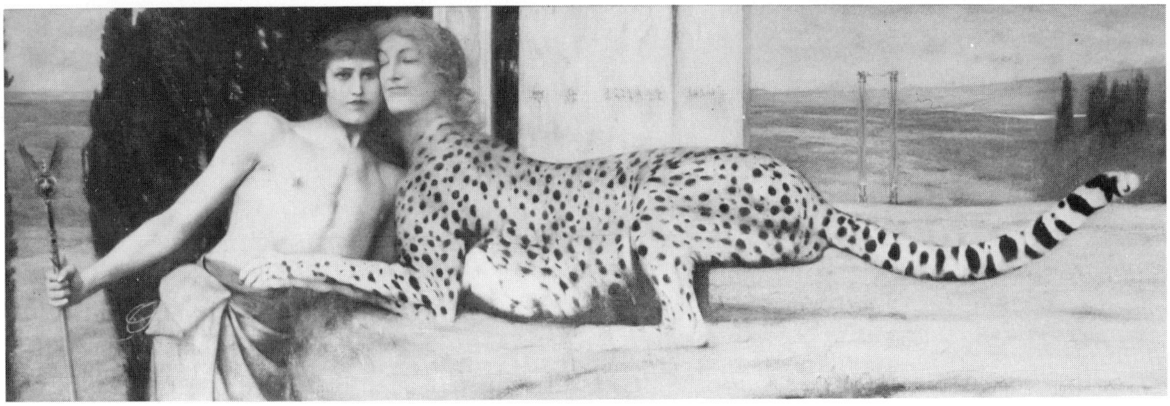

Fig. 9.4. Fernand Khnopff, *L'Art (Les caresses, Le sphinx)*, 1896. Brussels, Musées Royaux des Beaux-Arts de Belgique. © A.C.L., Brussels.

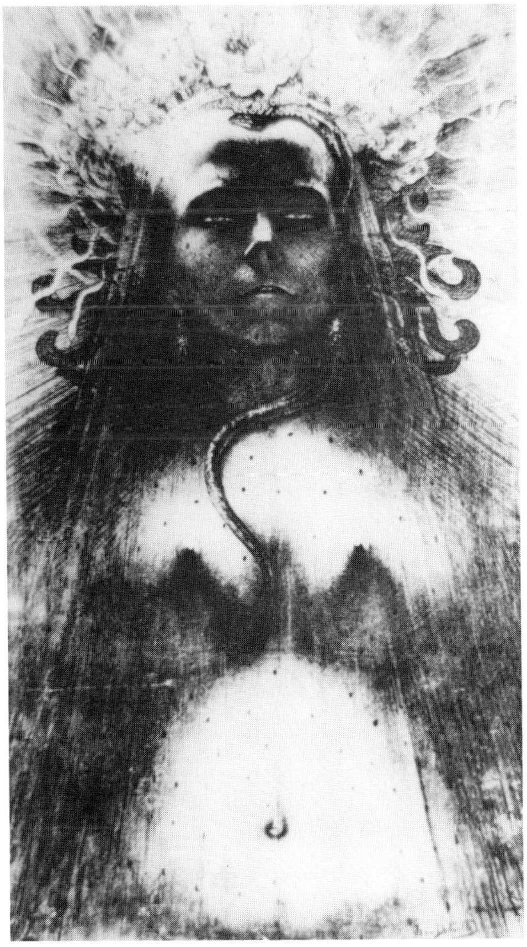

Fig. 9.5. Jean Delville, *The Idol of Perversity,* 1891, drawing. Munich, Galleria del Levante.

Tunaire"), which bore the ominous subtitle *The Rose of Hell.* Kundry and her sister seducers, Herodias, Artemis, and Medea, either gazed alluringly or glared forbiddingly from the canvasses of Delville, Khnopff, Point and others.

Delville's *Idol of Perversity* (fig. 9.5) was one of the most powerful expressions of negative femininity seen at the first salon of 1892. She is a modern Eve-Medusa whose sensual body is marred by sores, her thin, parted lips and cold, half-closed eyes cast in shadow. A snake writhes from between her breasts to the top of her forehead, where the rays of light in her shimmering halo assume the forms of twisting snakes. Péladan, who held Wagner's belief that the greater the power of the female in a culture, the greater the decadence, required his brotherhood to renounce sexual love before Leonardo.[40] It is easy to believe that the sight of Delville's *Idol of Perversity* could have turned many an ardent Rosicrucian heart to stone.

Also inherent in Wagner's music dramas and reflected in the philosophy of the Rose + Croix was a sense of racial pride based upon the events of an ancient mythical past.[41] Like symbolist art, Wagner's music and philosophy recognized myth and symbol as remnants of the collective unconscious of a culture—in Wagner's case, the German race, in Péladan's, the Latin. Both men desired a highly evolved humanity capable of receiving the ideas of the artist without ignorance or inhibition. Wagner, however, visualized a mass regeneration of society led and inspired by his example, whereas Péladan displayed no such optimism. To him, the impending new century signaled Armageddon for a race that traced its roots to the ancient Greeks. The purpose of the salons de la Rose + Croix was to stage a final brilliant demonstration before the doomed Latin race immolated itself and its traditions in an orgy of materialism and banality. Péladan chronicled the sorry state of society in his fourteen-volume work *La Décadence Latine,* where the loss of intellectual and racial aristocracy is mourned, and ignorance of tradition brings destruction. Both Wagner and Péladan worked under the guise of enlightened prophets; however, one believed that he was creating the art work of the future, whereas the other despaired of the future's ever arriving.

All of the Rosicrucian salons featured works bearing the titles of Péladan's novels, including several suffering *Patriciennes,* illustrating the Sâr's elitest, pessimistic views. Séon's frontispiece for Henri Nazel's *Crépuscule des dieux* (fig. 9.6) is a literal translation of Wagner's *Götterdämmerung (Twilight of the Gods),* the last of his *Ring* cycle which chronicles the demise of the gods and the destruction of Valhalla. The work shows the ruined torso of a classical god, whose toppled head is replaced by Péladan's disembodied face hovering like a spiritual apparition above it. Séon's image is Wagnerian in its vision of dead gods, and Rosicrucian in its depiction of those gods as Latin rather than Teutonic. The work also portray's the Rosicrucian belief that the Latin race, symbolized by the headless torso, would be supplanted by a higher ideal, represented by Péladan's luminous portrait.

Péladan's belief that decadence heralded the demise of Latin culture is echoed in Toorop's *The Young Generation* (fig. 9.7), shown at the salon of 1892. The work pictures an infant playing blissfully in the midst of frightful surroundings. A ghastly blood-red tree hovers menacingly over the innocent child while other sinister forms lurk in the dark background shadows. In startling contrast to the organic peril of the surrounding landscape, yet overwhelmed by it, are a railroad track and an electric light pole in the foreground. These represent the pride of the industrial age, yet they seem as fragile and threatened as the child. Barely visible behind the infant and barred

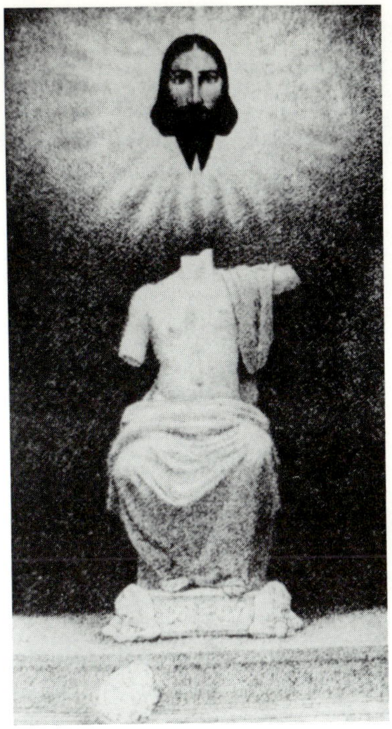

Fig. 9.6. Alexandre Séon, *Frontispice du Crépuscule des dieux de Henri Nazel,* 1893. *Catalogue Officiel Illustré du Salon,* No. 54.

from it by a ruined classical portal is a female figure, the previous generation,[42] who is both oblivious to the child's danger and powerless to assist. Péladan, echoing the universal sentiments of nearly every era concerning its young, railed against the deficiencies of fin-de-siècle youth. In the catalogue to the fourth exhibition, he wrote: "The philosophical education of our time is a true disgrace . . . the abominable universities pour forth words without ideas, and ideas without substance."[43] Toorop, drawing upon the natural concern of parents for their children, portrayed the young generation as victims of the carnivorous jungle of life, lacking the spiritual and intellectual skills required to survive. His painting echoes Péladan's warning, "Pitiful moderns—your course toward annihilation is fatal."[44]

Religion played an important part in the Rosicrucian revival of tradition as it did in Wagner's life and art. Péladan conceived the Rose + Croix "in Roman Catholic communion with Joseph of Arimathia, Hugh of the Pagans and Dante."[45] In imitation of Wagner, he elevated art to the status of a religion with artists as its clergy.[46] He believed that all great works of art were religious and that lack of religious sentiment in fin-de-siècle France signaled the end of civilization.[47] Consequently, the historical revivalism of the Rose + Croix revolved around the medieval and Renaissance eras, the glory days of the Catholic church. Studies emulating Botticelli and Memling were frequently exhibited along with armored knights and various *Florentines.* Among the Biblical subjects which dominated the exhibitions, the virgins and saints of Charles Filiger (fig. 9.8) are particularly illustrative of the theological and historical aura of the salons. Stylistically, these iconic, geometrically constructed images are reminiscent of cathedral stained glass. Their pure, sharply defined colors recall Péladan's dislike of avant-garde

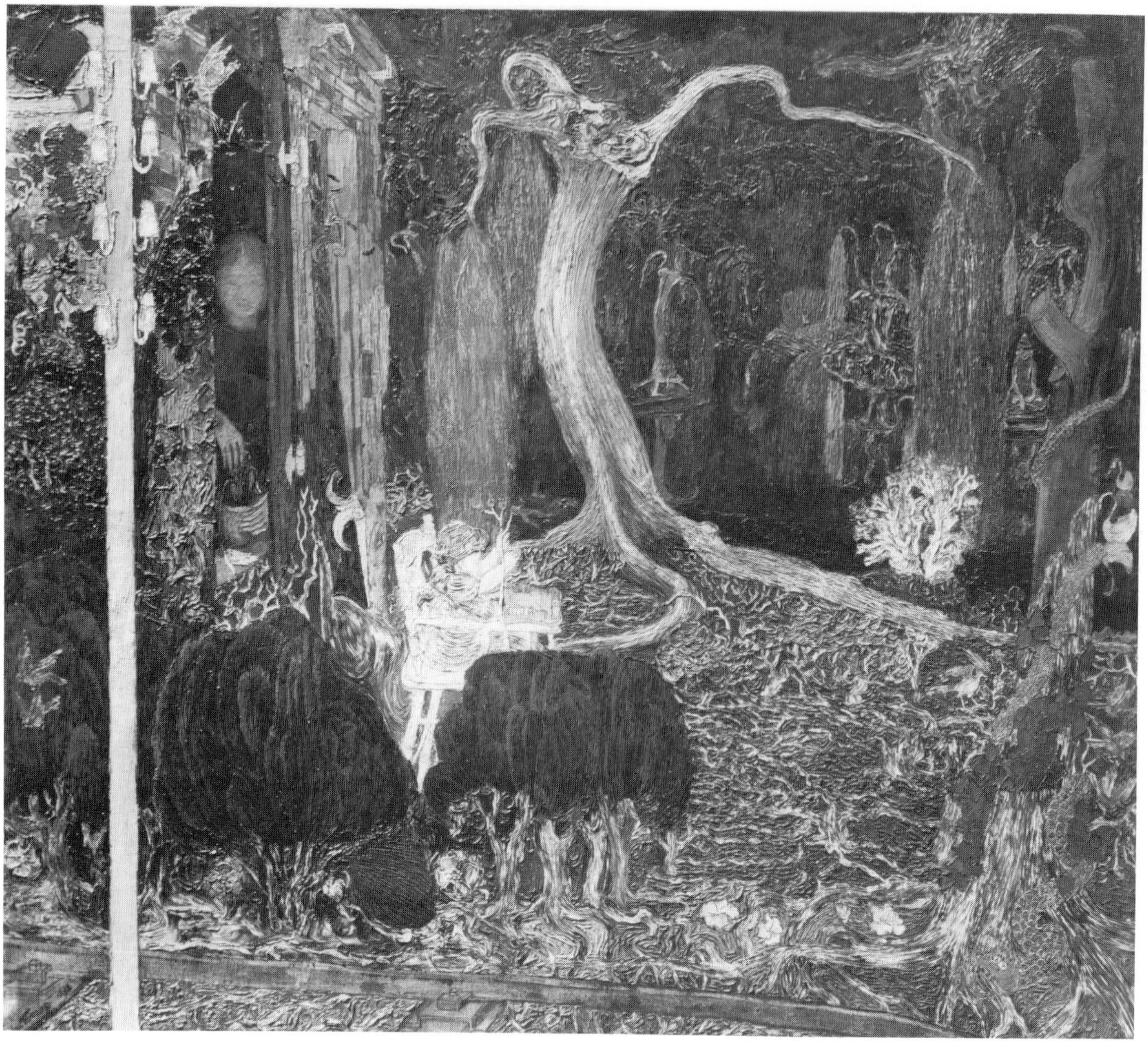

Fig. 9.7. Jan Toorop, *La jeune génération*, 1892.
Rotterdam, Museum Boymans-Van Beuningen.

experiments with optical mixing, and his insistence that "there is no such thing as a beautiful or ugly color, there are only beautiful or ugly combinations."[48]

It would seem, then, that Wagnerian philosophy provided ready-made themes which complemented the fin-de-siècle sentiments of the Rose + Croix. Indeed, the lessons of history teach us that retreat into conservative religious dogma, distrust of technology, ambivalence toward women, nostalgia for times past, cultural elitism, and fear of the future seem to be universal concerns of human beings poised at the end of a century, looking forward to the next. Exploitation of these topics was not limited to the context of the visual arts at the Salons de la Rose + Croix, but was also evident in the music which accompanied the exhibitions. The most surprising dominating musical

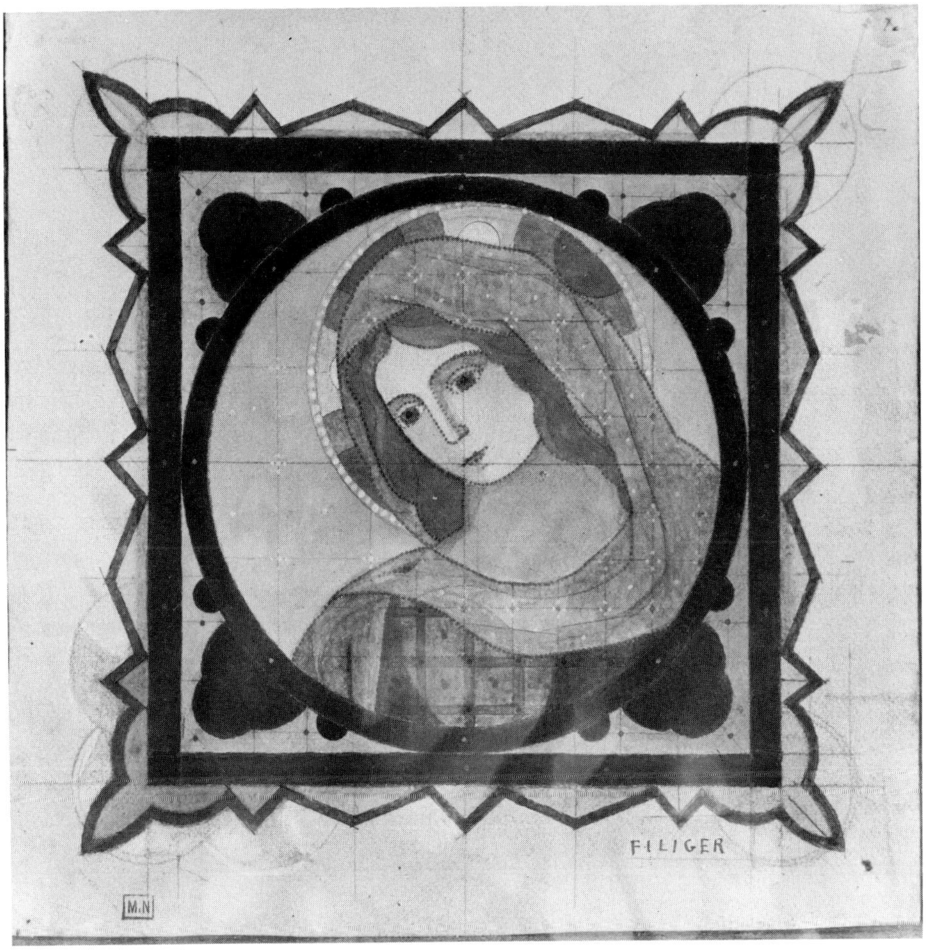

Fig. 9.8. Charles Filiger, *Head of the Virgin* (from *Four Chromatic Notations*), watercolor. Paris, Musée National d'Art Moderne.

presence at the first salon, apart from Wagner, was Erik Satie, who is credited by music historians with liberating French music from the clutches of Wagnerism.[49] His participation in the salons causes us to wonder if the Rosicrucian fascination with Wagner could have been almost entirely divorced from the actual sound of his music.

ERIK SATIE and the SALONS de la ROSE + CROIX

Unlike Wagner, who was appointed posthumously to the Rosicrucian Olympiad, Erik Satie's affiliation was voluntary. In his capacity as "official composer" of the Rose + Croix, Satie wrote several works, including music for Péladan's play *Le Fils des Étoiles*, a *Hymne au drapeau*, *Première pensée Rose + Croix*, and three *Sonneries de la*

Rose + Croix.[50] We must assume, then, that his sympathies lay with the idealist, Wagnerian aesthetic championed by Péladan and reflected in the salon exhibitions. Indeed, the events of young Satie's life before 1892 predisposed him to advocacy of the Sâr's philosophies. Having just ended a disastrous affair with the free spirit Suzanne Valadon, Satie was ready to relinquish the delights of feminine companionship. He harbored the belief that his ancestors came from an ancient line of aristocrats, lived in a state of self-imposed poverty and was rebaptized into the Catholic faith.[51] Erik Satie was fascinated with the mystic past, and, even before his Rosicrucian conversion, had composed several *Gymnopédies, Gnossiennes,* and *Ogives* in a pseudo-medieval style influenced by the writings of Flaubert and Péladan.[52] Debussy called him a "gentle medieval musician,"[53] while the humorist Alphonse Allais nicknamed him Esoteric Satie.[54]

Considering the godlike status that Wagner enjoyed with the Rose + Croix, one would expect the works of their official composer to sound at least vaguely Wagnerian. But such was not the case. To the modern ear, Satie's sparse, evocative Rose + Croix compositions seem diametrically opposed to the lush chromatic web of orchestral and vocal textures associated with Wagner. How was it possible that Satie's music could both embrace and undermine an entire philosophy? The composer himself explained his position, saying, "The orchestra should not grimace when someone enters a scene. . . . One must create a musical climate where the characters move and talk. No couplets, no leitmotifs—but suggesting a certain atmosphere of Puvis de Chavannes. . . . I am by no means anti-Wagnerian, but we must have our own music—without sauerkraut *(sans choucroute),* if possible."[55] In fact, Satie did serve *choucroute* to the Rose + Croix, but concocted it according to his own unique French recipe.[56]

Satie's Rose + Croix compositions share many structural and philosophical concerns with the art of the salons. A detailed analysis of all of this music would take many pages; however, the "Air du Grand Prieur" from the *Sonneries*[57] is representative of the group and can serve as a model for our purposes. Though in performance, this work has the calm, two-dimensional aura of a painting by Puvis de Chavannes,[58] the visual impact of the score is one of duality and opposition (fig. 9.9). It begins with static triad chords—some major, some minor—which, despite their harmonic ambiguity, suggest an air of spiritual assurance (fig. 9.9 A). These chords yield abruptly to a wandering melismatic line played in octaves, also constructed in rhythmic groups of threes (fig. 9.9 B).

The somewhat schizophrenic organization of this work has been explained as an attempt to replicate the effect of a medieval cantor and choir.[59] This is certainly true; but, more importantly, the bipartite nature of the *Sonneries* reflects the Rosicrucian fascination with the duality of flesh and spirit also characterized in Delville's painting (fig. 9.3). Satie isolates the static chords and the restless melody—musical equivalents of the opposing forces of male and female—spirit and flesh. The synthesis of opposites, the ultimate goal of Rosicrucianism, occurs in the middle section of the work, where the triads and the melody are played together—"married" into a unified whole (fig. 9.9 C). Satie is careful, however, to indicate the superiority of the male spiritual element by a reprise of the triad chord section without melismas at the end of the work. The *Sonneries* exist today only in piano transcription, but they were originally intended to be performed by harp and trumpet.[60] Satie's choice of the harp, a soft stringed instrument associated with angels and saints, coupled with the trumpet, a stri-

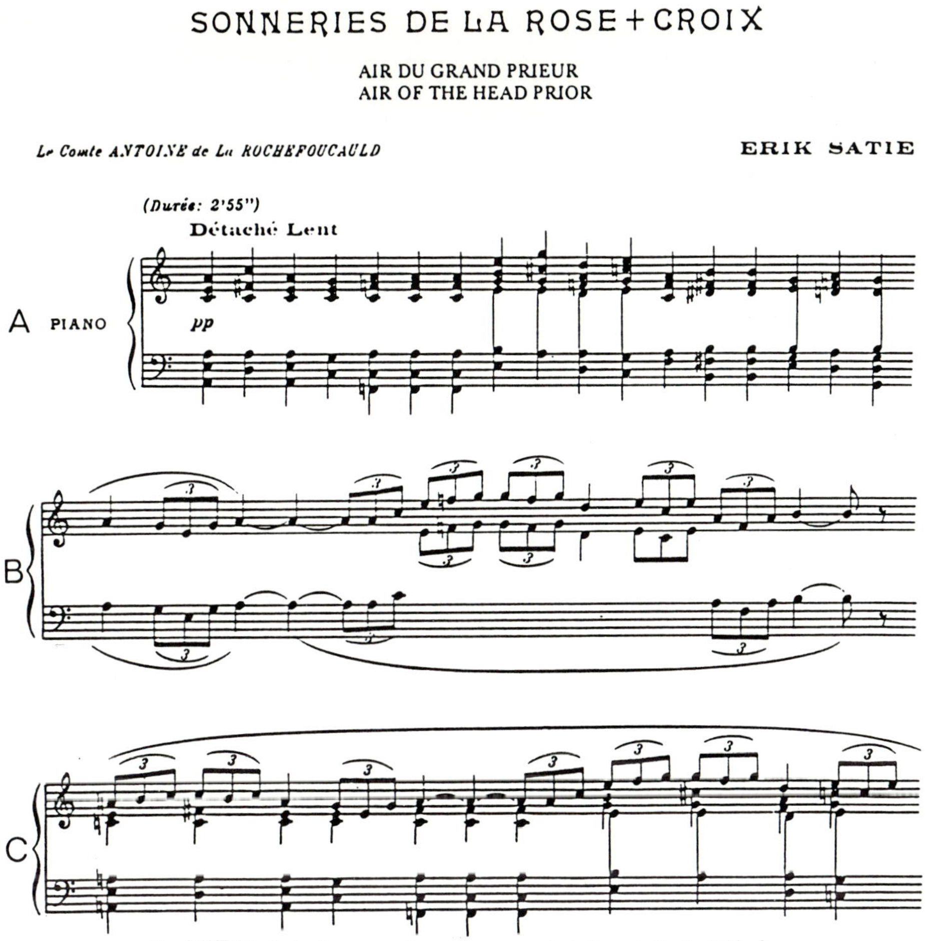

Fig. 9.9. Erik Satie, fragments from *Sonneries de la Rose + Croix*, "Air du grand prieur," 1891. Paris, Editions Salabert.

dent, brass instrument linked with battle and secular authority,[61] further reinforces the Rosicrucian preoccupation with the duality of flesh and spirit.

Satie's most extensive Rosicrucian music was written for Péladan's play *Le Fils des Étoiles,* which the Sâr subtitled *Wagnerie Kaldéenne.*[62] The play's scenario is ancient Chaldea, the hero a simple shepherd who, by overcoming material pleasures, becomes a priest and is rewarded by chaste marriage to his childhood sweetheart. The *Preludes* that preceded each of the three acts display the same binary opposition, symbolizing the conflict of flesh and spirit, as the *Sonneries.* Added to this is an upward movement of the chordal and melodic lines (fig. 9.10), reflecting the striving of Péladan's hero.[63] The concept of the struggle toward the "ideal" as an upward movement is also reflected in Carlos Schwabe's poster advertising the salon of 1892 (fig. 9.11).[64] Here, the human situation is visualized as a Platonic trinity of body, mind, and spirit embodied in three female figures. The darkly sensual representative of the flesh appears mired in a pool of muck at the bottom of a stair. She looks longingly up at a second figure, representative of the intellect, who is poised on the first step. This figure gazes

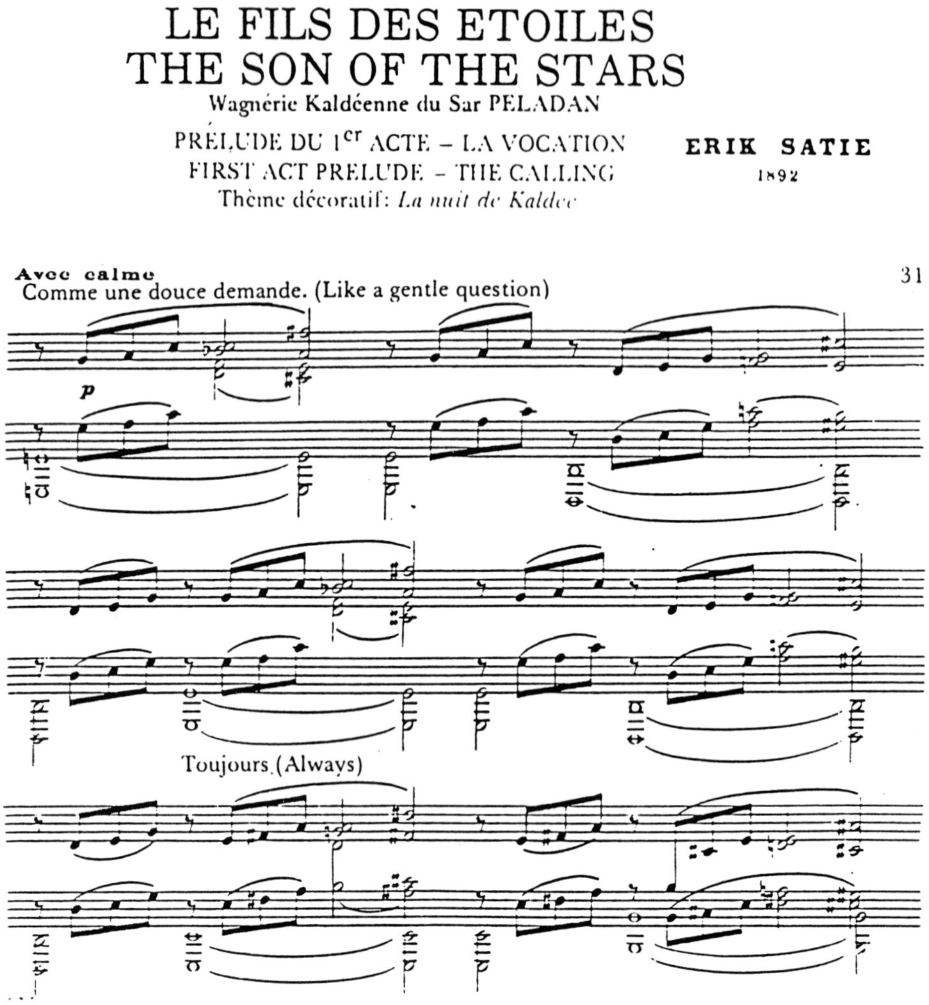

Fig. 9.10. Erik Satie, fragment from *Le Fils des Etoiles,* "Prélude du 1er Acte, La Vocation," 1892. Paris, Editions Salabert.

down over her shoulder while reaching toward the personification of the spirit, whose corporeality nearly dissolves in light at the top of the stair. Besides illustrating the upward movement from material to ideal, the poster shares its triple organization with Péladan's play and Satie's music. The number 3 was important to Rosicrucian philosophy, as the order itself was divided into three sectors—the Rose + Croix, the Temple, and the Grail—in reflection of the Catholic and Platonic trinities.

Péladan's play reflects the fascination with Indo-Chinese culture that swept France after Balinese music and culture were introduced via the Exposition Universal of 1889. Consequently, the *Gnossienne* (fig. 9.12), which Satie inserted in act one of *Le Fils des Étoiles,*[65] displays this awareness of Balinese music while satisfying the philosophical demands of the Rose + Croix. The modal melody (fig. 9.12 A) above a syncopated rhythmic base (fig. 9.12 B), one marking a constant pulse, the other floating

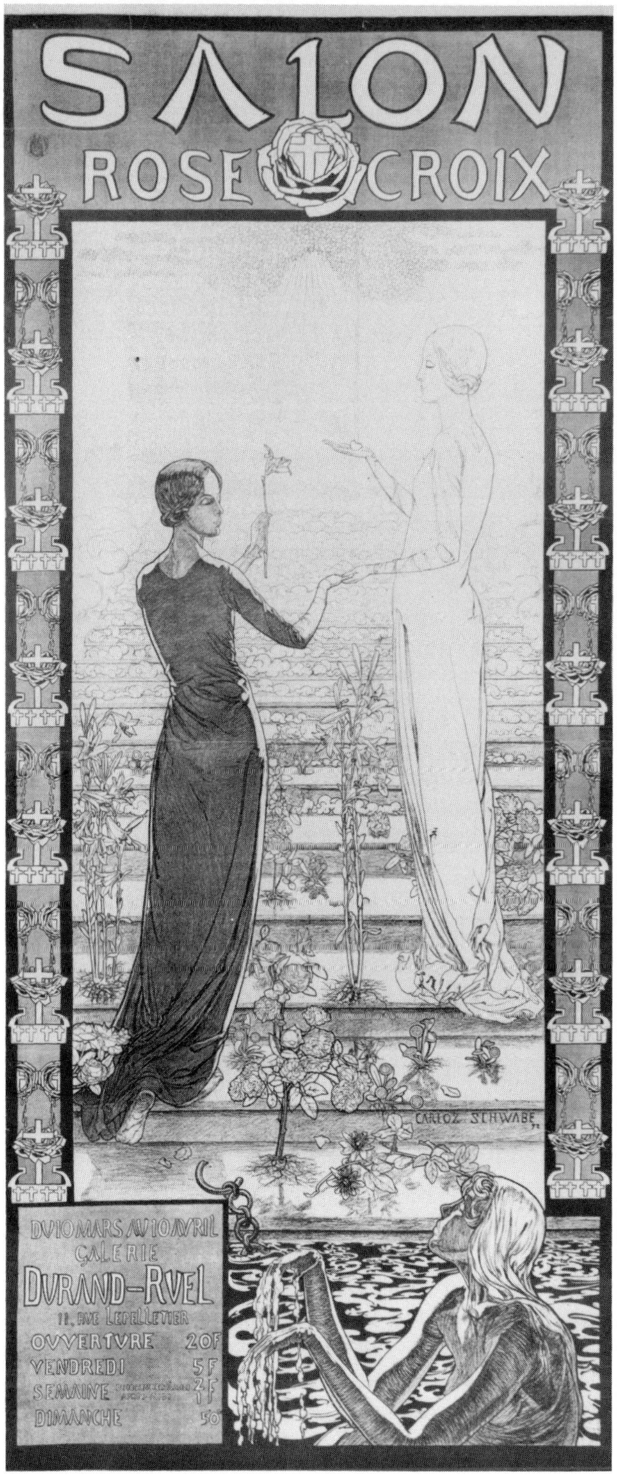

Fig. 9.11. Carlos Schwabe, Poster for the First Salon Rose + Croix, 1892. London, Piccadilly Gallery.

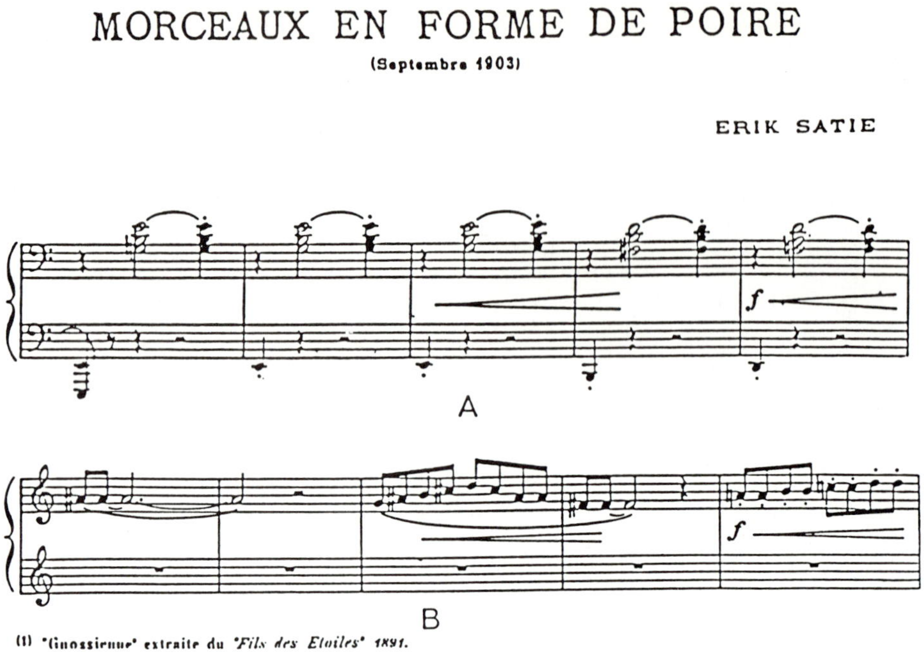

Fig. 9.12. Erik Satie, fragment of *Gnossienne* from *Le Fils des Étoiles,* 1891, published as part of *Morceaux en Forme de Poire,* 1903. Paris, Editions Salabert.

sinuously above, recalls Balinese music. At the same time, the separation of treble and base—rhythm and melody—illustrates the division of flesh and spirit at the core of Péladan's philosophy.

Of all the works by Rosicrucian artists, Toorop's *Three Brides* (fig. 9.13) is most closely allied both stylistically and philosophically to Satie's *Gnossienne.* Toorop, who was Javanese, imbued his works with a patterned decorativeness and undulating linearity reminiscent of native batiks from the Dutch East Indies. The *Three Brides,* like Satie's music, reflects the concept of the spiritual and sensual opposites united into a trinity. Toorop's trio of women consists of a virginal nun and a satanic temptress flanking a veiled bride who is both pure and sensual. The sinuous arabesques of hair and drapery which swirl around the three static figures also recall Satie's Oriental modal melody floating above chordal triads. Despite the loose and flowing auras of Toorop's *Three Brides* and Satie's *Gnossienne,* both painting and music are contained by an overall sense of symmetry and organization.

Satie indicated dominance of the spiritual element by instructions to the performer inserted in the score. Instead of the traditional Italian indications for tempo (such as *allegro* or *lento*), volume (such as *forte* or *piano*), etc., Satie wrote directions in French (such as *toujours,* or *comme une douce demande*) (fig. 9.10). These words and phrases do not apply to the physical mechanics of sound production but to specific spiritual states to which the performer should aspire when playing Satie's works. This emphasis on the spiritual rather than the physical aspects of musical performance, coupled with Satie's use of musical iconography that complemented the philosophies of the

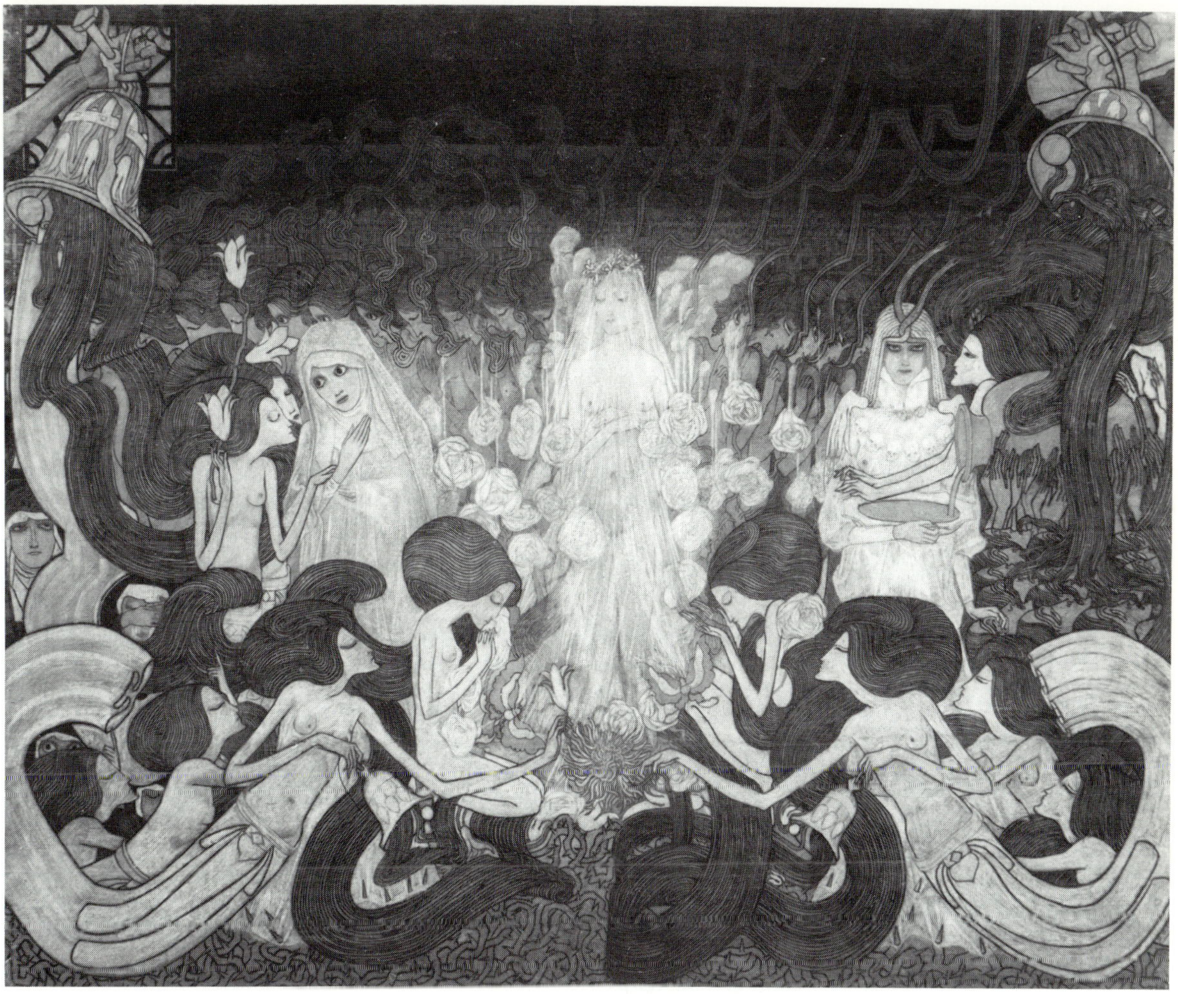

Fig. 9.13. Jan Toorop, *Les trois fiancées,* 1892.
Otterlo, Rijksmuseum Kröller-Müller.

Rose + Croix, must have given the exhibitions the air of a delicately-refined *Gesamtkunstwerk*. It appears that Satie's Rosicrucian music, though distinctly French, was closely tied by a subtle awareness of, and interaction with, the art of the salons, the philosophies of Péladan and, yes, the concept of symbolic music developed by Richard Wagner. Erik Satie succeeded in his goal of creating musical symbolism without employing a single leitmotif—a subtle *choucroute* indeed.

OTHER MUSIC at the SALONS de la ROSE + CROIX

Though Wagner was the guiding star of the Rose + Croix and Satie its official composer, the musical programs of the salons were by no means limited to the works of these two.

The concert advertisements in the catalogues of the first two exhibitions included composers of all eras (figs. 9.1 and 9.2). The list was not compiled indiscriminately but with an eye toward each composer's sensitivity to the themes reflected in the wider contexts of Rosicrucian art and philosophy. For example, the debt of Rosicrucianism to Freemasonery was acknowledged by the music of Mozart *(Sonata in A Major)*, whose opera *The Magic Flute* is an allegory reflecting the composer's involvement with the order. Mysticism and ambiguity were represented by the Musical "incantations" of Mme. Corrylange Moogenboom, which probably consisted of spontaneous improvisations inspired by the mood of the moment. Mme. Moogenboom also performed "two seances on the violin," conjuring up the spirits of Tartini, Bach, and Beethoven. The spiritual element was also reflected in the music of Schumann *(Berceuse)*, who was inspired by the German romantic mystic E. T. A. Hofmann. In contrast, the name of Bach was intoned as the embodiment of intellectual balance and harmony achieved by mathematical proportion. Indeed, the Rose + Croix endowed the *Well Tempered Clavier,* from which the *Prelude in B Major* comes, with the status of a musical Parthenon. In this connection, Mendelssohn *(Concerto in C Minor)* was revered for having led the rediscovery of Bach in the early nineteenth century.

The Rosicrucian belief in the omnipotence of the creative artist was represented by Beethoven, whose works (two waltzes, a bagatelle, the "Funeral March" from the *Eroica* Symphony, the "Allegro" from the *Apassionata* Sonata and the "Andante and Variations" and "Presto" movements from the *Kreutzer* Sonata) were performed at three concerts during the month of April 1893. Historians of the romantic era traditionally label the irascible Beethoven as the first composer to attain the status of "divine" during his lifetime. He established himself, thanks in no small part to the revolutionary spirit which gripped the world in the late eighteenth century, as an independent genius, above and beyond the petty demands of either royal patrons or unenlightened public. As a solitary bachelor who lived only for his art, Beethoven became a role model for members of the Rose + Croix. For similar reasons, the music of Chopin (*Nocturne in E Major, Mazurka in B Minor, Fantasie Impromptu,* three waltzes, *Scherzo in B-Flat minor,* and *Impromptu in B-Flat Major*) was also performed at Rosicrucian soirées. Like Beethoven, Chopin never married, but his long liaison with the literary dragon lady George Sand was perceived (wrongly in the nineteenth century) as having driven him to an early grave. Chopin's music, rarefied and elegant as was the man himself, also embodied Péladan's image of a fading aristocracy. In this connection, Chopin's famous "Funeral March" was heard in concert apart from the *Sonata No. 2 in B-Flat Minor,* to which it belongs.

Much of the music performed at the salons de la Rose + Croix reflected the concern with Catholicism and historical revivalism also demonstrated in its paintings. We have already spoken of the opening of the first salon, heralded by selections of a proper devotional nature from Wagner's Christian music drama *Parsifal.* Catholicism was further represented by César Franck (fig. 9.1), dead but two years in 1892. Franck's liturgical compositions written for the organ (he was employed as music director of Ste. Clotilde) reestablished the expressive capabilities of that instrument. In recognition of his contribution to French music, the third Rosicrucian performance of Palestrina's *Pope Marcello Mass* in 1892 was "consecrated to the students of Franck" and conducted by the most successful of them all, the young Vincent d'Indy. Though Franck's music seems not to have been performed at the salons, his spirit presided. Péladan exalted his memory with the title "archangel."

Aside from the homage to César Franck, much of the liturgical character of the Rosicrucian soirées arose from performances of early music. In this sense, the Rose + Croix continued the revivalism begun earlier in the century, to which we owe the rescue from obscurity of Gregorian plainchant and the music of Johann Sebastian Bach. Among the early composers to benefit from this revival spirit was Roland (Orlando) de Lassus, a sixteenth-century Flemish composer. Lassus' style, so reverently balanced in its counterpoint that it became known as the *ars perfecta,* demonstrated the sense of fervor tempered by discipline demanded of all contributors to the salons. His music, featured at the 1893 exhibition, affirmed Péladan's admiration for the early Netherlandish school of painters and enhanced those contributions to the salons that consciously emulated northern Renaissance masters. The music of the Italian High Renaissance was represented by Giovanni Palestrina, whom the Rosicrucians favored with three performances in one week of the *Pope Marcello Mass* in 1892. Palestrina led the Counter-Reformation movement toward conservative reform of church music in the sixteenth century, and his example inspired the Rosicrucians to do the same with regard to fin-de-siècle art and society.

In a sense, then, the art exhibited by the French Rosicrucian order, when considered alone, presents an incomplete picture of the salons. It is clear that the intended impact of these exhibitions was meant to be experienced on several sensate levels. Despite the old-fashioned romanticism displayed in some of the lesser products of the Rose + Croix, its synesthetic experiments would continue to be influencial beyond the short span of years devoted to the exhibitions. From Wagner to Péladan, to the Belgian symbolist salons via Delville, to Satie's later collaborations with Picasso and Diaghilev, to the motion pictures of today—the eye, the ear, and the word have combined to produce an art which, in its unity, becomes more than the sum of its separate parts.

NOTES

1. Alice Morse Earle, *Sun-Dials and Roses of Yesterday* (Norwood, Mass., 1902), 376.

2. For an examination of the Rose + Croix, its critics and its documents, see Robert Pincus-Witten, *Occultism in France: Joséphin Péladan and the Salons de la Rose + Croix* (New York: Garland Publishing, 1976). See also Paul Arnold, *Histoire des Rose-Croix et les Origines de la Franc-Maçonnerie* (Paris: Mercure de France, 1955); Bertholet, Dr. Ed., *La Pensée et les Secrets du Sâr Joséphin Péladan* (Lausanne: Genillard, Edition Rosicruciennes, 1952).

3. I wish to express my gratitude to Gabriel P. Weisberg and William Fleming for their preliminary readings of this study. Their generous expertise in the fields of art and music history has enriched it considerably. I owe both the initial inspiration for this study and my continuing interest in French nineteenth-century mysticism to my former teacher Elizabeth Holt. I dedicate this article to her in gratitude for her friendship and support.

4. For a modern history of seventeenth-century Rosicrucianism, see Francis A. Yates, *The Rosicrucian Enlightenment* (London: Routledge & Kegan Paul, 1972). For a nineteenth-century view, see Dr. Franz Hartmann, *Secret Symbols of the Rosicrucians* (Boston, 1888).

5. For a view of alchemy's practical origins, see John Maxon Stillman, *The Story of Early Chemistry* (New York: Dover Publishers, 1972); Laurinda S. Dixon, *Alchemical Imagery in Bosch's 'Garden of Delights,'* (Ann Arbor, Mich.: UMI Research Press, 1981).

6. See Laurinda S. Dixon, "Carloz Schwabe's *Spleen et Ideal*—A Study in 19th-Century Alchemical Revivalism," *Cauda Pavonis* (Spring 1987) n.p.

7. Some of the major occultist reviews of the 1880s and 90s were *Annales du Supernaturel, La Coeur, La Haute Science, L'Initiation, Le Lotus Bleu, La Lumière, La Voile d'Isis,* and *Psyché.*

8. This number was recorded at the sixth salon in 1897, held at George Petit's gallery. See Pincus-Witten, *Occultism in France,* 172.

9. The list of participants in the six-year history of the Rose + Croix included 193 contemporary artists, at least three anonymous contributors and thirty-five "old masters." See Robert Pincus-Witten, *Les Salons de la Rose + Croix* (London: Piccadilly Gallery, 1968), App.

10. The evening edition of *Le Figaro,* 2 September 1891, carried the following response by Puvis to Péladan's mention of his name in the morning edition of the same day: "I protest with all my strength against the mention that has been made of me in this morning's article, 'Le Salon de la Rose + Croix.' "

11. Joséphin Péladan, "Études de Sciences Mortes, Le Grand Oeuvre, d'après Leonardo da Vinci," *L'Artiste* (January 1883): 41–48.

12. Joséphin Péladan, *Salon de la Rose + Croix, Regle et Monetoire* (Paris, 1891), IV.

13. The Théatre de la Rose + Croix, which presented Péladan's plays at the salons, was financed by the English theosophical author Lady Marie Caithness.

14. Joséphin Péladan, *Salon de la Rose + Croix, Deuxième Geste Esthétique* (Paris, 1893), XXVII.

15. On the relationship of music and art in the philosophy of the Rose + Croix, see Leonardo da Vinci, *Traité de la Peinture,* Traduit intégralement pour la première fois en français sur le codex vaticanus (urbinas), 1270 par Jos. Péladan (Paris, 1928), 27–47.

16. This occurred in 1888, when Péladan, Stanislas de Guaita, and Antoine de la Rochefoucauld established the Rose + Croix Kabbalistique. Péladan's salons, beginning in 1892, marked his break with the original group and the establishment of the Rose + Croix + Catholique. For an account of the so-called "war of the two roses," see Pincus-Witten, *Occultism in France,* 70–82.

17. See program preface, "Soirées de la Rose + Croix," *Geste Esthétique,* 1892.

18. Péladan, *Deuxième Geste,* 165. With the loss of funds formerly contributed by Antoine de la Rochefoucauld, the Salons de la Rose + Croix steadily declined until their end in 1897.

19. Joséphin Péladan, *Le Théâtre Complet de Wagner, Ses XI Opéras Scène par Scène* (Paris, 1895).

20. The grail was the legendary chalice which caught Christ's blood at his crucifixion. According to Rosicrucian myth, it was taken by Joseph of Arimathea and passed down to Parsifal, last of the grail kings, who carried it to India. See Manly P. Hall, *An Encyclopedic Outline of Masonic, Hermetic, Cabbalistic and Rosicrucian Symbolical Philosophy* (Los Angeles: The Philosophical Society, 1977), XCIX, CLXXVII, CLXXX; Helen Adolf, *Visio Pacis. Holy City and Grail. An Attempt at an Inner History of the Grail Legend* (Philadelphia: The Pennsylvania State University Press, 1960).

21. See Lucy Beckett, *Richard Wagner: "Parsifal"* (Cambridge, England: Cambridge University Press, 1981).

22. The French fascination with Wagner did not take hold until after the composer's death in 1883. In 1885, the *Revue Wagnérienne,* devoted entirely to discussions of Wagner's philosophy, was established in Paris. By the 1890s, Wagner's music was regularly performed there. Since that time, the subject of Wagner's influence on cultural and historical events has consumed many volumes and cannot possibly be adequately summarized in a single footnote. See Henrik Barth, ed., *Internationale Wagner-Bibliographie* (Bayreuth: Editions Musica, 1968). For brief discussions of Wagner's influence on symbolist art see Philippe Jullian, *Dreamers of Decadence* (New York: Praeger, 1971); Francine C. Legrand, *Le Symbolisme en Belgique* (Brussels: Laconti, 1971); A. G. Lehman, *The Symbolist Aesthetic in France* (Oxford: Oxford University Press, 1968).

23. The events of Wagner's life and perceptive condensations of his writings and philosophy can be found in Albert Goldman and Evert Sprinchorn, eds., *Wagner on Music and Drama* (New York: E. P. Dutton & Co., 1964); Robert W. Gutman, *Richard Wagner: The Man, His Mind, and His Music* (London: Secker & Warburg, 1968); Ernest Newman, *The Life of Richard Wagner,* 4 vols. (New York: Knopf, 1933–46). For Wagner's writings see: *Richard Wagner's Prose Works,* trans. William Ashton Ellis, 8 vols. (1899; reprint, New York: Broude Brothers, 1966).

24. For a detailed discussion of the themes of Wagner's *Gesamtkunstwerk,* see Jack M. Stein, *Richard Wagner and the Synthesis of the Arts* (Detroit: Wayne State University Press, 1960).

25. Richard Wagner, *The Art-Work of the Future,* in Ellis, *Richard Wagner's Prose Works,* 1: 74–77, 132–41.

26. *Traité,* trans. Péladan, 27.

27. Ibid., 43.

28. Ibid., 27.

29. See Robert Donington, *Wagner's "Ring" and its Symbols* (London: Faber and Faber, 1976).

30. Wagner to Roeckel, 25 January 1854, in Goldman and Sprinchorn, *Wagner on Music,* 294.

31. Péladan, *Traité,* 46.

32. Ibid., 43.

33. *Salon de la Rose + Croix, Troisième Geste Esthétique* (Paris, 1894), 5.

34. See A. J. L. Busst, "The Image of the Androgyne in the Nineteenth Century," in Ian Fletcher, ed., *Romantic Mythologies* (New York: Barnes and Noble, 1967), 1–93.

35. For the alchemical tradition of the hermaphrodite, see Laurinda S. Dixon, "Water, Wine and Blood—Science and Liturgy in the *Marriage at Cana* by Hieronymus Bosch," *Oud Holland* 96 (1982): 73–96; and C. G. Jung, *Mysterium Coniunctionis,* trans. R. F. C. Hull, vol. 14 of *The Collected Works* (Princeton: Princeton University Press, 1970).

36. Quoted in Donington, *Wagner's "Ring,"* 269.

37. Hermaphrodites were featured in #1, *Le Vice Suprême;* #2, *Curieuse;* #7, *Coeur en peine;* # 8, *L'Androgine;* #9, *La Gynandre;* as well as in Péladan's play for the Théâtre de la Rose + Croix, *Le Fils des Étoiles.*

38. See Jeffrey Howe, "Mirror Symbolism in the Work of Fernand Khnopff," *Arts Magazine* 153 (September 1978): 112–18.

39. See Richard Wagner, "On the Womanly in the Human Race," in Ellis, *Wagner's Prose Works,* 6:335–37.

40. Joséphin Péladan, "Les Maîtres contemporains: Félicien Rops, Première Étude," *La Jeune Belgique* (1885; reprint, *La Plume,* June 1896): 15.

41. See Richard Wagner, "Art and Revolution," in Ellis, *Wagner's Prose Works,* 1:21–68; "The Art Work of the Future," in Ellis, *Wagner's Prose Works,* 1:69–214. Lehman, 222.

42. B. Polak, *Het fin-de-siècle in de Nederlandse schilderkunst, De symbolistische beweging 1890–1900,* Utrechtese bijdragen tot de kunstgeschiedenis IV (s'Gravenhage: M. Nijhoff, 1955), 352, quoting Toorop's explanation of this figure.

43. *Salon de la Rose + Croix, Quatrième Geste* (Paris, 1895), 18.

44. *Salon de la Rose + Croix* (Paris, 1896), 6.

45. Wagner, unlike Péladan, detested organized religion, preferring instead to make art a religion in itself. See Richard Wagner, "Religion and Art," in Ellis, *Wagner's Prose Works,* 6:211–284.

46. Péladan, *Deuxième Geste,* XXV.

47. *Quatrième Geste,* 14–15.

48. *Traité,* trans. Péladan, 203.

49. See Charles Koechlin, "Erik Satie," *Revue Musicale,* special number (1 March 1924): 193–207; Robert T. Laudon, *Sources of the Wagnerian Synthesis: A Study of the Franco-German Tradition in 19th-Century Opera* (Munich: Musikverlag Emil Katzbichler, 1979).

50. Satie's mystic music was dramatically different from that which he composed after 1895, when he became disillusioned with the occult scene. Other works written in the "mystical" style of the Rose + Croix, but not part of the salons, included *Deux préludes du Nazaréen* (incidental music, H. Mazel; *Upsud* (ballet chrétien); *Prélude d'Eginhard; Prélude de la porte héroïque du ciel* (drame ésotérique, J. Bois); *Messe des pauvres* (Latin Mass and psalms), *Fête donnée par des Chevaliers Normands en l'honneur d'une jeune demoiselle; Danses gothiques;* and *Gnossiennes* nos. 4–6.

51. For biographies of Erik Satie, see James Harding, *Erik Satie* (London: Secker & Warburg, 1975); Rollo Myers, *Erik Satie* (London: Dennis Dobson, 1948); Grete Wehmeyer, *Erik Satie* (Regensburg: Gustav Bosse Verlag, 1974).

52. See Léon Guichard, "Erik Satie et la musique Grégorienne," *Revue musicale* (15 November 1936): 334–35.

53. Quoted in Roger Shattuck, *The Banquet Years* (New York: Random House, 1968), 121.

54. Quoted in Harding, *Erik Satie*, 35.

55. The translation is mine. Quoted in Wehmeyer, *Satie*, 86.

56. For a discussion of Wagnerisms in Satie's music, see Wehmeyer, *Satie*, 73–95.

57. The three *Sonneries* are titled "Air de L'Ordre," "Air du Grand Maitre," and "Air du Grand Prieur."

58. Satie chose a fragment from a Puvis de Chavannes painting to decorate the first printed edition of the *Sonneries* (reproduced in Wehmeyer, *Satie*, 79).

59. Patrick Gowers, "Satie's Rose+Croix Music (1891–95)," *Proceedings of the Royal Musical Association* 92nd session (1965–66): 1–26.

60. See Péladan, *Regle et Monetoire*, XXVII.

61. Emanuel Winternitz, *Musical Instruments and Their Symbolism in Western Art* (London: Faber and Faber, 1967).

62. The work is subtitled thus in the *Deuxième Geste*, 1. *Le Fils des Étoiles* is organized in three acts. Satie's preludes which accompany each act are titled "La Vocation," "L'Initiation," and "L'Incantation."

63. Myers, *Satie*, 50.

64. The most recent discussion of this poster is Marla H. Hand, "Carloz Schwabe's Poster for the Salon de la Rose+Croix: A Herald of the Ideal in Art," *Art Journal* (Spring 1984), 40–45.

65. The *Gnossienne* written for *Le Fils des Étoiles* was published as part of *Trois Morceaux en Forme de Poire*, a work for piano, four hands. This is why the notation in fig. 9.12 appears on four staves instead of two.

10

KANDINSKY and "OLD RUSSIA"

An Ethnographic Exploration

PEG WEISS

His face is pale, but on the cheeks are two red spots. Likewise red are the lips. He has a great drum hung 'round and drums . . .

Kandinsky
Klänge, 1913

IN 1889 Wassily Kandinsky was elected to membership in the Russian Imperial Society of Friends of Natural History, Anthropology and Ethnography. He would successfully carry out an ethnographical investigation at the behest of the society, and the same year, the results of his work would be published as a nine-page article in the third issue of a new journal, *Ethnographic Review,* under the title "From Materials on the Ethnography of the Sysol- and Vechegda-Zyrians—The National Deities (According to Contemporary Beliefs)."[1] During the same period, another ethnographic essay by the young scholar, this one on Russian peasant law within the district of Moscow, would be selected for inclusion in a series of special ethnographic studies published by the Imperial Society.[2]

The first of these ethnographic essays was a summary of the research and interviews he had conducted during an ambitious trip into the still remote regions of the Vologda province in the summer of 1889. Then a 23-year-old student at the University of Moscow, Kandinsky had been selected in competition for this challenging assignment by the Imperial Society out of a field of many other competitors.[3]

Should this zealous pursuit of ethnological concerns by the man who would later be recognized as the father of abstract painting seem surprising, we have only to turn to his 1913 memoir, "Rückblicke," for confirmation of an interest that has, however, scarcely been mentioned in the voluminous literature on the artist. In several paragraphs devoted to an account of his university studies, Kandinsky recalled that he had studied national economy, Roman law, criminal law, the history of Russian law, most especially peasant law in which he took a great interest (and which appealed to him particularly as a Slav because, he wrote, of its "opposition" to Roman law). But, further, and "related to this," as he wrote, he had also studied "ethnography (from which I initially promised myself the soul of the people)."[4]

His actual trip to the Vologda region provided an experience that he ranked as among the most powerful of his student days, comparing it to the impression of his first sight of paintings by Monet and Rembrandt and his experience of a production of Wagner's *Lohengrin.* "My assignment," he wrote, "was double: to study peasant criminal law among the Russian citizenry (to discover the principles of primitive law), and to collect the remnants of pagan religion among the fishermen and hunters of the slowly disappearing Zyrians."[5]

In a passage as moving and poetic as any in the memoir, Kandinsky recalled that he had set out for the Vologda province by train with a feeling that he was traveling "on another planet." At the last station he changed to a steamer and spent several days gliding along the Suchona River ("deeply submerged in itself"), later making his way by primitive coach "through unending forests, between brightly hued hills." He traveled quite alone which, he reported, was good for meditation and for "immersing myself in the environment. . . . Days it was often burning hot, nights frosty." But it was the Zyrian people who captivated him with their "contrasting appearance"—now gray or yellow-gray from head to toe, then again appearing with "white faces, red-painted cheeks and black hair," clad in colorfully variegated costumes "like brightly-colored living pictures on two legs." The great two-storied wooden houses decked with carving likewise captured his attention.

In these "wonder houses" *(Wunderhäusern)* in which every surface was brightly painted, the walls hung with folk pictures—perhaps one "like a painted folk-song"—the traditional "holy corner" filled with icons shimmered with its eternal light. Here Kandinsky found himself immersed in an environment marvelously rich in color and symbol, moving him to exclaim that it seemed as if he had actually crossed a threshold and entered into a painting in which he could move and walk about. In the Russian version of the memoir, Kandinsky likened this moment to "a miracle."[6] It was an experience that would have long lasting reverberations not only in his art but also in his whole attitude toward the arts.[7]

There is still more information to be gleaned from Kandinsky's memoir pertaining directly to his interest in ethnography. In the Russian edition he added to his comment on the "frosty nights," an acknowledgment to a friend who had helped him procure suitably warm Zyrian clothing for the trip. This was his colleague N. A. Ivanitsky, whom Kandinsky described as a botanist, zoologist, and the "author of serious ethnographic studies." In a long note on Ivanitsky, in which he refers to him admiringly as a "noble hermit," Kandinsky also noted that his friend had been active in reorganizing the local cottage industry of handcrafted items made from native horn in an effort to protect the old folk art from exploitation by mercenary traders.[8]

We also learn from the pages of "Rückblicke" that Kandinsky had good personal reasons for being interested in ethnographic studies. Although he himself had been born in Moscow, his family comprised an interesting mix of Russian ethnic nationalities. Relatives on his mother's side stemmed from the German Baltic region, but his father had been born in Kyakhta, a city on what is now the border between Russia and Mongolia, southeast of Lake Baikal. His father's ancestors had moved to east Siberia, having been banished from west Siberia for "political reasons." This passage suggests the possibility that Kandinsky's trip into the eastern fringes of the Vologda area, bordering on the Ural Mountains and the beginning of western Siberia, was prompted by an urge to seek his identity in his ethnic heritage, to seek in the "soul of the people" his own roots.[9]

According to Nina Kandinsky's memoir, Kandinsky not only had Mongolian blood in his veins but often said with some pride that one of his great-grand-mothers was a Mongolian princess.[10] The peoples of the Lake Baikal area, the Buriats, were a Mongolic race whose traditions and heritage had already attracted the intense interest of several generations of travelers and ethnologists, so that, by the end of the nineteenth century, a substantial body of literature on the Buriats was available to the student of ethnology.

These few extracts from "Rückblicke" reveal a great deal about Kandinsky's interest in ethnography and its lasting effect on him. Indeed, that these memories were recorded with such immediacy and enthusiasm a quarter of a century after the fact lends substance to Wordsworth's insight that "the child is father of the man" and suggests that we art historians have been negligent in ignoring this perhaps most formative period of the artist's life experience. It has been little remarked in the literature on Kandinsky beyond a nodding reference here and there to his so-called Russian paintings. No attempt has been made to read his iconography in terms of his experience as a professionally trained ethnographer. In fact, neither of his 1889 articles has been published in English. This is all the more surprising in that, contrary to published reports, these essays are so dense with information and references that only a study far beyond the scope of this brief essay could begin to do justice to them. I will consider here only certain ramifications of Kandinsky's article on the Zyrians, today called the Komi, and even so, only a suggestion of the wealth and complexity of the issues raised can be offered here. Indeed, those early experiences reverberated in his work to the very end.[11]

Although art historians have overlooked this rich source for Kandinsky's later iconographic and aesthetic development, ethnographers have not been so remiss. Kandinsky's essay was in fact cited by the great Finnish sociologist and ethnologist Uno Holmberg in his monumental work *Finno-Ugric, Siberien,* volume four of *The Mythology of All Races.* Holmberg not only footnoted Kandinsky's essay but also referenced it in his extensive bibliography. Holmberg's work itself is still quoted and cited as authoritative by ethnologists around the world. The Hungarian folklorist D. R. Fokos-Fuchs also cited Kandinsky's work in his 1911 report of a student field trip among the Zyrians. Indeed, Kandinsky's essay has been cited as recently as 1964 by Ivar Paulson in his article "Outline of Permian Folk Religion" published in the *Journal of the Folklore Institute.*[12] Thus Kandinsky's observations on the Zyrians have passed into the ethnographic literature as accepted documentation.[13]

Before turning to Kandinsky's ethnographic publication itself, let us first recall some of those other events in his life and the obvious evidence presented in some of his works that relate to his ethnographic interest. There are, first of all, those "Russian paintings." Perhaps the most frequently reproduced and exhibited is the monumental *Motley Life* of 1907 (fig. 10.1), to which we shall return. Equally brilliant in coloring and conception are *Song of the Volga* of 1906 and *Riding Couple.* Others of importance include *Arrival of the Merchants* of 1905, *Early Hour* of 1907, *Troikas* of about 1906, and *Sunday Old Russia* of 1904. Although seldom reproduced, two others are also of interest: *Panic* and *Storm Bell,* both of 1907.

There were also tempera works on cardboard (such as the early *Russian Beauty in a Landscape* and *Bridal Procession*), as well as a number of watercolors and sketches, which have obviously Russian themes. But the medium which seems most frequently to have stirred his ethnic memories was that of the woodcut, in which time and again Russian costumes, Russian walled cities with gleaming cupolas, Russian churches, Russian boats, Russian heroes, and so on resound. The graphic work which

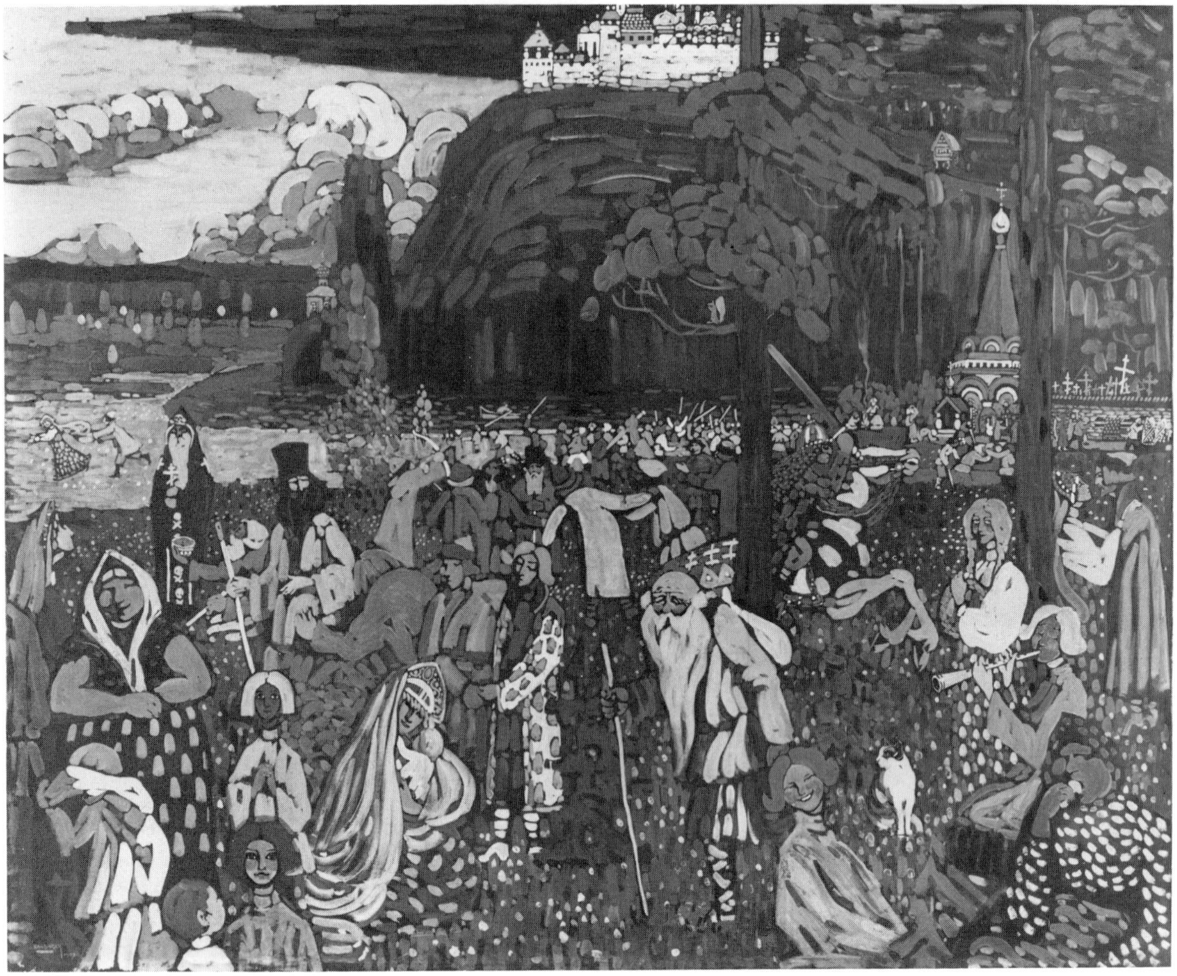

Fig. 10.1. Kandinsky, *Motley Life*, 1907. Tempera on canvas, 130 × 162.5 cm. Munich, Städtische Galerie im Lenbachhaus.

perhaps most nearly evokes the impression of his trip along the "serene and deeply-submerged-in-itself" Suchona River, bordered by its "wonder houses," is *Golden Sail* of 1903 (fig. 10.2). Here the wooden structures decorated with carving and brightly painted are set off against a dark ground that evokes the surrounding primeval forests of the ancient Zyrians.

There are other works of Kandinsky's Munich period with an ethnic flavor, namely those inspired by his 1904 trip with Gabriele Münter to Tunis, such as *Oriental* and *Arabs I (Cemetery)*, both of 1909. But there are also others of this period, such as the great *Picture with Archer* of 1909 and *Blue Mountain* (1908–09), that strike a strong ethnic note. Furthermore, in 1902 Kandinsky had personally invited the Finnish painter Axel Gallen-Kallela to exhibit in Munich with his Phalanx society. At the time, Gallen-Kallela was internationally known as the illustrator of the Finnish folk saga, *The Kalevala*, and his murals on the theme had adorned the Finnish pavilion at

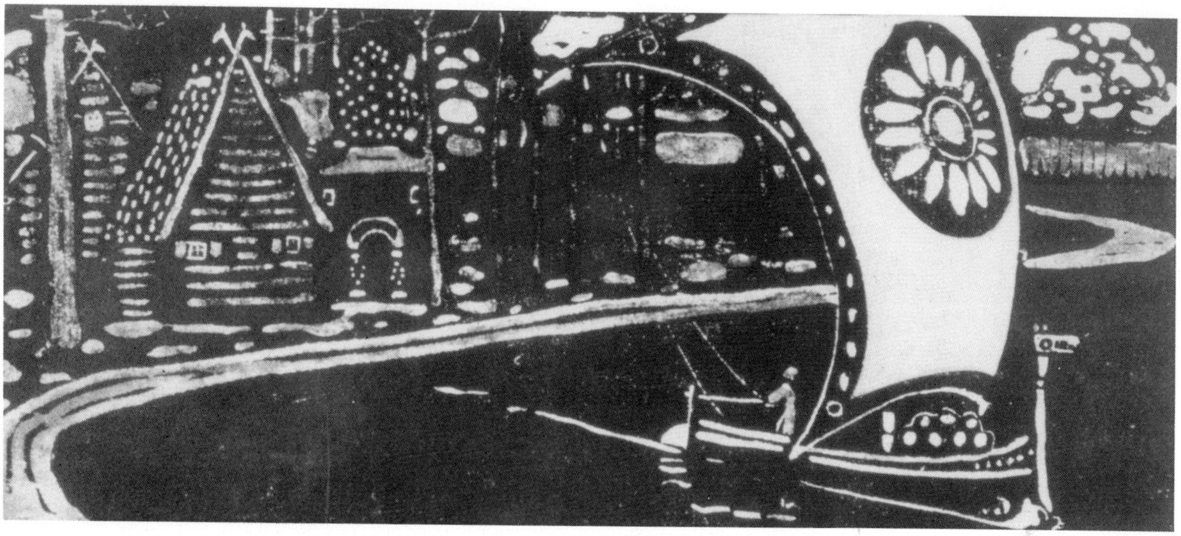

Fig. 10.2. Kandinsky, *Golden Sail,* 1903. Color woodcut, 12.7 × 27.7 cm. Munich, Städtische Galerie im Lenbachhaus.

the 1900 Paris World Exposition. Many of the works shown at Phalanx were based on themes of *The Kalevala,* an epic summarizing the mythology of the Finnic peoples (the Suomi and Karelians) who were, in fact, related to the Zyrians—all of them members of the broader linguistic category known as the Finno-Ugric.[14]

We also know that Kandinsky was an avid collector of folk art and that he not only delighted in the Bavarian folk art of *Hinterglasmalerei,* but also imitated it himself from about 1910 on, frequently casting the subject matter in Russian terms, as for example in *St. Vladimir* of 1911 (fig. 10.3).

But of course the most telling demonstration of Kandinsky's deep ethnographic interest was his inclusion of ethnic artifacts in the ground-breaking and influential *Blue Rider* almanac of 1912. A wide variety of ethnic objects was illustrated in the almanac, most having to do with themes of healing and salvation: Bavarian "miracle" paintings, a Ceylonese dance mask of the demon of disease, an Easter Island ancestor figure, and so on. As I have already suggested elsewhere, Kandinsky and his co-editor Franz Marc had consciously provided the almanac with a shamanistic theme, symbolizing their belief in the new art as a metaphor for cultural healing and salvation.[15]

In preparation for his ethnographic expedition Kandinsky marked a map of the area he was to visit (fig. 10.4) indicating that his route lay from Moscow to Vologda, near the fortieth meridian, and then east and north almost to the Urals. This corresponds roughly to what is today a territory combining parts of the Vologda and Arkhangel'sk Oblasts together with the Komi Autonomous Soviet Socialist Republic, a vast and still sparsely populated area of over 600,000 square miles still largely covered by dense taiga forest as it was in Kandinsky's day, stretching west to the crest of the Ural Mountains and north to the tundra of the Arctic circle. The major rivers, the Suchona, the Pechora, the Vychegda, and the Sysola, have been important transportation routes since the area was first settled in the tenth century. The central city of Syktyvkar, in Kan-

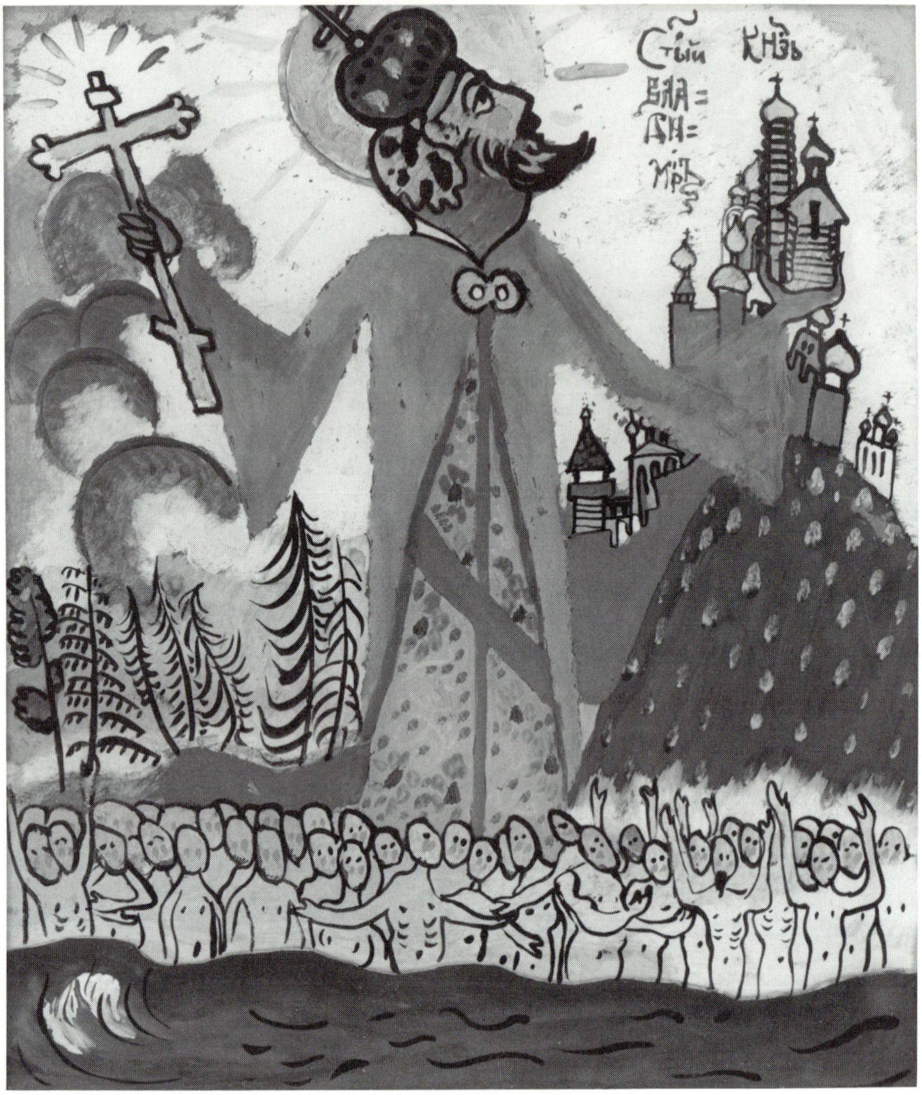

Fig. 10.3. Kandinsky, *St. Vladimir,* 1911. Glass painting, 29 × 25.6 cm. Munich, Städtische Galerie im Lenbachhaus.

dinsky's day known as Ust'-Sysol'sk, standing at the confluence of the Sysola and the Vychegda, was and is still an important center of trade especially noted for its fairs. Due to the density of the forests rich in game (especially squirrel and arctic fox) and the plentiful rivers, the native people, the Zyrians (or Komi), were hunters and fishermen.[16]

Kandinsky's ethnographic essay consists of three main elements: a critique of the established church in its relation to the Zyrians; a review of some of the major Zyrian deities and animating spirits; and an extended discussion of the Zyrian concept of *ort,* a palpable double or shadow. He had chosen this investigation of pagan beliefs, he wrote, "in view of the chaos of *contemporary* religious concepts."

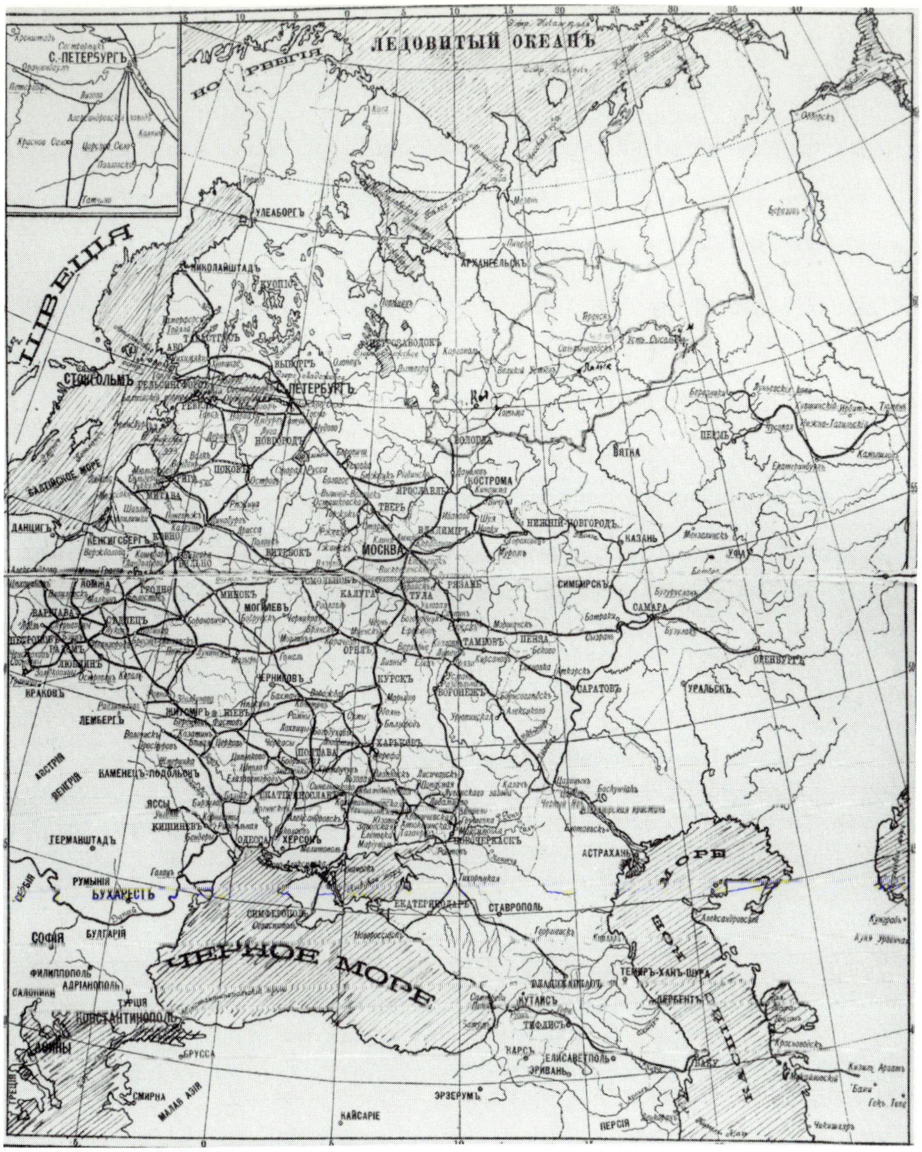

Fig. 10.4. Map marked by Kandinsky to indicate boundaries of the Vologda province, affixed to flyleaf of diary, 1889. Paris, Musée National d'Art Moderne.

Kandinsky's critique of the church for its role in the "reckless" and almost total eradication of ancient Zyrian beliefs and customs is sharp. He particularly notes that it was the missionary zeal of St. Stephen of Perm that had forced the Zyrian conversion and caused the utter destruction of another regional tribe, the Chuds (who, it was said, to avoid the Bishop's persecution, had fled into the forests where they buried themselves and their belongings).[17] As a result, the Zyrians had been taught to refer to their ancestors by the derogatory (Russian) term *poganyi*, a word suggesting something unclean, a meaning emphasized by its etymological association with the Russian *poganka,* a poisonous mushroom.

Among the various deities and legendary figures about whom Kandinsky sought information was the so-called Slata Baba or "golden woman" mentioned by the sixteenth-century Austrian diplomat and gadabout Baron Sigmund von Herberstein, whose famous chronicle of his Russian travels the young scholar had evidently consulted. Another was called Iomala, about whom only notions of evil or anger remained and another, Churila, who, according to one old man, was a principal deity of the ancient Chuds to whom this informant ascribed an animistic religion.[18] A deity named Voipel remained unidentified. Two other creatures who once animated the Zyrian world also survived only in fragments: the *leshak-mort* or "forest man," and Poludnitsa, a "midday-goddess" thought to protect the rye (in olden times, according to Kandinsky, no Zyrian would harvest the rye before St. Elias Day for fear of reprisal from her).[19] In his diary Kandinsky apparently recorded yet another deity, Vörsa, a water-spirit reputed to steal horses and children.[20]

The *domovoi,* however, a house-spirit imagined as a benevolent though sometimes mischievous protector of hearth and home, was still an active participant in Zyrian life. Associated with the hearth, the Zyrian *domovoi,* Kandinsky reports, refuses to move into a new house until the hearth is ready. Even then, no move to a new dwelling is made without some sacrifice for fear of disturbing the ancestors and thus provoking the *domovoi* to mischief, even to the extent of causing a death in the family. In this sense Kandinsky associates the *domovoi* with the Zyrian's ancestor cult, despite the Russian origin of the term.

As to natural phenomena such as the heavenly bodies, constellations, wind, fire, etc., Kandinsky found that somewhat stronger superstitions and remnants of pagan beliefs survived. The Zyrians still imagined the stars as "nailed" to the sky and the sun and moon as wanderers (a belief shared by the neighboring Samoyeds, who called the North Star the "nail of the sky").[21] Fearing to incur the sun's wrath, no one dared carry ice uncovered before St. Elias Day lest hail be sent in revenge, and old women still held "conversations with the wind." Various taboos concerning fire, such as prohibitions against spitting into it or stomping it out with the feet, and the use of fire for purification recalled the pagan veneration of fire.[22]

Kandinsky devotes most of his commentary to a consideration of remnants of the Zyrian's ancestor cult, especially as seen in their persistent although rather vague conceptions concerning an elusive being known as *ort.*[23] In so doing, his main concern is to demonstrate that the notion of *ort* is not to be misconstrued as "spirit" in the Christian sense of that term. Indeed, he sharply criticizes two scholars who had translated the Zyrian term *ort* by the Russian word *dukh* (meaning spirit in the intellectual Christian sense). Pointing out that all of the Zyrian forest spirits and water sprites are conceived of as corporeal, Kandinsky advances various testimony from his observations and interviews to show that *ort* was conceived of similarly.

Among the proofs of *ort*'s physical nature, Kandinsky reports, is its appearance before death when it is said sometimes to pinch the dying person so severely as to inflict blue spots. More often *ort* visits the dying person's relatives both before and for forty days after death, walking about in much the same form as the person of whom it is the double. Sometimes a towel is hung outside the home where a death has occurred so that *ort* and the dead person may dry themselves in the morning, but only *ort* is said to notice the towel.[24] In the case of a dead sorcerer *(koldun),* whose ability to transcend earthly bonds is especially suspect, Kandinsky reports that the Zyrians tie up the body so that relatives won't be disturbed by his *ort*'s nocturnal visits. It never occurs to anyone, Kandinsky observes, that the soul cannot be bound.

Such customs speak "loud and clear," Kandinsky says, against the exact identification of the *ort* with the dead person, not to mention his spirit or soul, about which no care is taken whatsoever. Interestingly enough, the young ethnographer calls upon that classic anthropologist and founder of the discipline, Herbert Spencer, to demonstrate that other primitive peoples may be more advanced than the Zyrians in respect to their understanding of the body-soul dichotomy. He cites a section from Spencer's multivolume work *The Principles of Sociology,* first published in 1876, dealing with the Indian Bhils who, it was said, left food at the grave for the dead person and at the threshold of his house for his "spirit" *(dukh).*[25] As to where the *ort* comes from and whence he goes after death, the Zyrians are mute. But, Kandinsky concludes, unquestionably the *ort* is not a spirit (in the sense of *dukh,* i.e., spirit, mind) and certainly not the *dukh* of ancestors.

As we shall see, these musings on *ort,* the discussion of the precise meanings of *dukh* (which shares the root of *dukhovnom,* the term Kandinsky would later use in the title of his treatise *O dukhovnom v iskusstve, On the Spiritual in Art*), and the references to practices concerning the burial of the *koldun,* the sorcerer or shaman, were to have important repercussions in Kandinsky's art and thought.[26]

Of primary concern to Kandinsky in composing his notes for this remarkable essay was his interest in the phenomenon of *dvoeverie* (or "double faith"), that is, the side-by-side existence of both pagan and Christian belief systems sometimes inextricably intertwined. We have already seen that in the artist's memory the moment of his immersion within a brightly painted decorated peasant house with its painted folk heroes and its "holy corner" was the apotheosis of his Vologda experience. Now, from the perspective of the ethnographic essay, one can imagine the overwhelming sense of presence in that room of the *domovoi,* perhaps even an *ort.* If perchance he had noticed an icon upside down, he would have been told that the saint was being "punished" for visiting an illness upon the family. Or, had he stayed on past St. Elias Day, he might have found a sheaf of rye or oats adorning the holy corner, representing the last sheaf of the harvest and laid there to assure a successful harvest the following season. On St. Elias Day itself, he might have followed the peasants out to the fields where they would appeal for a good harvest to their ancestors, whose spirits they imagined as residing among the grain.[27]

Viewed with the artist's ethnographic background in mind, the Russian paintings take on new meaning. *Motley Life,* with its bright medley of figures and action, is a prime example (fig. 10.1). Like *Arrival of the Merchants,* this painting presents a throng of people in old Russian costume converging on a town bordering a river. We need only recall that Ust'-Sysol'sk, the center of Kandinsky's activity as ethnographer, was at the confluence of two important rivers, and that it was therefore famous for its fairs, to recognize the setting. Clearly, both Christian and pagan imagery are present amidst this teeming multiplicity of life. The whole composition is built upon a series of contrapuntal contrasts: life and death, old and young, love and hate, peace and war, and so on.

Central to the composition is the figure of a long-bearded old man, a rucksack on his back, a staff in his hand. Is this the "old man" among Kandinsky's Zyrian informants who carried within himself the recollections of the Zyrian people? For assuredly we are back in Ust'-Sysol'sk in the midst of a fair by the Vechegda River. The squirrel in the tree about to be done in by the archer below is the "dead" giveaway, for the harvesting of squirrel pelts was then as central to the region's economy as the fir tree was central to its spiritual life.[28]

But the old man may have other connotations. His unrealistic green beard suggests an alliance with the supernatural and hence his possible identification as "old sorcerer." He carries a stave that points to the central vertical axis of the painting, leading the eye upward to the pair engaged in a life-and-death struggle and then on to the walled town (or monastery) with its church domes at upper center. Thus another counterpoint is set between upper and lower spheres, between pagan and Christian, an axis that turns about life and death.

An identification of the old man as old sorcerer is reinforced by the fact that among the Votiaks, another Finno-Ugric tribe with whose traditions Kandinsky was familiar, the being who instructs the shaman on supernatural matters is imagined in the form of an old man, and among the neighboring Cheremis the name for shaman or sorcerer is *kart* or "old man." Furthermore, the stave carried by the old man also suggests a reference to shamanic lore, for among several Siberian tribes the stave functions as the shaman's symbolic "horse" on which he rides to "other worlds" in the course of his duties.[29]

If we recall that *Motley Life* was painted in 1907 when Kandinsky was living in Sèvres, we should also recall that the artist was visited there by his father, who lived with him for some time. Since the elder Kandinsky would have been a source of Buriat lore, having lived near the Lake Baikal Buriat peoples much of his life, another interpretation of the old man is possible. The Balagask Buriats imagine the "owner of the whole earth," a personage called Daban-Sagan-Khatun, as a benevolent old man.[30] Then, too, it is primarily among the Buriats that the shamanic use of horse staves or horse sticks is common.

To return to the painting: immediately behind the old fellow, almost growing out of his back, is a tall tree—a pine, cedar, or fir, in any case symbolizing the home of the ancient pagan spirits. Dramatically opposing him across that vertical axis is the figure of an elaborately costumed mother and child flanked by a child in prayerful attitude, an obvious reference to orthodox veneration of the Virgin and child. Thus, horizontally across the central axis, we find yet another contrapuntal expression of *dvoeverie*. Examples of the pagan-Christian opposition can be found throughout the picture: the figure with stave, black beard, and tall black hat to the left of center suggests a black shaman, opposing the orthodox monk figure immediately to the left; just above right center, smoke from a fire (recalling pagan veneration of fire) opposes the church tower of a Christian cemetery, etc. A double meaning may in fact accrue to the mother-and-child image for, according to Fedotov, the cult of the Virgin (as Mother of God) was also allied with pagan veneration of Rozhanitsy, a goddess of childbirth, related doubtless also to the ancient myth of Slata Baba, the "golden woman." According to Herberstein's account and depictions in other old chronicles as well, Slata Baba was depicted with a babe in her arms and a small boy standing by her side. More observations could be made about this painting, but let these suffice to suggest that, indeed, this work has to do with the ramifications of *dvoeverie*.[31]

A somewhat later Munich work with ethnographic implications and a complex iconography that includes *dvoeverie* is Kandinsky's 1911 glass painting, *St.*

Vladimir (fig. 10.3). The work is an imitation of a Bavarian folk art known as *Hinterglasmalerei,* and in this sense then it is in the form of an ethnic artifact. The Cyrillic inscription translates as "Holy Prince Vladimir," recalling Vladimir's secular life before his baptism in A.D. 989 when he received the name Basil (Wassily), which was also Kandinsky's Christian name. The saint's position as founder of the Russian church is clearly symbolized by the cupolaed church held aloft in his left hand. The ranks of the baptized, white faced and red cheeked (like Kandinsky's recollection of the Zyrians), stand below him. But to the left of the picture, below the saint's right arm, stands a forest of fir or pine trees, recalling the sacred groves of the heathens and the homes of their former deities. Vladimir's identification in Russian lore with the ancient cult of the sun can be recognized in the halo behind his head, which is also a sun, with sun streaks emanating from it. St. Vladimir, in fact, was also known in the Russian epic poems as *Krasnoe Solntse',* "Ardent Sun" or "Radiant Sun."[32] Kandinsky's interest in the cult of the sun and his awareness of the loss of cultural heritage brought by Christianization led him to create in this modern icon a symbol of *dvoeverie.*

But it is in Kandinsky's self-identification with the image of the Russian folk hero St. George that we see the real meaning for him of his ethnographic studies and his awareness of *dvoeverie.* St. George, whose image adorned the cover of the *Blue Rider* almanac, came to be the carrier of Kandinsky's message of aesthetic salvation and healing, a fundamental theme of the almanac itself and one which recurred in his work throughout his life. In Kandinsky's mind, St. George epitomized the message of many of the ethnic artifacts illustrated in the almanac, each in its own way expressing a shamanistic appeal to the gods for health and eternal life.[33] The book itself was a metaphor for the social healing Kandinsky hoped the new aesthetic would bring. In fact, St. George, the ubiquitous *Egori Khrabry* (George the Brave or Hero) of Russian epic poetry, although a Christian saint, was endowed with shamanic powers.[34] As I have noted elsewhere, in Russia the saint's feast day on April 23 was also an important day in the agricultural calendar, celebrated with pagan rites as well as Christian ritual, and Kandinsky included in the almanac a Russian folk print from his own collection on this very theme, a typical example of *dvoeverie.*[35]

As a student of ethnography at a time when the discipline was growing by leaps and bounds, particularly in Russia where the lure of the mysterious Siberian tribes had been felt for centuries, Kandinsky would have been familiar with the literature on shamanism. He had obviously delved into the matter in his readings of Herberstein, Spencer, and Epiphanius (all referenced in his essay), and it can scarcely be doubted that he had read at least some of the burgeoning literature on the subject published in Russia and Germany from the middle of the century onward.[36] Indeed, Kandinsky would have heard relevant papers on shamanism read at meetings of the Imperial Society of Friends of the Natural Sciences, Anthropology and Ethnography at which he himself presented oral reports, and doubtless he would also have read essays on the topic published in *Ethnographic Review* to which he also contributed.[37]

When Kandinsky consulted Baron von Herberstein's famous account of his travels in Russia in the early sixteenth century, published as *Rerum Moscoviticarum Commentarij,* perhaps he had access to the Basel edition of 1556. He would have found the first full-page woodcut illustration in the book devoted to a seated portrait of the Russian Tsar Vasili III (resplendent in fur-trimmed robe and cap). He would also have noticed the inset heraldic emblem depicting St. George and the dragon (fig. 10.5). It is,

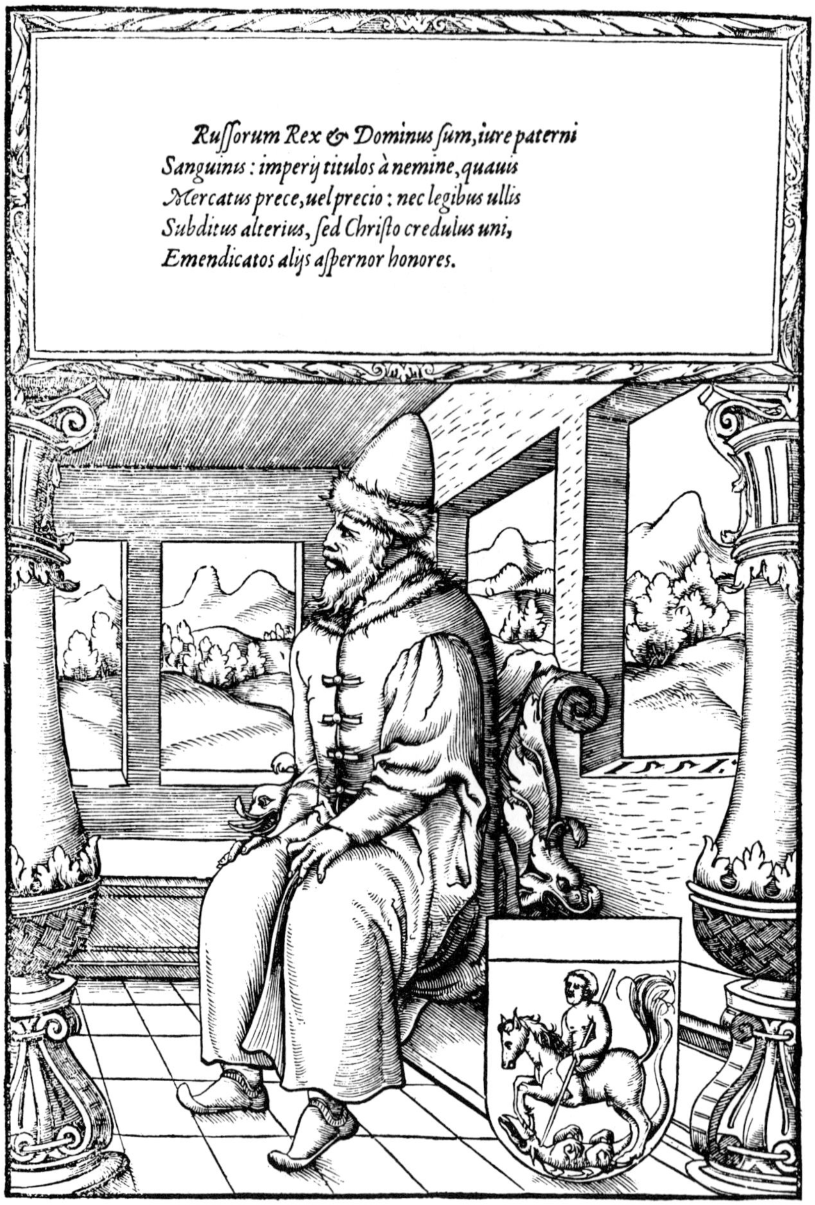

Fig. 10.5. Portrait of the Russian Tsar Vasily III from Sigmund Freiherr von Herberstein, *Rerum Moscoviticarum commentarij*... (1556). Photo Cornell University.

at any rate, a warrior astride a horse, directing his lance downward onto the throat of a vanquished dragon. But this saint has no Christian paraphernalia; indeed, he is short haired and quite naked—a pagan hero, Egori the Brave, carrying out the raw act that would lead to his canonization. As Egori the Brave was to Vasili III, so St. George and the dragon would become to "Vasili" Kandinsky. Surely we have come here upon the origin of that identification that would inspire the artist until the end of his life.

Other woodcuts in this edition suggest the original inspiration for later Kandinsky motifs. For example, one large woodcut illustrates the dress of Russian war-

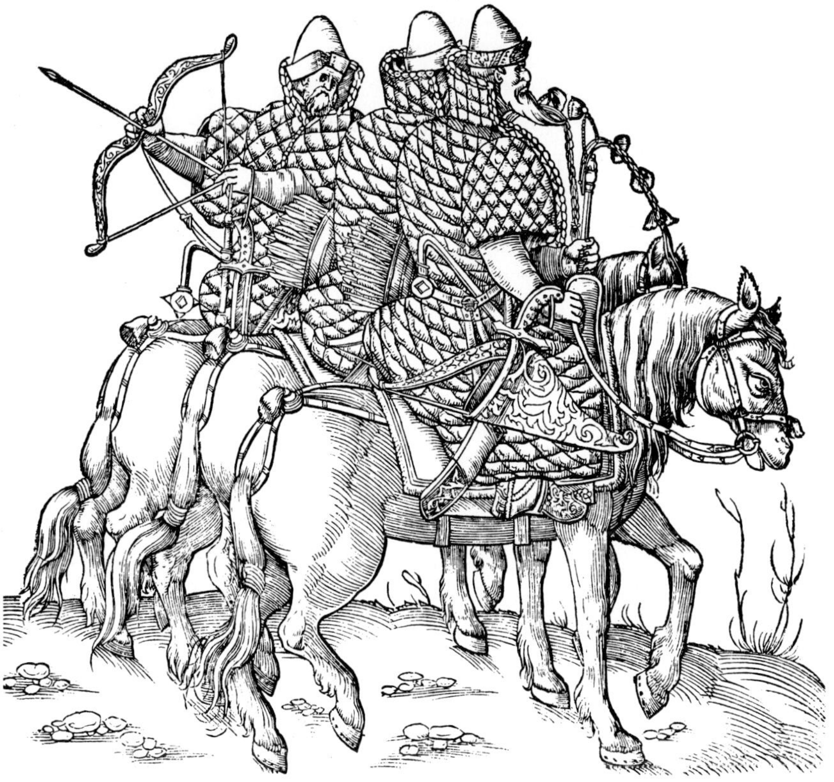

Fig. 10.6. Russian *Streltsy* from Sigmund Freiherr von Herberstein, *Rerum Moscoviticarum commentarij . . .* (1556). Photo Cornell University.

riors, or *streltsy.* Three warriors sit astride their fine horses. One raises his bow and arrow, turning to aim backward over the horse's rump (fig. 10.6).[38] Kandinsky recalled this marksman in an early tempera called *Russian Knight* (1902) and in *Picture with Archer* (1909).

St. George's Day also received Herberstein's attention. In the same section dealing with the legend of the "golden woman" to which Kandinsky referred in his essay, Herberstein related a tall tale of Russian natives who were said to "die" on the autumn St. George's Day, November 27, and to "rise again" on the spring St. George's Day in April.[39]

The SHAMAN ARTIST

For Kandinsky the step from identification with the role of St. George to assuming the role of shaman was easy enough: the Siberian shaman was also a "rider" whose calling was to heal. Indeed the shaman role may well have been the prior one in Kandinsky's experience.[40]

The role of the shaman in Russia's primitive tribes both east and west of the Urals was already well documented and understood by both European and Russian ethnologists by the 1880s. The term shaman is derived from an Evenk word, *saman,* which has been shown to have the etymological root of the Tunguso-Manchurian verb *sa,* "to know."[41] The shaman, then, was the all-knower who assumed the role of intercessor between humankind and the supernatural powers. Through his offices, physical and psychological ills could be healed, social problems of the clan solved, the future foretold, good hunting assured, and the lost found.[42]

The shaman—who had to be a person peculiarly predisposed to his calling—achieved his communication with the heavenly powers by leaving his body and journeying to other worlds (of which most tribes imagined there were several). He made this journey by means of his drum, which during his trance became his horse. On this magic horse he could fly above the treetops and mountains or descend to the underworld.[43] Among some tribes, notably the Buriats of the Lake Baikal area, he rode to his destination upon his horse stick.

Both the drum and the horse stick would have had special meaning for Kandinsky. For the drum provided a kind of canvas upon which the shaman drew pictograms of the upper and lower worlds and the creatures in those spheres who operated as his helpers (figs. 10.7, 10.8). The horse stick was an actual hobbyhorse cut from a birch tree (the birch being widely considered a sacred tree from west of the Urals to east Siberia). The upper end was sometimes crudely carved to suggest the horse's head, sometimes the middle was shaped to suggest the knee joint, and the lower end might be carved to suggest the hoof.[44]

We have only to turn to Kandinsky's memoir, "Rückblicke," to see how near was this shamanistic hobbyhorse to him. In the opening sentences he recalls that, like all children, he had loved to ride. He particularly recalled how his family's coachman used to carve for him just such a "horse" from the branch of a tree.[45]

Among Kandinsky's personal collection of folk art there was a wooden hobbyhorse—not of the stick variety but rather of the representational, rocking type—which seems to have had as rider a sorcerer or shaman (fig. 10.9).[46] The little figure was a bearded old man clad in a long robe and riding a spotted (piebald) horse; he wore a tall, pointed hat. It would seem that, odd as such a toy might be, this rider in fact represented a sorcerer or shaman. A similar shaman image in a tall, pointed cap figures in Kandinsky's painting *Storm Bell,* probably painted around the time of *Motley Life*. The piebald horse was particularly prized among the shamanistic tribes of Siberia, and we should note that Kandinsky also recalled in his memoir that the sight of such a horse in Munich had called up memories of his Russian past.[47]

But there is more that recalls shamanism in "Rückblicke." In speaking of the creative experience, Kandinsky echoed the sense of transport, the image of "riding" and "reining in" or "bridling" his inner resources in much the same language ethnographers have used to describe the shamanic experience. Expanding on the image of riding, Kandinsky writes: "The horse carries the rider with power and speed. The rider, however, guides the horse. Talent carries the artist to great heights with power and speed. The artist, however, guides his talent." He continues in the Russian edition: "The artist is perhaps in a position albeit only partially and by chance—to summon up within himself these states of inspiration by artificial means. Moreover, he can qualify the nature of those states which arise within him of their own volition. All the experience and knowledge that relate to this area are but one of the elements of 'consciousness.' "[48]

These confessions parallel to quite an astonishing degree the reports of

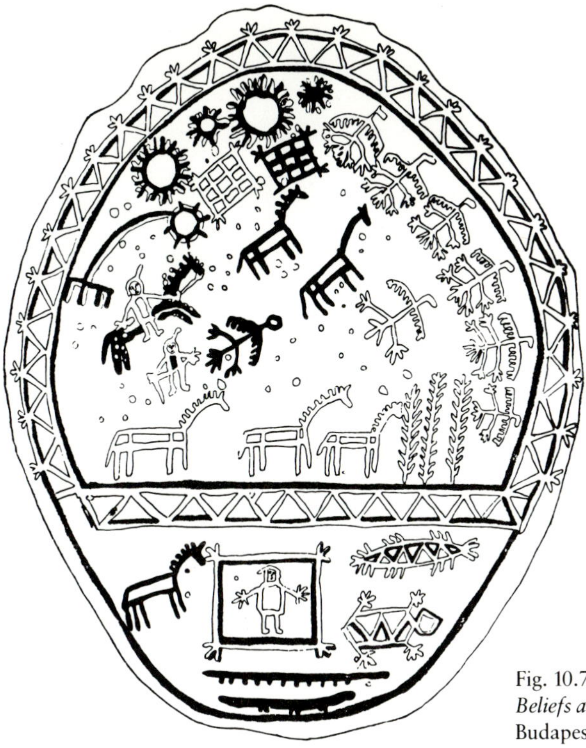

Fig. 10.7. Teleut Shaman's Drum. From Vilmos Diószegi, *Popular Beliefs and Folklore Tradition in Siberia* (Akadémiai Kiadó, Budapest, 1968), p. 493.

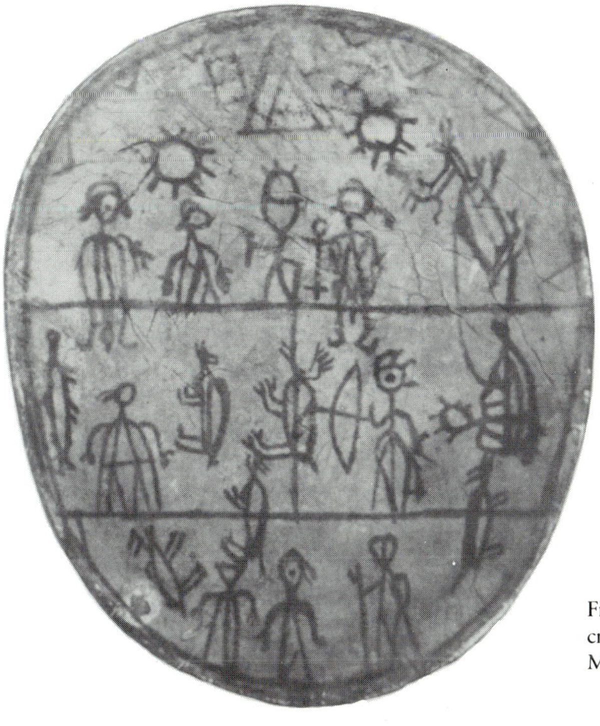

Fig. 10.8. Lapp Shaman's Drum. Bowl type, 37.5 × 32.9 × 9.4 cm., pine with reindeer skin membrane. Munich, Staatliches Museum für Völkerkunde.

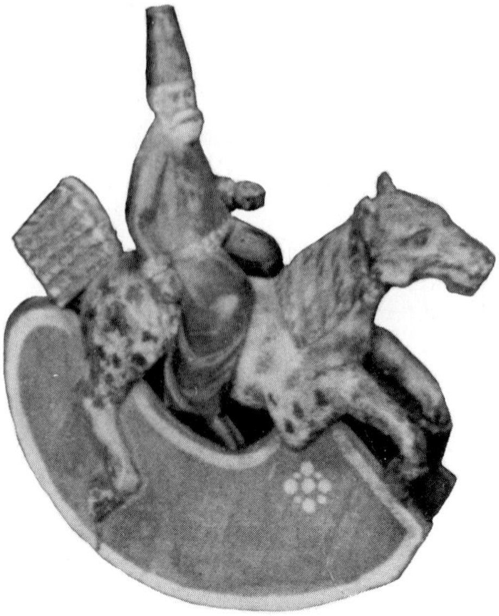

Fig. 10.9. Rocking horse toy with bearded figure, formerly collection of Kandinsky. Carved and painted wood.

ethnographers on the special psychological traits of Siberian shamans and their trance experiences. Shamans were almost universally marked by a special degree of sensitivity, often expressed in nervousness, excitability (sometimes to the point of hysteria), and innate creativity. For all that, they were required to keep themselves in check, to "rein in" their talent as it were, and to control their capacity to achieve various states of trance. Most authorities agree that the shaman was likely to be particularly intelligent and to have the capacity for special powers of memory and self-control. It might be "an inner voice" that would bid a likely candidate into communion with the supernatural.[49]

In Mikhailovskii, we read a description of a shamanic ritual in which the shaman *places the drum close to his host's ear,* blowing on his "sacred instrument," in order to drive into him the "spirit and power of his forefathers, thus preparing him to receive and understand the succeeding prophecies of the shaman." We are reminded here of Kandinsky's often-quoted introduction to the catalogue of the second Neue Künstlervereinigung exhibition—a passage that reverberates with shamanic analogy—in which he wrote of: "The calling. The speaking of secrets through secrets," and where he admonishes him who would turn *"the ear of his soul from the mouth of art"* (italics mine). He concluded by speaking of art as the means by which "man speaks to mankind about the supernatural."[50] It is the artist who holds the key to communication with supernatural powers—the artist in the role of shaman.

For the shaman, too, the creative act is a transport—in trance he imagines that he leaves his body and is transported to other realms where he sees figures and images of all kinds; upon his return, he reports what he has seen. As he drums and chants the tale of his incredible journey—for it has not been without struggle and hair-raising adventure—the drum becomes his vehicle, as the canvas or woodblock becomes the artist's vehicle, a concept Kandinsky tried to convey in naming his book of poems and woodcuts *Klänge,* "resonances." Repeatedly the shamanic experience is compared to a kind of "rebirth" or to a creation of "worlds," an analogy Kandinsky would apply to art.[51]

Kandinsky's metaphor of the artist riding his talent as a horse brings us back to the role of the drum/horse in the shamanist ceremony. In that ritual, which is found from the Finno-Ugric peoples of northwestern Russia to the far eastern tribes of Siberia, the shaman's drum plays the essential role. Without it he cannot make his journey either to retrieve the soul of a fatally ill person or to ask the gods for direction to the best hunting grounds. Drumming upon it he imitates the hoofbeats of his magic steed and upon its back he soars to those other worlds.

It would appear that, with the passage of time, Kandinsky's self-identification with the role of the shaman grew ever deeper. Not only do the signs and symbols of shamanic imagery appear in his works, but his writings, always visionary in tone, take on more shamanistic imagery as well. A striking example of this is his 1935 essay "Empty Canvas, etc."[52]

In his 1892 treatise on shamanism (published, as we have seen, by the same society that in 1889 had elected Kandinsky to membership), Mikhailovskii included a long extract that he had taken from accounts recorded and published by the German ethnologist Wilhelm Radloff in 1884 (a work that was doubtless accessible to Kandinsky, too). The documentation concerns the shamanizing ritual of an Altaian shaman attending sacrificial rites to the celestial deity Bai-Yulgen. Before undertaking his precarious journey into other worlds, the shaman must "enliven" or "animate" his drum. He does so by solemnly summoning his helping spirits. Drumming and chanting, taking on the roles of the spirits as they appear, he gathers them into his drum. As each one appears it calls, "Here am I!" As for example:

> You who rides amongst the thunder
> Who playfully with lightning comes
> Autumn cloud great with thunder
> Vernal cloud rich with lightning . . .
> Come . . .

Repeatedly after each new appeal, the spirit helper arrives with the call, "Here am I."[53]

Kandinsky begins his essay with an address to his "empty" canvas: he says it is only apparently empty and silent, but in actuality it is "full of tensions with a thousand soft voices, expectant." As each of the artist's elemental forms appears on the canvas, it announces *me voilà*, "here I am." "Each line says 'Here I am.' " "Black circle—distant thunder, a world for itself that seems to concern itself about nothing. . . . 'Here I am.' " All these voices come together in the total painting as a chorus, "HERE I AM." What "happens" in the painting shouldn't happen on the surface of the canvas, but "somewhere" in "illusory" space. In this way, the artist concludes, truth is born out of untruth—as indeed, we may add, the shaman often performs a miraculous deed through an apparent ruse. This truth, says Kandinsky, is called "HERE I AM."[54]

Almost universal across greater Siberia is the imagery of the cosmic tree (the sacred birch or sacred fir or pine), the ladder or ladder tree (by which the shaman ascends to the celestial sphere), the sacred path (river or road), and signs of the heavenly bodies (including moon, sun, the North Star, Venus, and the constellations), as well as a host of animal and bird spirits (which vary from place to place), and figures with special attributes representing various gods. Some of these images are physically present at the shaman rite. The cosmic tree, for example, is represented by the tree itself, some-

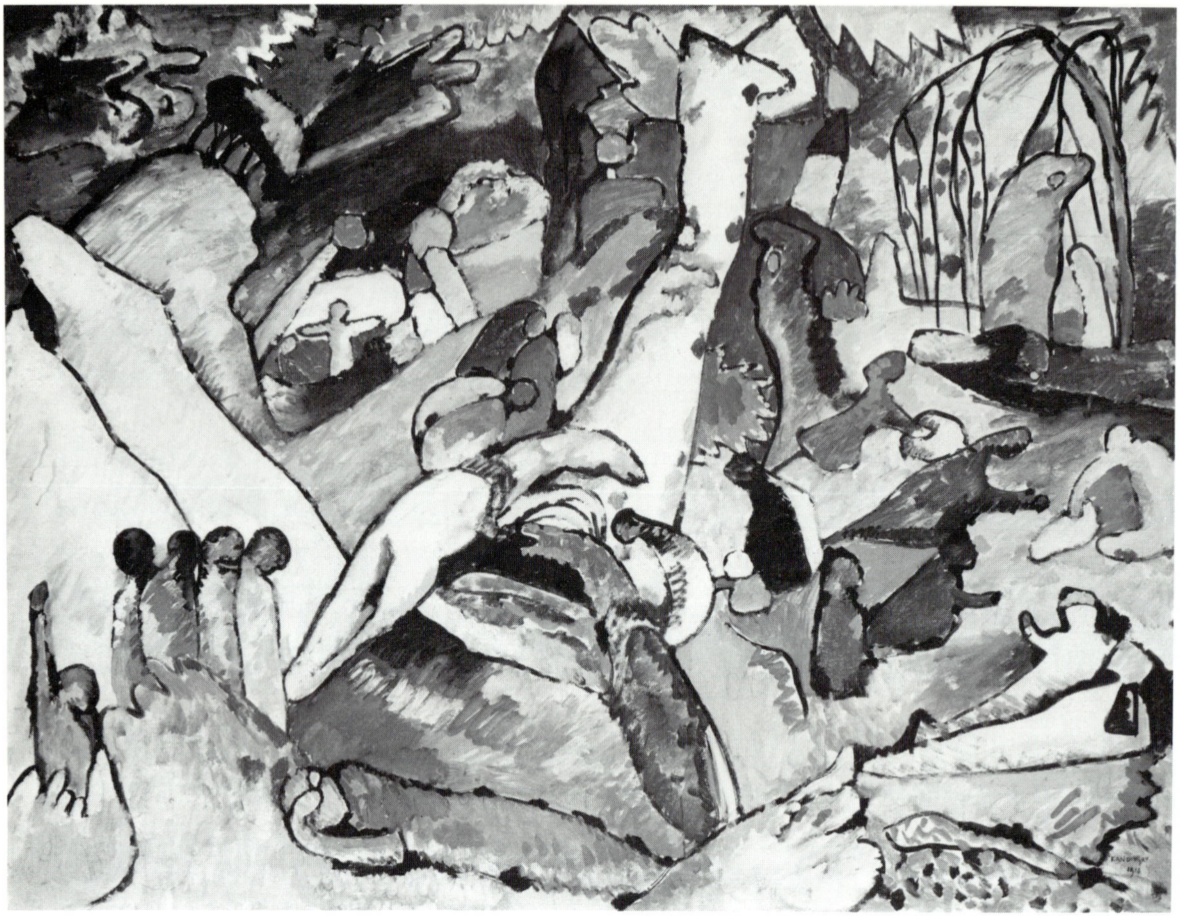

Fig. 10.10. Kandinsky, *Sketch for Composition 2*, 1909–10. Oil on canvas, 97.5 × 131.2 cm. New York, Solomon R. Guggenheim Museum. Photo Robert E. Mates.

times cut whole and set up in the tent or yurt; sometimes steps are cut into it to form the ascensional ladder.

We also find these elements represented on the surface of the shaman's drum (figs. 10.7, 10.8). As Mircea Eliade remarks, the drum "harbors a large number of ascensional symbols."[55] The surface of the Teleut drum shown in fig. 10.7 is divided into upper and lower spheres, corresponding to the celestial and nether worlds, which are separated by a zigzag line (the sacred path), also seen around the border of the upper half. Within are depictions of the sun and moon, the North Star and Venus, gridlike signs that may refer to the "Book of Divination," horses, riders, and birdmen. The celestial tree is to the left.[56] The zigzag line represents the road or path the shaman is required to follow to attain his goal, and the cosmic tree is his means of communication with the supernatural powers. Drum imagery is widespread and is found among the Lapps, the Ostiaks, the Yakuts, the Buriats, the Tungus, and the Teleuts, among others.

The Lapp drum depicted in fig. 10.8 is of particular interest to us because it is in the collection of the Museum für Völkerkunde in Munich and, indeed, was there as early as 1862. If we recall that it was in the collections of this museum that Kandinsky found most of the ethnic artifacts reproduced in the *Blue Rider* almanac, we can scarcely doubt that he was also aware of the presence of this drum. This speculation is further enhanced by the knowledge that the first issue of *Ethnographic Review,* the same one in which Kandinsky's first oral report to the society was noted and his field trip to Vologda province announced, carried a major article by N. N. Kharuzin entitled "On the Noids [Shamans] among the Ancient and Contemporary Lapps."[57] Remarkably well preserved (and accurately described in the museum catalog by 1904 as a Lapp shaman drum), the drum presents an array of figures relating to the Lapp pantheon of gods and to their world of reindeer, hunters, fishermen, and shamans. Of these, the image of the shaman-archer with his reindeer quarry and the central god of the upper region, corresponding to the heavenly sphere, with his hammer are perhaps the most striking. The hammer-carrying god is Tiermes or Thor, god of thunder; he is called Perun by other Finno-Ugric tribes and often associated since Christianization with St. Elias. The figure in the sled heading upward along the right edge toward the upper "celestial" zone may be an image of the shaman on his journey. Perhaps most striking of all is the mysterious double triangle at upper center. It has been identified variously as a sign for a mountain, a tent, or an encampment, most probably the home of Radien, the highest Lapp god—the world god who creates, structures, and orders all of life.[58]

Other symbols to be found on shaman drums include fantastic animals that seem to have no specific reference but look like strange microscopic amoebae. Besides the drums he may have seen in the collections of the anthropological museums in Moscow, St. Petersburg, Munich, Berlin, and Paris, Kandinsky would have encountered reproductions of them in the ethnographic literature with which he was familiar, including the ubiquitous Radloff.[59] These examples in no way exhaust the vast vocabulary of Siberian shamanic imagery. Besides the drum pictograms, many shaman costumes were hung with a multiplicity of signs in a great variety of materials (from forged pieces of iron, to conical copper "bells," to "snakes" of skin and fur). These also represented such entities as the heavenly bodies, as well as "helper spirits" in animal form—ribbons of fur or cloth to suggest snakes or dragons, kidney-shaped amulets associated with particular charms or spirits, etc.[60]

In the Russian edition of his memoir, Kandinsky recalled, "Once, in the throes of typhoid fever, I saw with great clarity an entire picture, which, however, somehow dissipated itself within me when I recovered. Over a number of years at various intervals, I painted *The Arrival of the Merchants,* then *Motley Life;* finally, after many years, I succeeded in expressing in *Composition 2* the very essence of that delirious vision." As I have suggested elsewhere, this is clear indication of an iconographic relation between these three pictures. Like *Arrival of the Merchants* and *Motley Life, Composition 2* (fig. 10.10) is crowded with figures and goings on. It has been described as a representation of the apocalyptic Deluge.[61] But might this work, again, be a testimony to Kandinsky's interest in *dvoeverie?* Might the giant figure in the foreground be the Zyrian Vasa, the water spirit who is imagined as clad in a green robe? It is said that when he throws himself from the shore into the water, a tempest arises.[62] Or, again, might this be a shaman figure in trance, with his spirit helpers flying on horseback above his head, ascending the "cosmic tree"? On the other hand, we seem to find the old man of *Motley Life* prone before a sacred tree in the upper right: a reference to the pagan custom of shaman burial in the sacred grove? Do the kneeling figures before him drum? To the left of the cosmic tree or pillar we see a figure in yellow standing in a boat. If we are dealing with a tempest brought on by Vasa, then perhaps here we have also to do with Numi-Torum, the principal god of the Voguls (neighbors of the Zyrians) who controlled all natural phenomena. His son, Yanykh-Torum, takes the form of a man, but it is said that "from the splendour of his raiment he shines like *gold*." It is he who descends to earth to respond to mortal appeals concerning atmospheric conditions. Is that, then, Yanykh-Torum in the boat?[63] Finally, both Finno-Ugric and Buriat legends concerning a great flood have been documented in the literature.[64] Perhaps here we have to do with Kandinsky's most complex statement on the phenomenon of *dvoeverie*.

A large watercolor entitled *In the Circle* (1911) with pictographic inclusions is particularly suggestive of the kind of pictographic elements on shaman drums. Suggestions of horses, ladders, and zigzag paths float about within a clearly circular drum form. Indeed, it is scarcely necessary to point out again the association in Kandinsky's mind between the horse and the circle. The shaman's drum is his horse, and for Kandinsky the representational horse became the circle, a round form closely analogous to that of the drum with which the shaman "shamanizes." Perhaps the most important work of 1911 was Kandinsky's *Composition 5 (Last Judgment)*. The Christian elements of this painting have been analyzed in some detail in the literature.[65] But within the present ethnographic context the similarity between the central double triangle and that on the shaman drum at Munich's Völkerkunde Museum is striking (figs. 10.11 and 10.8). The one-eyed figure in the upper left corner with black streaks signifying flying hair also recalls the one-eyed gods with flying streaks for hair as depicted in the drum pictograms. Further, the boat, the zigzag line reminiscent of those on shaman drums, and the iconographic remnant representing St. Elias—associated with Perun, the god of thunder—all suggest that here too the artist recollected his ethnographic experience.[66]

As I have suggested, shamanic imagery proliferates in Kandinsky's late work as well. In *The Arrow* (1943) the "skeletonized" figures, the arrow, the floating "drum" and "drumstick" (on the right shoulder of the right hand "skeleton") also call shamanic imagery to mind. *Figure Blanche* (1943) suggests a white shaman with his paraphernalia: an oval-shaped drum, a triangular "mask," various pendants common to the shaman's coat, feathered ornaments, and a boat (sometimes the shaman must forsake his horse for a boat). Certainly *On White* (1923), which must be considered part of the same series that includes *In the Black Square* and *Black Accompaniment*, seems to refer to shamanic lore in several of its figures: the black form streaking from lower right to upper left (toward heaven) is in the shape of the classic shamanic "horse stick," with a horse-head top and a bent knee midway. Kandinsky's hooked-curve symbol, upper left, to suggest horse and rider is presented threefold. The "cosmic mountain," "bird spirit," and cloud forms all attest to the shaman's flight to other worlds, and the kidney-shaped amulets of the shaman's coat can also be seen. The St. George figures of *In the Black Square* and *Black Accompaniment* may now be seen in this ethnographic light as fulfilling a shamanic role as well.[67]

In the shamanic literature we learn of the "black" and "white" shamans of the Buriats (the white associated with benevolent actions, the black, with evil), and we also find that in some shamanic rituals, the shaman is mysteriously endowed with the ability to speak words in strange tongues that sound like nonsense words. We also

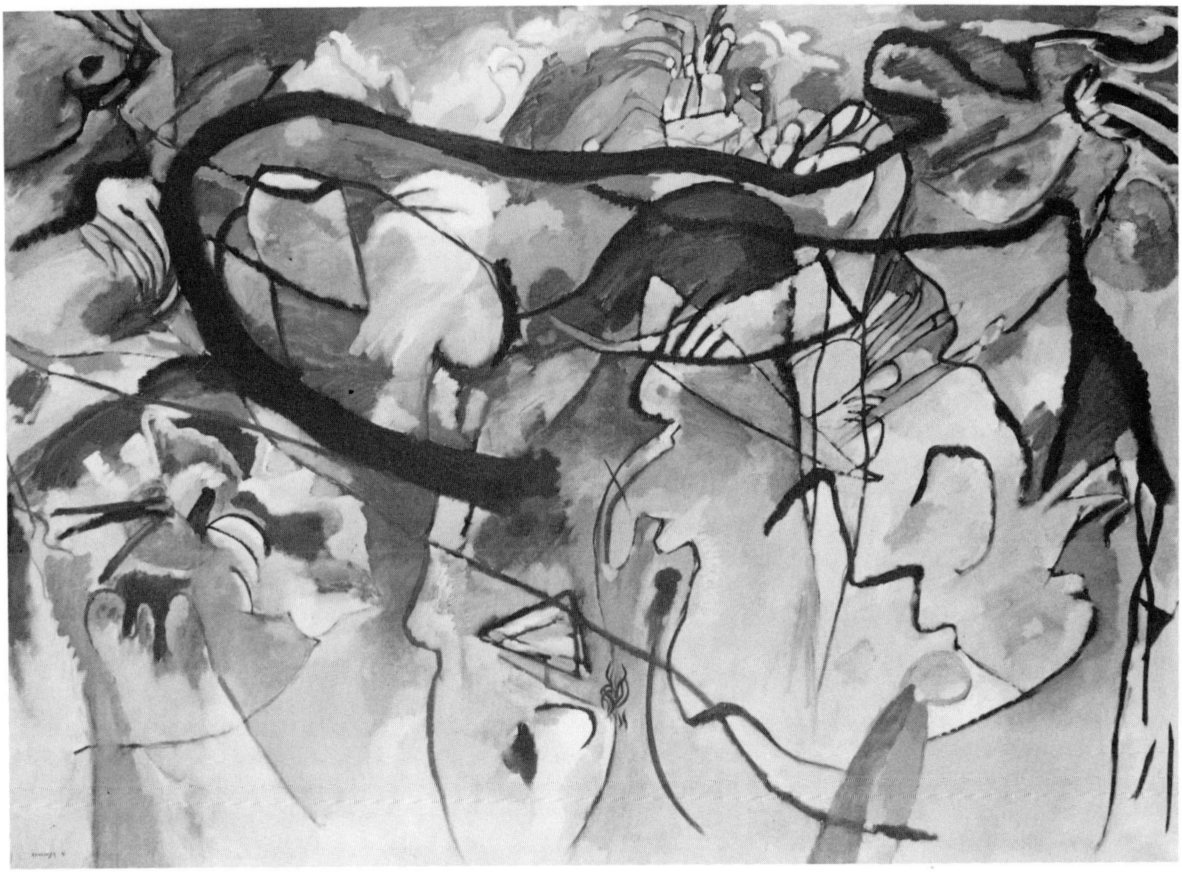

Fig. 10.11. Kandinsky, *Composition 5*, 1911. Oil on canvas, 190 × 275 cm. Switzerland, private collection. Photo Öffentliche Kunstsammlung Basel

read that in some areas, the observers at a shamanic ritual may act as a chorus to the shaman's song. Can we doubt then that Kandinsky's knowledge of such ethnographic lore informed the creation of his "color composition" or chamber opera *The Yellow Sound?* From this perspective, the dancer in white appears as a white shaman; the voice crying out *"undeutliche"* words such as *"Kalasimunafacola!"* may represent the shaman's voice; and the "black man" who appears on stage opposite a child in white suggests the role of the black shaman.[68]

It has been amply demonstrated that *The Yellow Sound* is steeped in orthodox Christian symbology.[69] But within its pages in the *Blue Rider* almanac are illustrations of ethnic artifacts, such as the Ceylonese demon mask of disease from Munich's anthropological museum side by side with Christian images. It may be recalled now that this very mask was reproduced in the pages of *International Archive for Ethnography,* the same journal that commented favorably upon Kandinsky's essay in *Ethnographic Review.* It may well be that we have here another case of *dvoeverie,* and that a second look at this stage composition from the perspective of Kandinsky's ethnographic training and experience would be rewarding.

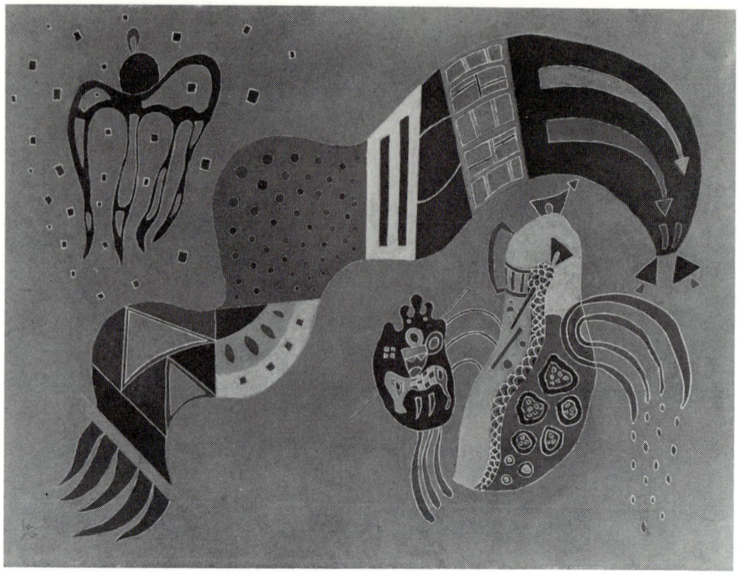

Fig. 10.12. Kandinsky, *Tempered Elan*, 1944. Oil on cardboard, 42 × 58 cm. Paris, Musée National d'Art Moderne.

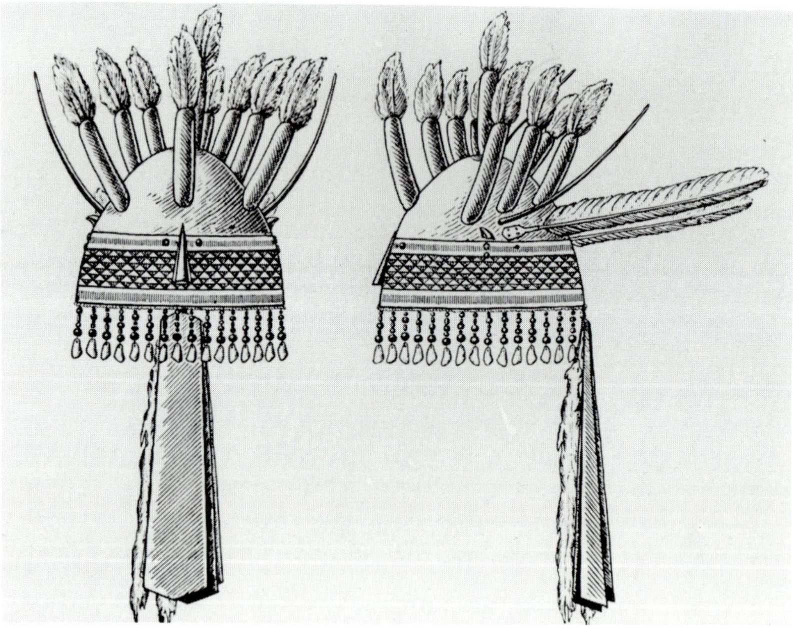

Fig. 10.13. Headdress of Tuva shaman. From Vilmos Diószegi and M. Hoppál, eds., *Shamanism in Siberia* (Budapest: Akadémiai Kiadó, 1978), p. 332.

As Kandinsky felt his life coming to its close, his paintings took a more somber turn. *Ribbon with Squares* (1944) sets its figures out upon some cosmic plane like nothing so much as a shamanic "icon." To the left is the head of the iron eagle who bore the shaman, below him the eternal snake (whose home, in Buriat lore, lies at the root of the cosmic tree in a lake of milk), above, the fire wheel—lighted by Russian peasants on St. John's night—symbolizing the ancient cult of the sun; below, the checkerboard of fate (perhaps associated with the so-called Book of Fates, which is represented by a grid on some shaman drums) and the ladder by which the shaman ascends to the heavenly spheres, while to the right, an ascending "soul" begins its journey beneath a square symbol of earth.[70] Another of the very late paintings, *Tempered Elan* (1944) returns to the St. George theme. Curiously St. George is presented as if inlaid within an emblematic palette or shield form, much in the same way that he appeared in that sixteenth-century edition of Herberstein's chronicles (figs. 10.5, 10.12).[71]

Apparently faced with a premonition of his death in February of 1944, Kandinsky's mind returned to his ethnographic experience, and in a work entitled *Le Lien vert* (fig. 10.14) he painted an almost representational image of himself assuming the shaman's role for his last journey. As we have seen, Mikhailovskii, in his 1892 paper on shamanism, recounts in great detail the ritual of an Altaian shaman in which, during the enlivening of the drum ceremony, the spirits called out as each arrived, "Here am I." At the climax of this ritual, as the shaman on his horse/drum reaches the zenith of his ride, he sings:

> Lord to whom three ladders lead,
> Bai-Yulgen, owner of three flocks,
> The blue slope which has appeared,
> The blue sky which shows itself,
> The blue cloud which whirls along.
> Inaccessible blue sky,
> Inaccessible white sky. . . .
> Who uses the hoof of the horse. . . .
> [Who] has created all men. . . .
> Thou who the starry sky
> Thousands and thousands of times hast turned,
> Condemn not my sins![72]

Le Lien vert provides a graphic depiction of this scene. On the right we see a conglomerate of forms hovering about three vertical stripes. In the shaman's song just quoted, the three ladders refer to the sacred tree or heaven tree, usually represented in the shamanic ceremony by three actual birch trees by which the shaman ascends to the celestial sphere.[73] At the foot of Kandinsky's triple tree trunk is a triangle, representing the cosmic mountain at the center of the earth. At the top, hovering just above the sacred tree, is a cloud symbol. Seen in this perspective, the hovering forms coalesce and metamorphose into the form of the artist shaman himself.

> But then I grasped
> My heaven tree grasped I
> How many are my colleagues
> May they bow down before me![74]

Here the shaman grasps the celestial tree wondrously with three arms (in Buriat legend, metamorphosis is characteristic of the shaman). His head is turned back over his shoulder and he wears, not the pointed cap, but a feathered helmet, another common type of shaman headdress (fig. 10.13).[75] Near his head, to the left, floats his drum. His coat is elaborately decorated, and he seems to wear his breastplate (a feature common among the Buriats and others) on his back. (The shaman's breastplate is often embroidered with "ribs" mimicking the shaman's skeleton.) His curved drumstick (ladle shaped, as is normal) floats just to the left of this ribbed breastplate. Floating about him are other small circles and pendants.

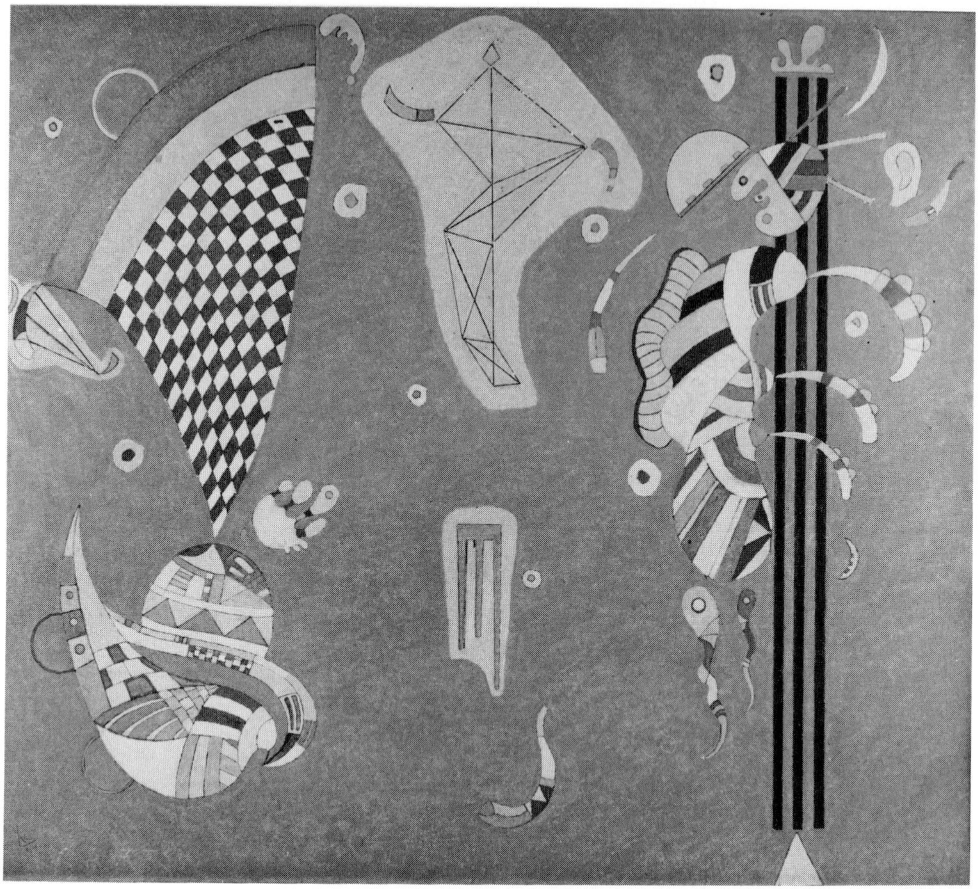

Fig. 10.14. Kandinsky, *Le Lien vert,* 1944. Oil on cardboard, 46 × 54 cm. Milan, private collection. © Galerie Maeght Lelong, Paris. Photo Claude Gaspari.

If we refer to the two drawings done in preparation for this painting (figs. 10.15, 10.16), we find, especially in the detail of the shaman alone, that these pendants and circles take on distinct similarities to the pictograms of heavenly bodies on shaman drums (cf. figs. 10.7, 10.8). They seem to represent the sun, moons, and planets. A comparison of the drum as depicted in the two drawings with its representation in the final painting reveals a progressively more accurate recollection of the drum in the Munich collection. In each case the edge of the drum is given a slightly different treatment. And in one, the decorative elements characteristic of the back side of bowl-shaped Lapp drums are suggested (fig. 10.15). But in the final painting, the stretched edge of the membrane pulled tight over the side of the bowl-shaped drum is indicated by geometric serrations, similar in their regularity to the more scalloped edge of the actual drum (figs. 10.14, 10.17).

On the left-hand side of the picture, we observe a hand-shaped form with more than the normal number of fingers. This, too, is most likely a reference to shamanic lore. The six-fingered hand is a common attribute of the shaman's costume (usually cut out of metal and appended, along with many other signs, to the back of his

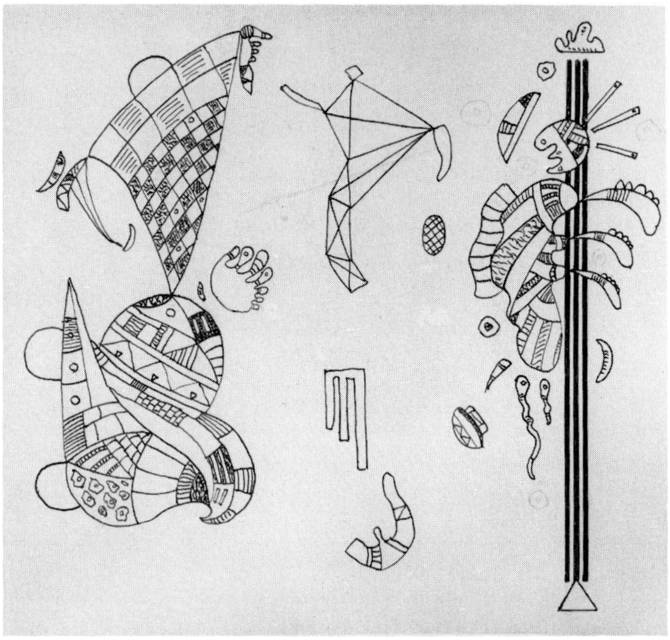

Fig. 10.15. Kandinsky, untitled drawing for *Le Lien vert,* February 1944, india ink and black lead, 19.6 × 21.1 cm. Paris, Musée National d'Art Moderne.

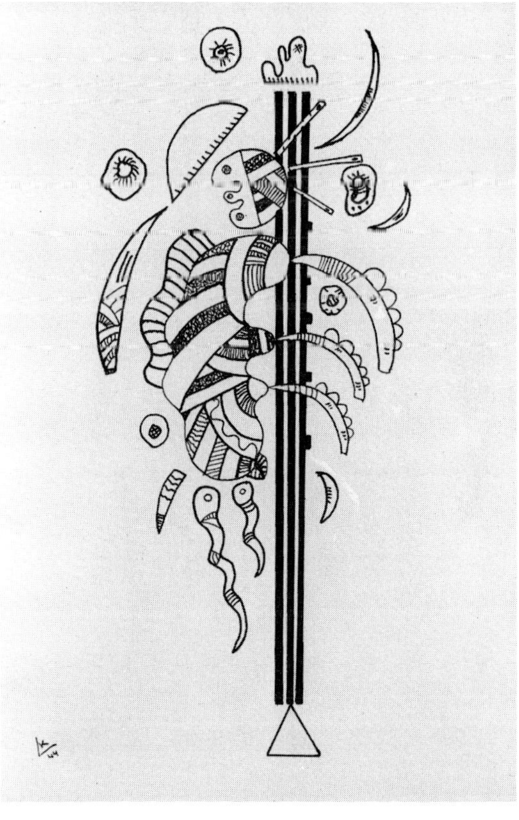

Fig. 10.16. Kandinsky, untitled drawing (of detail for *Le Lien vert*), February 1944, india ink, 27.3 × 17.2 cm. Paris, Musée National d'Art Moderne.

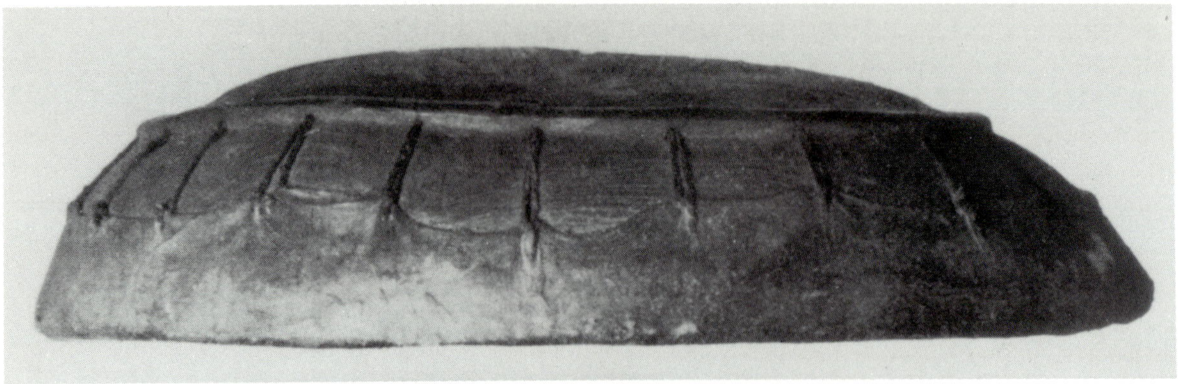

Fig. 10.17. Lapp Shaman's Drum, side view. Munich, Staatliches Museum für Völkerkunde.

coat). Its purpose is to distinguish the shaman from ordinary mortals. Kandinsky has improved upon the traditional design by adding one more finger to make seven, a number particularly important in shaman legend and lore.[76]

Hovering between the two richly decorative areas of the painting, and central to it, floats a figure consisting mostly of triangular forms. This seems to represent the skeleton or abstracted "double" in its shroud, perhaps the artist-shaman's *ort* tied up in accord with Zyrian custom.[77] In fact, the painting's original French title, *Le Lien vert* (used by Kandinsky in his own house catalogue), hitherto translated in the literature as *The Green Band,* offers an obvious clue. In the painting, the lines that form the horizontal axis and one side of the uppermost trapezium are *green* (as are two other lines of this geometric aggregate). This suggests that a more precise English translation would be *The Green Bond* (or cord or shackle).

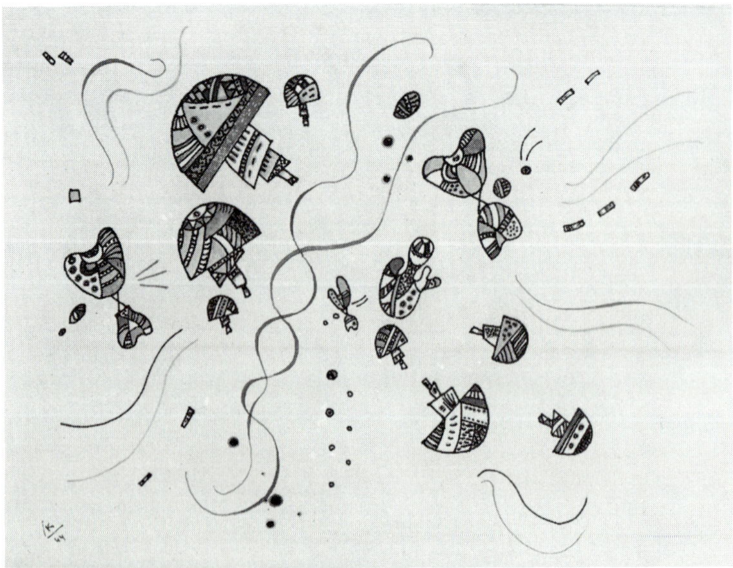

Fig. 10.18. Kandinsky, untitled watercolor ("last watercolor"), 1944, india ink, black lead, 25.5 × 34.6 cm. Paris, Musée National d'Art Moderne.

The most obvious figure in the almost Scythian conglomerate of forms rising to the left is the triangular grid or checkerboard. Its shape mimics the central skeletal *ort* to a certain degree, suggesting its position here as the second type of soul with which Zyrian belief endowed the human being, namely, the nebulous *lol,* literally the breath-soul, which upon death leaves the body as vapor. Its pattern adds a further interpretation relating to the "Book of Fates" or "Book of Divination" (often represented on shaman drums as a grid). This in turn is related to the deeply-rooted Russian belief that one's destiny is determined at birth. The dangling amulets suggest soul forms, perhaps here signifying rebirth. The mushroom-domed form below suggests the general shape of the Siberian yurt or dwelling, but it may have another association, as we shall see. The whole configuration seems to sail heavenward upon the back of a form resembling a bird, a frequent host of the soul among the Finno-Ugric, especially the Zyrian, peoples—and reminiscent of the fabulous "diver bird" associated in Finno-Ugric and Buriat myth with the creation of the world.[78]

There is, however, an important element missing from the final painting, a detail that was perhaps too close and too secret to expose to public view. In the large drawing (fig. 10.15), floating just below the shaman and to the left, is a mushroom-shaped form. In fact, I believe it is a mushroom and that it refers again back in time to Kandinsky's ethnographic essay. Kandinsky had reported that, with Christianization, the Zyrians had been forced to refer to their ancestors by the "insulting" name *poganyi.* As noted, etymologically related to *poganyi*—and sharing the implication of something dirty and inedible—is the Russian word *poganka,* a poisonous mushroom. But there is a further implication here. Widespread among the Finno-Ugric shamans was the custom of using the poisonous mushroom *amanita muscaria* (or *agaricus muscarius*), commonly known as fly agaric, to help achieve the state of trance and hallucination. In Zyrian Sysola dialect, exactly the area of Kandinsky's study, the word *pagalny (pagavny)* means to "lose consciousness," "to be poisoned," "to stagger," a reference to the ritual use of fly agaric. Neither the semantic nor the shamanistic associations would have been lost on Kandinsky, the trained ethnographer. In a watercolor of the same year as *Le Lien vert* Kandinsky filled the sheet with a veritable rain of mushrooms, together with some butterfly "souls" (fig. 10.18).[79]

Both *Motley Life* and *Composition 2* came to Kandinsky while he was in a state of hallucination from typhoid fever, according to the Russian edition of "Rückblicke." In the same edition he also remarked, "The artist is perhaps in a position—albeit only partially and by chance—to summon up within himself these states of inspiration by artificial means." He goes on to say that only years of experience train the artist to control these moments, to bring them up at will. We cannot know exactly what he meant by "artificial means," but in *The Green Bond,* he has left a suggestion that perhaps he envied the shaman's intoxication and ready trance. Perhaps he felt his own creative powers slipping away and gave expression to a dream of the past, of a time when he was in his youth and nothing was impossible.

If we turn once more to the lines of the opening poem from Kandinsky's *Klänge* with which this essay began, we realize that we are once again confronted with a reminiscence of his ethnographic experience. The man with the white face and red cheeks in the long black coat who drums his way along the road is a Zyrian shaman. Sometimes he drums "feverishly," sometimes "mechanically," sometimes he drums "like the white-furred toy rabbit, which we all so love." The white rabbit pelt is in fact of particular significance to the Buriat shaman (and the Altai as well), for it represents the spirit of the hunt and is widely considered a messenger or helper of the powerful forest spirit. The fur of the white rabbit is said to have fallen from heaven into a shaman's drum to aid the original hunter, and among the Altais it is also associated with the protection of horses.[80]

Kandinsky ends the poem by saying that he has seen all this "from above" and begs the reader to do likewise. The shaman artist, on his sounding drum, has taken wing and would indeed fly to other worlds.

> His magic drum they hung on him
> His magic drum pulled itself tight
> Again he shamanized
> The old one doesn't cease.[81]

ACKNOWLEDGMENTS

Although these acknowledgments must be limited to a mere list, I hope that my friends and colleagues who so generously shared their time and expertise will read between the lines the depth of my gratitude: Kenneth C. Lindsay (State University of New York at Binghamton); Angelica Rudenstine (Institute of Fine Arts, New York University); Olga Snegireff-Fedoroff Stacy; Agehnanda Bharati (Syracuse University); Michaela Appel (Staatliches Museum für Völkerkunde, Munich); Ed Evans (Tozzer Library); Syracuse University librarians Elizabeth Gardiner, Randy Bond, and Dorcas Macdonald; graduate assistants Alyce Jordan and Elisa Bob; also Anna Gorbatsevich and Gerry Greenberg (Syracuse University); and the late William Wasserstrom (Syracuse University), whose enthusiasm for my earlier "shamanist" interpretation of the *Blue Rider* almanac encouraged me to pursue this research.

NOTES

1. Wassily Kandinksy, "Iz Materialov po Etnografii Sysol'skikh i Vychegodskikh Zyrian—Natsional'nyia bozhestva (po sovremennym verovaniiam)," *Etnograficheskoe Obozrenie (Ethnographic Review)* no. 3 (1889): 102–10. See also Nina Kandinsky, *Kandinsky und ich* (Munich: Kindler, 1976), 29, where the implication is that his appointment to the society ensued immediately after his return from Vologda province in the summer of 1889. New evidence, however, indicates that his involvement with the society, and perhaps his membership as well, dates from the previous year (see Peg Weiss, *Kandinsky and "Old Russia"—An Ethnographic Exploration,* Yale University Press, in progress). An abbreviated version of the present essay appeared in the *Syracuse Scholar* 7, no. 1 (Spring 1986): 43–62. (Transliterations from the Russian generally follow Library of Congress standards except that in some instances German transliterations have been retained. Some Russian "ii" name endings have been rendered as "y.")

2. Wassily Kandinsky, "O nakazaniiakh po resheniiam volostnikh sudov Moskovskoĭ gubernii" (On the Punishments [meted out] in Accordance with the Decisions of the District Courts of the Province of Moscow), *Trudy Etnograficheskago Otdela Imperatorskago Obshchestva Liubiteleĭ Estestvoznaniia, Antropologii i Etnografii* (Works of the Ethnographic Section of the Imperial Society of

Friends of the Natural Sciences, Anthropology and Ethnography), vol. 9 (Moscow, 1889), 13–19. For further information on Kandinsky's activities with the society and on several hitherto unknown publications by the young ethnographer, see P. Weiss, *Kandinsky and "Old Russia,"* cited in note 1, above.

3. Nina Kandinsky, *Kandinsky und ich*, 29.

4. Kandinsky "Rückblicke," in *Kandinsky, 1901–1913* (Berlin: Der Sturm, 1913), viii (hereafter, Kandinsky, "Rückblicke"). See also Kenneth C. Lindsay and Peter Vergo, eds., *Kandinsky Complete Writings on Art* (Boston: G. K. Hall, 1982) in which this work is translated as "Reminiscences" (357–82). I have used here my own translations from the German unless otherwise indicated; when reference is made to the 1918 Russian edition of this memoir, I have relied entirely and gratefully upon Lindsay and Vergo.

5. Kandinsky, "Rückblicke," XI.

6. Kandinsky, "Reminiscences" (Russian version) in Lindsay and Vergo, *Complete Writings*, 891, n. 47, 48.

7. Peg Weiss, *Kandinsky in Munich—The Formative Jugendstil Years* (Princeton: Princeton University Press, 1979), 63, 111, passim. For a travel account written only 42 years earlier on an expedition into the same region, see August Freiherr von Haxthausen, *Studien über die innern Zustände, das Volksleben und insbesondere die ländlicher Einrichtungen Russlands* (Hannover, 1847), VIII–IX, "Abreise nach Wologda," 223–82. Although the Baron's trip was mainly to collect agricultural data, many of his observations strikingly anticipate Kandinsky's.

8. Kandinsky, "Reminiscences," in Lindsay and Vergo, *Complete Writings*, 891, n. 45. According to Kandinsky, Ivanitsky lived in Kadnikov, a town to the northeast of the city of Vologda.

9. Kandinsky, "Rückblicke," IV, XXVIII. In the Russian edition of his memoir, Kandinsky reported that his father hailed from Nerchinsk, still further to the east; presumably he did spend at least a part of his life there.

10. Nina Kandinsky, *Kandinsky und ich*, 22. According to biographer Will Grohmann, Kandinsky had also once accompanied his father on a trip into Russia's Kazan province, where, Grohmann reported, "he was struck by the diversity of the nationalities in that part of Russia." See Will Grohmann, *Wassily Kandinsky, Life and Work* (New York: Abrams, 1958), 29.

11. As late as 1937, at the age of 71 and nearly half a century after the fact, Kandinsky recalled the "violence" of the impression made on him by his Vologda trip. See the letter from Kandinsky to André Dézarrois, 31 July 1937, quoted in Christian Derouet and Jessica Boissel, *Kandinsky: oeuvres de Vassily Kandinsky (1866–1944)* (Paris: Collections du Musée National d'Art Moderne, 1984), 13. The essays were not included in Lindsay and Vergo's edition of Kandinsky's writings on art, but there is a summary by John Bowlt, who concludes his observations on Kandinsky's Zyrian essay with the remark: "But there is very little indeed that relates to Kandinsky the artist or thinker of later years" (p. 863). A translation into German is available in H. K. Roethel and J. Hahl-Koch, eds., *Kandinsky Die gesammelten Schriften*, vol. 1 (Bern: Benteli, 1980), 68–87, 194–98. Errors and omissions, however, render this version unreliable.

12. Uno Holmberg [Harva], *Finno-Ugric, Siberien*, vol. 4, *The Mythology of All Races* (Boston: Archaeological Institute of America, 1927), esp. 10, 164, 527, 536, 542, 576, and passim. Kandinsky's work was cited by Holmberg as early as 1913 in *Die Wassergottheiten der finnisch-ugrischen Völker* (Helsinki: Druckerei der finnischen Literatur-Gesellschaft, 1913), 107, 286. For other authors who have cited Holmberg's numerous writings see, among others, Vilmos Diószegi, ed., *Popular Beliefs and Folklore Tradition in Siberia* (The Hague: Mouton, 1968); Vilmos Diószegi and M. Hoppál, eds., *Shamanism in Siberia* (Budapest: Akademiai Kiado, 1978). See also D. R. [Fokos] Fuchs, "Eine Studienreise zu den Syrjänen," *Keleti Szemle* xii, no. 3 (1911). For Paulson's recent citation of Kandinsky, see Ivar Paulson, "Outline of Permian Folk Religion," *Journal of the Folklore Institute* 2 (1964): 174, n. 104. Notice of Kandinsky's work on the Zyrians was originally given to Western European scholarship in the journal *Internationales Archiv für Ethnographie*, vol. 3 (1890), when N. v. Seidlitz reviewed the third number of *Ethnographische Rundschau (Etnograficheskoe Obozrenie)*, providing the title and a brief summation of Kandinsky's article (p. 247). The journal is interesting also for the articles it ran on topics that would have special interest for Kandinsky both at the time and later in his career, as will be shown.

13. See, for example, Károly Rédei citing Fokos-Fuchs and using Kandinsky's words almost exactly in the definition of a Zyrian word in *Die Syrjänischen Lehnwörter im Wogulischen* (The Hague: Mouton & Co., 1970), 95, n. 19.

14. See Weiss, "Kandinsky in Munich: Encounters and Transformations," in *Kandinsky in Munich 1896–1914* (New York: Solomon R. Guggenheim Foundation, 1982), 47–48. See also Uno Holmberg, *Finno-Ugric, Siberien,* passim, and Peter Hajdu, ed., *Ancient Cultures of the Uralian Peoples* (Budapest: Corvina Press, 1976), 1–144.

15. See Weiss, "Kandinsky in Munich: Encounters and Transformations," cat. nos. 304–10 and pp. 67–82; Peg Weiss, "Kandinsky and the Symbolist Heritage," *Art Journal* 45 (Summer 1985): 137–45. Several of the actual objects originally illustrated in the *Blue Rider* almanac, located by Kandinsky in Munich's anthropological museum, were included in the 1982 Guggenheim Museum exhibition "Kandinsky in Munich," organized by the author. Interestingly enough, the Ceylonese dance mask of the demon of disease from the collection of the Staatliches Museum für Völkerkunde in Munich had been illustrated in full color and described in great detail in volume 6 (no. 3) of the *Internationales Archiv für Ethnographie* (1893), the same journal in which Kandinsky's essay on the Zyrians had earlier been reviewed (Albert Grünwedel, "Sinhalesische Masken," 82–88, plate VII); cf. n. 12 above.

16. See Theodor Shabad, *Geography of the USSR A Regional Survey* (New York: Columbia University Press, 1951), 154–69, and M. G. Levin and L. P. Potapov, eds., *The Peoples of Siberia* (Chicago: University of Chicago Press, 1964), 91, 100, 106–108, and passim.

17. Kandinsky reports that though the Zyrians claim to know the location of some of these sites, they refuse to dig them up out of superstitious fear of some calamity. The image of burial occurs in several later Kandinsky paintings (e.g., *Improvisation 18, with Tombstones* and *Improvisation 21,* both of 1911). As his source for the information on St. Stephen, Kandinsky refers to the *Life of St. Stephen, Bishop of Perm* by Epiphanius the Wise, famous for his literary style of "word-weaving." St. Stephen of Perm (1349–1396) destroyed the arbors of the spirits and the idol sheds of the heathen Zyrians, but he also learned their language and created their alphabet. Perhaps most famous of the deeds related by Epiphanius was the bishop's encounter on the shore of the Vychegda River with the powerful Zyrian sorcerer, Pam. See G. P. Fedotov, *The Russian Religious Mind* (Cambridge: Harvard University Press, 1966), 230–45. From the fact that the Zyrians sometimes referred to their ancestors as *yelniki* (from the Russian *yel,* for fir tree), Kandinsky concludes that St. Stephen had cut down a sacred fir tree rather than the more often cited birch. But the tree varies from tale to tale; according to Vernadsky, St. Cyril cut down the sacred oak (George Vernadsky, *The Origins of Russia* [Oxford: Clarendon, 1959], 34). Most authorities agree that among the Finno-Ugric peoples (and indeed most other Siberian tribes), the birch, pine, fir, and cedar trees were most often designated as sacred.

18. See Holmberg, *Finno-Ugric,* 217 and especially 260–61. Although Kandinsky found no traces of Herberstein's "golden woman," she was probably a goddess of childbirth venerated by the Khanty/Mansi (Vogul and Ostiak) peoples who lived mostly, but not exclusively, on the eastern side of the Urals along the Ob River. See also Z. P. Sokolova, "The Representation of a Female Spirit from the Kazym River," in Diószegi and Hoppal, *Shamanism,* 498. It is important to note that Herberstein's chronicle which, as we have seen, was known to Kandinsky, included images of the fabled statue of the Slata Baba. This imagery was the subject of an important article by K. F. Karjalainen, "Alte Bilder zur ob-ugrischen mythologie" in *Mémoires de la Société Finno-Ougrienne* 135, no. 5 (1914): 1–26. Karjalainen traced the imagery of Finno-Ugric mythology in several old illustrated chronicles which may also have been known to Kandinsky as a student of ethnography. As for Iomala, the reference may have been to Joma, a mean forest witch, or it could also be taken as a reference to Jumala, a principle deity of the Finns. See D. R. Fokos-Fuchs, *Syrjänisches Wörterbuch* (Budapest: Akadémiai Kiadó, 1959), 332. Holmberg has also found that peoples of the south Votiak area know of a forest spirit that is especially evil called Shurali which plays particularly evil tricks (Holmberg, ibid., 181). Cf. G. V. Jusupov, "Survivals of Totemism in the Ancestor Cult of the Kazan Tatars," in Diószegi, *Popular Beliefs,* 199.

19. *Leshak-mort* was probably Holmberg's *vörys-mort,* a forest spirit taller than the highest tree who rushes about like a whirlwind. Kandinsky's love of color comes out in this discussion as he links Poludnitsa to the cornflower, known as "Poludnitsa-Blue" or "Eye of the Midday Goddess." See Holmberg, *Finno-Ugric,* 181 and 247, where he again cites Kandinsky.

20. Kandinsky's *vörsa* might have been the forest spirit *versa* described by Fokos-Fuchs as a giant as tall as a tree and having magic powers. (See D. R. [Fokos] Fuchs, "Eine Studienreise," 236 and *Syrjänisches Wörterbuch,* 103.) But since Kandinsky apparently identified this creature as a "water spirit," the reference may have been to *Vasa* described by Holmberg as a giant water spirit with a big round head, imagined as either clad in a green robe or naked, who causes tempests by throwing himself into the water. See Holmberg, *Finno-Ugric,* 197–98. Our knowledge of Kandinsky's exact diary notes is hampered by the fact

that it remains unpublished and has only been inadequately referenced in Roethel and Hahl, *Gesammelte Schriften* (196, n. 32), in which a few pages of sketches have been reproduced (figs. 17, 19–23). The diary itself, which Kandinsky kept with him until his death, is now in the Kandinsky archive at the Musée National d'Art Moderne, Paris. Small but thick, the notebook (502 pages; ca. 15 × 10 cm) includes ethnographic observations, bibliographic references and notes on reading, sketches of costumes, decorative details of interiors, furniture, landscape, architecture, lists of expenses, etc. (See Derouet and Boissel, *Kandinsky*, 13, 15.) For a discussion of the forest and water spirits of the Zyrians and their neighbors, see Ivar Paulson, *Schutzgeister und Gottheiten des Wildes (der Jagdtiere und Fische) in Nordeurasien*, Stockholm Studies in Comparative Religion, vol. 2 (Stockholm: Almquist & Wiksell, 1961), 124–27. Interestingly enough, Paulson's discussion of the Russian water spirit suggests the possible source for Kandinsky's 1911 oil painting *Nude:* "The wife of the northern Great Russian waterspirit has the appearence of a woman with great, pendulous breasts and long hair. She often sits on a stone by the water and combs her hair." (p. 279). Waves lap at the knees of Kandinsky's *Nude* and although she seems to lack a comb, her other attributes are suggestive. Furthermore, in the background, details of architectonic structures suggest the characteristic roof finials of Zyrian (and other north Russian) houses. Similar finials are depicted in Kandinsky's woodcut *Golden Sail*, fig. 2.

21. Holmberg, *Finno-Ugric*, 221.

22. In an 1896 paper on the Yakuts, the Polish ethnographer W. Sieroschevski, discussed similar superstitions concerning fire. See "The Yakuts," trans. W. G. Sumner, *Journal of the Anthropological Institute of Great Britain and Ireland* 31 (1901): 106. Kandinsky's colleague Ivanitsky also wrote on the veneration of fire among peasants of the Vologda area (see n. 31, below).

23. Although Kandinsky felt that this creature was a purely Zyrian phenomenon not mentioned by other scholars among the related Permians and Votiaks, it has been shown by Holmberg and others to have been a rather widely-spread belief, relating to the concept of the double. See Holmberg, *Finno-Ugric*, who relates *ort* to the Cheremiss *ört* and Vogul *urt;* see also Karoly Rèdei, *Lehnwörter*, 95, n. 19, who also relates it to *urt* and *vurt*. See also Géza Roheim, *Hungarian and Vogul Mythology*, Monographs of the American Ethnological Society (Locust Valley, N.Y.: J. J. Augustin, 1954), 49, 59, 85. For another very similar contemporary discussion of *ort*, see F. J. Wiedemann, *Syrjänisch-Deutsches Wörterbuch*, Indiana University Publications, Uralic and Altaic Series, vol. 40 (reprint of 1880 edition, The Hague: Mouton & Co., 1964), 211.

24. Rédei confuses *ort* with "spirit" *(Geist)* but cites Kandinsky's testimony on the "blue spots" almost word for word (though without reference), *Lehnwörter*, 95, n. 19. See Holmberg, *Finno-Ugric*, 169–72, with respect to the Votiak spirit *ubyr*. On the towel custom, see Gustav Ränk, *Die Heilige Hinterecke im Hauskult der Völker Nordosteuropas und Nordasiens*, Folklore Fellows Communications, no. 137 (Helsinki: Academy of Sciences of Finland, 1949), 48ff.

25. See Herbert Spencer, *The Principles of Sociology* originally published in London, 1876–96 (3 volumes). In the edition of 1882 (New York: D. Appleton & Co., 1882, vol. 1), the exact citation appears on p. 171, whereas Kandinsky cites p. 172, possibly from another edition. Roethel and Hahl have confused the issue by giving the English title of quite another work by Spencer titled *Descriptive Sociology*, which was a tabular compendium of information on the world's races and to which Kandinsky does *not* refer. (Cf. Roethel and Hahl, *Gesammelte Schriften*, 72, n. 1.) Kandinsky seems to assume that the Bhil's symbolic gesture of placing food at the *grave* for the body but at the *threshold* for the spirit implies a conception of separation of body and soul (or spirit) without an implication that the soul might be expected to "consume" the offering. For more recent research on the number and types of spirit/souls recognized by the Zyrians, see Ivar Paulson, "Jenseitsglaube der finnischen Völker I: in der wolga-finnischen und permischen Volksreligion" in *ARV* 20 (1964): 125–64, and V. N. Chernetsov, "Concepts of the Soul among the Ob Ugrians" (originally published in 1959) in H. N. Michael, *Studies in Siberian Shamanism*, Arctic Institute of North America Anthropology of the North: Translations from Russian Sources, no. 4 (Toronto: University of Toronto Press, 1963), 3–45. Chernetsov posits multiple spirit/souls.

26. Kandinsky's careful scrutiny of the usage of the word *dukh* (German *Geist*) and his *rejection* of it for the concept of a palpable double or shadow (which he describes as "relief-like") lend further weight to my discussion of his use of the term *dukhovnom* (as in *O dukhovnom v iskusstve*, translated by him into German as *Über das Geistige in der Kunst*) as a conscious choice to emphasize its meaning as spirit/mind rather than as having any association with a meaning-range that might convey a sense of "spiritualism" or "spiritism." Cf. Weiss, *Kandinsky in Munich*, 139–41.

27. G. Ränk, *Heilige Hinterecke*, 23–29, 32–33, 59–62, and passim. Ränk describes in

detail the ways in which the "holy corner" came to symbolize the coexistence of pagan and Christian beliefs, particularly among the Finno-Ugric peoples.

28. Squirrel pelts are mentioned as a mainstay of the Zyrian economy in travel accounts as ancient as Herberstein's chronicle and as recent as 1926. See A. Radó, ed., *Guide-Book to the Soviet Union* (New York: International Publishers Co., c. 1926), 353 (two million squirrel pelts harvested in 1924). On the spiritual significance of the fir, pine, or cedar tree, see n. 17, above, and n. 31, below.

29. Kandinsky, "Etnografii," 103, 105, 106. The information on the Votiaks had already been published by Kandinsky's colleague P. M. Bogaevskii in 1888. It was then quoted by V. M. Mikhailovskii, who also cited the Cheremis term for sorcerer in his landmark work "Shamanstvo" (Shamanism), which was published in the proceedings of the Imperial Society of Friends of Natural History, Anthropology, and Ethnography in 1892, in the same series in which Kandinsky's essay on peasant law had been published in 1889. Mikhailovskii was vice-president of the Society's Ethnographic Section and may have known Kandinsky either as a student at the University or as a fellow member of the society. A partial translation of Mikhailovskii's work is available as "Shamanism in Siberia and European Russia," trans. Oliver Wardrop, *Journal of the Anthropological Institute of Great Britain and Ireland* 24 (1895): 62–100, 126–58. On the "old man" as shaman, see 153, 155. On horse staves, see Mircea Eliade, *Shamanism Archaic Techniques of Ecstasy* (Princeton: Princeton University Press, 1970), 467; M. A. Czaplicka, *Aboriginal Siberia A Study in Social Anthropology* (Oxford: Clarendon Press, 1914), 203–5, 224; Holmberg, *Finno-Ugric*, 522; and Mikhailovskii, "Shamanism," 81.

30. Czaplicka, *Aboriginal Siberia*, 284, citing an 1895 work by M. N. Khangaloff.

31. See G. P. Fedotov, *The Russian Religious Mind*, 2:349–62. For a general discussion of *dvoeverie*, see George Vernadsky, *The Origins of Russia*, 315. It is interesting to note that Kandinsky's friend Ivanitsky published some notes on the worship of fire and trees, as well as other folk beliefs, among the peoples of Vologda province in *Ethnographic Review* in 1891. See N. Ivanitsky, "Notes on Folk Beliefs in the Vologda Region" (Worship of Fire and Trees; Beliefs in Metamorphosis; History of Burial Customs), in *Etnograficheskoe Obozrenie* 10, no. 3 (1891): 226–28.) On the image of Slata Baba, see n. 18, above.

32. Vernadsky, *The Origins of Russia*, 109–10, 314–15, passim.

33. Weiss, "Kandinsky in Munich: Encounters and Transformations," 67–82.

34. H. M. Chadwick and N. K. Chadwick, *The Growth of Literature* (Cambridge: Cambridge University Press, 1936), 2:180, 199–202.

35. Weiss, "Kandinsky and the Symbolist Heritage," 137–45.

36. See, e.g., the extensive bibliographies in Diòszegi, *Popular Beliefs;* Diòszegi and Hoppal, *Shamanism in Siberia;* Czaplicka, *Aboriginal Siberia;* and Anna Leena Siikala, *The Rite Technique of the Siberian Shaman* (Helsinki: Finnish Academy of Science and Letters, 1978).

37. According to notes of the society published in the third issue of the journal (the same in which Kandinsky's essay on the Zyrians appeared), during one of the three meetings held by the society "since the 15th of October," Kandinsky presented his field trip report and, among others, V. M. Mikhailovskii presented a report "On Shamanism Among the North American Indians." See *Etnograficheskoe Obozrenie* 3 (1889 [late Fall?]), 212. Further, announcement was made of an important study on Lapp shamanism by N. N. Kharuzin, whose earlier article on the same topic had already been published in the journal's first issue. According to the notes section of that first issue, Kandinsky had already presented a preliminary report on the beliefs of the Zyrians, and Kharuzin had also presented an oral report on Lapp shamanism. See *Etnograficheskoe Obozrenie* 1 (1889 [Spring]), 177. In the same section field trips for the coming summer, including Kandinsky's to Vologda, are announced. As noted previously, Kandinsky also reviewed books for *Ethnographic Review* in which among other things, the subject of shamanism was discussed (see Weiss, *Kandinsky and "Old Russia,"* n. 1, above).

38. Sigmund Freiherr von Herberstein, *Rerum Moscoviticarum commentarij Sigismundi liberi baronis in Herberstain, Neyperg, & Guettenhag: Rvssiae, & quae nunc eius metropolisest, Moscouiae, breuissima descriptio....* (Basileae: Ionnem Oporinum, [1556]). These or similar illustrations also appear in other editions, e.g., Basel 1551, 1557; Vienna 1557. In Herberstein's book, scenic strips depicting typical Russian landscapes border the large maps. These, too, are recalled in such Kandinsky works as *Russian Village on a River with Ships* and *Russian Knight* (both of ca. 1902). Even more closely allied to the Herberstein illustrations are two watercolors of Russian hunting and winter scenes recently published in Derouet and Boissel, *Kandinsky*, nos. 223, 224.

39. This tale may represent a misunderstanding by Herberstein of a long-standing tradition by which Russian peasants were allowed the freedom to move from one feudal estate to another only once a year, namely during a period after the autumn harvest associated with the November St. George's Day (actually a law under Ivan the Terrible, ca. 1550). Serfs seeking re-employment then in the spring would, of course, turn up again around the time of the spring planting, i.e., near the time of the April St. George's Day. Cf. Michael B. Petrovic, "The Peasant in Nineteenth-Century Historiography," in Wayne S. Vucinich, ed., *The Peasant in Nineteenth-Century Russia* (Stanford: Stanford University Press, 1968), 218ff. The association is interesting, too, in that St. George would figure prominently in Kandinsky's later All Saints' Day (i.e., resurrection) paintings.

40. The many analogies between the roles of shaman and artist have often been remarked. See Andreas Lommel, *The World of the Early Hunters* (London: Evelyn, Adams & Mackay, 1967). Of particular interest is the essay by Odd Nordland, "Shamanism as an Experiencing of the 'Unreal,' " in Carl-Martin Edsman, ed., *Studies in Shamanism* (Stockholm: Scripta Instituti Donneriani, Aboensis I., 1967), 167–85. See also W. Sieroshevski, "The Yakuts," 105; A. Hultkranz, "Ecological and Phenomenological Aspects of Shamanism," in Diószegi and Hoppál, *Shamanism in Siberia*, 50–53; G. M. Vasilevich, "The Acquisition of Shamanistic Ability among the Evenki (Tungus)," in Diószegi, *Popular Beliefs*, esp. 343.

41. Siikala, *Rite Technique of Siberian Shaman*, 14; and Peter Hajdu, "The Classification of Samoyed Shamans," in Diószegi, *Popular Beliefs*, 155. Both reference Vilmos Diószegi, "Samán (The Etymology of the Word Samán)," *Magyar Nyelv* 43 (1947): 211–12.

42. Hultkranz, "Aspects of Shamanism," 33–37. Hultkranz defines the role of the shaman as threefold: as physician, diviner, and psychopomp. See also Siikala, *Rite Technique of Siberian Shaman*, 13–14, 18, where the social role of the shaman is emphasized. It is important to point out here that shamanism is not to be confused with what is commonly known as spiritism or the occult, in which a key concept is "possession." The shaman plays a distinctly social role, and it is he (or she) who possesses and controls the shamanic ritual and his or her own part in it. See V. Voigt, "Shamanism in North Eurasia as a Scope of Ethnology," in Diószegi and Hoppál, *Shamanism in Siberia*, 62–63; L. Krader, "Shamanism: Theory and History in Buryat Society," ibid., 188–90; Eliade, *Shamanism*, 93; and Hultkranz, "Aspects of Shamanism," 44–47.

43. Hultkranz, 35–36; Mikhailovskii, "Shamanism," 79–80 and passim; Czaplicka, *Aboriginal Siberia*, 203–205, 224, and passim; L. P. Potapov, "The Shaman Drum as a Source of Ethnographical History," in Diószegi and Hoppál, *Shamanism in Siberia*, 174–75; S. I. Vajnstejn, "The Tuvan (Soyot) Shaman's Drum, and the Ceremony of Its Enlivening," in Diószegi, *Popular Beliefs*, 331–38; and Eliade, *Shamanism*, 173–74, 467.

44. Czaplicka, *Aboriginal Siberia*, 224; and Vilmos Diószegi, *Tracing Shamans in Siberia: The Story of an Ethnographical Research Expedition* (Oosterhout: Anthropological Publications, 1968), 42. Diószegi noted having seen hundreds of horse sticks in the museum at Leningrad (St. Petersburg).

45. Kandinsky, "Rückblicke," III.

46. I photographed this toy horse and rider during a visit to Mme. Kandinsky's Neuilly home in 1980. It stood approximately 18 inches high; the rider was detachable from the rocking horse. Subsequently it was sold at auction in 1983, together with other ethnic artifacts from Kandinsky's personal collection. (See auction catalogue *Succession de Madame Nina Kandinsky*, 16 June 1983, Raymond Caron, Puteaux.) It was not purchased by the Musée Nationale de l'Art Moderne (letter to the author from Mme. Jessica Boissel, of the Centre Pompidou, 17 Oct. 1985). The hobbyhorse is clearly visible in a photograph of the artist's studio published in Nina Kandinsky, *Kandinsky und ich*, following p. 128.

47. Kandinsky, "Rückblicke," IV.

48. Ibid., XVI; and Kandinsky, "Reminiscences," in Lindsay and Vergo, *Complete Writings*, 1:370 and 2:892, nn. 54, 55, 57.

49. Czaplicka, *Aboriginal Siberia*, 169–75; Eliade, *Shamanism*, 29–30 and passim.

50. Mikhailovskii, "Shamanism," 76; Wassily Kandinsky, "Zu unbestimmter Stunde. . . . " in *Neue Künstlervereinigung München, II. Ausstellung* (Munich: Bruckmann, 1910–1911). Cf. G. M. Vasilevich, "Acquisition of Shamanistic Ability," in Diószegi, *Popular Beliefs*, 345.

51. Kandinsky, "Rückblicke," XIX. See also Eliade, *Shamanism*, 76.

52. Wassily Kandinsky, "Toile vide, etc." ("Empty Canvas, etc."), in *Cahiers d'art* 10, nos. 5–6 (Paris, 1935): 117.

53. Mikhailovskii, "Shamanism," 74–76; Wilhelm Radloff, *Aus Sibirien: Lose Blätter aus meinem Tagebuche,* 2 vols. (2nd ed. 1893; reprint, Oosterhout: Anthropological Publications, 1968), 2:21–23. These songs had actually been written down and published by V. Verbitskii (Verbickij) as early as 1864. Translation of this verse is mine, from Radloff. The refrain "here am I" is a translation of Radloff's *"da bin ich."*

54. Here the reference to a distant thunder that seems not to concern itself with external affairs recalls the Samoyed conception of the principal deity, Numi-Torem (often compared to the Scandinavian god of thunder, Thor) who is all-powerful over natural phenomena but who remains reserved and distant. The phrase "me voilà" might, of course, be translated "Here am I" or "I am here" or, as here and in Lindsay and Vergo, "here I am"; the meaning in any case is the same. Cf. Lindsay and Vergo, 780, where the editors compare this phrase to a similar phrase (used, however, in a different context) in *Ueber das Geistige in der Kunst* (Munich: R. Piper & Co., 1912), 103.

55. Eliade, *Shamanism,* 171.

56. Vilmos Diószegi, "Pre-Islamic Shamanism of the Baraba Turks and some Ethnogenetic Conclusions," and S. V. Ivanov, "Some Aspects of the Study of Siberian Shamanism" (on the book of divination) in Diószegi and Hoppal, *Shamanism in Siberia,* 83–167, 32.

57. N. N. Kharazin, "On the Noids among the Ancient and Contemporary Lapps," *Etnograficheskoe Obozrenie* 1 (1889), 36–76. The provenance of the Munich Lapp drum is confirmed in letters to the author from Frau Michaela Appel of the Staatliches Museum für Völkerkunde, Munich, 26 February 1986 and 17 March 1986. See also Ernst Manker's monumental study *Die lappische Zaubertrommel,* 2 vols. (Stockholm: Acta Lapponica, 1938 and 1950), 1:802–806 and 2:423–26.

58. See Manker, *Lappische Zaubertrommel,* 1:54–55, 803; 2:76–86, 423–26. On replacement of Perun by St. Elias, see G. Fedotov, *Russian Religious Mind,* 357–58. For further comments on the Munich drum, see Andreas Lommel, "Schamanistische Kunst," *Die Kunst,* Jubiläumsausgabe, Heft 10 (October 1985), 802–807.

59. See Diószegi, "Pre-Islamic Shamanism," 107ff; Mikhailovskii, "Shamanism," 79–80, 146–47; Radloff, *Aus Sibirien,* 2:18–19, pl. 1. Manker cites Christoph Gottlieb von Murr, *Beschreibung der vornehmsten Merkwürdigkeiten in der Reichstadt Nürnberg, in deren Bezirke, und auf der Universität Altdorf. Nebst einem Anhange,* 2nd ed. (Nürnberg, 1801), with reproduction of the drum now in the Munich Völkerkunde Museum and Johannes Schefferus, *Lapponia* (Frankfurt, 1673); German ed., 1675), also with illustrations, both of which Kandinsky could have known. See also Franz Weinitz, "Die lappische Zaubertrommel in Meiningen," *Zeitschrift für Ethnologie* 42, no. 1 (1910), 1–14.

60. Georg Nioradze, *Der Schamanismus bei den sibirischen Völkern* (Stuttgart: Strecker & Schröder, 1925), 66–74 and Vilmos Diószegi, "The Problem of the Ethnic Homogeneity of Tofa (Karagas) Shamanism" in Diószegi, *Popular Beliefs,* 286–324. See also Diószegi, "The Three-Grade Amulets among the Nanai (Golds)," ibid., 388.

61. Cf. Peg Weiss, "Books in Review," *Art Journal* 44, no. 1 (Spring 1984): 93 and Rose Carol Washton Long, *Kandinsky: The Development of an Abstract Style* (Oxford: Clarendon Press, 1980), 112–13, 132, and passim. According to Eichner's account, Kandinsky stated that *Composition 2* was painted "without theme"; on the other hand, Kandinsky also referred to the "tragic quality" of its composition and drawing. Johannes Eichner, *Kandinsky und Gabriele Münter von Ursprüngen modernen Kunst* (Munich: Verlag F. Bruckmann [1957]), 111–14. Cf. Kandinsky, "Reminiscences," in Lindsay and Vergo, *Complete Writings,* 890. Vergo uses the translation *Colorful Life* rather than *Motley Life.*

62. See n. 20 above and Holmberg, *Finno-Ugric,* 181, 197.

63. Czaplicka, *Aboriginal Siberia,* 289 and K. F. Karjalainen, *Die Religion der Jugra-Völker* II, Folklore Fellows Communications, no. 44 (Helsinki and Porvoo: Suomalainen Tiedakatemia and Werner Söderström Osakeyhtiö, 1922), 189–93, where the son of Torem (Torum) is linked not only with Christ but also with St. George, and the conflation of the legends is traced specifically to the influence of the Zyrians on the Ostiaks. In Votiak religious belief, the death of a shaman may also provoke a great storm. See I. Paulson, "Seelenvorstellungen und Totenglaube der permischen und Wolga-finnischen Völker," *Numen* 9, no. 3 (September 1964): 223. It may also be noted that this image of the boat figure with outstretched arms is very similar to many such images on the shaman drums of the Lapps (as in Manker, *Lappische Zaubertrommel,* esp. e.g., 32, 56, and passim).

64. F. G. Jackson, "Notes on the Samoyads of the Great Tundra," *Journal of the Anthro-*

pological Institute of Great Britain and Ireland 24 (August 1894–May 1895): 396. Czaplicka, *Aboriginal Siberia,* 290; Nioradze, *Der Schamanismus,* 91; Holmberg, *Finno-Ugric,* ch. 4, 361–70 (myths of destruction of the world).

65. On Kandinsky's horse/circle imagery, see Weiss, *Kandinsky in Munich* (Princeton), 128–35 and Weiss, "Kandinsky in Munich: Encounters and Transformations," 78–82. On *Composition 5,* see Eichner, *Kandinsky,* 114–15 and Washton-Long, *Kandinsky,* 113–16 and passim.

66. It is interesting to compare the imagery of the Chukchee drawings collected by the ethnographer Waldemar Bogoras in 1899–1900 with analogous details of Kandinsky works such as *In the Circle.* See W. Bogoras, *The Chukchee 1904–1909,* in Franz Boas, ed., *Memoirs of the American Museum of Natural History* 11, pts. 1–3, reprint from the Jesup North Pacific Expedition (Leiden: Brill, 1909; New York: G. E. Stechert & Co., 1909), esp. 277–377 (reprinted from vol. 7, pt. 2, 1907) and passim. An extended discussion of Kandinsky's use of this and other shamanistic imagery is included in Weiss, *Kandinsky and "Old Russia,"* n. 1, above.

67. As suggested in Weiss, "Kandinsky in Munich: Encounters and Transformations," 71–72. See also E. J. Kimball and Peg Weiss, "A Pictorial Analysis of 'In the Black Square,' " *Art Journal* 43 (Spring 1983): 36–40, and Peg Weiss, "Kandinsky and the Symbolist Heritage," *Art Journal* 45, no. 2 (Summer 1985): 140–41.

68. On the use of strange languages or nonsense words by shamans, see Mikhailovskii, "Shamanism," 65; Siikala, *Rite Technique of Siberian Shaman,* 21–21, 127, 134, 137; Peter Hajdu, "The Nenets Shaman Song and Its Text," in Diószegi and Hoppál, *Shamanism in Siberia,* 370–71. On the chorus, see L. Gáldi, "On Some Problems of Versification in Samoyed Shamanistic Songs," in ibid., 132.

69. See Susan Stein, "The Ultimate Synthesis: An Interpretation of the Meaning and Significance of Wassily Kandinsky's *The Yellow Sound,*" Master's thesis, State University of New York, Binghamton, 1980.

70. Holmberg, *Finno-Ugric,* 357, 505, 506; Vernadsky, *Origins of Russia,* 112–13 (on fire wheel).

71. Kenneth C. Lindsay, "Les thèmes de l'inconscient," *XXe Siècle* 27 (December 1966): 46–52; Weiss, "Kandinsky in Munich: Encounters and Transformations," 30; and Weiss, "Kandinsky and the Symbolist Heritage," 141. Lindsay interpreted the figure on which the St. George appears to rest as a feminine figure, identified as such by her triangular crown. However, although the triangle may be associated in Byzantine iconography with the feminine as Lindsay points out, in fact, the czar and other members of Russian aristocracy depicted in Herberstein's chronicles wear triangular (i.e., conical) caps. Lindsay then suggested that this female figure may represent the Virgin Mary who "weeps for mankind" and who protects St. George from "symbolic evil by means of her miraculous veil—the *pokroff,*" the form floating diagonally across the space. The concept of *dvoeverie* would account for the ambivalence of the motif as a conflation of symbols representing a nostalgia for both the shamanic and the Orthodox aspects of old czarist Russia.

72. Mikhailovskii, "Shamanism," 77–78.

73. Cf. Vilmos Diószegi, "Pre-Islamic Shamanism," 117–18; Hultkranz, "Aspects of Shamanism," 36; Mikhailovskii, "Shamanism," 74; and Holmberg, *Finno-Ugric,* 349ff. The theme of the cosmic pillar also appears in the well-known Russian folk tale of "The Seven Semyons" in which the eldest Semyon, a smith, forges a tall pillar from the top of which his brother becomes the shamanic "all-see-er." Because of their power over fire and metals, smiths were perceived as possessing a power, especially with respect to healing, second only to that of shamans. With the coming of Christianization, it is hardly surprising that the healing saints Cosmos and Damian became the patron saints of smiths. Nor is it surprising that the smith, an artist and craftsman, should be associated with shamanic powers, a connection Kandinsky would not have missed. Indeed, Kandinsky's friend Ivanitsky had published a report on folk medicine in the Vologda province in which Sts. Cosmos and Damian were also cited as those to whom one should pray for "enlightenment of the mind." (See N. A. Ivanitsky, "On Folk Medicine Province of Vologda," *Etnograficheskoe Obozrenie* 12, no. 1 (1892): 182–85. See also Vernadsky, *Origins of Russia,* 136, and Eliade, *Shamanism,* 370–74 and passim.) In this context it is also interesting that St. Simeon is the Stylite who spends his life in meditation upon a pillar; this saint—noted for having converted the pagans to Christianity—is to be found in Kandinsky's 1911 glass painting *All Saints II* along with a pair of figures I have previously speculated may be identified as the physician saints Cosmos and Damian. But this pair might also represent the reconciliation of pagan and Christian belief expected by many turn-of-the-century Russian intellectuals; the figure on the

left representing the pagan Finno-Ugric tribesman wearing his characteristic colorful stockings and the one on the right (who carries a cross in the watercolor sketch for the picture) representing the Christian. (See Weiss, "Kandinsky in Munich: Encounters and Transformations," 75.)

74. Shaman song collected by Castrén, ca. 1842 (song no. 19), quoted in L. Gáldi, "Samoyed Shamanistic Songs," 130; also in P. Simonsics, "The Structure of a Nenets Magic Chant," in Diószegi and Hoppál, *Shamanism in Siberia*, 388–89.

75. On the shaman's cap, see Vilmos Diószegi, "The Problem of Ethnic Homogeneity of Tofa (Karagas) Shamanism," in Diószegi, *Popular Beliefs*, 298, 306; but esp. G. N. Gračeva, "A Nganasan Shaman Costume." In Diószegi and Happál, *Shamanism in Siberia*, 333. See also Nioradze, *Schamanismus*, pl. 14 (feathered helmet).

76. See Nioradze, *Schamanismus*, 69, fig. 15, also 57, 65 (illustration of ribbed breastplates). A six-fingered hand is to be found in Kandinsky's 1943 painting *A Conglomerate*. Eliade reports that the Yurak-Samoyed shaman wears a glove with seven fingers, *Shamanism*, 278.

77. See Kandinsky, "Iz Materialov po Etnografii Sysol'skikh i Vychegodskikh Zyrian," 106–107. See also V. N. Chernetsov, "Concepts of the Soul among the Ob-Ugrians" in Henry N. Michael, ed., *Studies in Siberian Shamanism* (Toronto: University of Toronto Press, 1963), esp. p. 29, where Chernetsov describes the custom among some tribes of tying up the bodies of all deceased, and the use of a special "knot of the dead."

78. Conglomerate Scythian forms are found all across Siberia. For a typical such bird form discovered in the Vychegda valley, see G. M. Burov, *Arkheologicheskie pamiatniki Vychegodskoi doliny* (Syktyvkar: Komi kn. izd., 1967), 9 and Karl Jettmar, *Art of the Steppes The Eurasian Animal Style* (London: Methuen, 1964), 200. For many more bird-shaped and other conglomerate artifacts from this region, see Dmitri M. Anuchin, "K istoria iskusstva i verovaniy u priuralskoy chudi" (Contributions to the history of art and beliefs among the Ural Chuds), in *Materialy po arkheologii Vostochnykh guberniy*, vol. 3 (Moscow, 1899), 106, 112, 120, and passim, also plates I–III. Anuchin is of concern in the context of this study because he too was a member of the Imperial Society and contributed to *Etnograficheskoe Obozrenie*. A widespread Siberian belief (particularly among the Buriats) held that when the soul leaves the body, it may be reborn in an infant. See Holmberg, *Finno-Ugric*, 6–11 on the Zyrian *lul* (actually *lol*) and the bird soul, and 317–325 on the diver bird and creation myths. On the "Book of Fates," see Fedotov, *Russian Religious Mind*, 1:349–50, and Eliade, *Shamanism*, 272ff. See also M. Hoppál, "Folk Beliefs and Shamanism among the Uralic Peoples," in Peter Hajdu, ed., *Ancient Cultures of the Uralian Peoples*, 232.

79. For a thorough discussion of the etymology of the Finno-Ugric terms for fly agaric and the intoxication of the trance, see J. Balazs, "The Hungarian Shaman's Technique of Trance Induction," in Diószegi, *Popular Beliefs*, esp. 56–57; also Eliade, *Shamanism*, 400–401, where he particularly refers to the Zyrian's neighbors, the Voguls, and their use of the word *pankh* for this particular mushroom, meaning also "intoxication" (a related word is also used by the Mordwyns and Cheremis). See also Fokos-Fuchs, *Syrjänisches Wörterbuch*, 715 *(pagalni-pagavni)*, 806 *(poganei)*. For the concept of the soul in the form of a butterfly, also common among the Finno-Ugric peoples, see Holmberg, *Finno-Ugric*, 8–9.

80. See Ränk, *Heilige Hinterecke*, 156–57.

81. From a Samoyed shaman song recorded by Castrén in the 1840s, from L. Gáldi, "Samoyed Shamanistic Songs," 131.

IV

The Work of Art as Symbol Arising from a Historical Context

11

BOCCACCIO LOOKING at ACTUAL FRESCOES

CREIGHTON GILBERT

SOME REMARKS in the works of Bocaccio have always been noticed as among the most interesting contemporary written responses to trecento painting. Best known, of course, is the story in the *Decameron* about Giotto, along with those about more obscure painters. The long description in his early *Amorosa Visione* was introduced into the learned literature by Schlosser.[1] Here I would like to discuss passages in the *Genealogy of the Gods*, which seem not to have been considered in studies of *Kunstliteratur*, but which I would suggest are more revealing than the others about painting of the time. To be sure, one wants to avoid exaggerating the natural interest we feel in what a great writer says about painting, especially in a period when any writing on art is sparse. Often it does not have special value, for many writers in all periods have had as little concern about the visual arts as other narrow specialists, including art historians, evince about what is not their area. But the passages in the *Genealogy* seem to have been overlooked with less justification. They do not match what was being looked for in texts and documents by art historians of an earlier generation (who did most of the work in establishing the corpus of such writings), in that they give us no attributions or chronology, nor even an explicit statement of a large critical standpoint. But they perhaps tell us on other levels about how painting was looked at, in ways which we have assumed could not be ascertained in the trecento precisely because such writings were not before us.

The last parts of the *Genealogy of the Gods* have rightly been given much attention by historians of culture in the Burckhardt tradition, and thus have been supplied with splendid analyses both internal and with respect to their intellectual context.[2] These parts, Books 14 and 15, shift from the main theme of the work, which is a practical reference tool for writers wishing to refer to classical myths. They turn to the even more practical underlying need of campaigning for the permissibility of poetry, especially that of ancient Greece and Rome, against religious writers who taught that Christians should not read it. The theological attack is best known from the writings of a later Florentine, the Dominican Cardinal Giovanni Dominici, who argued that even if it did no harm, at a minimum it would take time away from what was better, such as scripture.[3] Some responses of Boccaccio's cannot but appear simpleminded, and these include the sections in which he alludes to painting. Responding to the complaint that poetry is lascivious, he invokes among other things the rotten apple argument: the sins of a few should not condemn all poets. Another is the argument that "it is allowed to others." It is unfair to condemn poets for what painters are permitted. This introduces Giotto:[4]

> If Praxiteles or Phidias, so well versed in sculpture, carved Priapus going toward Iole by night, rather than Diana who was so admirable for chastity, or if it happens that Apelles, or our Giotto to whom Apelles in his time was not superior, paints Mars in conjunction with Venus, rather than Jove giving instructions to the Gods from his throne, should we say these arts are to be condemned? It would be crazy.

To us the remark may first seem remote from what we know of the works of these artists and thus without interest, a mere flourish invoking their names. There seems indeed no basis for saying either Greek sculptor produced a work representing Priapus or Iole. We may think that Priapus was chosen because, being the extreme case of a figure involving sexuality, his name permits the deduction that any other image is all the more permissible when he is. Iole may be the best name available for a figure likely to be the object of sexual interest. Again, the theme linked to Giotto strikes us as very far from our well grounded knowledge of his work, with its religious narrative and tragic emphasis. I shall argue that it is not so far, but would like to go first to a second passage where the demonstration can be made in a simpler way. Some 25 pages later, Boccaccio in a similar argument calls it inconsistent to outlaw poetry when no one is forbidden to read the works of heretics (to learn their errors) or to watch performances of street jugglers, however unchaste, or to hear actors sing "evil things." Nor are we condemned to hell for having heard a pimp cursing. Similarly:[5]

> To painters, even in holy churches, it is permissible to paint the dog Cerberus, guarding the gate of Pluto, Charon the oarsman crossing the river Acheron, the Erinnys wreathed with snakes and armed with lit torches, and Pluto prince of the kingdom of hell tormenting the damned, but for poets to have written the same things in verse is a crime, and unforgivable sin for the reader. To the same painter it is permitted in the rooms of kings and noblemen to paint the loves of the ancient gods and the crimes of men, and every other invention of theirs without any prohibition, and it is permitted to all to see this as they please, but the inventions of poets.

Here again our very familiarity with the themes of trecento painting may make this text seem far from the reality of that art, and so not of interest. Used to inspecting polyptychs or fresco cycles of saints' lives, we naturally are not attuned to the notion of paintings by the same artists out of classical poetry and myth, Cerberus the dog, Charon with his boat, the Furies, and Pluto. It could very naturally be deduced that Boccaccio was drawing on his reading experience of the classics. And yet a second thought impels us to note that the list is not random at all. There is only one context in which all four of these figures appear together in major roles, and it is not from antiquity. The *Inferno* of Dante, where we find them, was of course immensely admired and studied by Boccaccio. At least in verbal form, these figures are not at all distant, but belong to the modern Florentine culture of the trecento.

This obvious link brings out an elegant irony in the latter part of Boccaccio's quoted remarks. When these classical personages are cited by poets, he notes, the poets are called criminals, and their readers sinners. He is pointing out that when theologians condemn this paganism, they are not simply stamping out the secular, but in their simplicity undercutting the *poeta theologus*. Even his silence about Dante's obvious name, as if providing him protection, enhances the point.

As to painting, it is evident that the listed pagan figures will also all appear together in illustrations of hell as viewed by Dante, thus again a real trecento figuration. Indeed they are not likely to appear together anywhere else. But Boccaccio further specifies that his reference is not to illuminated manuscripts, but to what we see in churches. The question thus arises as to whether the *Inferno* was the theme of church painting, in a place and at a date allowing Boccaccio to cite it. Of course, there is just one outstanding such work, the fresco by Nardo di Cione at Santa Maria Novella in Florence (fig. 11.1). It is normally dated in the 1350s, at a time when Boccaccio was working on the *Genealogy.* It is commonly noted in the literature that this huge wall scene, part of a Last Judgment cycle, is the first known to us that adopted Dante as the authority on the topography of hell. It modifies the earlier imagery of Last Judgments, such as Giotto's in Padua and that in the Campo Santo in Pisa, to follow Dante's arrangements, a procedure that was to be retained more or less precisely by many later images.

It will be recalled that in the preface to the *Decameron* Boccaccio tells of a group of friends meeting in this same church of Santa Maria Novella, in 1348. Nardo's fresco, even in its present very overpainted state, makes especially conspicuous precisely the persons listed by Boccaccio. At the top, Charon with his large boat shares the center with Cerberus. Closest to the very middle the main group shows the Furies with their snakes, while Pluto is the big figure at the bottom center.

Knowing now what Boccaccio had in mind as he was writing, we can again appreciate the ironic purpose. Of course this was a theme not only allowed to a painter in a church, but demanded: the story of salvation. It belongs of right and preference in the great Dominican center, which was cultivating the preaching of orthodox faith. Unless the preachers failed to notice that they were presenting pagan images, they were using them for their own goals. What nonsense, then, for them to condemn the poet who was doing just the same.

The significance of Boccaccio's allusion for our studies reaches to the most mundane. In a catalogue raisonné citing the bibliography of Nardo's fresco, Boccaccio would have now to be inserted as the earliest item, by far. Thus the traditional art historian who only assembles literal materials (if any such survives) is no less involved than those who explore interdisciplinary links with poetry or the history of the consuming of art, *Rezeptionsgeschichte.* In all of Boccaccio, including the *Decameron,* this appears to be the most recently executed work of art to be cited. Elsewhere he refers most to Giotto, and to Giotto's contemporaries Buffalmacco and Calandrino. These were now part of established tradition. Only here we see him taking note of the very contemporary. To be sure he does so, like most people, because of the ax he himself has to grind.

However stimulated, what Boccaccio spotted in the fresco was a series of classical figures. No one would have predicted that; we do not look at Nardo's work and register a *rinascimento dell-antichità.* It is not like the *Visitation* at Reims or the so-called *Hercules* of Nicola Pisano, which jump out from the context as classical. Did these figures jump out in this way for Boccaccio? Perhaps instead we might apply Panofsky's famous formula according to which in the Middle Ages images may show classical form or classical subject but not both, grouping Nardo's figures with the latter. And yet a full synthesis of classicism emerged in Florence by the end of the trecento, conspicuously in the *Hercules* of the Porta della Mandorla. In general, the trecento masters up to that point relate transitionally to classicism, as Panofsky elsewhere argued, as *i primi lumi.*[6]

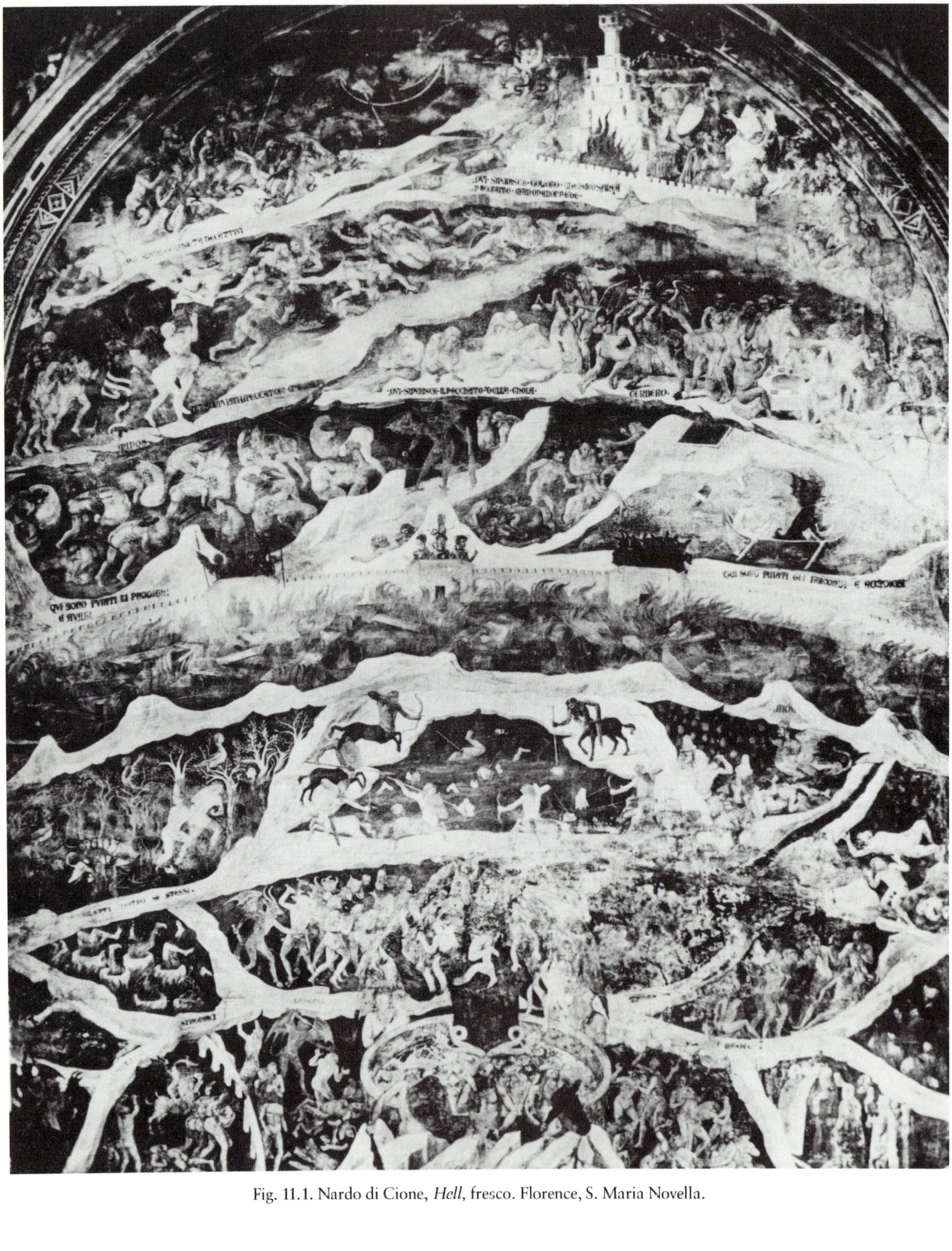

Fig. 11.1. Nardo di Cione, *Hell*, fresco. Florence, S. Maria Novella.

If we think of the specific dates of Nardo's work and Boccaccio's comment, we are in the years right after the Black Death and have here what must count as *the* one richest text responding to a contemporary work of art from that time. Despite the fact that the theme of the painting is damnation, the way it is here being seen does not correlate with the Meiss conception of the period, which was based strongly on views of how the art public was behaving and used less direct data than this. Explicitly accepting Meiss's findings and extrapolating further, Panofsky reported a "regression or recession of an active interest in the Antique" which "fits in with the general trend of events in Tuscan painting after about 1350." He particularly cites "the Florence of Orcagna."[7] We must now query that finding. To be sure, despite quoting Meiss on a change not only "of style" but also "of taste," Panofsky here is mainly talking about style, the relations between plane and space and between line and mass. But when he then proceeds to such other aspects as a denial of individuality and a magnifying of the divine and reducing the human, the conclusions do seem to be plainly in conflict with Boccaccio's approach. We may then be led also to look stylistically at such images as Nardo's Charon to ask whether they correspond to the descriptions of a post-1350 change. Certainly Meiss's concept has in recent years tended to be contravened from many different points, indeed finding its chief retention today among generalists.

This text is perhaps most surprising in that Boccaccio's remarks on painting are not ekphrasis on imaginary images, as has generally been assumed about similar references by writers of his tradition. He gives us a particular allusion to a major painting he saw. With hindsight, it is obvious that to do so gives strength to his argument against the theologians that an ekphrasis could not, and so it was probable that he would do this. It was also probable from such a perceptive and affectionate observer of his own immediate world. Elsewhere I have offered grounds to show that the same is true of his description of one fresco in the *Amorosa Visione;* there, Boccaccio is describing a secular painting by Giotto. He is, I would propose, describing two others in two other passages in the *Genealogy of the Gods.*

As already remarked, his assignment to Giotto of an image of "Mars and Venus conjoined" is so distant from our idea of Giotto that we might not even pause over it. And yet it happens that the reference matches with a precision that is almost comic a lost work of Giotto which was, in fact, the largest fresco cycle ever produced by the master, now virtually forgotten. This is the work in the Palazzo della Ragione in Padua that was destroyed by fire in 1420 and soon thereafter replaced by the cycle that survives there today, reflecting the same iconography. The source references to it have been fully assembled. The most important report is that of about 1340 by Giovanni da None, an official who spent his working years in that very palazzo. He wrote in his essay on the glories of the city that the "twelve heavenly signs and the seven planets with their attributes shone on that ceiling, marvelously executed by the great painter Giotto."[8] As Mars and Venus are two of the planets, Giotto did paint what Boccaccio said he did. That he is alluding to this specific fresco cycle is confirmed elegantly by his word choice, saying the two are "conjoined." That word has of course its most precise sense as a term in astrology, referring to planets or stars being immediately adjacent and occupying the same part of the sky, which then influences people on the earth. Giotto's fresco was astrological in its references, as we know both from the citation of the "twelve signs"—of the zodiac—and the present fresco cycle on the ceiling. It in fact shows Mars and Venus adjacent on the short south wall. It also shows Jupiter, but of course *not* "giving instructions to the Gods from his throne." It is tempting to think that Boccaccio might even be alluding to the cycle in this last part of his remarks too, in saying what is not shown by the artist who paints Mars and Venus.

However that may be, the remark that "Giotto paints Mars and Venus in conjunction" undeniably refers to this painting by Giotto which does so and needs to be added to the list of early citations of the work. It is one of only three that cite it before it was destroyed, and thus cannot but be notable for Giotto studies. (Besides the text of Giovanni da None, the third reference is the early but very summary mention by Riccobaldo da Ferrara.)

Here again Boccaccio makes the painting an item in his own argument, as his specific phrases delightfully show us. He might have picked any two planets if he wanted to mention their conjunction. In choosing these two he of course is exploiting the pun in 'conjunction' to suggest Mars and Venus sexually joined. If there were any doubt of that, it is removed by his parallel with Priapus and Iole. But if we the readers or the theologians were to object to such an improper image, he is ready to point out that his allusion is perfectly chaste, from astrology. He has tricked us into thinking he was prurient and therefore can call us so; the critics of poetry can be shown to be on shaky ground, forbidding too what is perfectly acceptable.

Our quoted passages include still one more reference written as if about a recent painting, when Boccaccio writes that "to the same painter it is permitted in the rooms of kings and noblemen to paint the loves of the ancient gods and the crimes of men." Is this again a reference to an actual work he had seen? There is an immediate argument that it is not, because again that whole kind of subject is not typical of the works of Boccaccio's time or the previous centuries. Seznec, speaking of the pagan gods and basing himself on a previous, more quantitative survey, remarks that "scenes of seduction or rape, of love or drunken revelry" are typical of Italy from the fifteenth century on, but "admittedly no parallel to these had been seen since the end of the ancient world."[9] This would evidently tell us that here we do have an ekphrasis. But there are two factors which might make us hesitate to say so. First, as already noted, Boccaccio is involved here in a very real fight against the theologians who want to block poetry, and it is part of his counterargument to have cited real paintings in both the other cases we have explored. Thus it would be not only inconsistent for him to fall back on ekphrasis here, but weak and against his own interests; he might better have omitted this example. Yet that still would leave us with the difficulty that scenes of gods making love were not produced. However, there too our previous examples may make us look at the matter differently. When Boccaccio talked of Mars and Venus, he let us think he was describing them making love, but he was playing a sly rhetorician's trick on us. Here he again talks of the gods in love—should we not think that he is playing that same trick, the more as it would again be to his advantage? In this more probable case, we would not be stopped by Seznec's point and need not assume ekphrasis. We may then hypothesize a real fresco seen by Boccaccio in a royal or noble palace that could on one level be described as about the loves of the gods but which was *meant* to present some other concept.

That does not seem easy, but we are helped in that one element in this reference to a painting is, unlike the rest of it, less vague than in Boccaccio's other two. That is the reference to location, the royal or noble hall. Boccaccio lived mainly in Tuscany, which has no such places, and he was really familiar with only one city having a king and court. That was Naples, and so we might first look in that court for a painting that matches his specifications, holding the possibility of others in reserve. A royal hall in Naples was, it happens, painted by Giotto, who in fact painted none anywhere else. As noted above, Giotto was Boccaccio's favorite painter; Boccaccio's admiration was certainly generated in Naples, where he spent his teens and twenties at the court and which is the only place where he may (very probably) have had contact with the then distinguished artist. So we can be sure he was acquainted with that decoration of a royal hall; did he mention it in this passage?

This work of Giotto's has been even less studied, not surprising for a work by him that is lost and also secular. We owe our awareness of it essentially to a passing phrase by Ghiberti, who says that Giotto painted famous men in a *sala* of the King of Naples. Vasari elaborated on the point, adding correctly that the work was destroyed when King Alfonso remodeled the castle in the mid-fifteenth century (and also adding some less convincing anecdotes.)[10] Luckily one other source supplements our knowledge richly. This is a series of nine sonnets, surviving in six manuscripts in whole or in part, among which one includes the heading: "Sonnets composed by [blank] who, being in the *sala* of King Robert of Naples, saw these famous men painted, and he made a sonnet for each one, as follows." Though Giotto is not named, the link to him is firm through Ghiberti. This richer source, in a way that seems typical of the neglect of this large project by Giotto, has been presented in print only once, in a journal of small circulation in the year 1900.[11] Later writers on Giotto have cited from this the names of the nine famous men and sometimes other details, introducing errors. It may thus be worth while here to explore a bit further what we can learn from this text toward reconstructing Giotto's cycle—and we can learn a surprising amount—even if some of it will not bear directly on the issue of whether Boccaccio was citing it. Among other things, it emerges that the paintings anticipate some formulations of Boccaccio's own, and that most but not all of the men were shown with women they loved.

The editor of 1900 reported the nine sonnets in the following order: Alexander, Solomon, Hector, Aeneas, Achilles, Paris, Hercules, Samson, Caesar. The order of these names simply follows that of one manuscript which contains eight names, and adds the missing one, Caesar, at the end. So it would hardly seem to have a claim to follow the original intent. Yet that manuscript turns out to be the most faithful, I shall argue, and it happens that the order can be confirmed. I am indebted to Gino Corti and Philip Mattox for inspecting all the manuscripts and giving me key information. Mr. Corti reports that they are all datable, through handwriting, between 1380 and 1450. Two of them are not useful for us, since they include only three or five sonnets and mix them with other material (Laurenziano-Strozziano 174 and Magliabecchicano II 40). The others, with seven or more, are: (1) Laurenziano-Rediano 184, first half of the fifteenth century; (2) Magliabecchiano II I 157, same dating; (3) Magliabecchiano II IV 114, 1380–90; and (4) Laurenziano Mediceo-Palatino 119, 1430–40. They arrange the names in the following order:

(1)	(2)	(3)	(4)
Alexander	Solomon	Solomon	Solomon
Solomon	Hector	Hector	Hector
Hector	Achilles	Achilles	Achilles
Aeneas	Aeneas	Aeneas	Aeneas
Achilles	Samson	Samson	Samson
Paris	Paris	Paris	Paris
Hercules	Hercules	Alexander	Hercules
Samson		Hercules	Alexander
			Caesar

At first these lists seem to mix partial likeness and random divergence. Yet significant patterns are present. Only (4) shows all nine names;[12] the rest omit one or two. In all of them the omissions are the same, Caesar (all three times) and Alexander (once); the other seven names always appear. Further, Caesar and Alexander also account for the irregularities of order, appearing either at the beginning (Alexander in [1]) or end (both names in [4]) or—the only small variant—as next-to-last (Alexander in [3]). The other seven names not only always recur but generally keep the same order. In three lists these seven are in exactly the same order—a fact only apparent when we extract Alexander from that list in (3). The remaining list, (1), shows a different order for the seven only in interchanging the third and fourth names and in putting Samson seventh rather than fifth.

List (1) differs from the others in both these ways, in the small shifts in order of the seven names and in the different placing of Alexander as the first name, whereas the others put him and Caesar at or almost at the end. So there seem to be two redactions. The three-manuscript redaction does not have a claim to being more reliable on the basis of having more examples, since all of them are likely to follow one prototype, from which indeed their modifications would be slight. The redaction surviving only in manuscript (1) has the better claim. It is the only one with the heading alluding to the *sala;* hence it cannot be derivative from the other version, but the reverse could be true, in which case the differences would represent errors in the three-manuscript group.

But both agree in most things, starting with the distinction between two subgroups of names. The small subgroup with Alexander and Caesar, sometimes omitted, put in different positions in sequence, and always at the outer ends, deserves to be called marginal to the whole. Conversely the seven names, always present, tending strongly to stay in the same order, seem to be the primary subgroup. Another difference is that the two subgroups refer to different phases of world history. Alexander and Caesar are much later than all those in the list of seven, who belong either to the Trojan War, to even earlier Greek myth, or to the Old Testament chronicle books. This type of difference in epoch was understood in Boccaccio's time, as is easily seen from the similar series of famous men in histories of the six ages of the world. Further, Alexander and Caesar form a natural pair; as imperial conquerors, they have a claim to fame of a different type from the other seven. The position of Caesar and Alexander as each other's obvious counterparts is most obvious in their being so presented in Plutarch's parallel lives.[13] And they differ from the other seven in still another, rather surprising, independent variable: the sonnets describe the other seven as being accompanied in the paintings by women, but those describing these two do not.

The seven comprise Solomon, who in his sonnet introduces us to "this accursed creature, enemy of the male species"; Hector, pointing to "her who here gazes on me fixedly"; Achilles pointing to "this damsel"; and Achilles saying "this is Polyxena"; along with Aeneas, Paris, and Hercules, who do not point but give many of their lines to Dido, Helen, and Deianira. The other two sonnets do not give a single word to women; the concurrence with the other differences noted for the same two cases makes that less likely to be coincidence. The visual suggestion is of seven frescoes each showing a male and a female figure, and two 'marginal' ones each with one male only. The latter might be 'marginal' in being narrower as well, or in some other way.

The fact that the two redactions differ in placing the marginal figures at the beginning or the end of the list would seem to suggest that one is in error. But if so, it would be a larger error than otherwise appears, and another hypothesis can explain the difference without error. We may then invoke the principle that, where one hypothesis imputes error to the source on which we otherwise are depending and the other does not, it is unreasonable to opt for the theory of error. Frescoes in a *sala* normally cover all four walls. It is a common experience to have difficulty deciding where such a sequence starts. We usually count on its being beside a door or perhaps a corner, which is enough to know in the case of a single level, as here. It is still harder when there is no narrative. Those preparing the two redactions of the lists may then have made differing assumptions, one starting with the marginal figures and going around, the other starting after them and arriving at them as the last. If so, we can deduce the usual all-around scheme. It is notable that the lists differ only as to the marginal figures, which thus evidently signaled a "bordering" quality. We may assume that relatively weak signals of beginning appeared on both sides of them.

Since two figures are marginal, we must ask whether the start is before the two, after the two, or between them, in the original intention. Help on this comes from considering two other men who make an obvious pair, Solomon and Samson. They are the only nonclassical heroes of any kind, besides sharing their Old Testament origin. As an unexpected independent variable, they also are the only two men whose accompanying women are not *named* in the sonnets. That is understandable in the case of Solomon's idolatrous wife who is unnamed in the Biblical source, but conversely most peculiar in the case of the famous Delilah. Further, in the one-manuscript redaction (which has seemed the better one) they come first and last on the list of seven, suggesting a symmetrical pairing. The oddity of Delilah's namelessness in the sonnet would be explained through reference to the ordinary namelessness of Solomon's wife, making a pairing in itself, if the fresco (naturally) provided the latter with no inscription, and for symmetry's sake none was provided for Delilah. This fits the list's indication of the symmetry of the two heroes as first and seventh on the wall. (The three-manuscript redaction relates Solomon and Samson in a way that is not readable in any form of symmetry, but irregular; this seems then a further token of the superiority of the one-manuscript version.) This symmetrical location for the two Old Testament figures, then, would suggest an analogous pairing of the two conquerors Alexander and Caesar, also at the two ends of the cycle, which would then start in between them.

Indeed the middle five figures between Solomon and Samson just as readily make symmetrical pairs. Hercules, second of the seven, is the figure in Greek myth whom we automatically tag as "strong," and Hector, sixth of the seven, is the one we pick for the same quality among Trojans. So does the sonneteer, making them say "Hercules was I, strongest" and "I was the famous and strong Hector" in their opening lines; no other sonnets contain that epithet. So too Aeneas, third of the seven, and Paris, fifth, are the two heroes in whose lives love stories outweigh their military careers by far; the sonneteer tells how Dido on seeing him "was heated in her heart" and how Paris "became eager for Helen in his heart." Such suggestions, to be sure, are legitimately subject to the criticism that one can find something in common between any two given items, but I believe that can be overridden here in that these are the *main* qualities of the men in every case, hardly found in any of the other men.[14] We are then left with Achilles as the chief hero in the middle. As we started with an apparent row of equals, that may seem surprising but also has a good basis. One need only recall the *Iliad*, which also

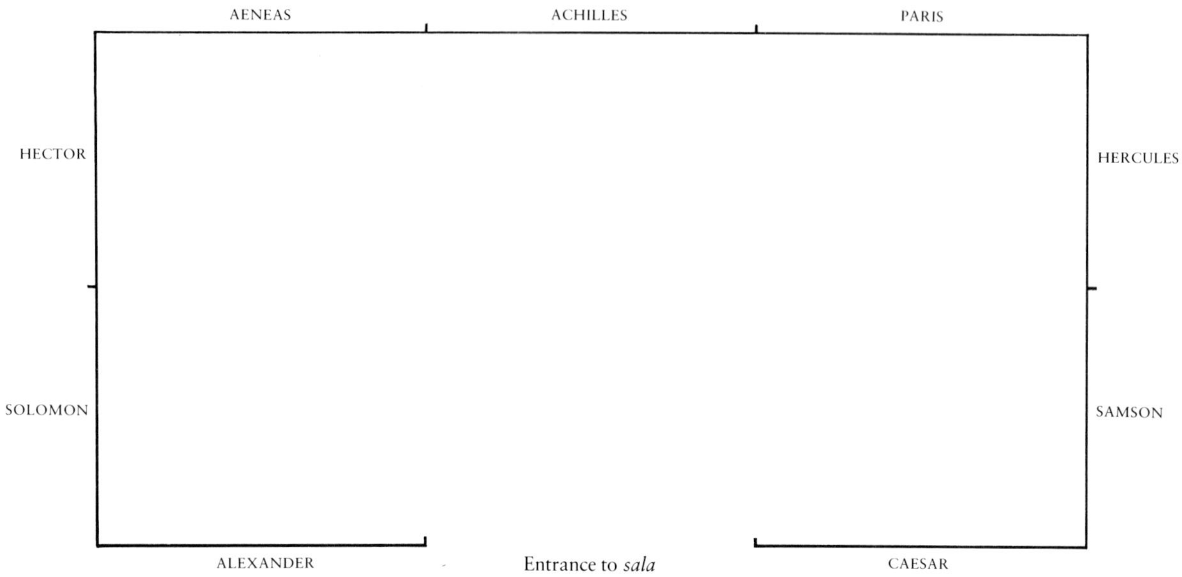

Fig. 11.2. Reconstruction of the arrangement of frescoes by Giotto in the *sala* of King Robert of Naples.

may give the effect of having many coequal heroes, but tells us in its first line that it is really the story of Achilles.

It seems possible, then, to suggest the layout of the frescoed walls, omitting windows and the like. The cycle runs all around, on one level. It starts between Alexander and Caesar, but in a way that could let one think it started before or after the pair of them. Figure 11.2 seems to be the only simple system that provides for all this. Further, it underlines all the paired symmetries noted above, not only in concept but also visually, since the two imperial conquerors, the two strong men, the two lovers, the two Old Testament figures, all are either directly opposite each other or flank a single intermediate central figure or door; we do not have to find symmetries at any distance. The one puzzle is as to the two interchangeable positions possible for Caesar and Alexander, for which there is little evidence since Caesar is only on one list. I have relied on the point that Caesar has much that is obviously in common with Samson but not with Solomon; the former two share their violent deaths in spectacular public assemblies—and we shall see further that the deaths of the heroes are a chief motif for all. Neatly enough, Alexander has much that is obviously in common with Solomon, but not with Samson, the former two both being the great kings of their lands, ruling wider realms than any before or after them. Thus I have placed the similar figures side-by-side.[15]

But what is odd is the choice of these nine figures as the set, which is surely unique. It seems unlikely that any other program picked, as its representatives of the Old Testament, Samson and Solomon and only them. By that very token they may explain the general purpose. These two would seem to be the only Old Testament figures outstanding for the fatal effect women had on them, again emphasized in the sonnets. With Samson this goes without saying; Solomon's sonnet, after reporting his glories, goes on to tell how the "accursed creature" so affected him that we cannot say whether he is in heaven or hell.

Plainly too, that kind of thematic focus dovetails with the fact that the heroes in the frescoes are accompanied by the women. And in the others besides Solomon and Samson we continue to find that the women led the heroes to death. This would be obvious with Hercules, even if the sonnet did not tell us how he killed Nessus for taking his wife and as a result "my death came about." Paris tells us that Helen was "the cause why the Trojans died, and I died with them." The Achilles we know from the *Iliad* would not fit this pattern. But in the sonnet he is accompanied by his bride Polyxena and tells us that "at her word I died." This is the story of Achilles used by Dante, who puts him in the circle of the lustful; Boccaccio also makes it the point of his life of Polyxena, in his book on famous women. It was first developed in the Troy romance of Benoit de Saint-Maur. Achilles enters Troy by night, tempted by a promise of seeing her, and Paris with others ambushes him.

Aeneas is a little different. He has of course a relationship with a woman that leads to death, but it is her death, and the sonnet says, "I was to blame." This same shift is present in the case of Hector in an even more puzzling way. Nothing happens to Hector along these lines in the *Iliad,* yet in the sonnet he tells us that the Amazon queen Penthesilea, who "here gazes fixedly on me," "for me died." By great luck the life of Penthesilea, again in Boccaccio's book on famous women, helps us. He remarks that, in the opinion of some, she loved Hector and joined him in battle in which she was killed. The recent editor[16] notes that there is no trace of this in Boccaccio's source on Penthesilea, nor have I been more successful in finding a literary source. But now we do see a precedent for what he wrote, a recent one known to him, in this fresco cycle by Giotto.

This pattern does not appear in usual cycles of famous men. It seems that Giotto's cycle may not belong to that genre, as Ghiberti said it did. It suggests, rather, the genre most commonly known as the imagery of the power of women. Best known in German prints of the fifteenth century, this includes Solomon and his idolatrous wives; a marvelous drypoint by the Housebook Master shows him with one of them. The literature on the genre is slight, with respect to general surveys including earlier phases; a helpful summary is provided by Vizketely, under the better rubric "Slaves of Love."[17] In rare cases, he notes, these may be women; Dido is his only firm example. The motif first emerges in French thirteenth-century sculpture (a context with links to Angevin Naples) in sets of only two figures, either Aristotle and Virgil or Aristotle and Samson. The first known larger set is at Konstanz, dated either 1306–16 or ca. 1350.[18]

Though Konstanz is far from Naples both in culture and space, there are reasons to think there is a connection of some kind with Giotto's series. Not only are these the only known treatments of the motif between the end of the thirteenth and the late fourteenth century; both shift to the medium of fresco, both are in secular buildings and accompanied by poems. They are also, as noted, the first to include a larger number of slaves, and of Giotto's nine heroes five are in Konstanz too, only one of them, Samson, having appeared earlier. (The other four in common are Solomon, Achilles, Paris, and Alexander.)

The Konstanz set illustrates a short poem, a *Spruch,* by the delightfully named contemporary Frauenlob. He gives each hero a line, or in a few cases half a line. These are inscribed on the fresco, in circular frames around each image. The paintings show not only the heroes but the women they loved, not mentioned in the poem. Can that have been the case with Giotto too? The groups form graphic narrative scenes, rather than being standing icons.

The analogy to Giotto may seem less strong in that Konstanz offers fourteen heroes, so the overlap of five with Giotto may seem less marked. However, of the fourteen, a number are subtypes of love slaves who might be unlikely choices for Giotto, and the comparison even sharpens our understanding of what Giotto was saying. Thus Frauenlob's Arthur and Percival are heroes of northern poetry who are very rare in Italian imagery, and his Aristotle and Virgil are love slaves in a context of low comedy, whereas Giotto's heroes are all bound to seriously tragic fates. Holofernes, the only villain in Frauenlob's set, points up that Giotto's heroes are all to be admired. So is David, but love was not fatal to him or any woman he loved, as it was for all Giotto's heroes. Absolom and Azahel are not known in any tradition as slaves of love; Frauenlob's inclusion of them as such, it has been suggested,[19] shows the influence of earlier German love poetry in which they were named, in a group with Samson and others, as supreme in their specialties. The poets declared that they would not exchange their love to have the strength of Samson, the beauty of Absolom, the swiftness of Azahel, or the qualities in which Aristotle and others were preeminent. Frauenlob then swept all these into his poem and called Absolom and Azahel love slaves like the rest, without any specifics. In the Konstanz fresco Azahel is duly accompanied by a woman. (The fresco of Absolom is lost.) This explanation of the presence of the two is evidently correct, despite the rather capricious causation, in view of the recurrence of the long list of names. At the same time, the absence of these figures from Giotto's set is not at all surprising.

Thus just the remaining six of Frauenlob's heroes are of the kinds that Giotto's scheme would seem to have called for, and of these Giotto includes five, all but Adam. The agreement in the inclusion of Alexander is the remarkable factor. Of him Frauenlob wrote: "Though so powerful, to him befell the same" (i.e., as to Absolom, whom "a woman betrayed"). It was noted that the Naples sonnet mentioned no woman in the case of Alexander (and Caesar), and indeed the usual legends about him involve no fatal love. Yet the link from Giotto's figure to the Konstanz figure requires us to ask whether Giotto too might have attached such a tale to him. Since almost all the seven Naples sonnets which do allude to the heroes' fatal love do so in their final climaxes, such an association with Alexander may first be sought at the end of his. There, following a series of his successes, is the quite puzzling passage: "I entered the sea, in a closed tin, and saw the bottom and the fish; reader, if you are lazy, take my example." This still seems remote from fatal love, but by luck the legends of Alexander's descent into the sea have been the theme of an excellent monographic study by D. J. A. Ross.[20] The tale emerged in thirteenth-century Germany. The great king, when he made his descent, entrusted his air tube and rope to the woman he loved, but her true lover persuaded her to drop them, almost killing Alexander until another turn in the story rescued him. Since this tale of love and a near escape from death is indeed the reference of the final lines of the Naples sonnet, we must accept that in Giotto's cycle Alexander was, after all, though a marginal figure, as much a slave of love as the central seven heroes.

This somewhat complex chain of inferences (presented in the version of this study given as a public lecture) received a surprising and neat confirmation when the unpublished image of Alexander in the Konstanz set became available in a reproduction. The artist shows Alexander inside a bell jar, with fishes, connected by a tube to the hand of a lady standing on a tower. This image of the story, far older than any noted by Ross, shows that in Konstanz and Naples not only did Alexander appear as a slave of love, as he never seems to do elsewhere, but that in both cases the same rather unusual tale about him was the basis. Besides tightening the proof that Giotto's Alexander was such a slave, this tightens the linkage between the two cycles greatly. One is reminded that the most famous work of Giotto for the trecento, his Navicella, also had as its theme people in danger of drowning. Was his Alexander shown in a secular version of that image? Here only speculation is possible.

This makes it inevitable that Caesar, the other of the two marginal figures, must have been thought of too as a slave of love. In his case it is still harder to see how, and no clues emerge. The last line of his sonnet mentions his death, but no connection with fatal love is obvious. A possibility involves a tale which was, at least, a famous one, so much so that it is the only entry under Caesar in the vast *Motif Index of Folk-Literature* of Stith Thompson. Shakespeare also used it. It is the incident in which his wife, on the basis of a dream, urged him not to go to the Senate on the Ides of March.[21] In some versions he yields to her at first, but then goes when the conspirators mock him for doing what a woman says. To be sure, love by or for Calpurnia was not fatal to him; might we say that her action led to his death because it involved a woman's role? It remains a mystery how Caesar's being a slave of love led to death, but we can hardly doubt that he was here so regarded.

Giotto did his painting in Naples around 1330. Boccaccio was then a boy in the same royal court. In 1355 he began his book on famous women, which he first planned to dedicate to the Queen of Naples, but in the end offered to the sister of the Florentine royal counselor there. We have seen that his book shares with Giotto the novel story of Penthesilea. He surely saw much more in this cycle by the artist he most admired. His preface to this same book explains that he chooses few Jewish or Christian women, emphasizing those of Greece and Rome. Again, he includes not only virtuous women but those who had "strong but destructive characters." He boasts his book had no precedents. And yet these general patterns are foretold in Giotto's painted cycle.

The title Ghiberti gave to it, "famous men, in the king's *sala,*" evidently calls for basic alteration.[22] Is it then the case that it is the cycle Boccaccio in the *Genealogy* called "loves of the gods and crimes of men, in a royal hall"? It indeed is focused both on loves and on crimes, since almost all the loving couples shown include one who acted criminally against the other. And it is in a royal hall. Thus the description is more cumulatively apt than could have been guessed, and few other candidates to fit Boccaccio's terms are likely to appear. But of course it seems wrong as to one term, the gods. To be sure, one could recall that Caesar was declared a god,[23] that Hercules was a demigod, and that Boccaccio's precise phrase does not demand that all the figures be gods. However, to learn how Boccaccio would define a pagan god one should, after all, turn to this very book as a whole; to write a genealogy of the gods is not different from writing up their loves. In his preface he expands and qualifies his title, saying he will report "the pagan gods and the heroes who, according to the ancient stories, are descended from them." One is not surprised that he then gives full space to all the early Greeks and Trojans in our cycle, Achilles, Aeneas (whose mothers indeed were divine), Paris, Hercules, and Hector. On the last page of Book 13, the last that is genealogical, he speaks of Alexander, who, claiming to be a son of Zeus, marks for Boccaccio the end of the era, when "that ancient madness, by which the famous gloried in being inscribed as progeny of the gods," ceased. Here too Alexander is a marginal figure. That Boccaccio, with the polemical irony that informs his other descriptions of paintings, should in the context of his book have called Giotto's cycle a picture of love and crime among gods and men is not demonstrated, but is well within the limits of the plausible.

APPENDIX

ALESSANDRO

Sono Alessandro, e mostro in questa storia
    Signor del mondo, e non senza cagione,
    Chè, combattendo in ver settentrione,
    Di tutto l'universo ebbi vittoria.
Sazia non fu l'ardita mia memoria:
    Avendo vinte tutte le persone,
    Oltre all'umana abitazione
    Insino all'Uzian mostrai mia gloria.
Ancor più fece l'animo mio magno:
    Salii nell'aria e mostrai ch'io non volli
    A mia gran signoria par nè compagno.
Quivi, cresciuto il mio voler sui colli,
    Entrai nel mare, e nel più chiuso stagno,
    E vidi tutto il fondo e pesci molli.
Lettor, se pigro sei, mio esemplo tolli.

SALOMONE

Io fui ultramirabil Salamone,
    Di cui saver riluce tutto il mondo:
    Molte question solvetti di gran pondo,
    E 'l tempio edificai per mia ragione.
Tengon le genti elloro opinione,
    S'io sono in cielo o s'io gravai giù al
        fondo:
    A questo punto, lettor, non rispondo,
    Ma vo' che 'l ver ne sia mio testimone.
Molti libri scriss'io di mia dottrina:
    Trattai di Re e recai in figura
    El cielo, el mondo e ciò che ne diclina.
Ma questa maledetta creatura,
    Nemica della spezie masculina,
    Mi fe creder per mia disavventurs:
Onde mia fama luce assai più scura.

ETTORE

I' fui illustre e forte Ettor troiano,
    Che contro a Greci fei si ab antico,
    (Benchè a me non lece quel ch'io dico),
    Ch'io n'uccisi migliar colla mia mano.
E s'al seren mio padre il re Priamo
    Rimaso fosse un altrettale amico,
    No l'avria morto Pirro empio nimico,
    L'onor di Troia non sarebbe a piano.
È costei qui, che si fiso mi mira,
    Pantesilea, magnanima reina,
    La cui fama ancor nel mondo spira.
Per me mori e qui meco confina,
    E solo un braccio ci diè a Persepina:
    Meco mori in una medesima ira,
Ma no'n una medesima mattina.

ENEA

Son per Enea qui figurato e scorto,
    Per quel gran duca egregio troiano,
    Che tanto corsi per lo mare oceano
    Fin ch'al lito di Dido presi porto.
La qual, come dagli occhi suoi fui scorto,
    Del mio piacer s'accese nel cor vano;
    E poi s'uccise con sua propria mano,
    Quando partimi: e certo io ebbi il torto.
Poi gii in Italia per voler divino;
    Prima vidi lo inferno e Proserpina,
    Turno, Camilla e vinsi il re Latino,
E disposai la sua figlia Lavina,
    Avendo tutta Italia a mio domino:
    Fei crescer Roma, ch'era piccolina;
Posile nome, regola e dottrina.

ACHILLE

Io fui il magnifico d'Achille,
Che tanto d'arme fe'contro a Troiani:
Pantesilea mori per le mie mani,
E 'l fortissimo Ettorre ancor sentille.
Degli altri uccisi più di mille e mille,
Gente minuta, e cavalier sovrani
Della città, ed altri più loutani,
Che per atarli abbandonar lor ville.
E questa è Polisena, la mia sposa,
La quale io miro ancor con grán diletto,
E certo che l'amai sopr'ogni cosa.
Finite fur le nozze nel mio letto,
Palese fu a quella fresca rosa
Fuor della mia persona ogni difetto,
Ben ch'al suo dir mori nel suo cospetto.

PARIDE

I' son Paris dell'alto re Priamo
Qui figurato e fui 'l suo quinto figlio:
Più bello assai che non fu mai il giglio;
Ma di prodezze mie non ragioniamo.
Trova'mi si nel cor d'Elena bramo,
Che 'n Grecia io passai, per mio consiglio,
E non pensando al fururo periglio
Che 'l mio legnaggio e me fe venir gramo.
Quivi fec'io del mio parer ragione,
Siccome i' fe di dar la poma d'oro,
Diella a Venus e disservi' Giunone.
Cosi trass'io del real concistoro
Quella reina; di che fu cagione
Che moriro i Troiani ed io con loro.
Cosi rimaso foss'io a guardar al toro.

ERCOLE

Ercole fui, fortissimo gigante,
Il quale molti adorar per iddeo;
Quasi la terra mi sottomis' eo,
E 'l mar segnai ove non va più avante.
Tutte le bestie insino al leofante
I' vinsi colle pugne e anche il leo,
E strangolai il fortissimo Anteo,
Ch'era maggior di me, ma non si atante.
E molto fe' per amor di Dianira,
Che tanto a me fu bella e si mi piacque,
Si com 'l sa a cui mostrai mia ira.
I' Nesso uccisi perchè seco giacque,
Il quale ancora all'inferno s'aggira
Intorno al sangue delle boglienti acque;
Benchè per lui la mia morte nacque.

SANSONE

Voi, che mirando andate i greci e ebrei
Famosi antichi per la sala bella,
Mirate me che, con una mascella
D'asino, uccisi mille Filistei.
Ancor glorificar più mi potrei;
Se non che, io inamorai d'esta donzella,
La quale, artata, con falsa favella,
Mi parlò si che mi scopersi a lei.
E preso dall'amor che ragion torce,
Al sonno mi legò, com' saper puoi;
Poi mi levò i crin colle sue force.
Allor fur presti li parenti suoi
E fecermi orbo, andando con iscorte,
Fin ch'io gridai: *moia Sanson co' suoi!*
Allor tirai per mille par di buoi.

CESARE

Io fui l'ardito Cesare imperiers;
D'ogni paese volli esser signore;
L'animo mio fu di tanto valore
Che ad ogni affanno volli esser primiere.
Regi, signori e tutte lor bandiere
Per mio comando givan dentro e fore;
Ed ebbi in me tanto valente core
Ch'io non temetti di niun suo potere.
Non ebbi mai paura di morire,
Nè già temetti mai un grande storno,
Anzi mi confortava a ringioire.
Il cor me ne sentia, avendo attorno
I franchi cavalier, pien d'ogni ardire
Nelle battaglie, senza far soggiorno.
E tutto il mio poter mori in un giorno.

NOTES

1. J. V. Schlosser, *Quellenbuch zur Kunstgeschichte des abendländischen Mittelalters* (Hildesheim, 1896; reprint 1976), 352–67.

2. The classic studies are those of C. Osgood, *Boccaccio on Poetry, being the 14th and 15th books . . .* (Princeton, 1930), on the essay itself, and of A. Buck, *Italienische Dichtunglehren vom Mittelalter bis zum Ausgang der Renaissance* (Tubingen, 1952), on the context.

3. G. Dominici, *Lucula Noctis,* ed. E. Hunt (Notre Dame, 1940).

4. The lines are in Book 14, approximately a quarter of the distance from its beginning. In this paper I am especially pleased to follow the Holt model in presenting the texts in a close English translation. My edition is the Renaissance Italian translation by M. G. Betussi, *Della Geneologia degli Dei* (Venice, first ed. 1547; reprint 1627, Venice), 217v.

5. This passage is a little more than one-third from the end of Book 14. In the edition cited in the previous note, it is p. 230r.

6. E. Panofsky, *Renaissance and Renascences in Western Art* (New York, 1960; reprint 1969), ch. 3, *I primi lumi.* The author restates the formula of "disjunction" between classical form and subject earlier, on p. 84.

7. Ibid., 155.

8. P. Murray, "Notes on Some Early Giotto Sources," *Journal of the Warburg and Courtauld Institutes* 16 (1953): 62–63.

9. J. Seznec, *The Survival of the Pagan Gods,* first French edition 1940, English reprint 1961, Introduction, p. 5.

10. L. Ghiberti, *I Commentari,* ed. O. Morisani (Naples, 1947), 33; G. Vasari, *Le Vite,* ed. G. Milanesi (Florence, 1878), 390–91.

11. G. De Blasiis, "Immagini di Uomini Famosi in una sala di Castelnuovo attribuite a Giotto," *Napoli Nobilissima* 9 (1900), 65–67. See Appendix.

12. De Blasiis reported that no manuscript has the full set; he described (4) as lacking Samson. However, he is included there, as Mr. Mattox reports, providing also the explanation of why De Blasiis missed him: he was also omitted from the index provided by the eighteenth-century compiler. Samson's presence, in fifth place, makes much difference to our chances of analyzing the various texts, as will be obvious in the following discussion.

13. Plutarch's *Lives* had not been translated from the Greek in Giotto's time. I mention the analogy simply to suggest the extreme obviousness of a parallel between Alexander and Caesar, which could occur to anyone. It is of course possible that the Greek traditions in southern Italy, not so much from Magna Graecia as from ties to Byzantium, made Plutarch available there in the fourteenth century. If his lives of Alexander and Caesar had indeed been a factor in this cycle, Giotto would certainly have learned with interest of a remark on the first page of the life of Alexander, explaining why these two biographies are not thorough. It is because these two heroes did so much: "Therefore, as portrait-painters are more exact in the lines and features of the face, in which the character is seen, than in the other parts of the body, so I. . . . "

14. Certainly one would think of strength as Samson's main quality, but to pair him with either Hector or Hercules one would have to ignore the separate classical subgroup within which the latter are paired, and the absence of an allusion to his strength in his sonnet.

15. Support for this layout seems also present in the Samson sonnet, which begins: "You who are going about the beautiful *sala* admiring the famous Greeks and Hebrews." This conspicuously omits the Roman, Caesar. In the layout here offered, that would be all right, since we have not yet got to Caesar, at the end of the set. It might be argued contra that the omission of Trojans from the quoted phrase makes it valueless for this purpose. However, it is not unusual to subsume Trojan heroes with the Greeks in such cases. Thus B. Degenhart describes the set as consisting of Hebrew, Greek, and Roman heroes. (B. Degenhart and A. Schmitt, *Corpus der italienischen Zeichnungen 1300–1450* [Berlin, 1968], Teil 1, vol. 2, 594.)

16. G. Boccaccio, *Concerning famous Women,* trans. and notes by G. Guarino (New Brunswick, N.J., 1963), 65.

17. A. Vizketely, "Minnesklaven," in E. Kirschbaum, *Lexikon der christlichen Ikonographie* (Freiburg, 1971), vol. 3, 270, with bibliography. A further reason why it is less good to classify the set as

Uomini famosi is that it would then be earlier than any known instance. While its untypical character might seem consistent with that status, this classification has also led to such confusion as calling it a "variant of the type of the nine worthies" though that type did not yet exist, its literary origin being of just this time. (Degenhart, as in note 15, 619, n. 25).

18. H. Schmidt-Pecht, "Alte Hausmalereien in Konstanz," *Das Bodenseebuch*, vol. 27 (1940), 32–39, with repr. of six of the fourteen figures; F. Maurer, "Der Topos von der 'Minnesklaven,' " *Deutsche Vierteljahresschrift für Literaturwissenschaft und Geistesgeschichte*, vol. 27 (1953), 182–206, with text of the poem by Frauenlob (see *infra*) p. 197; A. Knoepfli, *Kunstgeschichte des Bodenseeraumees*, I (Konstanz, 1961), pp. 129–130; M. von Claparede-Crola, *Profane Wandmalerei des 14. Jahrhunderts zwischen Zurich und Bodensee*, diss. (Munich, 1973), pp. 82–83. Of these, only Schmidt-Pecht has any illustrations. The originals are lost, and known from nineteenth-century drawings. The work was dated before 1316 by Schmidt-Pecht on the basis of a document showing that in that year the house passed from lay to clerical use. Knoepfli dated it ca. 1350 on the basis of costume comparisons. However, since he did not address the argument for the other date, and since copies dilute the value of costume comparisons, which in this period are sparse and show gaps between dated examples, the other proposal may still be considered. I am greatly indebted to the courteous and prolonged efforts of Dr. Fromm, Konstanz, Dr. Marcel Baumgartner, Zurich, and Mr. Garry Apgar, New Haven, through whom I obtained reproductions of the unpublished roundels and copies of the recent publications.

19. Maurer, as in n. 18, p. 194.

20. D. J. A. Ross, *Alexander and the Faithless Lady, an inaugural lecture* (London, 1968), 20 pages.

21. The version by Valerius Maximus, in his group of stories about dreams (I, 7, 2) appears to be the earliest on record.

22. The only study to have dealt with the thematic idea of Giotto's cycle as an issue is, as the author rightly claimed, F. Bologna's *I pittori alla corte angioina di Napoli* (Rome, 1969), p. 220. Since it is also fairly recent and likely to be consulted, explicit notice of its doubtful aspects may be required. After naming the heroes, the author writes: "From certain allusions in the sonnets one can deduce that they were accompanied . . . precisely by Roxane, the Queen of Sheba, Andromache, Dido, Polyxena, Helen, Deianira (or Iole or Omphale), Delilah and Cleopatra." This list, which appears also in earlier commentators, is so erroneous—four (and also the alternates to Deianira) out of nine being wrong—that one must inquire how it happened. It would appear that it was first taken for granted that *all* the heroes were so accompanied, and then, since no woman was named in the first sonnet, a name was picked that is commonly associated with that hero, and the same method was then used throughout. Bologna goes on to note that the criterion of selection is difficult to understand, but that there was some sort of effort to show a concordance between the Biblical and classical worlds; he cites Alexander and Hercules as compared with the two Biblical figures. There was simultaneously a contrast between examples of virtue and their contraries; he cites Hector and Aeneas for one, Achilles and Aeneas for another instance. But the presence of Caesar, "autonomous from other comparisons," evokes a more historic order, departing from the medieval encyclopedic traditions of the others. It is striking that these efforts to analyze the theme ignore the women who appear in it. While that might be an advantage in view of their erroneous identifications, it would seem unlikely to lead to an adequate solution. As is often the case, the most unusual elements of a scheme are good clues to its purpose.

23. The suggestion that the fatal love connected with Caesar was that of Cleopatra, suggested in the preceding note, at first glance seems to have much to be said for it. Cleopatra's love did lead to death, and she is the most famous person so affected who is connected with Caesar. On the other hand, the love that was fatal to her was not for Caesar; if the tale of her death was the one meant, it would seem reasonable that Anthony would have been represented. Further, the sonnet in which Caesar speaks of his career and death does not mention her or even allow for implying her, as all the sonnets otherwise do mention or imply the women in question. Thus this hypothesis seems to encounter even more difficulties than the one presented above.

12

The SPECIAL ORDERS of ROBERT MILLS

ROBERT L. ALEXANDER

THE WINNING OF MAJOR COMPETITIONS for a church and a monument established Robert Mills (1781–1855) as an architect of national standing. The two resulting works, his Monumental Church (1812–1817) in Richmond and his Washington Monument (1814–1829) in Baltimore, are recognized today as significant steps in the development of the Greek Revival style.[1] Each one, moreover, demonstrates his determination to adapt models of other times and places to a personal statement with symbolic meaning. During the second decade of the nineteenth century, relatively early in his career, he made such adaptations in the architectural orders, sometimes applying symbolic ornament and at other times employing parts that bore generally recognized meanings.

An example of the first approach appears in the Monumental Church, an octagonal structure with a portico-like monument on one side housing a sarcophagus with the ashes of the victims of a disastrous theater fire (figs. 12.1, 12.2). Inside the church, rows of pews on either side of the central aisle and in the horseshoe-shaped gallery face the chancel screened by two tall Ionic columns between antae faced with pilasters in the same order. To the Ionic columns, of the Erechtheum type, Mills applied appropriate mortuary symbols (fig. 12.3). For the palmettes and anthemions in the necking of the ancient model, he substituted stars and inverted torches, which he described as "Sarcophagic emblems." This character extends to the capital itself where the star reappears, and below it the folds of a winding cloth replace the curving lines of the cushion between the scrolls in the ancient Greek example. To the Doric columns supporting the gallery he added corner acroteria and a pediment, recalling Roman cippi and sarcophagi, as another form of commemoration of the victims of the theater fire (fig. 12.4).[2]

In evoking specific meanings through symbolic ornament, Mills participated in an activity that interested a number of architects of the age. In America some notable examples appeared during the Federal period, including Major Pierre L'Enfant's American orders for Federal Hall (1789) in New York City and the cotton, corn, and tobacco orders (1809, 1815) in the national Capitol in Washington by Benjamin Henry Latrobe, Mills's architectural mentor.[3] In this atmosphere Mills's application of "Sarcophagic emblems" to the columns of the Monumental Church is understandable.

Mills's competition design of January 1814 for the Washington Monument shows a great deal of symbolism to be applied as bronze decoration. Inverted torches and stars, providing a commemorative aspect, and honorific emblems, such as wreaths and armorial shields, appear on the rectilinear base, while seven bands of reliefs

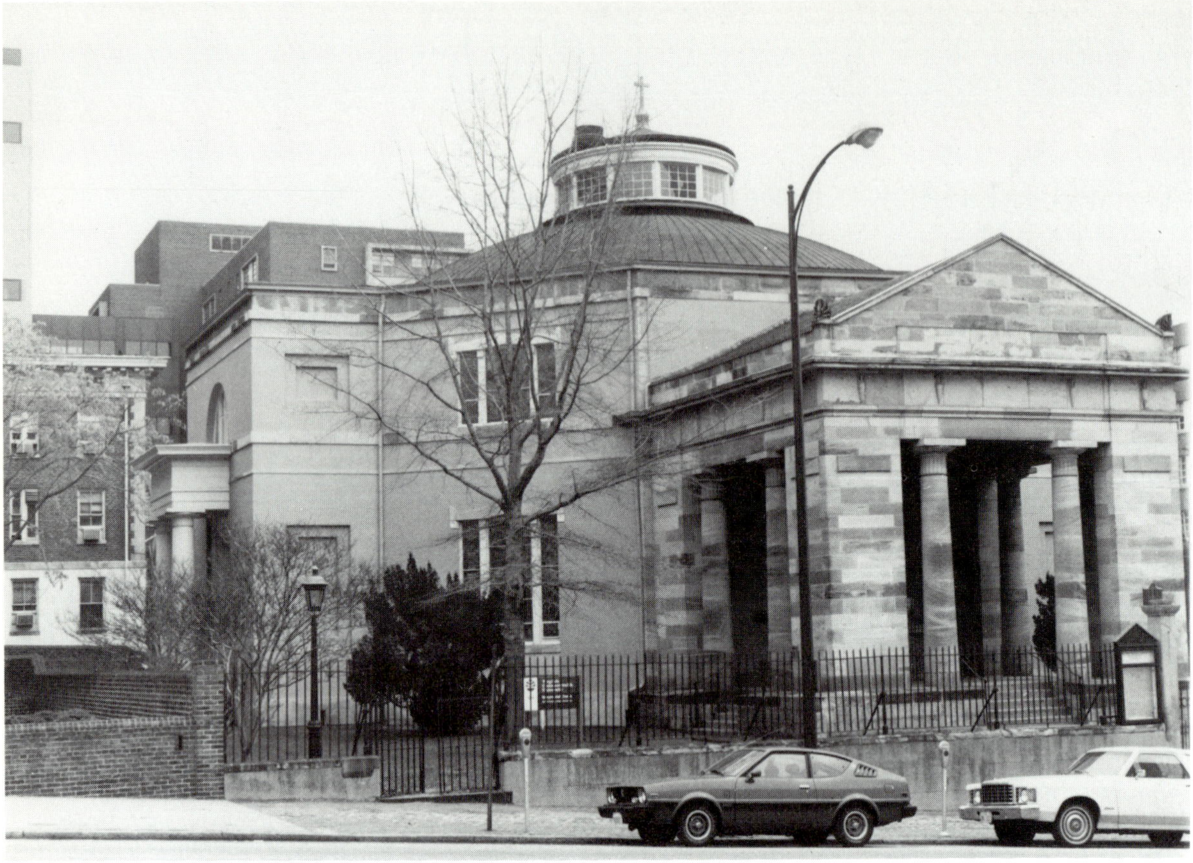

Fig. 12.1. Robert Mills, Monumental Church, Richmond, Virginia, 1812–17.

and inscriptions dealing with significant events in the life of George Washington surround the great column. Although he still hoped many years later to retain one or two bands of decoration—shields and spears, stars—by 1816 most of the bronze was eliminated, and eventually the lack of money left the monument with no sculpture beyond the huge statue of Washington at the top (fig. 12.5). Mills, however, had already indicated the alternative way—employing generally recognized meanings in architectural parts—to endow expressive meaning upon the enormous Greek Doric column. In an essay that accompanied the competition drawings, he described the order itself as "masculine" and possessing the "solidity and simplicity of character emblematic of the illustrious *personage* to whose memory it is dedicated."[4]

Mills took another opportunity to achieve meaning in the order which, in the early design, was a Doric of the archaic period derived from the temples at Paestum, with a smooth shaft to receive the bronzes. The broad curve of the echinus signaled to the age that the architect turned to the origins of Greek architecture, to the time when it was closer to nature. As constructed, the column was related to examples found at the Temple of Apollo at Delos, where narrow bands of fluting at the neck and foot of the shaft were to guide workmen in finishing the column. Ignorant of the ancient archi-

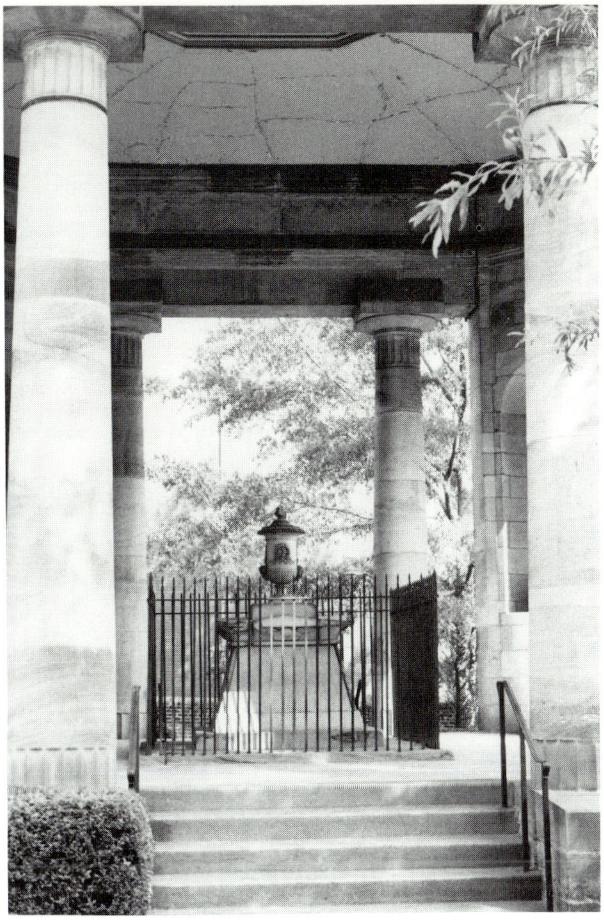

Fig. 12.2. Robert Mills, Monumental Church, detail of monumental porch.

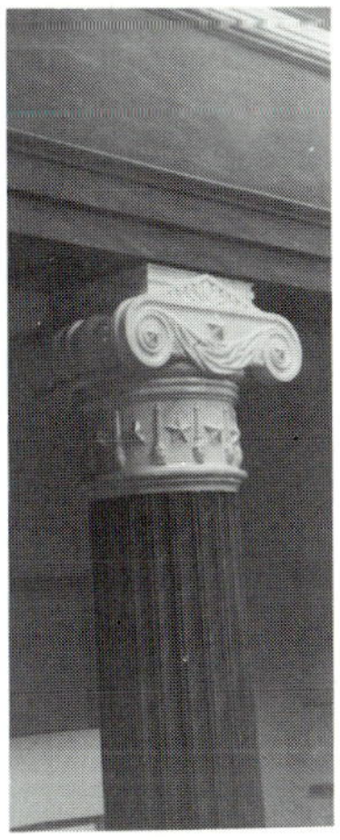

Fig. 12.3. Robert Mills, Monumental Church, detail of interior Ionic order.

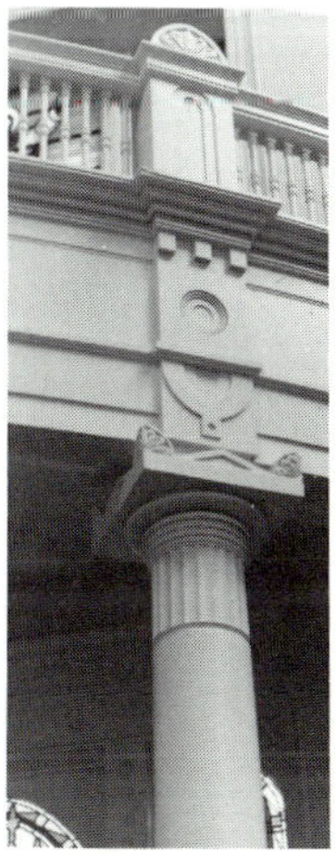

Fig. 12.4. Robert Mills, Monumental Church, detail of interior Doric order.

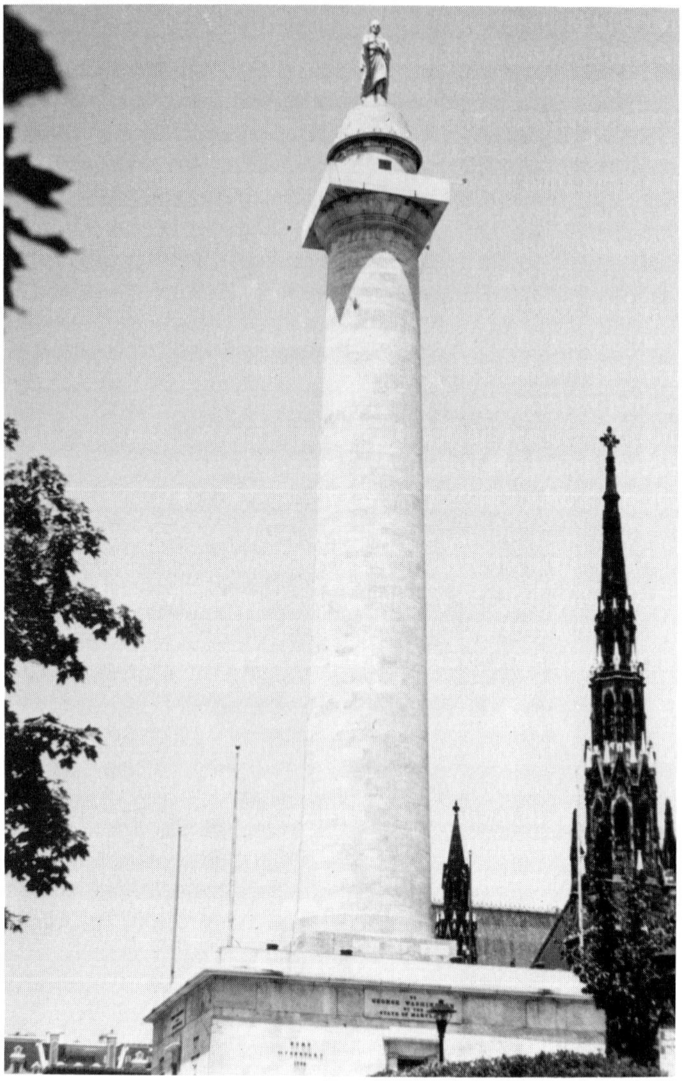

Fig. 12.5. Robert Mills, Washington Monument, Baltimore, Maryland, 1814–29.

tect's intention to have the channels completed, some theorists of Mills's day considered this shaft closer to the origins of architecture than a fluted Doric. At the cornerstone ceremonies on 4 July 1815 a large painting showed the intended appearance of the monument, and the column was clearly of the Delian type.[5] Thus, during the year and a half when revisions stripped the bronze ornament for the sake of economy, Mills strengthened the connotations of the bare architectural element by combining the Delian form with the Paestum order. Although he never commented on this point, Mills probably saw the combined order as reinforcing the reference to the fundamental strengths admired in the character of Washington.

In employing the orders for their expressiveness, Mills drew upon a tradition that had ancient origins but excited much interest during the Age of Reason. Jacques-François Blondel, in the publication of his teachings, summed up and enlarged upon ideas of Vitruvius in his general, metaphorical assignment of each order to a typical use according to its character. So that the viewer might immediately understand the nature and function of a structure, he assigned the Tuscan order for use in military works, Doric for sacred edifices, Ionic for elegant houses, Corinthian for royal palaces, and Composite for public, festival architecture. His slightly younger contemporary, Sir William Chambers, less verbose and systematic, pressed similar ideas through the late eighteenth century and was a source for Asher Benjamin who adapted the orders for American use. Mills knew this tradition from several sources: James Hoban whom he assisted at the White House, Thomas Jefferson who granted Mills the use of his library, Charles Bulfinch to whom Mills was introduced in 1802, and Latrobe for whom Mills worked from 1803 to 1808; through Latrobe's friendship with Maximilian Godefroy, he may have had a fairly direct link to French sources.[6] Against this background, the Doric order of the Washington Monument was "masculine" for Mills and his contemporaries; as a sacred building and for its seriousness, the Richmond monument also required Doric.

The shared commemorative function of the two monuments and the lengthy period of work on the Richmond structure (as late as 1817) undoubtedly played a part in Mills's decision to strengthen the meaning of the Baltimore column by the alteration of the shaft. He had, in fact, already employed a variation of the Delian column on both the exterior and interior of the Monumental Church. It appears in stone on the monumental porch and the two smaller entries to the building and in wood as the supports for the interior gallery (figs. 12.2, 12.4). A broad echinus, based on the type from Paestum, provides another archaizing touch in the stone column; for the wooden column, the capital is simplified into a broad disk above a graduated series of three torus moldings.[7] A ring of fluting surrounds the upper and lower ends of the shaft, but the upper ring is considerably taller than the Delian type and an astragal molding separates it from the rest of the shaft. For these columns, then, Mills used the ancient model from Delos, substituted the echinus of Paestum, and enlarged the upper row of fluted channels.

Sources for the variant orders appear in rediscovered antiquity, but they include also some modern works. The French scholar Julien-David LeRoy made the Delian Doric available in the mid-eighteenth century, and although it rarely appeared on the continent, a number of architects employed it in the last decades of the century, beginning with Nicholas Revett about 1776; and in the 1790s Latrobe combined it with the Paestum proportions and capital, a form close to that employed by Mills on the Monumental Church. Conversion of the upper row of fluting into an elongated necking, on the other hand, began with Robert Adam who introduced the fluting in the 1760s and George Dance Jr. who lengthened the fluted necking about 1768, both of them using this variation in Ionic. Sir John Soane employed the form several times in the 1780s, and Bulfinch introduced it to America in his Tontine crescent of 1793–94. Mills extended the process of alteration in fusing this necking with the Delos-Paestum Doric of Latrobe. Further, but more speculatively, the process may have been facilitated by the visual impact of the customary abbreviation of the column in representations of the orders where most of the shaft was omitted; the section of a fluted column below the capital resembles Mills's elongated necking. For Mills the addition of the element used by Dance, Soane, and Bulfinch probably was a means of modernizing the ancient order.[8]

Even before Mills met Bulfinch and apprenticed with Latrobe, he knew

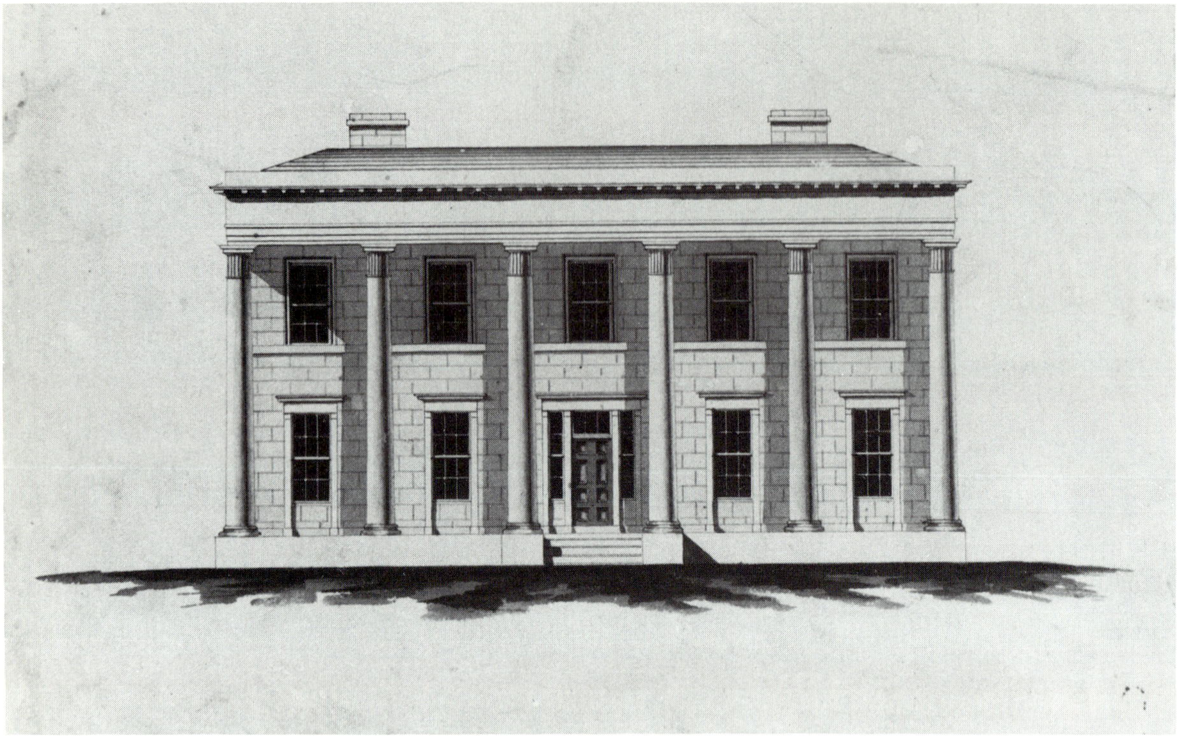

Fig. 12.6. Robert Mills, design for Didier house, 1817. From the collections of the South Carolina Historical Society.

that international theory and practice endowed the orders with characteristic meanings. During his twentieth year (1801–02), his architectural training began when he joined Hoban in the construction of the White House. He clearly engaged in reading such works as the treatise of Chambers, for in an essay on the Tuscan order written at this time, Mills followed the tradition of assigning the order to uses where its "apparent Solidity and Simplicity" were appropriate, e.g., "at the Entrance of Cities, Magazines, Etc." By 1813, as his education and experience grew, he employed symbolic ornament to endow greater specificity of meaning upon his compositions. Although he employed special orders for only a few years early in his career, the interest remained alive. A note from his readings as late as 1838 shows how deeply ingrained these ideas were: "Temple of Apollo at Delos, has flutes at the neck & foot of column."[9]

Mills employed his form of Doric in domestic works as well as for public monuments. In a design of 1817 for the mansion of a Baltimore merchant, Henry Didier Jr., he created a five-bay house with a high portico across the front, its roof supported by six two-story columns (fig. 12.6). Although the column has a base rather than fluting at the bottom and the shape of the echinus is not indicated clearly, at the top of the shaft fluting fills an elongated necking and stops at a molding. With its tall proportions, eight diameters high, this column exemplifies the Federal attenuation of the orders rather than the ancient Greek stockiness and stability. Perhaps Mills wanted to lessen the solemnity of the Doric by giving it proportions closer to the Ionic, an order that was recognized as appropriate for private houses.[10]

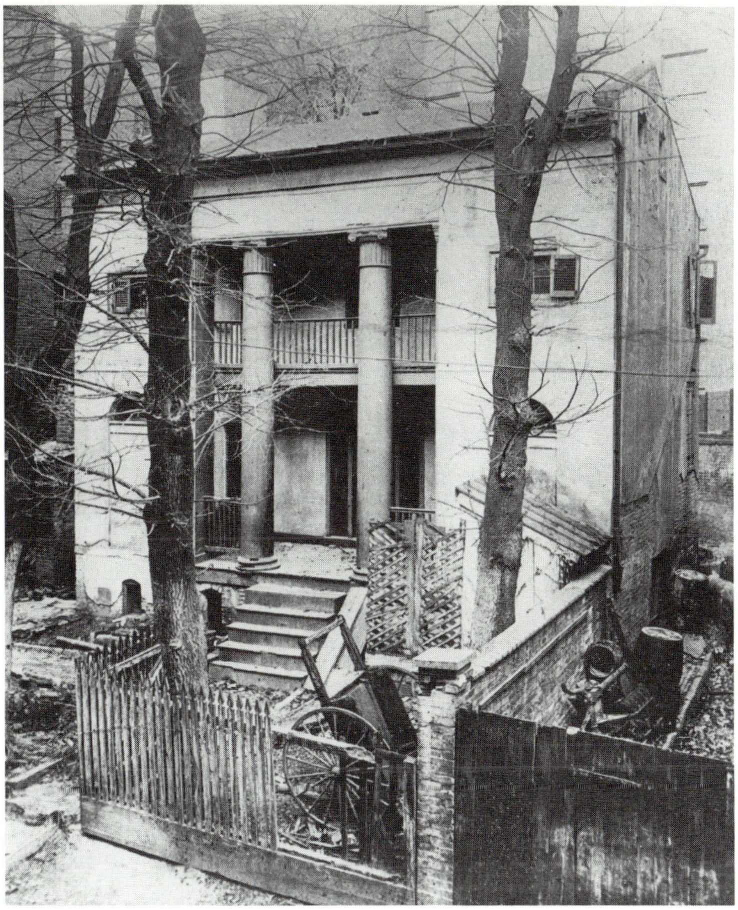

Fig. 12.7. Robert Mills, Tusculum, William Gwynn house, Baltimore, Maryland, 1816. Courtesy of the Maryland Historical Society, Baltimore.

An Ionic order with the tall fluted necking appeared in Mills's designs during the same decade. In 1815 he did some minor work in the home of William Gwynn, editor of the Baltimore *Federal Gazette,* but in the spring of 1816 he undertook more extensive alterations. With Gwynn he discussed a drawing of the proposed changes on 20 June, and over the rest of the year he supervised the construction. A sketch made in September shows the order of the new front that was to be distinguished by a two-story recessed vestibule with two columns in-antis (fig. 12.7); the column was 16 feet 10 inches high, with a lower diameter of 21 inches. As the time approached for completing the columns, on 13–14 December he detailed the capital for the carpenter, making a small sketch in his journal as a record of its form (fig. 12.8).[11] It was modern Ionic, that is, Renaissance rather than antique, with four diagonal volutes and no cushion over the egg and dart molding between the volutes. Fillets rather than arrises separated the flutes of the tall necking.

The year 1817 is the terminus for Mills's designing with these special orders, as shown by the Didier house and the date of completion of such a work as the monumental porch (1815–17) of the Monumental Church. Early prints of the church indicate the order and other parts in a general way that is at variance with the completed structure.[12] Thus, its design in 1812 is probably not the beginning of his use of the spe-

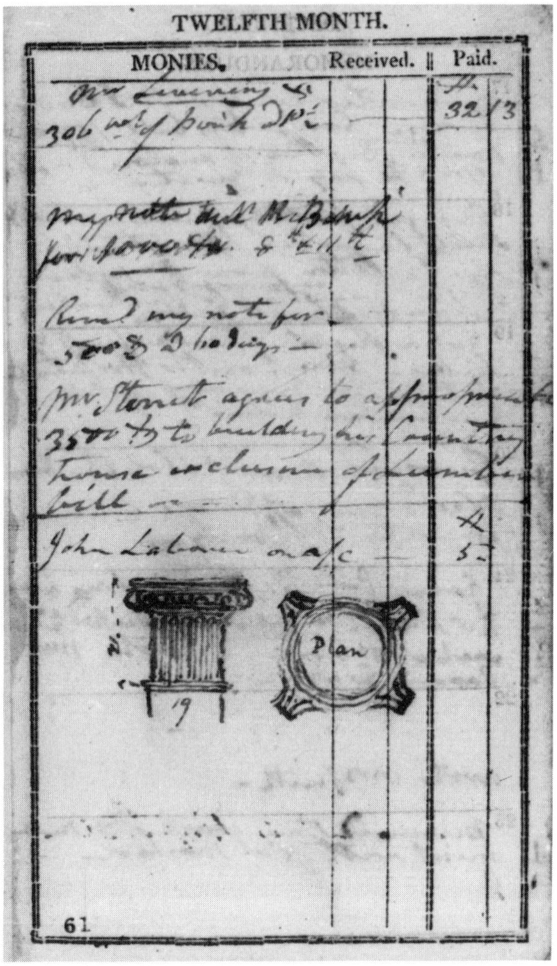

Fig. 12.8. Robert Mills, sketch of capital for Gwynn house. Courtesy of the Library of Congress.

cial orders. In keeping with the practices of many architects, including his master, Latrobe, Mills often began construction well before establishing details that could be finished later in the process of building. His alterations of the Gwynn house, for example, were planned in the spring of 1816, but the capitals were not detailed until December, and Mills gave the working drawing to the carpenter immediately. Although the church was begun in 1812, the first service took place on 4 May 1814, so that his thinking and drawings for the interior Doric and Ionic orders probably dated from late in 1813, time enough for the building committee to give approval and for the workmen to fashion the columns. All the other works and special orders discussed here date within the period 1813 to 1817.

The variety in the orders of this limited number of works demonstrates the way Mills developed his skills in design. He separated the Doric and Ionic into parts, base, shaft, capital, and the enlarged necking, which then became elements for combining in various ways. An unworked surface on the shaft enhanced the decorative effect of the necking and perhaps underlay his preference for the unfluted shaft. This exploration

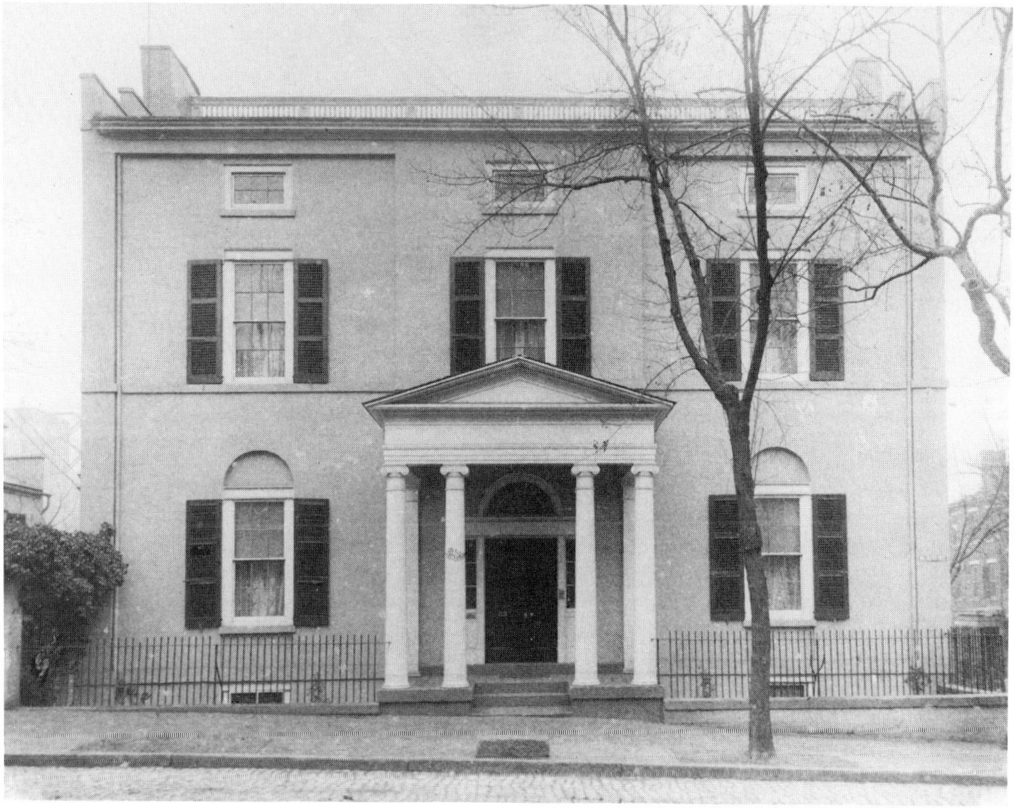

Fig. 12.9. Robert Mills, Cunningham-Archer house, Richmond, Virginia, 1814–15. Courtesy of the Valentine Museum, Richmond, Virginia.

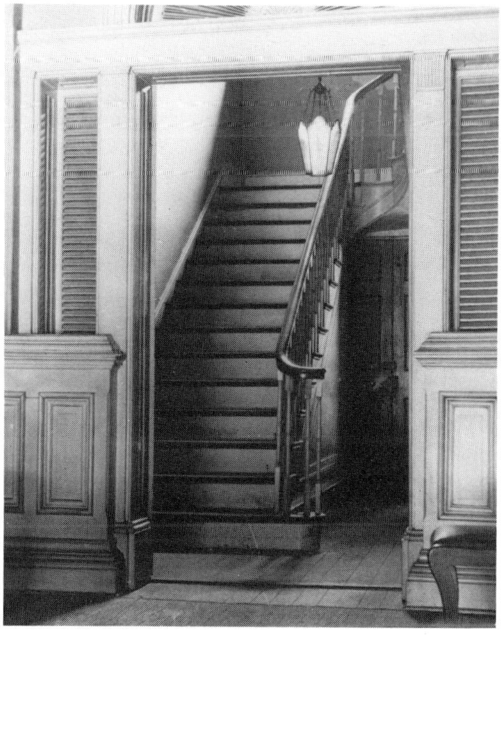

Fig. 12.10. Robert Mills, Cunningham-Archer house, hallway screen. Courtesy of the Valentine Museum, Richmond, Virginia.

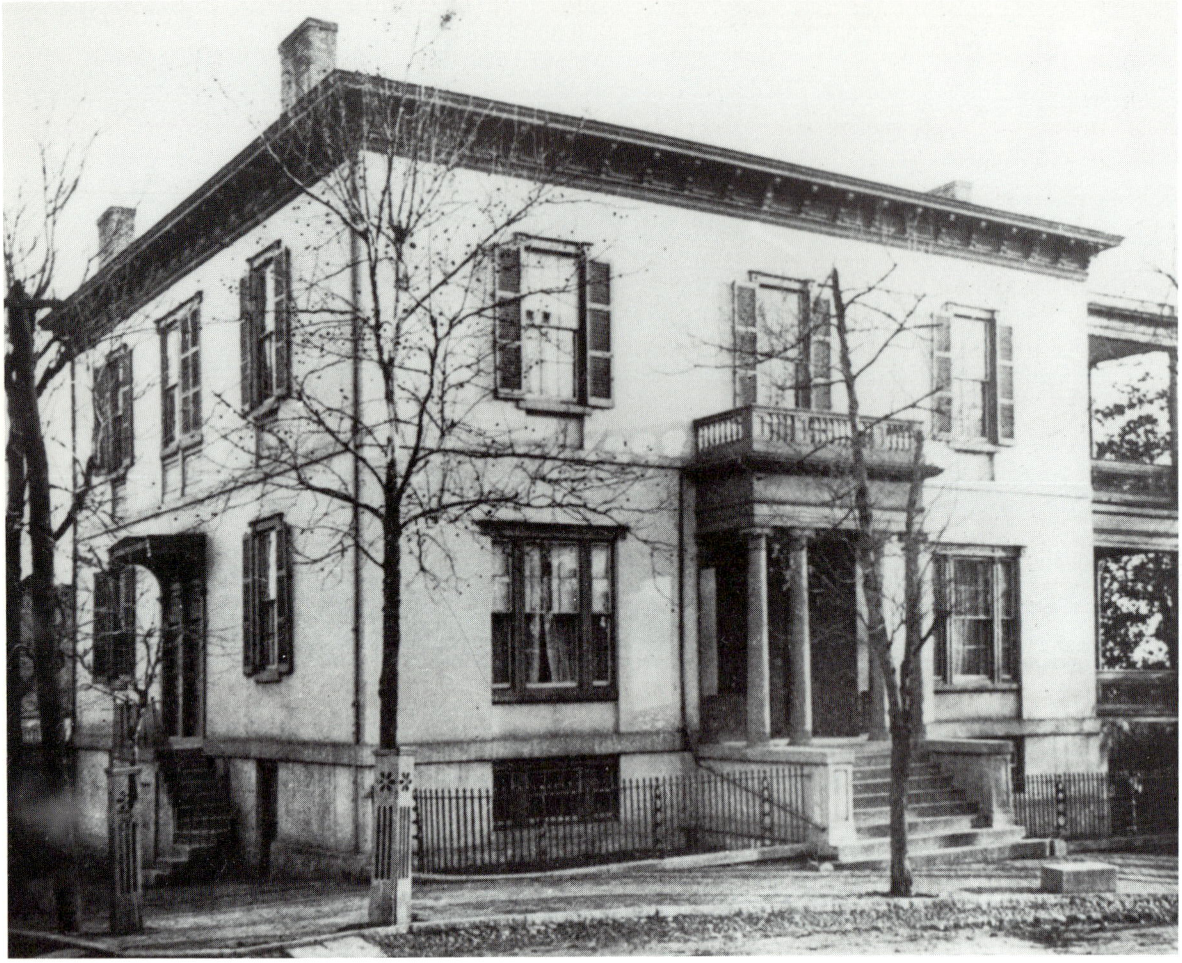

Fig. 12.11. Robert Mills, Hanover House, Joseph Marx house, Richmond, Virginia, c. 1813–15. Courtesy of the Valentine Museum, Richmond, Virginia.

of the possibilities for combination in the orders occurred at just the time when Mills was seriously concerned with the problems of architectural composition in a larger sense. In 1816–17 he brought to culmination a system of design that organized a block-long front.[13] In houses and especially rows in Philadelphia and Baltimore, he employed a limited vocabulary of forms including arched recesses and single and triple windows and doors. Each opening sat upon or hung from one of the continuous horizontals (water table, string course, cornice), with a vertical alignment of the door and window frames; the block-long facade was covered by a network of verticals and horizontals. Repetition and alternation of arched and rectangular forms of different sizes produced a counterpoint of rhythms and accents within the network. The strict alignment of verticals and horizontals is especially evident in the design for the Didier house.

Early stages in the formation of this vocabulary and system appear in the two houses in Richmond that have long been attributed to Mills. On the basis of his interest in these variant capitals and columns, the attributions can be strengthened. The Cunningham-Archer house was begun probably in 1814 and was essentially finished when it was insured on 7 November 1815 by its owner, Edward Cunningham, who was a businessman with interests also in several manufacturing firms (fig. 12.9). It was a broad structure, its three wide bays emphasized by the lateral recesses. A pedimented portico projected from the middle bay, with two Ionic columns on either side of the wide central intercolumniation. Here was the Roman arrangement of volutes, parallel on front and back of the capital, and between them was a graded sequence of torus moldings as on the interior Doric of the Monumental Church. They had also the elongated, fluted necking at the top of the shaft and a shorter row at the bottom and stood on a simple base composed of a single torus molding. These forms were echoed, without the volutes, in the two pilasters against the wall of the house as well as those used as framing elements throughout the interior (fig. 12.10). In addition to these columns, the traditional attribution to Mills is supported by the similarity with the Gwynn house in the use of stucco over brick, string course at the second floor level, form of window in arched recess, and small mezzanine window in the top story. In addition, one documentary reference links Mills with this house; in 1816 he noted that he had ordered $270 worth of marble mantlepieces from a firm in Philadelphia for Mr. Cunningham.[14]

Hanover House, another attribution to Mills, was built by Joseph Marx, an immigrant from that German city who became one of Richmond's wealthy merchants (fig. 12.11). Its construction occurred perhaps in 1813–14, though the owner delayed insuring it until 20 October 1817; its evaluation of $23,000 made it one of the most expensive in the city. A large, almost square block, it had colonnaded entrances on the east and west sides and a two-story portico along the south. The Ionic columns of the west porch (and their spacing) were identical with those of the Cunningham-Archer house, but a balustraded deck rather than a pedimented roof covered the entrance. Other elements, too, were parts of Mills's vocabulary at this time—stuccoed walls, water table and string course, tripartite windows, simple door and window frames, recesses. For Mr. Marx, also, he ordered a number of marble mantlepieces.[15]

Except for the instance in the work of Bulfinch, in this country the elongated, fluted necking seems to be the mark of Mills. He employed it for just a few years, 1813–17, at a time when he was much concerned with specifically architectural problems. Recently developed in England, its principal function probably was to modernize the classical or archaic, Greek, Roman, or Renaissance orders, and thus the structures in which they appeared. Just as Palladio employed the architectural forms he deemed suitable for "Persons of different Conditions," Mills incorporated appropriate messages in the buildings he designed for the gentlemen who were his clients.[16]

NOTES

1. The basic work on Mills is H. M. Pierce Gallagher, *Robert Mills, Architect of the Washington Monument, 1781–1855* (New York: Columbia University Press, 1935). For the church see Margaret Pearson Mickler, "The Monumental Church," Master's thesis, University of Virginia, 1980; for the monument see J. Jefferson Miller II, "The Designs for the Washington Monument in Baltimore," *Journal of the Society of Architectural Historians* 23 (1964): 19–28; unless otherwise noted, information on these struc-

tures comes from these sources. It is a privilege to offer this work to Elizabeth Gilmore Holt in respect, affection, and thanks for many years of warm friendship.

2. The star and inverted torch appear also in the designs for the Washington Monument, and in the description of this work Mills called them "Sarcophagic emblems"; the description accompanied the original drawings in the competition and has been published in William D. Hoyt Jr., "Robert Mills and the Washington Monument in Baltimore," *Maryland Historical Magazine* 34 (1939): 154–57. Mickler has made a careful study of the symbolic decoration in "Monumental Church," 38–41.

3. For L'Enfant's orders see H. Paul Caemmerer, *The Life of Pierre Charles L'Enfant, Planner of the City Beautiful, The City of Washington* (Washington: National Republic Publishing Company, 1950), 113, 116, quoting from *The Massachusetts Magazine,* June 1789. For Latrobe's orders see Talbot Hamlin, *Benjamin Henry Latrobe* (New York: Oxford University Press, 1955), 270–71, 532–33, pl. 23; and Paul F. Norton, *Latrobe, Jefferson and the National Capitol* (1952; New York & London: Garland Publishing, 1977), 219–21, 247, pls. 40, 54. Perhaps because the alterations consisted largely of decorative enhancement rather than significant changes of form, Asher Benjamin belittled this kind of order; at the least, his criticism shows how widely known these efforts were. For Benjamin's opinion see *The American Builder's Companion* (1806; 6th ed., 1827; reprint ed., New York: Dover Publications, 1969), 32; and idem, *The Rudiments of Architecture* (1814; reprint ed., New York: Da Capo Press, 1972), 44.

4. The statue measures about sixteen and a half feet high. The characterization of the Doric appears in Mills's description; Hoyt, "Washington Monument," 155.

5. For the orders of Delos and Paestum, see Dora Wiebenson, *Sources of Greek Revival Architecture* (London: A. Zwemmer Ltd., 1969), ch. 4, 47–74; this study provides the historical and intellectual background for the modern use of Greek orders. For an engraving of the eight-foot-high painting of 1815 by Henry Warren, see Miller, "Washington Monument," fig. 9. The column, in fact, was never intended to have the lower row of fluting; instead, a narrow projecting band to provide visual support for the bronze ornament appears in many drawings and on the actual monument.

6. Jacques-François Blondel, *Cours d'architecture, ou Traité de la décoration, distribution & construction des bâtiments,* text 6 vols., plates 6 vols. in 3 (Paris, 1771–77), 1:410. Sir William Chambers gave appropriate uses as he discussed each order; for Doric and Ionic see his *A Treatise on the Decorative Part of Civil Architecture,* 3d ed. (London, 1791), 52, 56. Benjamin virtually quoted Chambers in his assignment of the orders; for the Doric and Ionic see his *American Builder's Companion,* 34, and *Rudiments of Architecture,* 46–48. While traveling in 1802 to study the architecture of the northern states, Mills carried a letter of introduction from Jefferson to Bulfinch (Gallagher, *Robert Mills,* 8). For Godefroy's knowledge of Blondel, see Robert L. Alexander, *The Architecure of Maximilian Godefroy* (Baltimore and London: The Johns Hopkins University Press, 1974), 31–34 et al.

7. For a possible source for the graduated wooden rings see Benjamin, *American Builder's Companion,* pl 10 lower left, and *Rudiments of Architecture,* pl. 10 lower left.

8. For LeRoy and eighteenth-century use of the Delian Doric, see Wiebenson, *Sources of Greek Revival Architecture,* 70, pls. 39, 45; for Latrobe's use, see ibid., 71, pl. 53, and Talbot Hamlin, *Benjamin Henry Latrobe* (New York: Oxford University Press, 1955), 44–46, 101 n, pl. 2. For the alteration of the Ionic necking, see Robert Oresko, ed., *The Works in Architecture of Robert and James Adam* (London: Academy Editions; New York: St. Martin's Press, 1975), 126, see also 22; Dorothy Stroud, *The Architecture of Sir John Soane* (London: Studio, 1961), pls. 17, 25, 44–45; and Harold Kirker, *The Architecture of Charles Bulfinch* (Cambridge, Mass.: Harvard University Press, 1969), pl. 34. Soane may have gotten the form from George Dance Jr., who used an Ionic with a tall necking in an "Adamesque looking" room at Pitzhanger Manor (1768–70), where Soane did his first architectural work; the shape of the fluting is not clear (Pierre de la Ruffiniére du Prey, *John Soane's Architectural Education, 1753–80* [1972; New York & London: Garland Publishing, 1977], 21–22, fig. 4. On Soane's admiration for Adam, see ibid., 40.

9. For the essay on the Tuscan order see Gallagher, *Robert Mills,* 153–54. The later observation appears in a notebook used by Mills in 1837–40, 42, now in the Manuscript Division, Library of Congress. Undoubtedly the note on the Delian order arose from Mills's recent use of it in a more archaeological form in his design for a marine hospital for 100 patients (Gallagher, *Robert Mills,* 59, illus. opp. p. 62). Late in his life (1852) Mills planned a change in the circular colonnade he designed to surround the base of his monumental obelisk to Washington; for the original Doric he wished to substitute an "American order," the details of which are indecipherable (Pamela Scott, "Robert Mills's Washington National Monument," Master's thesis, University of Delaware, 1985, 30–32).

10. This design is usually known as the Dedian house, following Mills's identification on the drawing (Gallagher, *Robert Mills,* 96, illus. opp. p. 98; for the drawing, 1827–28, see Gene Waddell, "Robert Mills's Fireproof Building," *South Carolina Historical Magazine* 80 [1979]: 116 n.). In the records of Baltimore, I have found only one reference to a "Henry Dedean"; he was given notice on 5 September 1818 to repair the footways of his property on Franklin Street between Park (then North) and Cathedral Streets (City Commissioners, RG 3 S 1 Box 24, 1818/389, Baltimore City Archives, Baltimore, Maryland). The name is wrong, for this property belonged to Henry Didier Jr. in 1816–17. A wealthy merchant, Didier had been in London in 1816 where Sir Thomas Lawrence painted his portrait (Eugene L. Didier, "The Social Athens of America," *Harper's New Monthly Magazine* 65 [June–Nov. 1882]: 30). On 12 October 1816 he joined with other property owners in petitioning for establishment of the northeastern corner of Franklin and Cathedral Streets, which was done on 28 October (*Records of the City of Baltimore: Eastern Precincts Commissioners, 1812–1817; Western Precincts Commissioners, 1810–1817* [Baltimore: City Library, 1909], 242, 244). A petition for the establishment of official boundaries usually preceded any construction in new areas of the expanding city. Instead of building, however, Didier sold part of the property to John Oliver on 12 May 1817 ("Land Records," 122–23, Robert Oliver Papers, MS 626, Manuscript Division, Maryland Historical Society Library, Baltimore, Maryland), and the rest to Nathaniel F. Williams on 5 December 1817 (Indenture, 25 May 1819, John Campbell White Papers, Box 1, MS 1005, Manuscript Division, Maryland Historical Society Library). Inasmuch as Mills did not mention this design in his 1816 journal, he probably drew it early in 1817 before Didier decided to sell the property (Robert Mills, "Pocket Memorandum Book, or Daily Journal for the Year 1816," Manuscript Division, Library of Congress, Washington, D.C.; published in part: Robert Xavier Evans, ed., "The Daily Journal of Robert Mills. Baltimore, 1816," *Maryland Historical Magazine* 29 [1934]: 257–71).

11. Mills, "Pocket Memorandum Book," fols. 6, 38, 43, 45–47, 51, 53, 55, 58, 61, 63v, 76v and under dates 6, 8 Apr.; 20 June; 22, 24, 25, 28, 29 Oct.; 1, 14 Nov.; 13, 14 Dec.; the sketch of the column appears on fol. 47, of the capital on fol. 61. Mills received $200 in July for expenses of construction (fol. 38), and at the end of the year Gwynn still owed him $150 (fol. 63v). The house, called Tusculum, was built about 1812 by Robert Cary Long Sr. (Clare Wittler Eckels, "Baltimore's Earliest Architects, 1785–1820" [Ph.D. diss., The Johns Hopkins University, 1950], 97–100). Its evaluation for tax purposes was $400 (perhaps ten percent of its market value), and the construction of 1816–17 added $80 ("Tax Appraisor's Book," 1813, Ward 3, p. 247, and 1816, Ward 3, pp. 34, 48, RG 4 S 2, Baltimore City Archives). Gwynn described his house shortly after it was enlarged.

> My place of residence, though no more like Cicero's Villa than I like Hercules, is called Tusculum—all for the sake of mystery. It stands in a part of the town where it would require an Ariadne to find it:—Since I am upon the Subject I will describe it. The situation is all I could wish, central and retired. My principal front is upon an alley, and a gate intervenes between the door and the narrow pavement. It is a little palace, resembling in appearance some of those delicate, princely pasteboard castles from which our playhouse kings stalk forth to take the air. Sid, when he is inclined to be merry with me, says the building is of the bird-cage order, and he calls the architecture *composite,* not to be sure in the technical sense, but as composed of all the prettiness displayed in the classical school of our long steeple builder, who, he swears, has exhausted all the magnificence of his genius in the design. I beg it, however, to be understood that the plan is entirely my own, and that the aforesaid long steeple builder is no more guilty of the beauties of my Tusculum, than he is innocent of the defects of———. I have two most lordly pillars which sustain my out-spreading roof—a ballustrade, architrave, frieze, cornice—aereostyle, all *secundum artem.* On either side of a large and majestick glass door, which opens the adytum of my temple, are two small rooms:—one, my study, the other my hall of audience.

(John Pendleton Kennedy, "From the Tusculum," *The Red Book* 1 [5 November 1819]: 59–60). The expression "long steeple builder" was current in Baltimore as a reference to Robert Cary Long Sr., who build a very tall steeple on St. Paul's Church (1814–17). For knowledge of the photograph of Tusculum (razed 1891), I am indebted to Carleton Jones (see his *Lost Baltimore Landmarks* [Baltimore: Maclay & Associates, 1982], 28).

12. For early prints of the church, see Gallagher, *Robert Mills,* opp. p. 82, and Mickler, "Monumental Church," pls. 37, 38.

13. Mills experimented also with the upper portion of the orders; the architrave might have two or three bands, and the frieze and cornice varied in dimensions, moldings, and other details. On occasion he introduced appropriate symbols here, e.g., the lachrymal vases in the frieze of the Richmond monument (fig. 12.1). Mills perfected his compositional system in Waterloo Row, designed in December 1816, in Baltimore (Robert L. Alexander, "Baltimore Row Houses of the Early Nineteenth Century," *American Studies* 16 [1975]: 74–75).

14. Mary Wingfield Scott, *Houses of Old Richmond* (Richmond, Va.: Valentine Museum, 1941), 118–21; the house was demolished in 1927. Policy no. 1694, 7 November 1815, Mutual Assurance Society, Virginia State Library, Richmond, Virginia. For the mantlepieces see Mills, "Pocket Memorandum Book," fol. 68v. Mills also employed the hallway screen (fig. 12.10) at the Hampton-Preston house (1818) in Columbia, South Carolina; one stood on the main floor and another still stands on the second floor.

15. Scott, *Houses,* 112–14; the house was razed in 1891. Policy no. 916, 20 October 1817, Mutual Assurance Society. At $554.25, the mantlepieces ordered for Marx probably included some for another house he was building at the same time (Mills, "Pocket Memorandum Book," fol. 68v).

16. Mills was acquainted with Palladio's work; see Waddell, "Robert Mills's Fireproof Building," 121–22. The quotation is from the Preface of Palladio's *The Four Books of Architecture,* as rendered in Elizabeth G. Holt, *A Documentary History of Art,* 2 vols. (Garden City, N.Y.: Doubleday & Company, 1957–58), 2:50.

13

Le CHEMIN SYMBOLIQUE

Ferdinand Hodler's Symbolic Path of *Autumn Evening*

SHARON HIRSH

IN FERDINAND HODLER'S LATE LANDSCAPES, the forms and colors of his native Swiss scenery came to represent the structure and meaning of life itself. Although Hodler continued to work from nature and to attend to descriptive detail, he emphasized above all else the underlying order of nature; this uniformity he called "parallelism." According to his theory, the repetition of human and earthly nature—their parallelism—would dominate any superficial idiosyncracies. Furthermore, "parallelism" was less a visual phenomenon of nature than what Hodler termed "a world law of universal validity"[1] that maintained, in spite of apparent external differences, an important commonality in all living things. "When I am on the sea," he wrote, "I can see only the sky and water, a long line of infinite horizon. When I see a dead man, the eternity of his silence moves me, impresses me deeply. For twenty years I have noted similar phenomena and reproduced those resemblances, those similarities."[2] For Hodler, because nature was a beautiful model of underlying truths, the landscape was less a view of nature than a symbolic vision of the supernatural.

The origins of symbolic landscape in Hodler's work can be seen in *Autumn Evening* (1892, fig. 13.1), in which a central, strongly foreshortened path beckons the viewer toward a horizon, there to meet with a brilliant infinite sky. The path is obsessively direct and aligned on a perspective learned from dramatic baroque landscapes, such as Hobbema's well-known *Avenue at Middelharnis* (1648, London National Gallery), which had influenced many Swiss romantic landscapes earlier in the century. Certainly, Hodler's traditional artistic education and training—his studies in the École des Beaux-Arts in Geneva had been under the Barbizon-related painter Barthelemy Menn—had encouraged the constant study of earlier masters for models of figural proportion, points of technique, and especially composition.

Autumn Evening's compositional debt to baroque landscape had already been anticipated in several earlier landscapes; *Road from Evordes* (c. 1890, fig. 13.2) in particular presents another version of Hobbema's strikingly centralized path. *Autumn Evening* is, however, in other respects very different. In the *Road from Evordes*, the fullness of the green trees and the inclusion of naturalistic shadows on the road domesticate the scene, much as Hobbema's dramatic landscape is softened by the inclusion of farmland to the right, a hamlet in the background, and a man with his dog on the road. In *Autumn Evening* no such incidental or human-related details remain. Although it probably derives from the earlier *Evordes* view (similarities include the stepped grass line on either side of the road, the placement of the trees, and the ditch on the right side

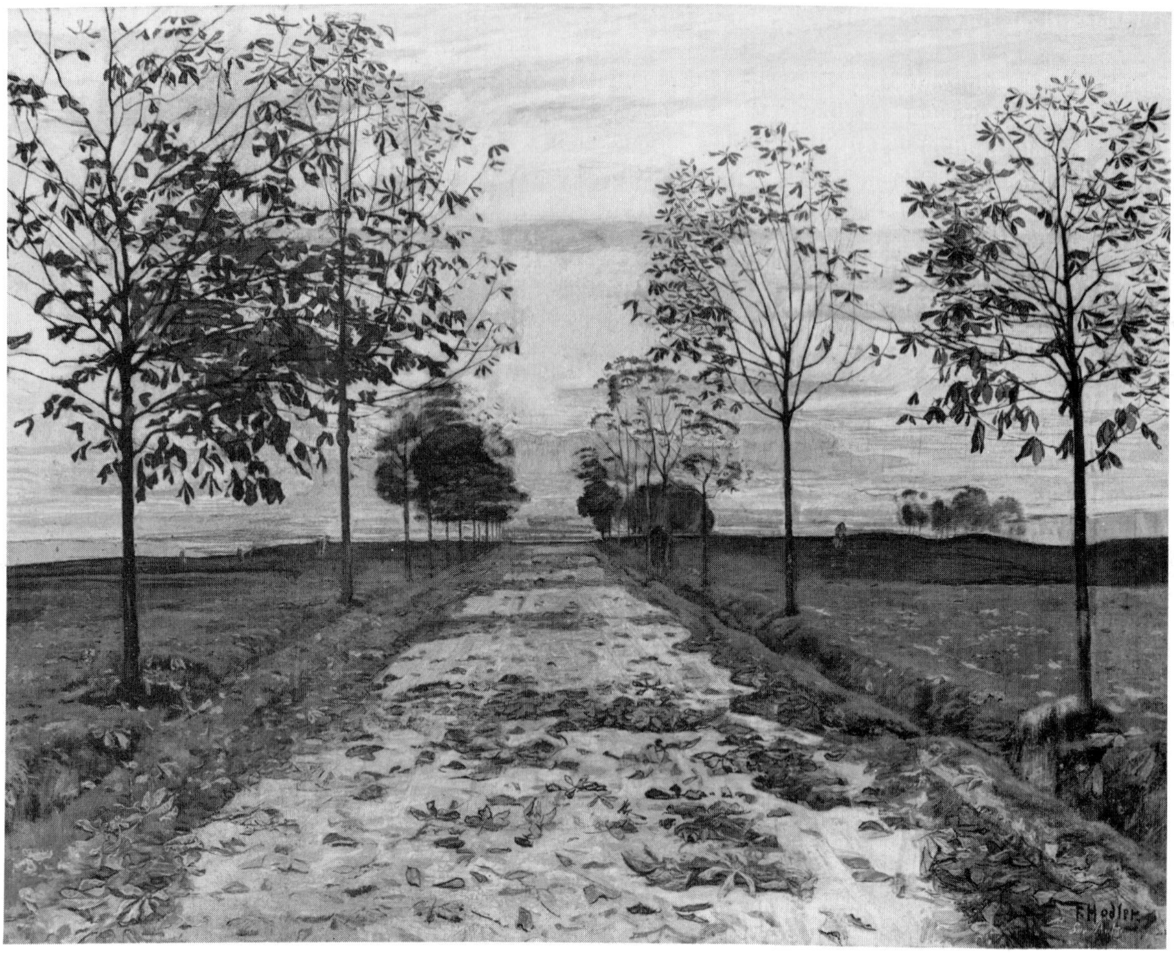

Fig. 13.1. Hodler, *Autumn Evening,* 1892. Oil and tempera on canvas. Musée d'Art et d'Histoire, Neuchâtel. Photo Jean-Marc Breguet.

of the road), it is remarkably bare. The shift in season from spring in the *Road* to fall in *Autumn Evening* justifies some of this bareness, of course, but it does not explain the notable excision of the mountain, a deletion which was made at a late stage in the painting; the outline of a mountain and much of its peak are still visible beneath light overpainting.

This was an important change, since the mountain dominates the earlier view and made a finite, tangible end for the painting. The path of *Autumn Evening* leads to an ethereal sky, with clouds that stretch beyond the boundaries of the frame to a seemingly endless world. As viewers stand on the path in *Autumn Evening*—and there is no other possible approach—they are forced by the steepness of the perspective and the bareness of the autumn scene to concentrate on a hauntingly warm, enveloping sky. Rather than inviting a passive observation of a particular scene, as had the earlier *Road from Evordes, Autumn Evening* encourages meditation—on the warm autumn dusk,

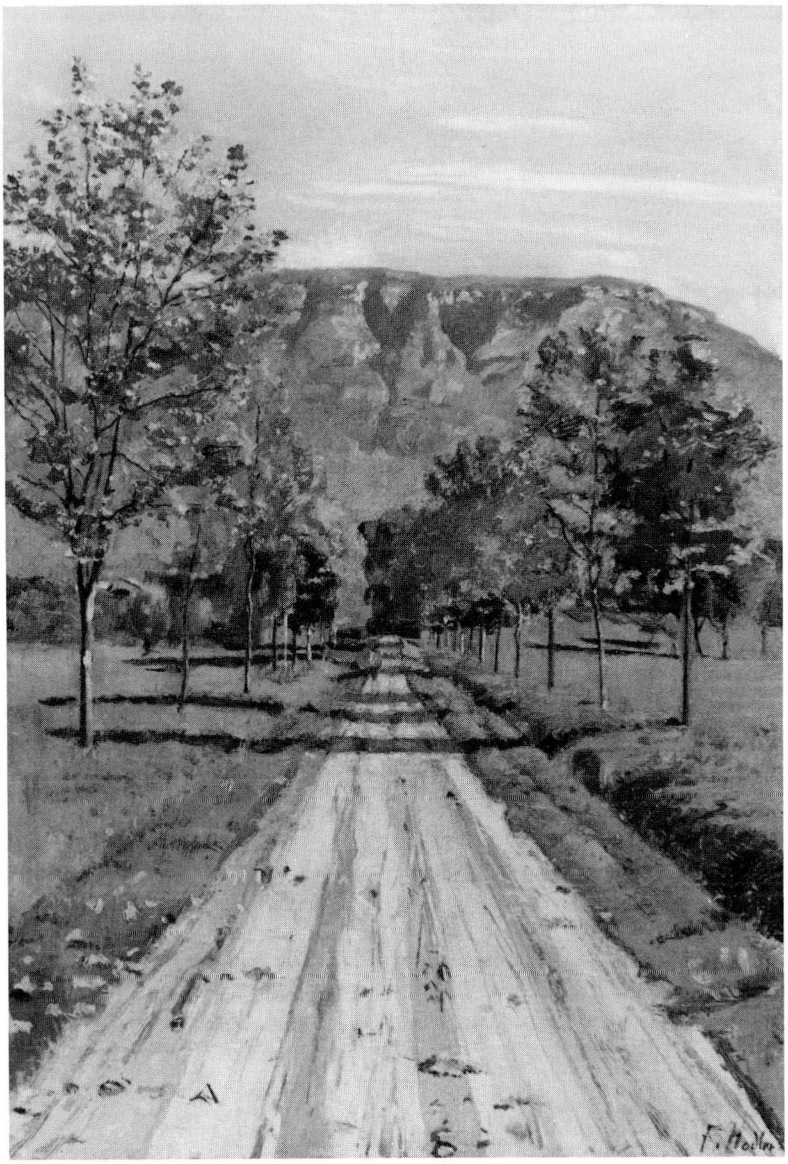

Fig. 13.2. Hodler, *Road from Evordes*, c. 1890. Oil on canvas. Stiftung Oskar Reinhart, Winterthur.

the infinite stillness, and the resonance of the transient earth to the eternal world. Since the path leads to infinity, *Autumn Evening* is intended to signify the coming of death.

In its use of landscape to lead us not to the mountainous end of the road but to meditations on the basic questions of existence, *Autumn Evening* represents a major breakthrough for Hodler. The concern of this, his earliest Symbolist landscape, with the cycle of nature as symbolic of cycles of life is very much in keeping with other fin-de-siècle symbolic expressions of the life cycle that regularly inundated the annual salons. Typical of them is Lauritz Anderson Ring's *Evening: The Old Woman With*

Death (1887, Statens Museum for Kunst, Copenhagen), in which a tired old woman is seated on the side of a road, while above her and seeming to emerge from the clouds is the skeletal figure of death with a scythe. The rolling landscape in the background is shown not only in the evening but also in autumn coloration. Ring's and Hodler's equation of fall with the autumn of one's life has as its common source the nature symbolism of the earlier romantics. Philipp Otto Runge and Caspar David Friedrich, in particular, drew correlations in their work between the diurnal and seasonal cycles and the cycles of human physical and spiritual life.[3]

That Hodler's association between the seasonal and life cycles was precisely the same is evident in a painting executed about the same time as *Autumn Evening*. Titled simply *Autumn* (1893, Musée d'Art et d'Histoire, Geneva), the old man in it represents life's passage. We learn that Hodler made the connection from his notebooks, where he writes that he wants to execute an entire series of paintings that together will represent the basic cycles of existence: the times of day, the seasons of the year, the times of life and of spiritual awareness.[4] In *Night* (1890, Kunstmuseum Bern), he paints not only the darkness of night but also the bleakness of winter, which reinforces the menacing appearance of death. The message of autumn and the end of life is clear in the simplified but still indicative, fall setting of Hodler's *Weary of Life* (1891–92, Kunstmuseum, Bern). In 1892 an optimistic note in the series is introduced by a female figure in *Communion with Infinity* (fig. 13.3), who appropriately achieves her spiritual revival on a hill that glows with the bright green grass of spring. Finally, in his *The Consecrated One* (1893–94, Kunstmuseum, Bern) it is again spring, clearly indicated not only by the setting but also by the spring flowers held by six guardian angels, here equated with a chosen child's promised growth to maturity and enlightened spirituality.

In light of the clarity and consistency of Hodler's equation between the seasons and the stages of physical and spiritual growth in these figural paintings, the presentation of pure landscape in *Autumn Evening* may seem at first to be a radical departure. Although we are tempted by the repetition of the seasonal motif to consider *Autumn Evening* to be a rare, nonfigural component of the series, the other paintings seem to have little else in common. Like many other artists of the 1890s, however, Hodler thought in terms of major exhibition statements; he showed his public only the single finished canvas that was the result of a long evolution of preliminary and, in many ways, explanatory drawings and sketches.

To find the connection between *Autumn Evening* and the other paintings of his symbolic figural series, then, we must turn to the many sketches and drawings that led up to it. Like many of the Symbolists, Hodler developed the iconography as well as the style of the final work in his drawings. His sketchbooks dating immediately prior to a major painting such as *Autumn Evening* therefore disclose a kind of plot, as one iconographic idea and image is gradually developed over the course of several successive sketches into a new idea or theme. Although the relationship was not apparent when the paintings were exhibited in 1893, and remains hidden today in the canvases themselves, the preliminary drawings reveal that *Autumn Evening* was not, after all, a departure from Hodler's other figural works, but rather had gradually emerged as a new image from them.

The key to this fuller understanding of *Autumn Evening* is its original existence in Hodler's notebook sketches as *le chemin symbolique* (fig. 13.4). The de-

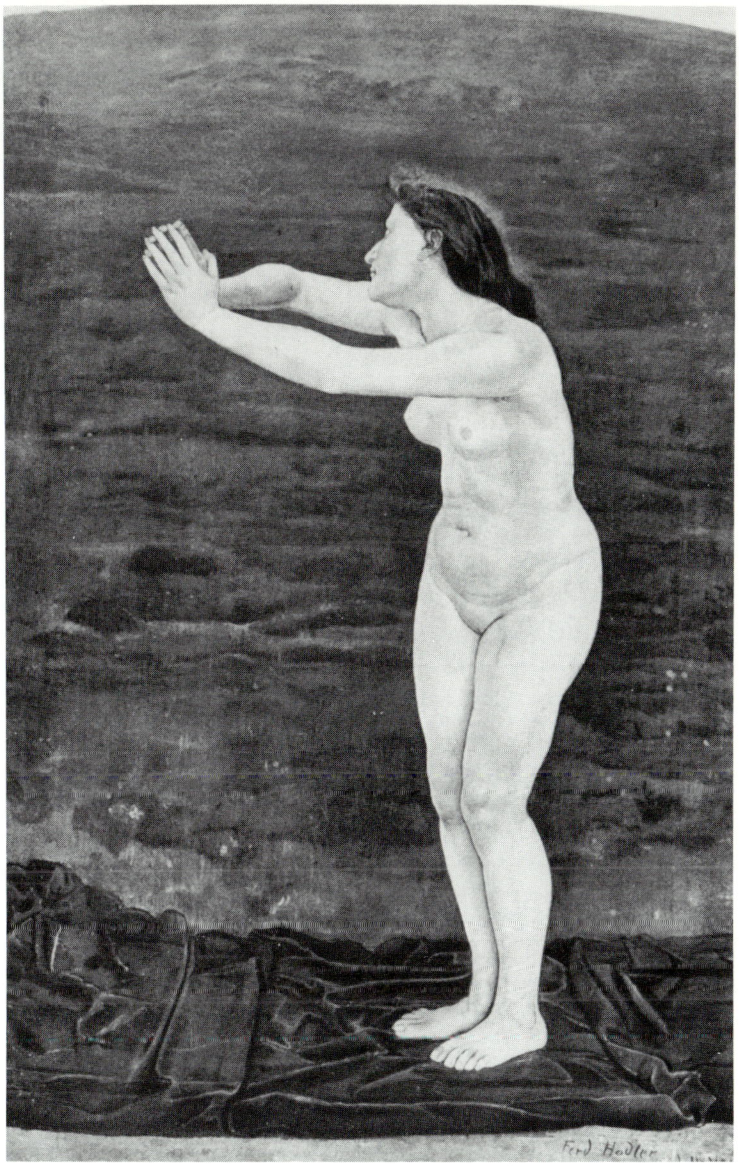

Fig. 13.3. Hodler, *Communion with Infinity,* 1892. Oil on canvas. Oeffentliche Kunstsammlung Basel.

signs for this "symbolic path" already show the centralized, sweeping perspective and emphatic horizon line of *Autumn Evening*, but differ from the final presentation in two significant additions: a figure or figures that stand on the "symbolic path" (fig. 13.5), and a hill or mountain to which the path leads, reminiscent of the mountain that rose at the end of Hodler's earlier and naturalistic *Road from Evordes*. The hill of the *chemin symbolique* drawings appears in some as a separate, distant hill and in others as the final rise of the path itself. Both the background hill and the figures on the path reveal their iconographic relationship to Hodler's predominantly figural series and, in-

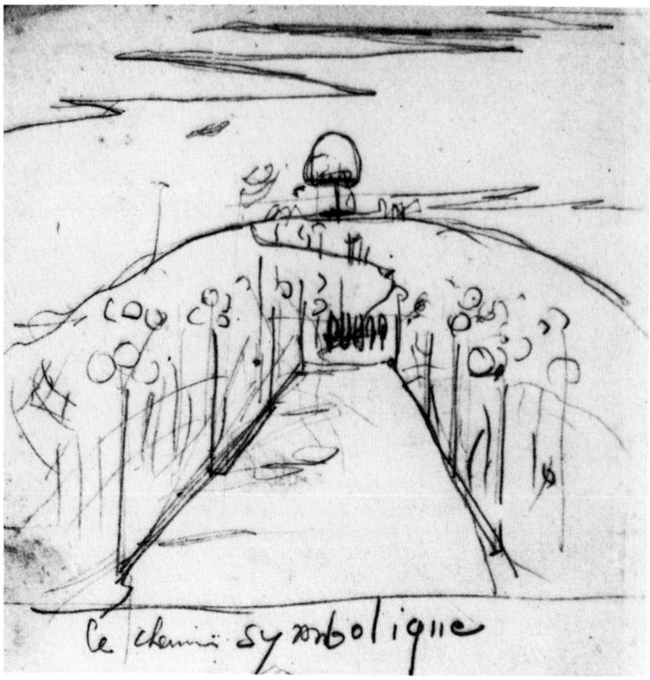

Fig. 13.4. Hodler, *Le chemin symbolique*. Pencil. Musée d'Art et d'Histoire, Geneva, Notebook 1958.176/8, p. 12.

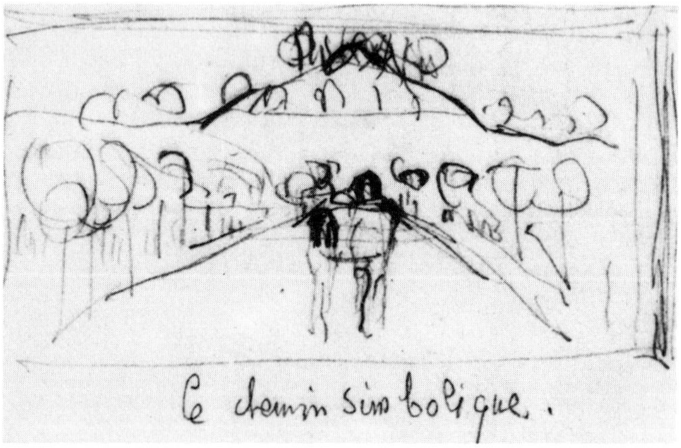

Fig. 13.5. Hodler, *Le chemin symbolique*. Pencil. Musée d'Art et d'Histoire, Geneva, Notebook 1958.176/4, p. 6.

triguingly, to the one painting most contemporary and seemingly most opposed to *Autumn Evening:* the *Communion with Infinity* (1892, fig. 13.3).

This relationship can also be discovered in other Hodler drawings of 1892, including several of a woman lying on the ground with her head dejectedly cradled in her arms that Hodler titled "Sadness unto the Soul" (fig. 13.6). The figure is an earlier version of the woman in the *Communion with Infinity;* the two figures are similar in proportion and appearance (the model for both was Augustine Dupin, Hodler's companion at the time), and are included side by side in many drawings.[5] Although the upward-struggling woman of the *Communion with Infinity* and the woman "saddened

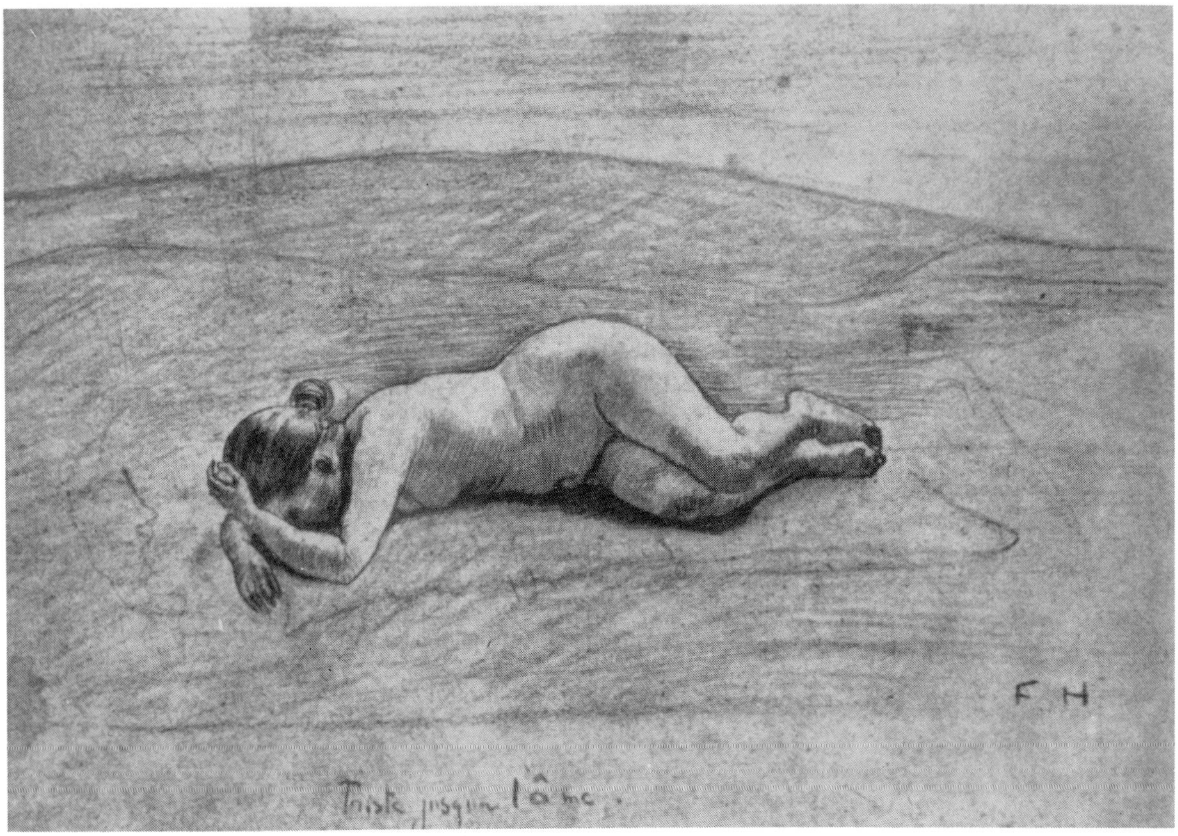

Fig. 13.6. Hodler, *Triste jusqu'à l'âme*, 1892. Lead pencil and blue crayon on chamois paper. Private collection, Switzerland.

unto the soul" hopelessly bound to the earth are visual opposites, they were meant to show the same soul in two stages—the dejected beginning and the ecstatic end of spiritual enlightenment. This progression appears in another sketch (in the Zurich archives) in which the dejected one is approached by two women, guardian figures who gaze down on her in sympathy. In at least one other drawing, Hodler provides the title *You Will Not Remain on Earth (vous ne resterez pas sur la terre,* fig. 13.7); the "saddened" woman eventually escapes her earthly cares and becomes one of the select figures whom Hodler called "the souls who flee the earth" (fig. 13.8).

In other sketches, the saddened person has already arisen. In this pose, she is standing on a rectangular cloth and is easily recognizable as a prototype for the woman of *Communion with Infinity.* In still other drawings from the period, the woman from *Communion with Infinity* appears in a landscape populated by black-draped malevolent figures, one of whom Hodler would elsewhere identify as a "Dark Genius."[6] The addition of these dark geniuses, versions of the phantom in Hodler's earlier *Night* that now appear as obstacles to a *Communion with Infinity,* proves the complexity of Hodler's symbolic series, since they also occur in the drawings of the symbolic path (fig. 13.9). These sketches showing the symbolic path populated by dark geniuses

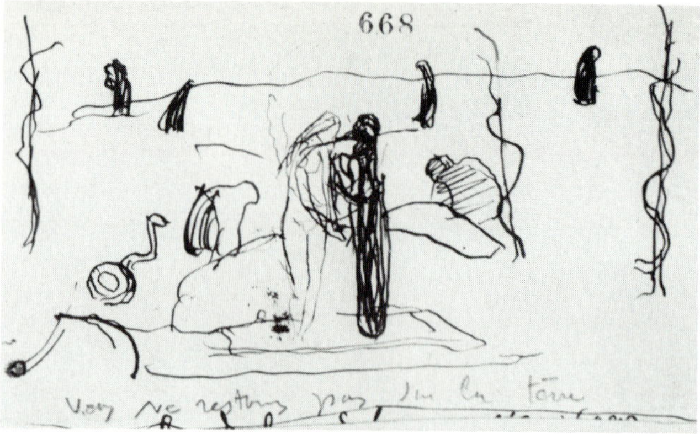

Fig. 13.7. Hodler, *Vous ne resterez pas sur la terre.* Pencil and ink. Kunsthaus Zurich, Inv. 668.

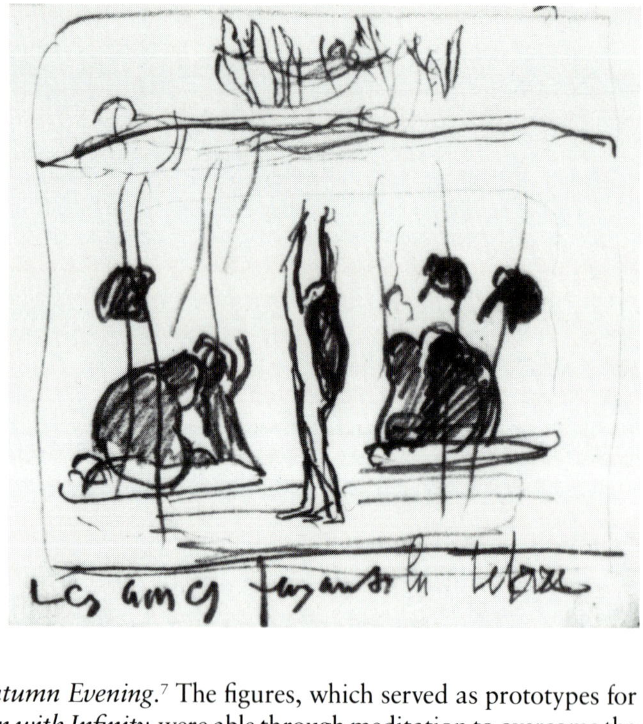

Fig. 13.8. Hodler, *Les âmes fuyant la terre.* Musée d'Art et d'Histoire, Geneva, Notebook 1958.176/9, p. 63.

clarify the meaning of *Autumn Evening.*[7] The figures, which served as prototypes for the woman of *Communion with Infinity,* were able through meditation to overcome the dark genius of the *Night,* ascend the hill, and "flee the earth"; they are the same figures that stand on the symbolic path. Several transitional drawings show these figures reclining or standing on unfurled cloths next to the symbolic path of *Autumn Evening* (fig. 13.10). The connection between the two paintings is further substantiated by Hodler's titles written in his own hand on some of the drawings: "Path of the Delighted Souls" and "Path of the Exceptional Souls."[8]

In another drawing (fig. 13.11), Hodler incorporated all of his 1892 imagery into a single thematic composition. In the foreground a couple face the viewer and appear little interested in the landscape behind them, small fields with the suggestion of a path on either side leading to a symmetrical line of trees that outlines the ridge of the

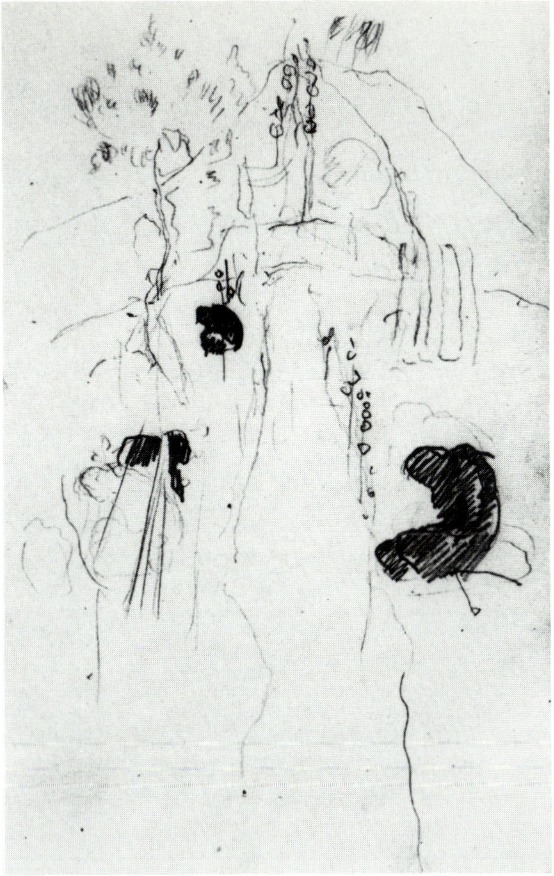

Fig. 13.9. Hodler, *Le chemin symbolique*. Pencil and ink. Musée d'Art et d'Histoire, Geneva, Notebook 1958.176/9, p. 29.

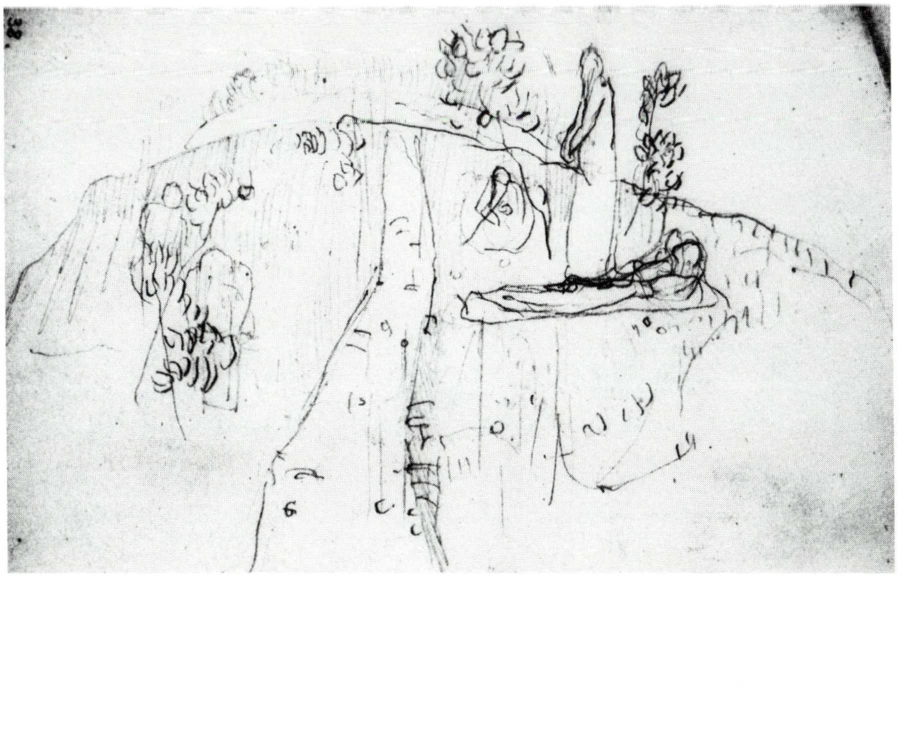

Fig. 13.10. Hodler, Untitled drawing. Musée d'Art et d'Histoire, Geneva, Notebook 1958.176/9, p. 38.

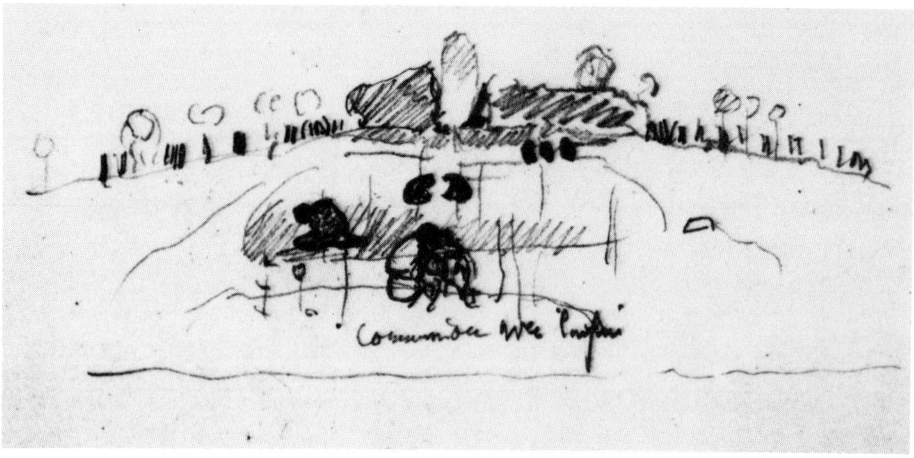

Fig. 13.11. Hodler, *Communion with Infinity.* Musée d'Art et d'Histoire, Geneva, Notebook 1958.176/9, p. 30.

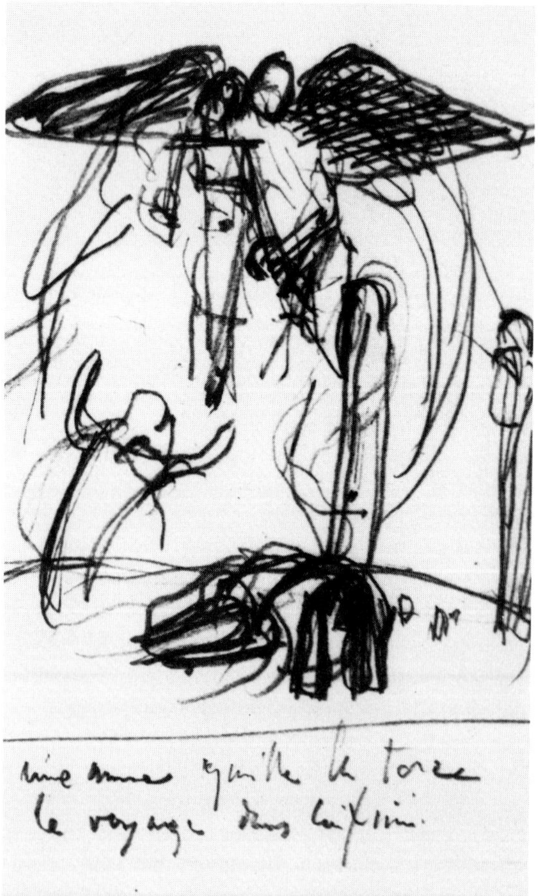

Fig. 13.12. Hodler, *Une âme quitte la terre/le voyage dans l'infini.* Musée d'Art et d'Histoire, Geneva, Notebook 1958.176/7, p. 25.

hill. The path that the couple would have to follow to reach that ridge, symbolic of the higher realm to which they must aspire, is already lined with unenlightened dark geniuses. Although the composition is reminiscent of *Autumn Evening*, Hodler's title makes another connection. He calls it "Communion with Infinity."

In light of this evolution of interrelated imagery in Hodler's drawings of 1892, it is clear that although the final paintings in his symbolic series are finished statements in themselves, they are thematically connected in Hodler's own notebooks with the progression of the saddened soul of *Night* beginning its journey up the symbolic path towards a communion with infinity. The connection between this somewhat pantheistic theme and Christian resurrection and redemption seems to have been a direct one in Hodler's mind, although it never surfaced in the final paintings of *Communion with Infinity* and *Autumn Evening*. In a small hurried sketch in one of his notebooks from this time (fig. 13.12), Hodler draws figures reminiscent of Mary Magdalen, the Virgin, and St. John in a Crucifixion who all lead the viewer's eye to a winged figure above. This figure either carries or accompanies another limp rising figure, recalling Renaissance Last Judgment scenes in which angels appear to escort the rising bodies of the saved to heaven. Hodler's caption below the sketch identifies the meaning of the drawing in typically universal terms: "A soul leaves the earth/the voyage into infinity" ("Une ame quitte la terre/le voyage dans l'infini").

In its iconographic complexity and in its correlation of nature symbols to more traditional religious symbols, such as the robed and winged figures that often appear in the drawings, Hodler's *Chemin Symbolique* reveals the influence of his participation at that time in the Parisian Salon de la Rose + Croix. This salon, the showcase of an exotic and esoteric exhibition society dedicated to the revival of spirituality in art, had been founded in 1891 by Joséphin Péladan, a writer who had already named himself, in emulation of Russian royalty, the Sâr. Hodler, for whom critical acceptance in Paris was a personal priority at that time, was pleased by the Sâr's invitation to exhibit in the first Rose + Croix exhibition in 1892 and sent works to that as well as to the second exhibition the following year. In his sketchbooks, which also served as personal notebooks, Hodler records not only the exhibition dates and address but also mentions its illustrated catalogue, which must have been sent to him in Geneva.[9] That Hodler carefully studied this catalogue is clear from the numerous correlations between the Rosicrucian illustrations and Hodler's own imagery at that time, including the *chemin symbolique* and *Autumn Evening*.

The catalogue of the first Rose + Croix Salon featured the work of Alexandre Séon, one of the Sâr's own illustrators, whose design for *A Troubled Heart* (fig. 13.13) was remarkably close to Hodler's saddened soul. Séon's imagery, however, is much more explicit and more identifiably Christian than Hodler's. So also was Felix Oudart's *On the Path* (present location unknown), which was included in the Rose + Croix Salon and catalogue of 1893. Again, although close in concept to Hodler's *chemin symbolique* in its representation of malefic obstacles besetting the human who seeks enlightenment, Oudart's imagery is more figurative and even obvious, with snakes actually curling to attack the worshipper on the path.

Certain little-known sketches make it apparent that Hodler did consider relatively self-evident, traditional Christian symbolism for the *chemin symbolique*. In one particular drawing, an extremely foreshortened path leads to and then becomes the hill of enlightenment, now capped with a cross and carrying what must have been direct

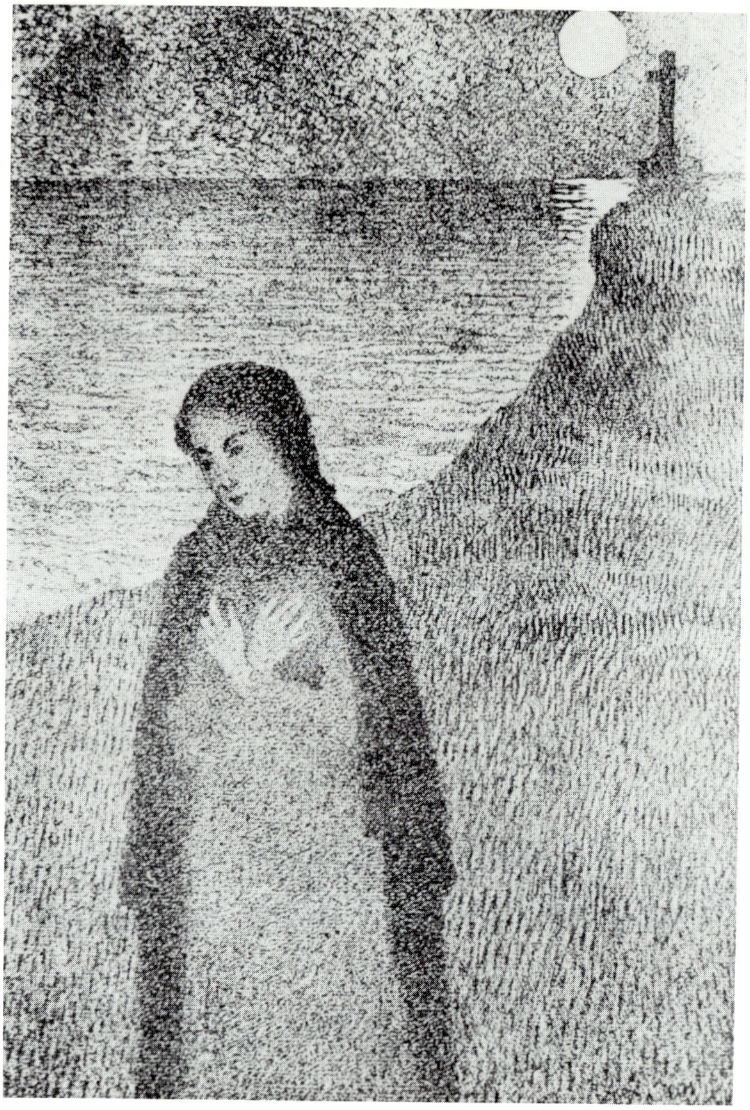

Fig. 13.13. Alexandre Séon, *A Troubled Heart*, c. 1892. Illustration, *Salon de la Rose + Croix Esthétique*, 1892.

reference to the Latinophile leanings of Sâr Péladan's own writings—a Latin dictum beginning with the word "credo" scrolled into the clouds above.[10] Hodler's temporary fascination with the Rosicrucian imagery resulted in one painting, now rarely seen, titled *Path of the Chosen Souls* (Private Collection, Basel), which depicted in Easter tones of lilac and yellow a grassy and beautifully-flowered path leading to a redemptive cross above. Usually attributed to 1894 but probably dating from the time of Hodler's closest association with the Rose + Croix in 1893, this painting confirms with its obviously Christian cross Hodler's adherence to traditional symbolism during the year following *Autumn Evening*. The design was also figural, however, and therefore differs sharply from the unpeopled and entirely symbolic landscape of *Autumn Evening*.

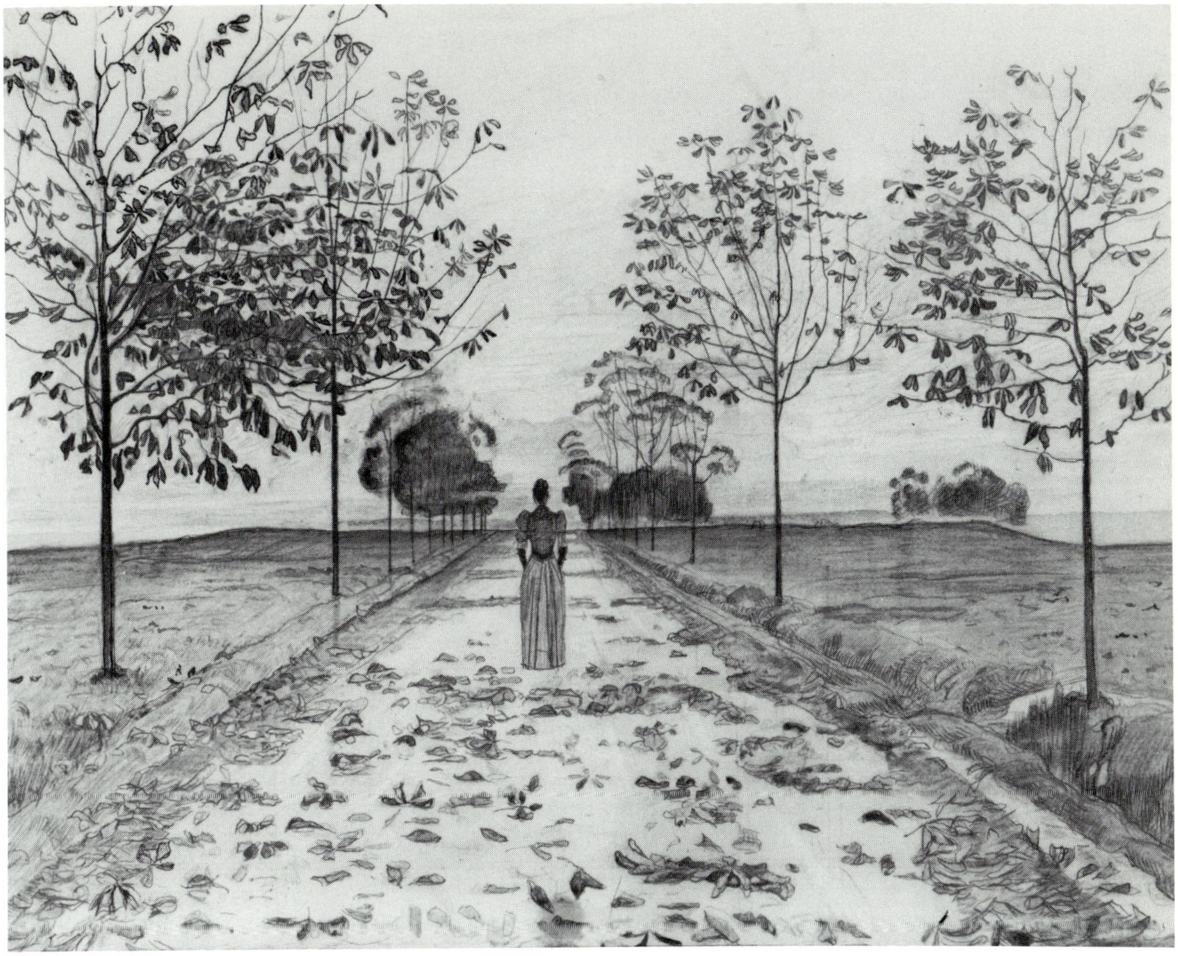

Fig. 13.14. Hodler, Sketch for *Autumn Evening*, 1892. Lead pencil, water color, gouache, oil, and varnish on beige paper. Musée d'Art et d'Histoire, Geneva.

Originally even *Autumn Evening* had figures in it, however. In a finished drawing of the same time (fig. 13.14), a woman viewed from the back dominates the path; and in the finished painting, a dark outline has begun to bleed through the overpainting and to rise to the surface as a blue outline of the woman in its center. A similar outline, only recently identified, suggests that at some earlier time, at least one other figure stood at the lower right of the path. This side figure is also female; her three-quarter profile faces the horizon.[11] Had these figures remained, Hodler's painting would have complied with the requirements of the Concours Calame (a competitive Genevan exhibition) of 1893: "a landscape with figures or animals representing an autumn sunset."[12] *Autumn Evening*, which was awarded a second prize at the Concours, was painted over, therefore, only after the exhibition, held in early 1893. With that change, however, Hodler created a very different, and ultimately very Symbolist, landscape.

By means of the sketch that still includes the central female figure (fig.

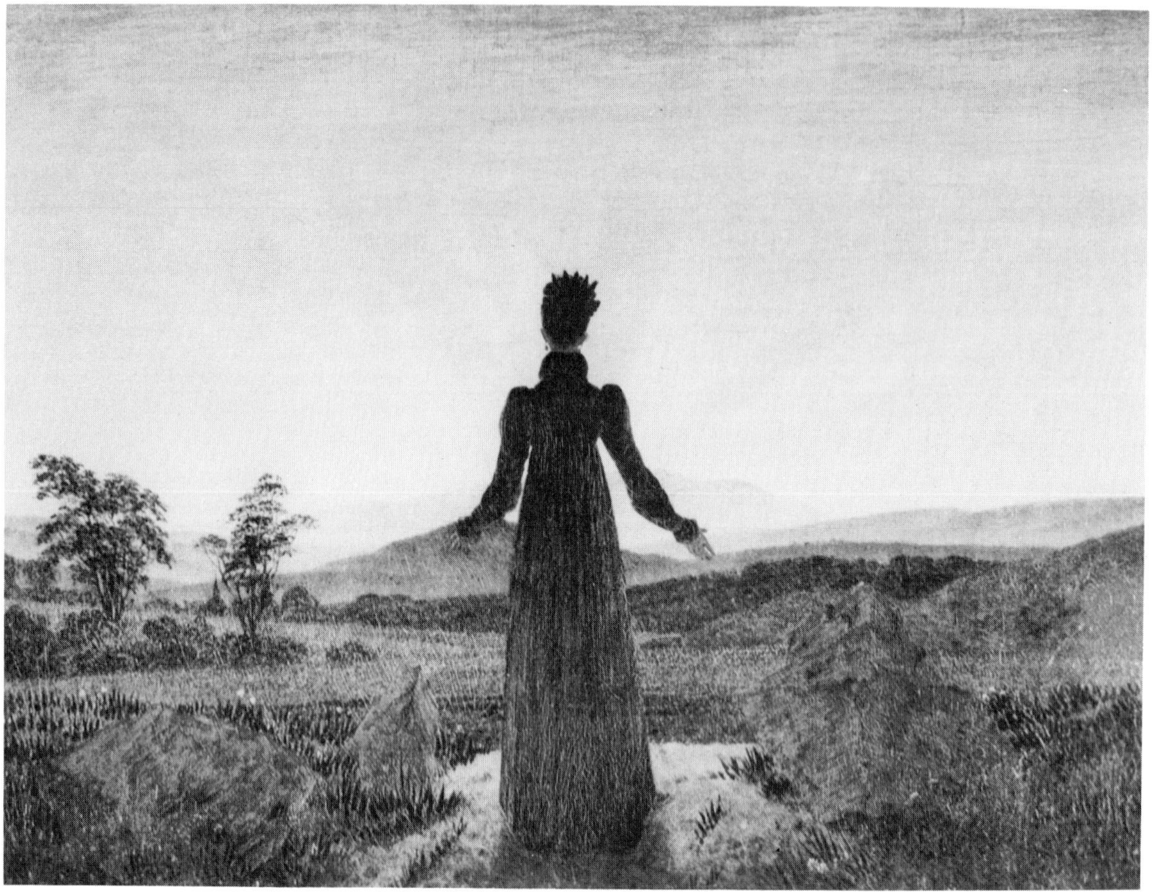

Fig. 13.15. Caspar David Friedrich, *Woman Before the Setting Sun*, c. 1818. Oil on canvas. Museum Folkwang, Essen.

13.14), we are reminded of the closeness of Hodler's original conception to that of German romantic works, such as Caspar David Friedrich's *Woman before the Setting Sun* (fig. 13.15). In both the drawing and the Friedrich painting, nature is presented as the romantic mirror of emotion; the figures serve as focal points, but, with their backs to us, also as intermediaries to the vista that spreads out before them. They also effectively cut, however, the continuity of the horizon and the insistent central lines of the path.

Hodler's later overpainting on *Autumn Evening* therefore had far-reaching effects. As was clear from the earlier comparison to Hodler's own *Road from Evordes* (fig. 13.2), the *Autumn Evening* is contrived to be more supernatural than natural.[13] By painting the trees in winter starkness rather than in leaf or bloom, and by changing the naturalistic lighting that produces real shadows in the earlier scenes to an inner glow that emanates uniformly from the painting itself in the later work, Hodler switches from an illusion of nature to an allusion to it.[14] Furthermore, by belatedly eliminating the mountain range and figures in the painting and widening the viewer's foreground view of the path, Hodler emphasized the triangular form of the path as the single most important and insistent element in the painting. The result is that, while *Autumn Evening* maintains enough specificity to remind us of a particular scene, and to indicate to us its origins as the *Road from Evordes,* it nevertheless transcends these specific identifying details to become a symbolic path. For, as Hodler commented in a notebook in 1892, he was most interested in a "realistic translation of the soul of nature," and this artistic "translation" could become "more real, more striking than reality itself."[15] In its final state, *Autumn Evening* presents not a realist view but a Symbolist vision of nature.

Abstracting landscape in this manner combines elements of neoclassical and romantic theories generally considered to be opposites, as Rosenblum has pointed out: "Neo-classical theorists had taught artists to look beneath the face of common nature and reveal in their pictures the underlying order of the universe, . . . Romantics were to find that superficial appearances concealed not so much order as impenetrable depths of inexplicable mystery."[16] In *Autumn Evening,* the forceful and almost geometric ordering of the lines of the landscape, already evoking Hodler's own theory of "parallelism," but also echoing a classicist's understanding of the landscape, serves nevertheless to lead the viewer towards the infinite and unfathomable sea of sky beyond. And yet, Hodler's work is not simply neo-romantic. In *Autumn Evening,* one cannot easily progress from one image to another, as one does even in the Friedrich painting (from the woman to the bushes to the trees and rolling hills beyond), to understand the dual role of nature as both a mirror of human emotions and catalyst of transcendent thoughts. Instead, the viewer of *Autumn Evening* is forced to accept the total composition of stark, flattened, and abstracted forms as a recreation of nature that suggests, rather than metaphorically represents, states of the soul. As such, it illustrates the Symbolist poet Gustave Kahn's definition of Symbolism as different from romanticism by means of its obverse relationship between feeling and form. Rather than beginning, as the romantic still did, with the tangible world and then subjectifying it according to one's feelings, the Symbolist instead objectified the idea or feeling by giving it a tangible form.[17]

Once *Autumn Evening* is understood as a Symbolist expression of a state of the soul, then the degree to which it is similar to, and even more radical than, its figural counterpart, the *Communion with Infinity,* can be appreciated. In the latter, similar subtle deletions, generalizations, and abstractions from earlier Hodler works[18] had resulted in an arrestingly stark and flat composition of female form against a green backdrop, intended to evoke through tangible imagery an intangible state of the soul. Because we now know the common origins of this work and *Autumn Evening*—both were, in fact, evocations of a communion through nature with infinity—we realize that their seeming difference is superficial and based primarily on distinctions between figural and landscape format. But if *Autumn Evening* began as a symbolic path, complete with complex and multifigural symbols, we must remember that the original figure of the symbolic path, "saddened unto the soul," eventually became the woman of *Communion with Infinity.*

One final reminder of this interrelationship is commonly overlooked in *Communion with Infinity:* Hodler presented the scene at sunset. In a letter to his friend Büzberger in 1892, he explained: "My main work of this summer . . . is a medium-sized painting that portrays a nude female figure standing on a black cloth and in an open field. The lighting is *after sunset* and the nude body reflects the color of the illuminated atmosphere."[19]

Hodler's *Autumn Evening* therefore not only equates with *Communion with Infinity* as a major statement in his symbolic series of the 1890s, but also stands as a uniquely nonfigurative one. For Hodler, it represented the "road of life" in a way very similar to that of other Symbolists.[20] But for Hodler, it also represented a spiritual *chemin symbolique* the traversing of which would lead to an ultimate oneness with nature and divinity, toward a "communion with infinity."

Of course, Hodler's figural works with these themes attracted more critical attention than the landscape. The *Communion with Infinity,* for example, was derided as much as it was praised, but it never failed to encourage analysis as an idealistic or, to use the term offered in 1891 by the critic G.-Albert Aurier, "Ideist" painting.[21] *Autumn Evening,* on the other hand, was rarely mentioned. In fact, in 1892, the year when both the *Communion with Infinity* and *Autumn Evening* were finished, Hodler was praised for exhibiting a few "innocuous" landscapes and thereby avoiding too much "symbolism." Reviewing Hodler's one-man show in Geneva that year, Charles Boniface wrote:

> Mr. Hodler has not sent this time these grand "machines" in which his talents are without doubt evident, but where he [usually] puts a philosophical or sentimental intention which too often perplexes us and escapes us; [here] he has only studies whose themes do not exceed their presentation. . . . At least it charms us today, it makes us feel a penetrating and prolonged emotion which we have not experienced before, or not in the same manner before the more or less obscure allegories of which we constantly speak.[22]

Little would Boniface have guessed that within a year Hodler would again be presenting these "perplexing philosophical intentions" in the form of a landscape.

Only one contemporary critic, Hodler's constant champion and friend, the Symbolist poet Louis Duchosal, suspected that Hodler's landscapes along with his figural work were becoming increasingly Symbolist. In a review of Hodler's landscape contributions to the municipal exhibition of 1893, Duchosal suggested that the viewer, although inevitably appreciating the "rigorous construction and the impeccable drawing" of a Hodler landscape, might find something more: "If he is not absolutely foreign to things of the dream, he will finish by understanding that with Mr. Hodler the imagination and vision function together and that this [landscape] . . . of such beautiful truth of order, assumes the penetrating character of symbolism."[23]

His first such fusion of vision and imagination in nature, *Autumn Evening,* represented not only a breakthrough in landscape for Hodler in 1892 but also a model for future, increasingly expressive and symbolic landscapes. Although Hodler later reincorporated his original notions of the symbolic path with symbolic figures in paintings such as *Emotion* (1902, Kunsthistorisches Museum, Vienna) and *Silence of the Evening* (1904/05; Kunstmuseum, Winterthur), *Autumn Evening* also strongly affects his twentieth-century landscapes. In their placement of the viewer in direct confrontation with a landscape focused on a distant point, these landscapes refer back to his crucial decision in 1892 to paint out the mountain and figures and to emphasize instead the wide-angled approach to the viewer's path. In *Eiger, Monch and Jungfrau* (1908, private collection, Switzerland) the perspective lines of the *Autumn Evening* path are replaced by the lines of a mountain peak. Here, the viewer is led not to a horizon but to glowing background clouds, causing the sensation of hovering mysteriously before the view.

Hodler's late landscapes take *Autumn Evening*'s use of the horizon as a major structural and symbolic element to further conclusions. In *Autumn Evening* the road and the trees focus the perspective, but it is the strong, sweeping line of the earth itself that is most compelling, suggesting that the two human-made lines, however forceful, lead finally to a natural line of earth and sky. The suggestion of cosmic proportions made by this contrast in *Autumn Evening* adds to its symbolic effect. In Hodler's later landscapes, which he called *paysages planetaires*,[24] this cosmic line is emphasized in scale and definition, often to the point of dominating the entire composition as it does in his broad views of *Sunset on Lake Geneva* from around 1915.[25]

Finally, the overriding and almost overwhelming symmetry of view became, with *Autumn Evening*, an important symbolic indication of the underlying harmony and order of Hodler's parallelistic, cosmic universe. As he later said, his approach was twofold: he would first deliberately seek out those natural phenomena and the views of them that most emphasized symmetry. He would then manipulate this natural harmony by means of a bilateral composition full of repetitive forms and colors, simplified by the deletion of extraneous details, in order to lead the viewer not so much to an understanding of nature as mirror of divine power, as to a recognition of its essential mystery. This is precisely the evolutionary history of *Autumn Evening*. From its origins as both a descriptive landscape in the *Road from Evordes* and an overtly symbolic path in Hodler's notebook sketches, the canvas now known as *Autumn Evening* was gradually transformed into a compelling vision of a spiritual state of the soul.

NOTES

1. C. A. Loosli, *Ferdinand Hodler* (Bern: R. Sluter, 1921–24), vol. 1, 75. All English translations, unless otherwise noted, are mine.

2. Manuscript notebook, Geneva Musée d'Art et d'Histoire, Inv. no. 1958. 176/231.

3. Runge's *Tageszeiten (Times of Day)* of 1802–10 included, for example, *Morning* (1808, Kunsthaus Hamburg), which was intended as a depiction of not only dawn but also spring, infancy, and the nativity of Christ. Philipp Otto Runge, *Hinterlassene Schriften* (Göttingen: Vandenhoeck & Kuprecht, 1965), 2:176.

4. Hodler's intentions for a complete cycle of works based on the times of day were first noted by Hans Muhlestein and Georg Schmidt, *Ferdinand Hodler, 1853–1918, sein Leben und sein Werk* (Zurich: Eugen Rentsch Verlag, 1942), 312. Hodler's final presentation of these transcending themes was neither as codified as Runge's *Times of Day*, nor as programmatically complete as Edvard Munch's *Frieze of Life*, also of the 1890s; some of Hodler's times, like *Twilight*, never evolved from their sketched beginnings. (See "Le Crépuscule," c. 1890, notebook, Geneva Musée d'Art et d'Histoire, 1958, 176/8, 30: Ill. S. Hirsh, *Ferdinand Hodler* (New York: Braziller, 1982), 23.

5. Most notable is a graphed sketch of 1892, Kupferstichkabinett Basel, Inv. 1952.4+5, which depicts Augustine as the poor person on the left side margin of a page otherwise filled with facial and figure studies for *Communion with Infinity*.

6. "Genie Sombre," c. 1889–90, Kunsthaus Zurich.

7. This image recurs in several of Hodler's notebooks of the 1890s. The most precise identification of these dark beings by Hodler occurs in one notebook of c. 1899. Here, the artist describes the black-draped figures, who would soon appear as souls afraid of *Truth* (1904, Kunsthaus Zürich), as "sinister human beings" who are "the unhappy, fleeing the day" ("des êtres humains sinistre . . . des malheureux fuiant le jour"). Notebook, Geneva Musée d'Art et d'Histoire, 1958.176/23, p. 7.

8. "Chemin des ames délites," notebook sketch, Geneva Musée d'Art et d'Histoire,

1958.176/2, 8. "Le chemin des âmes exceptionelles," notebook sketch, Geneva Musée d'Art et d'Histoire, 1958.176/9, 11.

9. Notebook list, Geneva Musée d'Art et d'Histoire, 1958.176/76, n.p. Hodler also noted Péladan's name, along with plans to travel to Paris for the Rose + Croix exhibition (there is no evidence of the trip being accomplished), in a notebook of 1893, Geneva Musée d'Art et d'Histoire, 1958.176/76, n.p.

10. This unknown drawing in a notebook of c. 1894–95 (Geneva Musée d'Art et d'Histoire, 1958.176/123, 7) accompanies several sketches portraying the woman of Hodler's *Emotion* (1894, Kunstmuseum Bern), with hands clasped before her, striding above the clouds in a heavenly realm focusing on a cross. Such sketches reveal not only Hodler's fascination at this time with the neo-Catholic imagery of the Salons de la Rose + Croix, but also suggest his recourse to past religious painting for compositional inspiration.

11. I observed this second figure for the first time when the painting was included in "The Mystic North" exhibition (Art Gallery of Ontario) in 1984. Visual evidence of dark blue outlining, similar to that of the central figure, which is easily visible, is just beginning to show under Hodler's overpainting in lighter, often white paint. Recent X-rays (Cincinnati Art Museum, 1984) of this area of the canvas failed to reveal any specific underlying form. For firmer confirmation of the right-hand figure just now emerging, infrared studies may prove helpful but have been unavailable to date.

12. As noted by the *Journal de Genève,* 21 September 1892, p. 3.

13. Roald Nasgaard, *The Mystic North* (Art Gallery of Ontario, 1984), 125–26.

14. I am indebted to Reinhold Heller for his suggestion of these comparative terms.

15. "La traduction realiste d'âme de la nature. Cette traduction devient plus realiste, plus frappant, que le réalité elle meme." Notebook, Geneva Musée d'Art et d'Histoire, 1958.176/7, 18.

16. Robert Rosenblum, *Romanticism* (New York: Harper and Row, 1979), 34.

17. Gustave Kahn, *L'Evenément,* 1886, translated by Herschel B. Chipp, *Theories of Modern Art* (Berkeley: University of California Press, 1970), 50.

18. In particular, the *Dialogue with Nature* of 1884 (Kunstmuseum Bern).

19. "Meine Hauptarbeit diesen Sommers . . . ist ein mittlegrosses Bild, das line nackte weibliche Figur auf einem schwarzen Tuch und auf freien Feld stehend darstellt. Die beleuchtung ist nach Sonnenunterganz und der nackte Körper reflektiert die Farbe des so beleuchtung Luftreises." (italics mine) Letter from Hodler to Büzberger, 17 September 1892. C. A. Loosli, *Ferdinand Hodler: Leben, Werk, und Nachlass* (Bern, 1924), 4:334–35.

20. A series of drawings by Edvard Munch executed in the early 1890s are particularly comparable; all incorporate the sweeping, lonely perspective of a frontal path leading towards an infinite, empty sky. In one untitled drawing (c. 1893, Munch Museum, Oslo), in Ill. Reinhold Heller, *Munch: The Scream* [New York, 1972] (fig. 27), Munch portrays a solitary man, seen from the back who walks down the barren path towards a tree-lined horizon remarkably similar to those of Hodler's sketches.

21. G.-Albert Aurier, "Le Symbolisme en peinture: Paul Gauguin," *Mercure de France* 2 (Paris, 1891): 164.

22.

> "M. Hodler n'a pas envoyé cette fois ces grandes machines dans lesquelles ses qualités sont évidentes sans doute, mais où il met une intention philosophique ou sentimentale quit trop souvent nous déroute ou nous échappe, il n 'a que des études dont la donnée n'excède pas le cadre. . . . Et quand meme cette déclaration est bien un peu profane, nous n'hésitons pas à avouer que nous le préférons tel quel. Au moins, il nous charme aujourd'hui, il nous fait éprouver une émotion pénétrante et prolongée que nous ne ressentons point, ou pas de la meme façon devant les allégories plus ou moins obscures dont nous parlions tout à l'heure."

Charles Boniface, "Exposition Hodler," 1, 2, *Tribune de Genève,* 5–6 Feb. 1892. Hodler regularly held such a one-man exhibition in early winter months of the year.

23. Louis Duchosal, "Exposition Beaux-Arts 1893," *Journal de Genève,* 26 March 1893, suppl. 73, 1.

24. Johannes Widmer, *Von Hodlers letztem Lebensjahr* (Zurich: Rascher, 1919), 9.

25. E.g., *Sunset on Lake Geneva* (1915 Kunsthaus Zurich) in Hirsh, *Ferdinand Hodler,* 127.

14

TATLIN'S MONUMENT to the THIRD INTERNATIONAL as a SYMBOL of REVOLUTION

CHRISTINA LODDER

VLADIMIR TATLIN'S MONUMENT TO THE THIRD INTERNATIONAL (fig. 14.1) has long been acclaimed as one of the most potent symbols of political revolution in general and of the Russian Revolution in particular. Tatlin's contemporaries acknowledged this. For example, the architect, Konstantin Mel'nikov, is reported to have said, "Our revolution is dynamic. Tatlin is making the spiral a modern symbol."[1]

That Tatlin consciously conceived the tower as an expression of the aspirations of the Revolution and of the revolutionary period is quite clear and implicit, for example, in the following statement that he made several years later to A. Begicheva in Kiev in 1925: "My monument is the symbol of the epoch. Unifying in it artistic and utilitarian forms, I created a kind of synthesis of art with life."[2]

The monument was completed three years after the Revolution. It was initially commissioned in 1919 as part of Lenin's Plan for Monumental Propaganda, which was inaugurated in the spring of 1918 to furnish the main cities of the new socialist state with monuments to great men and revolutionaries.[3] Lenin's intention, both to educate the population and to inspire them with revolutionary feelings, undoubtedly reflected an element of visionary idealism. Moreover, it seems that Lenin himself acknowledged an influence from the utopian writings of the Renaissance scholar Campanella. According to Lunacharsky, Lenin stated:

> Campanella in his *City of the Sun* says that the walls of his fantastic socialist city are covered with frescoes, which serving the youth as a graphic lesson in natural science and history, arouse civil feelings and, in a word, participate in the business of raising and educating the new generation. It seems to me that . . . with certain changes this could be adopted by us and put into operation now . . . I have called what I am thinking of monumental propaganda.[4]

As head of the Moscow Department of Fine Arts within the Commissariat for Enlightenment, Tatlin was responsible for implementing the plan in Moscow, for commissioning statues, and for organizing their delivery, erection, and unveiling. Reporting on his experience to the Committee of People's Commissars, Sovnarkom, in the summer of 1918, Tatlin criticized current practice and asserted that the monuments erected should express the new relationship between the state and society that had been established by the October Revolution, and that they should embody the new role that artists now oc-

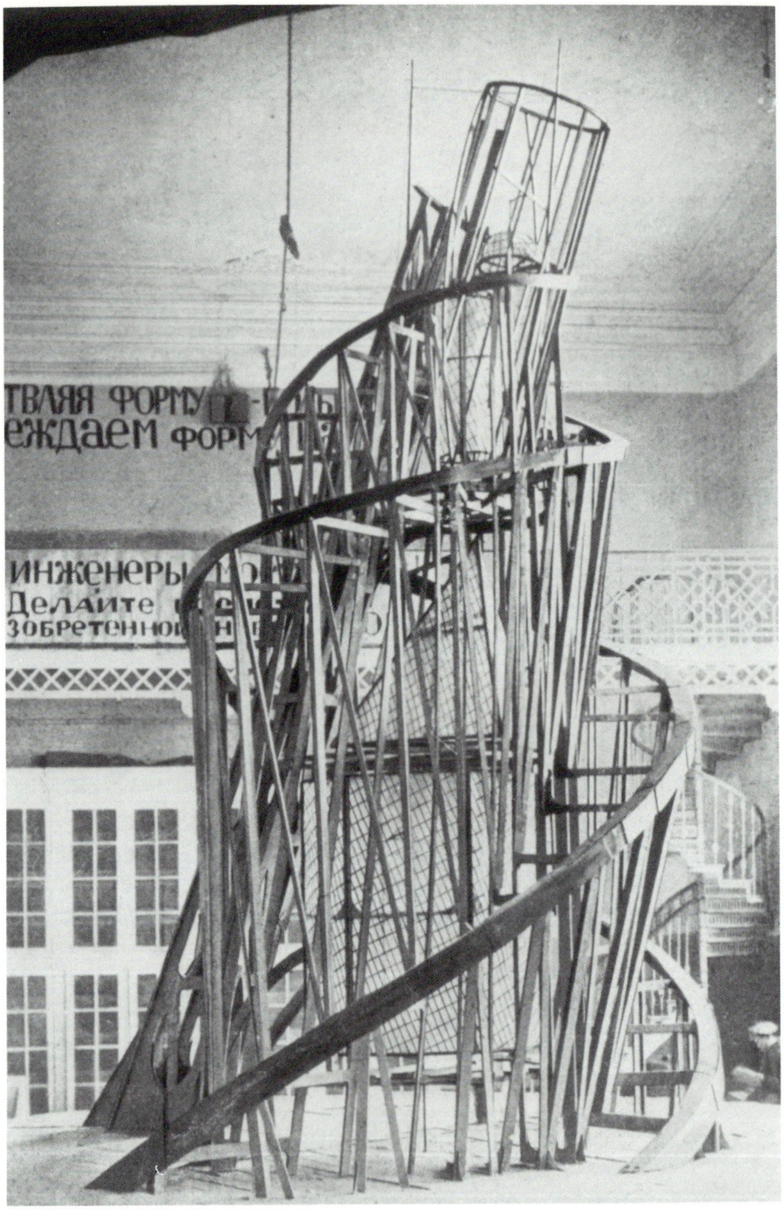

Fig. 14.1. Tatlin's Model for a Monument to the Third International.

cupied within the new social structure. Tatlin emphasized that such monuments should be "free creations in a socialist state" and that in addition to traditional "monuments depicting influential individuals," there should also be "monuments to the Revolution, to a relationship between the state and art which has not existed until now."[5]

Tatlin's new conception of public revolutionary monuments, as expressed in his report of 1918, would undoubtedly have conditioned his own interpretation of his task when, six months later, he himself became a participant in the plan. Tatlin's observations in the 1918 report suggest that he would have regarded the expression of the new social relationships as of prime importance in the formulation of his design.

Furthermore, what we know of the evolution of the Monument's form would tend to confirm this supposition. Nikolai Punin's description of the tower published in 1919 indicates clearly that by this stage Tatlin had totally rethought the idea of what a monument should be in the new society and decided that "all the elements of the monument should be modern technical apparatuses, promoting agitation and propaganda."[6] Tatlin's proposal replaced the traditionally static statue with a dynamically functional building, "a place of the most intense movement." Apparently he had not yet finally determined the precise form that would be appropriate to express this new conception, although he did envisage different geometrically shaped structures, linked by lifts, that would be allotted to specific functions. Presumably the determination of the monument's purely functional considerations preceded the definition of its form. Yet, when it was finally decided, the form was highly innovative and constituted a very deliberate juxtaposition of visual elements.

The Monument to the Third International was unveiled in Tatlin's Petrograd studio on the third anniversary of the October Revolution. A month later it was moved to Moscow where it was on display during the eighth congress of the Soviets in December 1920. The model (fig. 14.2) was made of wood and stood about seven meters high: a prototype for a structure that was to dominate the Petrograd skyline, straddle the Neva, and rival the Eiffel Tower in height and importance. Its form consisted of two converging spirals which moved in the same direction around a thrusting diagonal supported by a series of girders. This skeletal structure supported four glazed volumes: a cube, a cylinder, a pyramid, and a hemisphere (fig. 14.3). Punin described it:

> The monument consists of three great rooms of glass, erected with the help of a complicated system of vertical pillars and spirals. These rooms are placed on top of each other and have different, harmonically corresponding forms. They are to be able to move at different speeds by means of a special mechanism. The lower storey rotates on its axis at the speed of one revolution per year. This is intended for legislative assemblies. The next storey, which is in the form of a pyramid, rotates on its axis at the rate of one revolution per month. Here the executive bodies are to meet (the International Executive Committee, the Secretariat, and other administrative bodies). Finally, the uppermost cylinder which rotates at the speed of one revolution per day is reserved for information services: an information office, a newspaper, the issuing of proclamations, pamphlets and manifestoes—in short all the means for informing the international proletariat; it will also have a telegraphic office and an apparatus that can project slogans on to a large screen. These can be fitted around the axes of the hemisphere. Radio masts will rise up over the monument. It should be emphasised that Tatlin's proposal provides for walls with a vacuum (thermos) which will help to keep the temperature in the various rooms constant.[7]

This description emphasised that the tower was indeed to be a functional building, created to actively participate in the making of revolution, to function as a machine promoting world revolution by acting as the administrative and propaganda center for the recently resuscitated international communist organization, the Third International.

At the same time Tatlin, in accordance with the objectives of Lenin's Plan, obviously wanted to inspire the public with revolutionary thoughts and to sym-

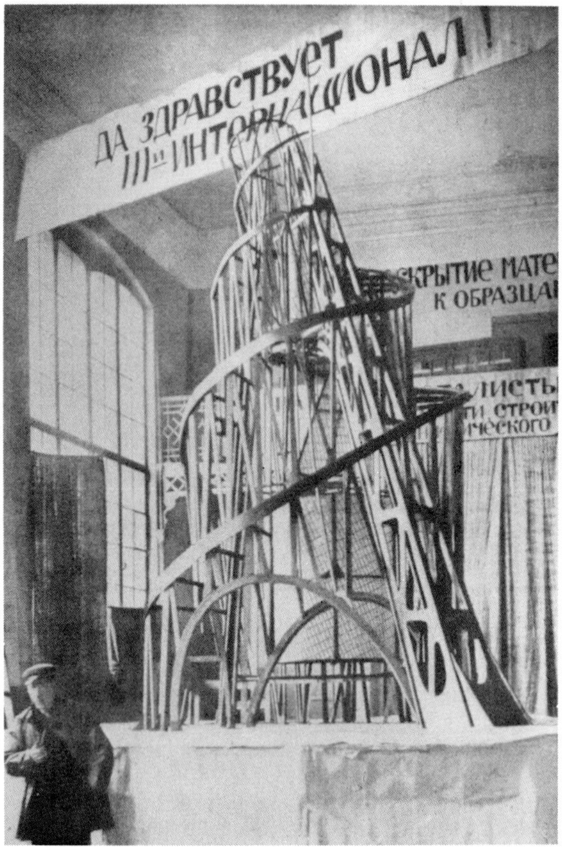

Fig. 14.2. Tatlin's Model for a Monument to the Third International with Tatlin in front (with pipe).

bolize the heroic quality of the period through the external form of the tower. If Tatlin's own assertion is to be believed, the component structures, both separately and collectively, expressed a clear symbolism. The internal glazed geometric volumes may, on one level, have been intended to epitomize the new visual vocabulary of the contemporary avant-garde. Punin's 1919 report on the monument had stressed that "the form of the monument will correspond to all invented artistic forms at the present time. In the current artistic situation these forms will obviously be cubes, cylinders, spheres, cones, segments, spherical surfaces and fragments of these."[8] This catalogue of precise euclidean geometric forms comprising the fundamentals of the new artistic language does not relate directly to the prerevolutionary, three-dimensional work of Tatlin. His counter-reliefs were concerned with "material, volume, and construction" and "the complicated investigations and demonstrations of material as such, and its consequences—movement, tension and their inter-relationship."[9] The geometric vocabulary seems rather to be extrapolated from the contemporary achievements of the avant-garde in general and especially from the Suprematist paintings of Kazimir Malevich, with their pure geometric shapes in primary colors floating against a white background.

Although the model was made of wood, the final monument was to be made of iron and glass, which Tatlin called "the materials of modern classicism."[10] If credence is to be given to El Lissitzky, the new materials were themselves expressive of the new ideology. Lissitzky declared, "Iron is strong like the will of the proletariat. Glass is clear like its conscience."[11] That Lissitzky's identification was neither eccentric nor inappropriate to the intellectual currency of the period is confirmed by the contemporary poetry of Aleksei Gastev, which extolled and emphasized the industrial nature of the working class, its roots in an industrial culture, and its links with the machine. Moreover, in his 1920 brochure on the monument, presumably written with Tatlin's cooperation, Punin suggested that the meetings were to be held in the glass chambers to emphasize the honesty and openness of the new processes of administration. He wrote that by "being raised into a higher level of space ... and through the material (glass), the purity of the initiatives, their liberation from material constraints, and their ideal qualities are stressed."[12]

The skeletal structure supporting the rotating volumes consisted of the two spirals supported by the strident diagonal (see figs. 14.3 and 14.4). This created, in Punin's words of 1920, "a dynamism of unsurpassed greatness."[13] Moreover, Punin saw the spiral as being expressive of the new dynamism of social progress. He asserted, "The spiral is the movement of liberated humanity. The spiral is the ideal expression of liberation: its base set in the earth, it flees from the ground and becomes a symbol of the suspension of all animal, earthly, and groveling interests."[14] Hence Tatlin's tower could indeed be seen to be translating "an ancient concept of form" into "a new material for a new content."[15]

Traditionally, the spiral derived from the notation for water, the life-giving properties of which led the spiral to be regarded as a symbol of life, continuity, and development. In Greek thought time was conceived as a cylindrical spiral that wound up and then wound down again. Such a spiral conception of time emphasized the continuities of history and represented history as an endless sequence of advances and recessions. Such a spiral was not necessarily the clearest illustration of the Marxist belief that history comprised a logical and inevitable progress from primitive forms of social organization, such as feudalism, to capitalism and finally reaching an apex of perfection in communism. An open-ended, cylindrical spiral ultimately implies a degree of reversibility. Such reversibility was and is inconceivable to the Marxist.

Tatlin's two spirals are not cylindrical; they are conical. They start at a wide base and become dramatically narrower at their apex. This suggests a finite, nonreversible movement. It implies that the spirals are moving towards a defined objective and point of ultimate development. Tatlin himself made this explicit in his own statements about the tower.

> I placed at its basis the screw, as the most dynamic form—a symbol of time, energy, lucidity, striving. The transparent construction from metallic forms has the form of a spiral—inclined at the angle of the earth.[16]

Such a spiral adheres far more closely to the dialectical conception of history. That this spiral could indeed express the Marxist idea of revolutionary development is demonstrated by the fact that the revolutionary leaders themselves used the image of the spiral during the years 1917–20 as a visual analogy for the revolutionary process. In 1918 no less an authority than Lenin wrote in his preface to his pamphlet on Karl Marx that:

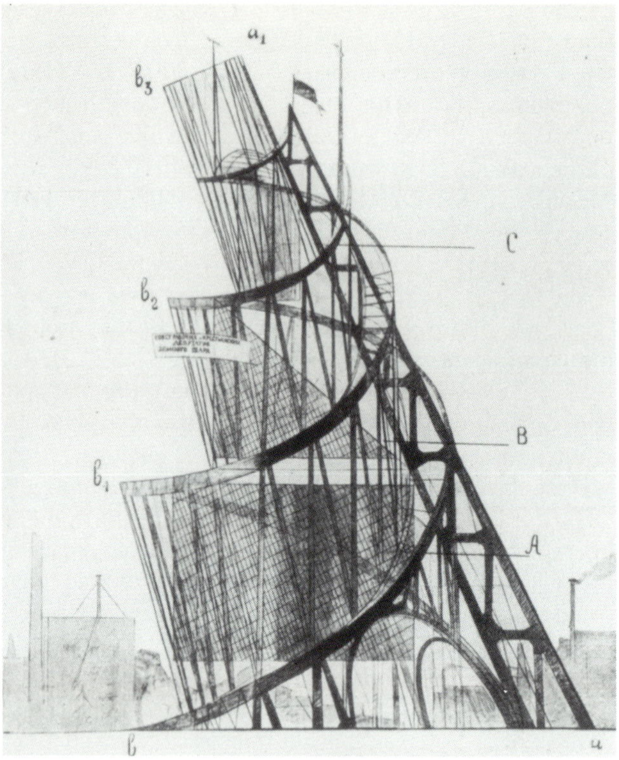

Fig. 14.3. A drawing of Tatlin's Monument to the Third International.

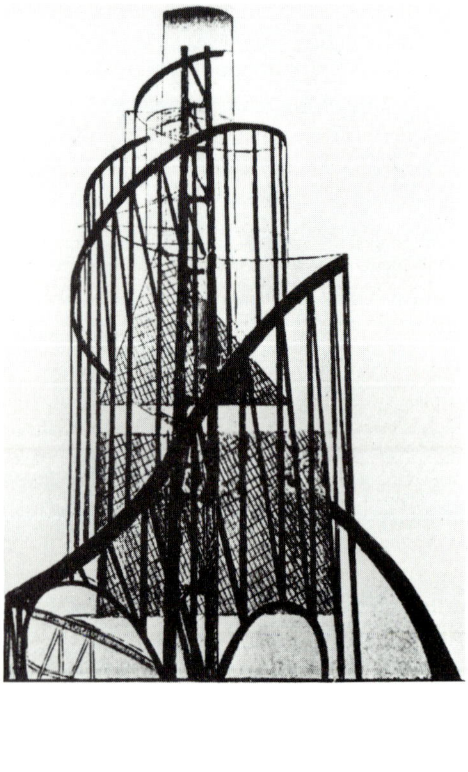

Fig. 14.4. A drawing of Tatlin's Project to the Third International published.

> Nowadays, the idea of development, of evolution has penetrated the social consciousness almost in its entirety, but by different ways, not by way of the Hegelian philosophy. But as formulated by Marx and Engels on the basis of Hegel, this idea is far more comprehensive, far richer in content than the current idea of evolution. A development that seemingly repeats the states already passed, but repeats them otherwise, on a higher basis ("negation of the negation"); a development, so to speak in spirals, not in a straight line; development by leaps, catastrophes, revolutions, "breaks in continuity"; the transformation of quantity into quality; the inner impulses of development, imparted by the contradiction and conflict of the various forces and tendencies acting on a given body, or within a given phenomenon, or within a given society; the interdependence and closest, indissoluble connection of *all* sides of every phenomenon (while history constantly discloses ever new sides), a connection that provides a uniform, law-governed, universal process of motion—such are some of the features of dialectics as a richer (than the ordinary), doctrine of development.[17]

In this popular publication of 1918, Lenin was expressing an idea which he had explored earlier in 1915 when writing "On the Question of Dialectics." There he had remarked:

> Knowledge is represented in the form of a series of circles, both by Hegel (see Logic), and by the modern "epistomologist" of natural science, the eclectic and foe of Hegelianism (which he did not understand!), Paul Volkman. . . . Human knowledge is not (or does not follow), a straight line, but a curve, which endlessly approximates a series of circles, a spiral. Any fragment, segment, section, of this curve can be transformed (transformed one-sidedly) into an independent, complete straight line, which then (if one does not see the wood for the trees) leads into the quagmire, into clerical obscurantism (where it is anchored by the class interests of the ruling classes). Rectilinearity and one-sidedness, woodenness and petrification, subjectivity and subjective blindness—voila the epistomological roots of idealism.[18]

Moreover, in employing the spiral metaphor, Lenin was expanding on its use by Engels in his *Dialectics of Nature,* which was not published until after Lenin's death but which Lenin is reputed to have known.[19] In this work Engels made the following statement:

> Dialectics as the science of universal inter-connection. Main laws: transformation of quantity and quality—mutual penetration of polar opposites and transformation into each other when carried to extremes—development through contradiction or negation of the negation—spiral form of development.[20]

The spiral form of development has now become an accepted element of Soviet Marxist philosophy, and it is usually cited in relation to the law of the negation of the negation, which is the third of the three main laws of dialectics. A contemporary definition, for instance, reads:

> *Spiral in Development:* a figurative description of the outcome of development employed by Engels and Lenin in elucidating the law of the negation of the negation. The process of development produces in phenomena an "apparent return to the old" (Lenin), in the course of change; this implies a repetition at a higher level of some features of a lower level. This may be depicted graphically as a Spiral in which each new turn repeats the preceeding one, but at a higher level. The general impression of ascendant and progressive development is thus created. De-

> velopment in a spiral form is at once opposed to the typically metaphysical idea of development as being motion along a closed circle, without any new elements.[21]

Statements of this kind suggest that Tatlin's use of the spiral in the monument was directly related to political ideology, and that for Tatlin, as for Lenin, the spiral served as a powerful visual metaphor for revolution. Although it is unlikely that Tatlin's knowledge of dialectics was very advanced, it is possible that he read Lenin's pamphlet on Karl Marx, particularly in view of his duties in implementing the Plan for Monumental Propaganda. Naturally, it is difficult to ascertain, especially from this distance, the precise nature of Tatlin's political beliefs. He undoubtedly did identify with the Bolshevik Revolution of 1917 and the concomitant political, economic, social, and cultural reorganization of Russia. He later wrote, "To accept or not to accept the October Revolution? There was no such question for me. I organically merged into active, creative, social, and pedagogical life."[22] The evidence of his own involvement with the Department of Fine Arts and his work in the proletarian cultural organizations (Proletcult) indicate that this is no post hoc justification. Yet it is unlikely that Tatlin had any profound understanding either of the nature of the political realities of the period or of the political ideology of Lenin. In December 1920 in his declaration "The Work Ahead of Us," Tatlin made a very simplistic equation between the political and cultural revolutions, stating that "What happened from the social and political aspect in 1917 happened in our work as artists in 1913." This identification between the political and artistic revolutions was scorned by Trotsky, who stated that the avant-garde or the "futurists" had no real understanding of the anatomy of revolution or of the revolutionary tradition.[23] The priority that Tatlin here gave to cultural developments, in contrast to political and economic realities, accords far more with Aleksandr Bogdanov's ideas of the three autonomous paths to socialism (the political, economic, and cultural), a theory which Lenin opposed and moved against in 1921 when he abolished the independence of the Proletcults set up by Bogdanov.[24]

There is other evidence to indicate that the tower's relationship to Bolshevik ideology is far from straightforward. One feature that aroused comment and criticism in 1920 and that remains very puzzling about the Monument to the Third International is not the incorporation of an element of dynamism, but rather the precise nature of that dynamism: the use of the rotations of one revolution a year, one revolution a month, and one revolution a day, distributed among the glazed volumes so that the speed would increase towards the apex of the monument.

The complexity of the volumes and their rotations does imply very strongly a symbolic intention: the incorporation of the rotating structures answers no discernible technological, functional, or structural requirements. As Trotsky pointed out, Tatlin's design was far from presenting a pragmatic utilization of current technological possibilities:

> The Soviet state will take up the problem of gigantic constructions that will suitably express the monumental spirit of our epoch. Tatlin is undoubtedly right in discarding from his project national styles, allegorical sculpture, modelled monograms, flourishes and tails, and attempting to subordinate the entire design to a constructive use of material. But Tatlin has still to prove that he is right in what seems to be his own personal invention, a rotating cube, a pyramid and a cylinder all of glass . . . meetings are not necessarily held in a cylinder and the cylinder does not necessarily have to rotate.[25]

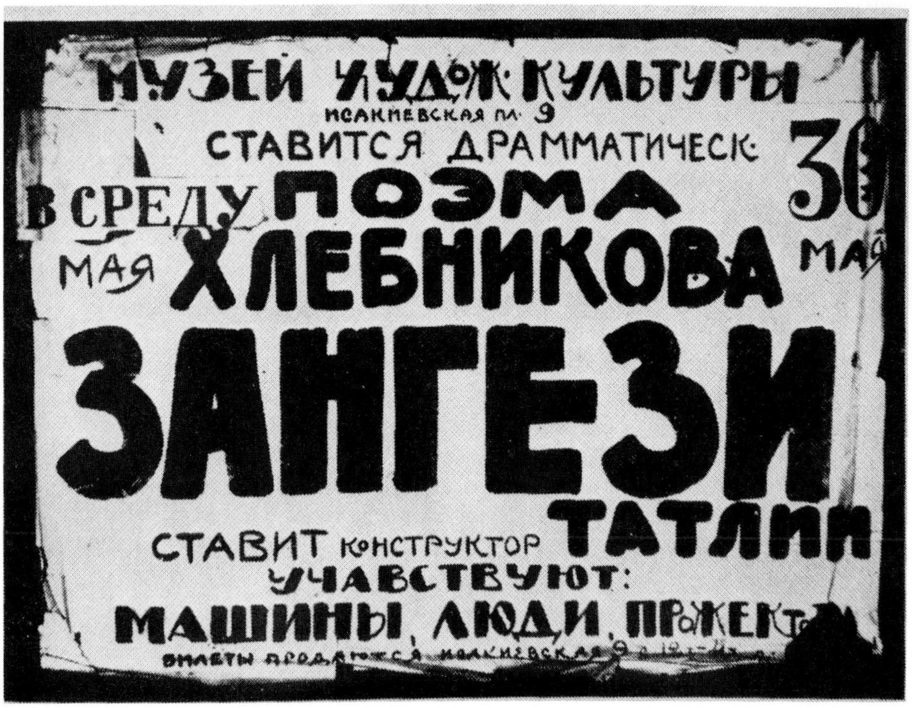

Fig. 14.5. Poster for Tatlin's production of *Znagesi.*

It is possible to regard the rotations of the glazed volumes as an illustration of the relationship of the three stages of social development: the long period of primitive social organization or feudalism, the briefer period of capitalism that in turn engenders its own demise by giving rise to the proletariat which will overthrow capitalism and institute the third and final stage of social organization, communism.

An alternative interpretation is, however, perhaps more probable. During the debate about the tower in December 1920, a fellow artist, Naum Gabo, argued that the monument was "technically out of the question," and added, "It is not that it cannot be built, but that it never will be built. You don't turn a six or seven storey building to follow the sun."[26] Despite Gabo's hyperbole, he highlighted an important aspect of the tower: that the rotations of the internal volumes are regulated, as he implied, by natural rhythms. The emphasis is on universal and natural time, rather than mechanical or narrowly human time. As Louis Lozowick observed: "Why these different velocities? Cosmic symbolism perhaps (romanticism slipping in by the back door): the earth moving around the sun (a year), the moon orbiting the earth (a month), the earth rotating on its own axis (a day)."[27]

To extend the argument that Tatlin fused other concepts of the space-time continuum with a Marxist metaphor for revolutionary change, I should like to propose that Tatlin's symbolism in the tower may also have been influenced by the futurist poet, Velimir Khlebnikov, and by his ornate, all encompassing theories of time.[28] Tatlin almost certainly had some knowledge of Khlebnikov's numerical theories of historical development when he began working on the design for the tower. Tatlin knew Khlebnikov, admired him greatly, considered him a genius, and recited his poetry throughout his life. Tatlin was evidently well acquainted with Khlebnikov's poetic and linguistic theories since the two artists collaborated in 1917 on a production of three of Khlebnikov's plays (*Death's Mistake, Madame Lenin,* and *Thirteen in the Air*), which unfortunately never materialized. In 1923 after the poet's death, Tatlin produced Khlebnikov's play *Zangezi* (fig. 14.5). Basing the production on the principle that "the word is a unit of construction—material is a unit of organized volume," Tatlin explained that "Khlebnikov took sounds as elements. . . . To reveal the nature of these sounds I have taken surfaces of different materials which have been treated in different ways."[29] The actors carried boards which were approximately one meter high and half a meter wide. These were prepared in the same way as icons and were painted, probably in different color combinations. One of the panels, which survived into the 1970s but has since disappeared, comprised a reddish border containing a blue rectangle on which numbers were inscribed in white paint.[30] It is the presence of these numbers that suggests quite clearly that at least by 1923 Tatlin was well enough versed in Khlebnikov's theory of numbers to implement those ideas in the production of *Zangezi.*

Yet it is clear that Tatlin already knew of Khlebnikov's theory of time and numbers by 1919, when he himself first referred to them in a set of theses, "The Initiative [or Initiative Taking] Unit in the Creativity of the Collective," which represented his own formulation of the new relationship between the artist and society. The "initiative unit" *(initsiativnaya edinitsa)* was the term that Tatlin adopted to describe the new type of artist produced by the artistic response to the political and social revolution of 1917. The term was explicitly intended to convey the collective, nonindividualistic essence of the new creative activity which Tatlin envisaged, which he called "invention." He wrote:

> The initiative [or initiative taking] unit is the collector of the ENERGY of the collective, which is directed towards cognition and invention. The initiative unit serves as the link between invention and the creativity of the mass.
>
> The viability of the collective is confirmed by the number of initiative units selected by it. . . . Invention is always the solution of the impulses and wishes of the collective and not of the individual.
>
> The world of numbers as that nearest to the architectonics of art gives us (1) confirmation of the existence of the inventor, (2) a full organic union between the [initiative taking] unit and the collector of numbers. There are no mistakes in Khlebnikov's example.[31]

Tatlin stressed his conception of the artist as a catalyst and focusing lens for natural and societal processes and minimized his significance as an autonomous personality. Describing the artist as merely a manifestation of the collective's creative powers, he emphasized the organic relationship existing between the artist and society. On the one hand, he reduced the individual importance of such a creative unit. Yet, on the other, he imbued that unit with the collective power and elevated it as the embodiment of the collective's creativity. In evoking Khlebnikov's analogy between word and number, Tatlin emphasized his own idea of design (or invention) as a maximal distillation of patterns found initially in natural phenomena. At the same time, Tatlin evidently considered his own activity as an "initiative taking unit" to parallel Khlebnikov's work with numbers and to be organically linked to it. This identification, which Tatlin made in 1919, may have been of crucial importance in determining the way he approached designing the tower.

Khlebnikov first published his ideas about the rhythms of time and the role of numbers in governing historical events in 1912 in the futurist book *A Slap in the Face of Public Taste.* Two years later he devised a government of time which consisted of "Presidents of the Globe," designated himself "First President of the Planet Earth," and adopted the title "Velimir I, King of Time." His interest in the numerical patterns of history was intensified by the advent of the First World War, and in 1915 and 1916 he elaborated his ideas in two major publications: *Battles 1915–1917: A New Teaching About War* and *Time is the Measure of the World.*

Fundamentally Khlebnikov considered that there were several significant numbers, comprising modules of years, which governed the sequence of historical events. One of these numbers was 365, the number of days in the year as the earth moved round the sun. Another was 48. As Khlebnikov explained:

> The number 365 is the basic number of the planet earth, its "number of numbers." As the most ancient of the relations of the planet Earth it has led to this that all the rest is constructed according to it and in this way the government of numbers arose. Subsequently the planet Earth must be understood as the ultimate creation of the pure art of sounds; where Skryabin is the planet Earth, the strings are a year and a day, and the ruling consonance, [*sic*], set at the head of all work are the numbers 365, 1, 25 (the sun's day is taken as 25 Earth days); the earth's day equals "a," the sun's day "M"; 48 = 2(M – a)/a.[32]

$$48 = \frac{2(M - a)}{a}$$

Moreover, these two basic numbers of 365 and 48 could be combined to produce two further modules: 317 (48 subtracted from 365) and 413 (48 added to 365).[33] In applying these modules to the analysis of history, Khlebnikov saw a basic unity between the fate of the individual and the state: the module "for a state is a year but for the individual soul a day."[34] In other words, he wrote, "The spirit of mankind relates to the spirit of man as a year to a day, giving in particular (the voice of the earth), the number 365."[35] The importance that Khlebnikov gave to 365 seems to be reflected in the significance that Tatlin gave to the lowest cube rotating at a speed of one revolution a year. It is the largest of the glass chambers and the most visually prominent of the three rotating volumes, and being the lowest, it also acts as the foundation for the other two.

Furthermore, Khlebnikov identified another important historical module in the number 28. Khlebnikov argued that generations are governed by 28 years and that "when a truth is born in year 'n,' the opposite truth is born in year 'n' plus 28."[36] Thus 28 is the number that links the generations. From this it would follow that if the unity between the individual and the state, or between the individual and mankind, is expressed in the number 365, then the relationship of both the individual and the state to subsequent generations is expressed in the number 28. Thus, the 28 days of the lunar month, the speed at which the next volume in the tower was intended to rotate, can also be directly related to Khlebnikov's theories.

For Khlebnikov the number one was also significant. Therefore Tatlin's uppermost volume rotating at one revolution a day may not only express a fundamental unit of earthly time but also the unity of cosmic and historical time. Furthermore, the day comprises 24 hours, and this number doubled produces 48 which, of course, was another of Khlebnikov's modules. In this way the uppermost volume may have been intended to reinforce the interrelationship of the volumes as representations of the numbers governing significant historical events. The number 48 subtracted from 365 would produce the number 317, which Khlebnikov argued was of immense significance in the fate of empires and nation states. Khlebnikov had attempted to prove this contention with a formidable array of examples derived from the history of Europe, Asia, and North Africa. He produced numerous tables correlating such events as, for example, the fact that the Romans settled Africa in 202 B.C. and that in 1066, 1268 years later, that is, four times 317, the Normans invaded and occupied England.[37] He drew numerical links between related but distant phenomena, for example, between the promulgation of the Justinian legal code in 533 and the issuing of the Napoleonic legal code in 1801, 1268 years later (again, four times 317).[38] Furthermore, arguing on the basis of the fact that the war of 1281–1293 heralded the end of the expansion of the Mongol Empire, Khlebnikov predicted that the present spate of wars (which he thought would take place over the period 1915–1927) would coincide with the decline of Europe or of a European state. Moreover, citing the wars of 534 and 555, Khlebnikov predicted that such an event would occur in 1917.[39] The verification of that prediction by the Revolution must have had an immense impact on Tatlin, who was already Khlebnikov's devoted admirer when the Revolution took place.

The significance of Khlebnikov's prediction for Tatlin would not have diminished by 1919 when Tatlin started designing his monument. This was, after all, the period when Tatlin was also formulating his ideas about art within the new political structure and was writing so emphatically, "There are no mistakes in Khlebnikov's example."

In this way it can be seen that the erudite, not to say bizarre, theories of Khlebnikov and the imagery of contemporary political rhetoric were for Tatlin complementary rather than contradictory forces in the processes of thought which crystallized into his design for the Monument to the Third International. The complex layers of symbolism which that structure embodies do not detract from its final rightness and simplicity as a visual image.

NOTES

I am most grateful to Dr. Julian Cooper for his invaluable help in advising about the presence of spiral analogies in Marxist writings, and to Alina Vasil'evna Povelikhina and Martin Hammer for their comments on earlier drafts of this paper.

1. Quoted in T. Andersen, *Vladimir Tatlin* (Stockholm: Moderna Museet, 1968), 63.

2. A. Begicheva, "Vospominaniya o Tatline: Do Kontsa ne razdagai," MS, private archive, Moscow, p. 10. The meeting and conversation referred to are said to have taken place on 25 August 1925 (ibid., 16).

3. "O snyatii pamyatnikov vozdvignutykh v chest' tsarei i ikh slug i vyrabotke proektov pamyatnikov Rossiiskoi sotsiatlisticheskoi revolyutsii" (The removal of monuments erected in honor of the tsars and their servants and the production of projects for monuments to the Russian Socialist Revolution), *Pravda,* 14 April 1918. For a discussion of the plan in more detail, see J. Bowlt, "Russian Sculpture and Lenin's Plan of Monumental Propaganda," in H. A. Millon and L. Nochlin, eds., *Art and Architecture in the Service of Politics* (Cambridge, Mass. and London: MIT Press, 1978), 182–93; and C. Lodder, "Lenin's Plan of Monumental Propaganda," *Sbornik* no. 6/7 (Leeds, 1981) 67–82.

4. A. Lunacharskii, "Lenin o monumental'noi propagande" (Lenin on monumental propaganda), *Literaturnaya gazeta,* no. 4/5 (29 January 1933). Reprinted in A. Lunacharskii, *Vospominaniya i vpechatleniya* (Moscow, 1968). See also S. Konnenkov, *Moi vek* (Moscow, 1972), 214, for the text of Lenin's letter.

5. V. Tatlin, Letter to Sovnarkom, end of August 1918, reprinted in *Lenin i Lunacharskii: Peripiska, doklady, dokumenty* (Moscow, 1971), 80.

6. N. Punin, "O pamyatnikakh" (About monuments), *Iskusstvo komunny,* no. 14 (9 March 1919).

7. N. Punin, "Tour de Tatline," *Veshch',* no. 1/2 (1922).

8. N. Punin, "O pamyatnikakh."

9. V. Tatlin, T. Shapiro, I. Meerzon, P. Vinogradov, "Nasha predstoyashaya rabota" (The work ahead of us), *VIII s'ezd sovetov: Ezhednevnyi byulleten' s'ezda VTsIK,* no. 13 (31 December 1920): 11.

10. Ibid.

11. S. Lissitzky-Küppers, "New Russian Art: a lecture" in *El Lissitzky: Life, Letters, Texts* (London: Thames & Hudson, 1968), 331.

12. N. Punin, *Pamyatnik tret'ego internatsionala* (Petrograd: Otdela Izobrazitel' nylch Iskusstv, N.K.P., 1920).

13. Ibid.

14. Ibid.

15. El Lissitzky, *Russia, An Architecture for World Revolution* (London: Lund Humphries, 1970) 29.

16. A. Begicheva, "Vospominaniya."

17. V. I. Lenin, *Karl Marks* (Moscow, 1918). Translation taken from V. I. Lenin, *Karl Marx* (Peking, 1967), 12–13.

18. V. I. Lenin, *Collected Works: Vol. 38 The Philosophical Notebooks* (Moscow and London, 1961), 362–63.

19. F. Engels, *Dialectics of Nature* (Moscow, 1972), 11.

20. Ibid., 17.

21. M. Rosenthal and P. Yudin, *A Dictionary of Philosophy* (Moscow, 1967), 129.

22. V. Tatlin, "Kratkii obzor" (Short summary), MS, private archive, Moscow.

23. L. Trotsky, *Literature and Revolution* (New York, 1925), 43.

24. See C. V. James, *Soviet Socialist Realism* (Oxford, 1975), 62ff.

25. Trotsky, *Literature and Revolution,* 246–47.

26. N. Gabo in S. F. Starr and K. Frampton, "Russian Art in Revolution and Emigration: An Interview with Naum Gabo," edited transcript, 1969, Beinecke Rare Book and Manuscript Library, Yale University, 9.

27. L. Lozowick, "Tatlin's Monument to the Third International," *Broom* 3, no. 3 (1922): 234.

28. The relationship between Tatlin and Khlebnikov has been treated in some depth in J. Milner, *Vladimir Tatlin and the Russian Avant-Garde* (New Haven and London: Yale University Press, 1983). With reference to the tower see pp. 166, 170. See also C. Lodder, *Russian Constructivism* (New Haven and London: Yale University Press, 1983), 208–9. In 1917 Tatlin had drawn a portrait of Khlebnikov (private collection, Moscow).

29. V. Tatlin, "O Zangezi" (Concerning Zangezi), *Zhizn' iskusstvo,* no. 18 (1923): 15.

30. This is based on information supplied by Alina Vasil'evna Povelikhina.

31. V. Tatlin, "Initsiativnaya edinitsa v tvorchestve kollektiva," MS, Central State Archives for Literature and Art, Moscow, Fond 665, opus 1, edinitsa khraneniya 32, list 11.

32. V. V. Khlebnikov, *Vremya mera mira* (Petrograd, 1916), reprinted in V. V. Khlebnikov, *Sobranie sochinenii* (Munich, 1972), 3:445.

33. Ibid., 428.

34. Ibid.

35. Ibid., 443.

36. V. V. Khlebnikov, *Bitvy 1915–1917gg: Novoe uchenie o voine* (Petrograd, 1915), reprinted in *Sobranie sochinenii* 3:433.

37. Ibid., 414.

38. Khlebnikov, *Vremya* in *Sobranie sochinenii* 3:440.

39. Khlebnikov, *Bitvy* in *Sobranie sochinenii* 3:410. This present study does not exhaust the subject of the possible influence that Khlebnikov exerted on the evolution of Tatlin's design for the Monument to the Third International. The fact that the tower contains three revolving glass volumes may refer to the importance which Khlebnikov gave to the number three. Khlebnikov asserted: "It is enough to contemplate the first three numbers, the really brilliant sphere, in order to construct the eternal. The laws of the world correspond to the laws of accounting [numbers]." ("Iz zapisnykh knizhek" [From the notebooks] in *Sobranie Sochinenii* 3:266). Moreover, the spiral form itself may be related to the emphasis which Khlebnikov gave to curvilinear organic form both in his architectural projects and in his poetry (see Lodder, *Russian Constructivism,* 207–8). In addition to his mathematical studies, Khlebnikov was also profoundly interested in Eastern philosophies and religions. He was deeply mystical in his approach to natural phenomena, and it is possible that for Khlebnikov the number three had mystical associations connected with the Christian trinity. This also may have exerted an influence on Tatlin and found reflection in the three large glazed structures of the tower that revolved.

V

The Historiography of Art History

15

The VALUES of the BYZANTINE TRADITION

A Documentary History of Goethe's Response to the Boisserée Collection

E. H. GOMBRICH

Any progress from a rigid, obsolete and artificial state toward a free and vital realism also implies a loss which can only be made good by and by, and frequently not before some time has elapsed.

THIS COMMENT BY GOETHE on the artistic revolution of the van Eycks and on their departure from the medieval traditions of art occurs in his account of the Boisserée collection published in 1816 in *Aus Kunst und Altertum*. The text of this essay, "From a Journey to the Rhine, Main and Neckar in the years 1814–15," can be found in all editions of Goethe's collected works[1] and has also been made available to English readers in the anthology by John Gage, titled *Goethe on Art*.[2] But though this text cannot be called unfamiliar, it is hoped that Elizabeth Holt will accept a comment on this comment as a tribute to her, for she, if anyone, must know how original were the opinions quoted in their time and how far-reaching were their consequences on the historiography of art. The carefully worded statement, judiciously attempting to balance the gains and losses of an artistic innovation, turns out to be the result of Goethe's determination not to be swept off his feet by the enthusiasm of the two German collectors of northern fifteenth-century painting who had become his friends but whose medievalizing tendencies he distrusted and resisted.

For facts and documents this study is wholly indebted to the monograph on the Boisserée Collection by Eduard Firmenich-Richartz of which only the first volume came out during the first World War in 1916.[3] But while that work concentrates on the acquisitions and social contacts of the two brothers, I propose to describe mainly the human story, which, as it will turn out, also explains the nature of Goethe's response. If the response will be found to exhibit a strong dose of ambivalence, the reasons must be traced to the beginnings of the two brothers' intellectual formation.

Sulpiz Boisserée (1783–1854) and his young brother Melchior (1786–1851) were the sons of a wealthy Cologne merchant. As a consequence of the Revolution of 1789, Cologne had moved into the French political orbit, and when Sulpiz (with whom we shall be mainly concerned) was twenty, Bertram, an older friend, suggested that the brothers should visit Paris. It was there in 1803 that they became the disciples and followers of the leader of the German Romantics, Friedrich Schlegel (1772–1829), a man Goethe heartily disliked, a dislike which was mutual. Having married Dorothea, the daughter of Moses Mendelssohn, Schlegel had gone to Paris a year earlier mainly to escape the disabilities that were still imposed on Jews in German lands. It was there that he learned Sanskrit and secured for himself a permanent place in the history of Indian studies, and it was there, also, that visits to the Musée Napoleon opened his eyes to the beauties of preclassical art which he expounded in his journal *Europa*.[4] The fertile mind and the personality of this versatile man so impressed the two brothers that they chose him as their guru; they lived in his house and attended his private lectures on literature. A year later they persuaded their master to accompany them to Cologne, using the opportunity for looking at the ancient cities and buildings in Belgium and the Netherlands, paying special attention to Gothic architecture.

It is well known that the new enthusiasm for these formerly neglected monuments was fed by two equally potent factors: the reaction against the anticlericalism of the French Revolution and the upsurge of German nationalism in the face of French cultural hegemony. By the time Friedrich Schlegel arrived in Paris, the first of these movements was well under way. In 1802 there had appeared François Renée Chateaubriand's seminal book *Le Genie du Christianism*, which asserted the superiority of the Age of Faith over the Age of Reason. The roots of German cultural nationalism, of course, go back much further. None other than Goethe had celebrated the greatness of the Strasbourg Cathedral in 1772 in his first publication, *Von Deutscher Baukunst*, in which he naively challenged the French to point to anything they had created which would equal this masterpiece.[5] The erroneous belief that the Gothic style was the national style of the German derived of course from its designation, which had been popularized by Vasari in the sixteenth century; but it needed Germany's humiliation during the Napoleonic wars to turn Gothic architecture into the symbol of a political movement. The incomplete cathedral of Cologne, which Sulpiz Boisserée first undertook to measure and record and later also to restore and complete, became the most potent embodiment of German aspirations.

In considering the career of this gifted amateur, a third historical factor must be taken into an account, one equally connected with the aftermath of the French Revolution and the Napoleonic wars: the dissolution of the monasteries and the secular administration of the Rhinelands had led to the sale or removal of many church furnishings, including altars and figures of saints dating from medieval times. This was a golden opportunity for collectors with antiquarian interests, among whom the brothers Boisserée became prominent after their return from Paris to Cologne.

They soon found, however, that it was one thing to admire the engaging piety and honesty of these relics of a Christian age, but a very different thing to assign them a place in a historical context. The history of German medieval art was a complete blank; next to nothing was known of the date and sequence of styles. No wonder that the meager facts to be found in the earlier writers, notably Giorgio Vasari and Carel van Mander, were used as points of reference against which to plot the development of the newly discovered school of German art. Vasari, of course, had described the rise of Italian Renaissance painting against the foil of the *maniera Greca*, the "ugly and clumsy" style of Byzantine art which had nevertheless prevented art from becoming altogether extinct during the Dark Ages. In one of his rare references to northern art he had also celebrated the achievement of Giovanni da Brugia [Jan van Eyck] as the inventor of oil painting, a new technique that had superseded the tempera painting of the Greeks and their followers. These ideas had gained currency among art lovers and were to form the cornerstone of their historical reconstruction. The process is reflected in the fragments of an autobiography from the pen of Sulpiz:

> So far those paintings were considered to date from an earlier period, which were found to be somewhat similar to those of the brothers van Eyck, but less perfect in design and execution. In general one inferred their greater age merely from their greater imperfections rather than from a wholly different conception and formation of heads and draperies. But when we first encountered paintings of apostles in the entrance hall of the St. Laurence church, in which the heads were rendered with broad forms, soft hair and beards and the drapery with simply rounded folds, all executed with a soft fluent brush, we did not hesitate at first to consider them Italian. They seemed to us to resemble the half-length paintings of apostles on golden ground from St. Luigi in Rome which we had seen in the restoration workshop of the Italo-Byzantine manner. . . . It did not last long however till we found several such paintings which were doubtlessly of local origin from the 14th and 15th centuries. At the same time we found that paintings with inscriptions and dates, which, because of their imperfections, had formerly been considered to be earlier than the van Eycks, actually belonged to their school. So we had to convince ourselves of a fact of which nobody had so far had the slightest inkling, the fact that the earlier painting of Cologne before the van Eycks, no less than the contemporary Italian school, relied on an old tradition of Byzantine models and that it had emerged from the same foundations of that traditional art, although with distinct individual characteristics.[6]

The modern art historian may here be tempted to connect these vague historical intuitions with the fact that there was indeed an "international Gothic style" that dominated the arts of Europe around the year 1400 before the emergence of the new realism. But subsequent utterances by Sulpiz indicate that he was far from such detailed knowledge of the history of art and that most of his opinions were wildly off the mark.

When in 1808 the brothers succeeded in acquiring the greatest treasure of their collection, Rogier van der Weyden's triptych from the monastery of St. Columba, (fig. 15.1) they had no doubt that they here had an example of the art of van Eyck who was seen to have wholly broken with the Byzantine tradition.

Sulpiz responded to Friedrich Schlegel's request for advice in matters of medieval art and set out his ideas in much more detail.[7] He refers to the opinion his correspondent had expressed himself in his journal *Europa* (vol. 4, pp. 5, 30, 109), the opinion "that at first painting among Italians and Germans was bound to have originated from the same point, . . . and that the earliest Christian paintings exemplified the Greek manner":

> It is precisely this continuous and exclusive persistence of the Greek style and manner in the old German schools of painting and sculpture from the earliest times to those of van Eyck which, due to our discoveries, has become the main foundation of our new understanding of our national art history.
>
> That the appearance of a contrasting, wholly nationally German manner which we had thought to be of earlier origin, is entirely due to the van Eycks is the second point; the third and most difficult point of our changed conception concerns the transition to that style from the earlier, wholly Greek manner.

Accustomed as we are to illustrated handbooks, it requires an effort to imagine how difficult it must have been, in the absence of any reliable illustration, even

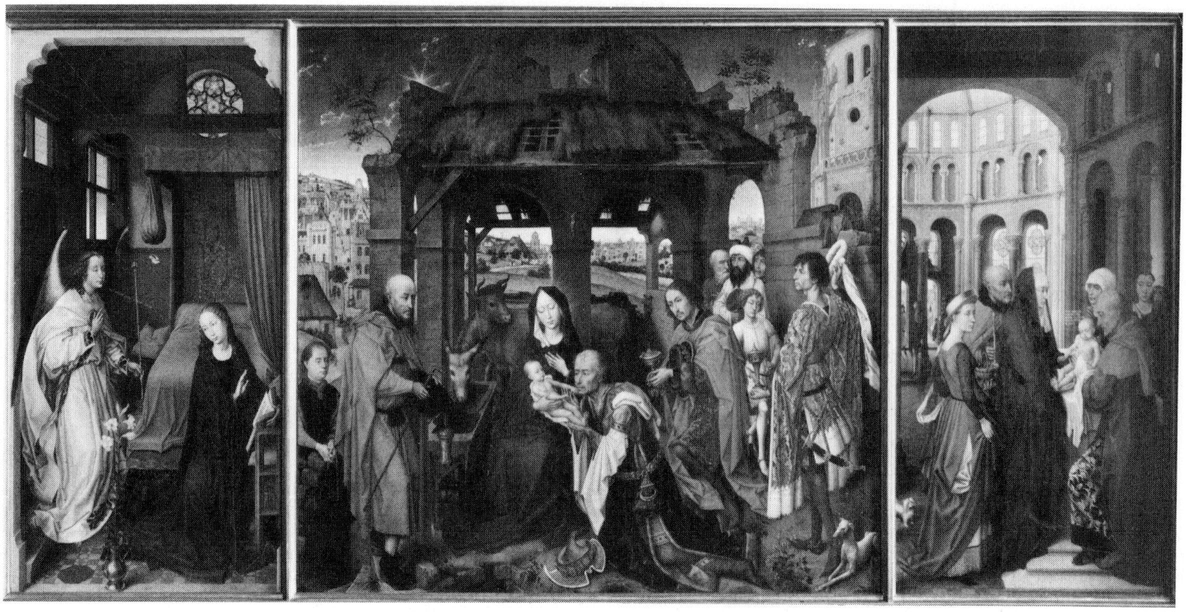

Fig. 15.1. Rogier van der Weyden, *Columba Altar.* Munich, Alte Pinakothek.

to attempt the construction of a historical picture of medieval art. It was only in the year in which Sulpiz wrote this account that the situation was at least partially remedied by the appearance of the first installment of Seroux d'Agincourt's *Histoire de l'Art par les Monuments depuis sa décadence au 4me siècle à son renouvellement au 16me* (Paris, 1811–20). Before that the only publication from which Sulpiz could derive any idea of the characteristics of the Byzantine style was the edition by Cardinal Albani of the *Menologium of Basilius II* (fig. 15.2), a richly illustrated manuscript in the Vatican library dating from the period around 1000. How much, however, they had to rely on hearsay is revealed in the incidental remark that "art lovers who had seen the neo-Greek paintings by Giotto" had assured them that certain German panel paintings were "very much like them in color and design."[8]

The brothers had no more luck in clarifying what they considered the most difficult point in their new view of medieval art history, the transition from the ubiquitous Byzantine style to that of the van Eycks. The misreading of an inscription had led them to the belief that the principal monument of the School of Cologne, Stephan Lochner's *Dombild,* was dated 1410 (instead of c. 1440) and had thus to be fitted into this transitional period.

Even the most skeptical art historian must admit that we have made a little progress since those days. And yet it will be seen that it was on these shaky foundations that Goethe based his important insight about the inherent values of the Byzantine tradition.

The strange concatenation of circumstances which opened the way for these young collectors to approach the virtual dictator of taste in German lands is worth relating.[9] Sulpiz had been asked by a retired French diplomat who had left the service of Napoleon, Karl Friedrich Reinhard, to find him a country retreat in the Rhineland for

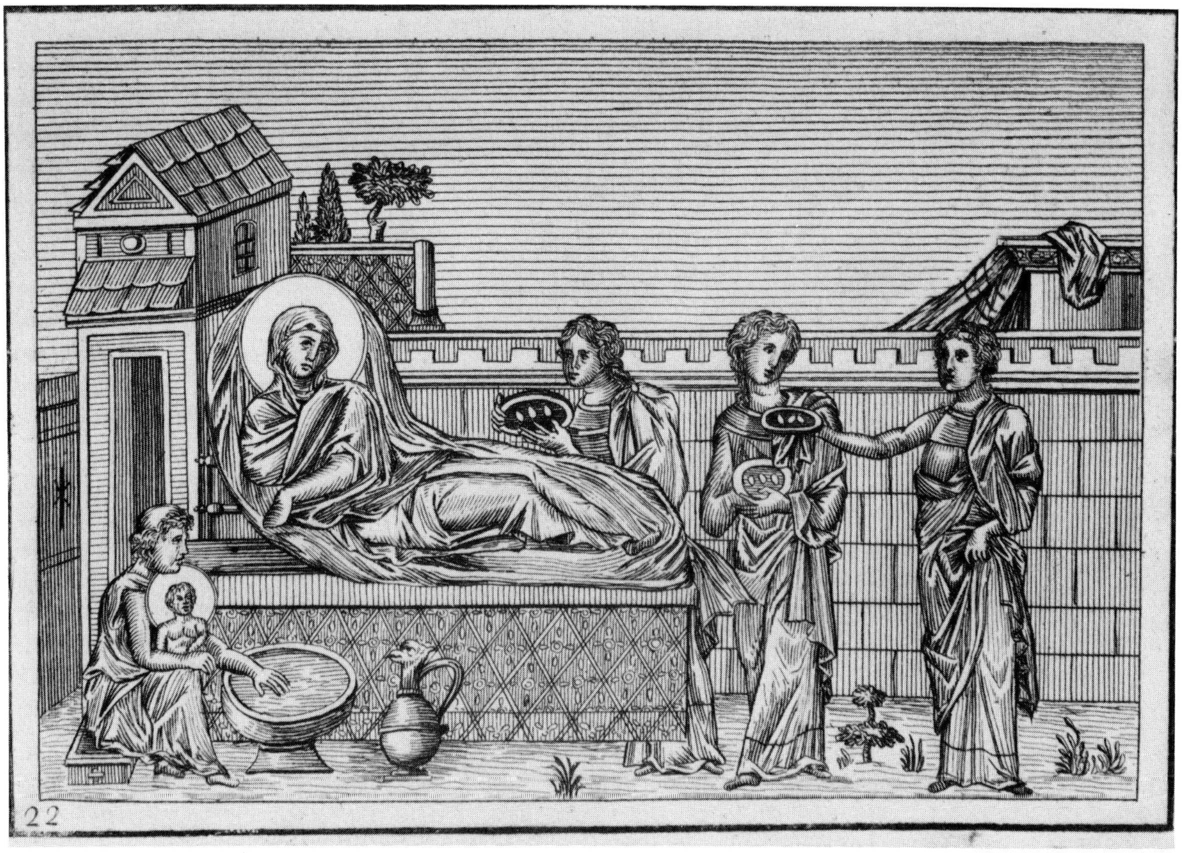

Fig. 15.2. *The Birth of the Virgin* from Cardinal Albani's edition of the *Menologium of Basil II* in the Vatican Library, Urbino, 1727, vol. 1, p. 24. By permission of the British Library.

the years of his retirement. But in these turbulent years he was abducted by the Russians, taken to a castle by the Dnieper, and only set free after diplomatic intervention. In need of rest, Reinhard went to the famous spa of Karlsbad where he met Goethe, who took a liking to this highly cultured man of the world.

Thus on 16 April 1810, Reinhard wrote a carefully worded letter to Goethe, mentioning that Sulpiz, who had recently moved to Heidelberg, was the owner of a very remarkable collection of old German paintings that he had rescued from perdition. But what would certainly interest Goethe was a project Sulpiz had conceived of publishing a description of Cologne Cathedral and its antiquities together with its history. The drawings were ready, and Sulpiz would dearly love to show them to Goethe and to make his acquaintance: "I can wholly recommend him to you as a well-behaved, upright and good natured person. . . . I respect and love this young man and am in contact with his house and his family."[10]

Goethe's reply was by no means encouraging. He would not advise the young man to undertake the journey to Weimar; he was much under pressure; and if the visitor came at a time of so much turbulence, he would have even less pleasure and profit than could otherwise be expected: "For as you must feel yourself, a disciple of Friedrich Schlegel would have to remain for a considerable time in my proximity and benevolent spirits would have to inspire both of us with special patience if anything enjoyable and constructive is to result from this encounter." However, having got this off his chest, Goethe felt it necessary to add that Reinhard's recommendation was certain to prepare a friendly reception for the visitor, "indeed in points which are generally hostile to me he will find me more patient and forgiving than I am usually."[11]

Sulpiz was well advised not to come before he had sent the drawings. Having looked at them, Goethe sent a more conciliatory letter to Reinhard, dated 14 May 1810: "One cannot prescribe to anyone to what he should turn his interest and how to cultivate his innate gifts. Moreover everything is very praiseworthy that brings to mind again the meaning of past times, especially when it is done in a truly faithful and critical manner. Accordingly the efforts of the young man which resulted in these drawings are highly laudable." And after discussing details of the drawings and of the cathedral, Goethe continues:

> Let this be, then, the sincere and unqualified praise that is due to the art lovers of Cologne. Admittedly it needs this kind of passionate limitation to produce something of this kind. Earlier in my life I was also interested in these matters and I indulged in a similar kind of idolatry of the Strasbourg Cathedral, the facade of which I still consider to be superior as an invention to that of Cologne Cathedral.
>
> What strikes me as strangest of all is German patriotism that wants to represent this obviously saracenic plant as sprung from its own soil. On the whole, however, the period in which this taste spread from South to the North remains truly interesting. I look at the whole thing as on a state of caterpillars and chrysalis in which the first Italian artists were also still confined till at last Michelangelo, in conceiving the Church of St. Peter, broke through the shell and presented himself to the world as a miraculously splendid bird.

After returning to more general expressions of benevolence, Goethe added a postscript asking Reinhard not to communicate to the "excellent young man" any of the utterances in the letter that could hurt him.[12]

Meanwhile Sulpiz had written a long and deferential letter to Goethe, declaring it to be his duty "to ask for the judgment of the man whose approval could guide and encourage my work more than that of any other and is also bound to have a most decisive influence on the completion of the work itself." After detailed discussion of the project concerning Cologne Cathedral he turns to an account of his collection:

> We possess not merely remarkable works but paintings which are at least in their expression more noble and more beautiful than can be usually seen in works of the old masters. . . . But the most important point remains our discovery, due to our collecting zeal, of a style of painting extending as far as the age of Jan van Eyck which continuously shows the traces of Greek influence, such as we hear it described in Italy before Raphael and which no one had expected up to now to have existed in Germany. The most recent of these works from the late 14th and early 15th centuries exhibit this manner in the great beauty of heads and draperies . . . the treatment of design and color is very different and more pleasing than we have expected so far of the German character and its frequently clumsily imitative art. There must be obviously the same foundations, and the early works resemble more and more the clumsy figures known from the Byzantine miniature paintings of the *Menologium* and other manuscripts.[13]

In his brief but courteous acknowledgment Goethe promised the writer that he could be sure of a most friendly welcome. Reinhard, the faithful intermediary, was not deceived. He wrote to Goethe on June 27, implying that it was probably a mistake not to let him pass on Goethe's misgivings for now the young man immediately thought that Goethe looked at these matters with his eyes. Whereupon Goethe hurried to ask him to enlighten the young friend in Heidelberg sufficiently, because otherwise the impending visit might lead to an unpleasant situation if he had not learned earlier what Goethe's real opinion was. No doubt the young man had done excellent work, but Goethe still thought that the subject was only praiseworthy as documenting a stage of human culture. Admittedly, Goethe concedes, if these nice young men did not consider this transitional state the highest, they could not summon the courage and energy for their labors.

> If the knight did not think of his lady as the most beautiful and unparalleled, he would not fight monsters and dragons for her sake.
>
> In my life I have experienced a sufficient number of similar situations with young people, which has prompted me recently to keep away entirely even from the better ones. They concede that we have influence, but they think it is they who have the insights and their silent intention is really to make use of the first for the sake of the latter. There is no true confidence to be established here. I don't take this amiss, but I prefer not to deceive myself in a good-natured way nor to further other people's purposes against my conviction.[14]

It is important to keep this frank avowal in mind, if we want to understand what followed. Goethe's fear that he might allow himself to be seduced to support a cause he really detested explains the ups and downs that characterize his behavior toward Sulpiz Boisserée and also its subsequent inconsistencies, which occasionally bordered on duplicity.

When, on 3 May 1811, the young man of twenty-eight stood at last before the great poet, then in his sixty-second year, he was to experience this ambivalence to the full. The account of this meeting he instantly gave to his brother is heartwarming in its immediacy and deserves to be quoted at some length:

> I just come from Goethe who received me stiffly and coldly, I was not to be put off and was also formal and not deferential. The old gentleman let me wait a little, till he came in with powdered hair, the ribbons of his decoration on his jacket. The address was as stiffly unbending as possible. I brought him many greetings. "Very nice," said he. We immediately came to talk about the drawings, the engravers, the difficulties, the publishers Cotta, and all those external matters. "Yes, yes, fine, hem, hem." Then we touched on the work itself, on the fate of the art of old times and its history. I was determined to counter aloofness with just the same aloofness, I talked as briefly as possible of the high beauty and excellence of the art in the Cathedral, and pointed out that having looked at the drawings he should have been able to convince himself—during all that he pulled a face as if he wanted to eat me. Only when we talked of old painting he somewhat thawed; hearing the praise of neo-Greek art he smiled, he asked about van Eyck, and confessed that he had not yet seen anything by him, asked about painters between him and Dürer and about Dürer's contemporaries in the Netherlands. He accepted my view that we had such beautiful paintings because the art of the Netherlands had been much more refined and pleasing than that of the rest of Germany. I was as accommodating in all these matters as you know me, but also as

> determined and free as possible and did not allow myself to be put off by his silence or his "yes, yes, nice, strange." I generously offered him my ideas about the development of painting through the influence of the van Eyck, but very cautiously, and allowed him to sense very clearly that one did not like to express one's thoughts about the fresh discoveries which we have been lucky enough to make. I only gave them in general outline, and he took all this in with pleasure.[15]

Only after the conversation had turned to Reinhard and other personal matters Goethe became more affable, "his smiles became more frequent and he invited me to his table tomorrow."

On the next day, 4 May 1811, Sulpiz was able to report a striking change of mood. He had brought Goethe Cornelius' illustrations to *Faust,* which earned applause, after which Goethe showed his visitors the *Four Seasons* by Philipp Otto Runge that hung on his wall and which he praised with genuine enthusiasm. "What, you don't know that? Look what kind of stuff that is, to drive you crazy, beautiful and mad at the same time."

At the next visit, Goethe even offered to come to Sulpiz the following morning "so that we can talk under four eyes, we must make use of the time we are together. By word of mouth and with the drawings at hand one can understand each other really." Sulpiz declined the honor of acting as host to Goethe, but his conquest was by then complete. Not that Sulpiz had any illusions:

> One must not forget over these brief spells of youthful enthusiasm that he is an old man and that one cannot expect of him any really active sympathy.
>
> All the arguments of the old man against the belief that Gothic architecture was invented by our nation have fallen silent, and everything he said about the Strasbourg Cathedral he soon dropped. Tuesday when I was alone with him with the drawings, he actually growled occasionally like a wounded bear, one saw how he struggled with himself and blamed himself ever to have misjudged such greatness.

Describing their next tête-a-tête at table, Sulpiz reports that hearing Goethe's praise he felt uplifted by the feeling of a great and beautiful cause having remained victorious over the prejudices of one of the most intelligent men "with whom I had to fight a real battle during the last few days. . . . I said what came to my mind, I don't know what words I used, they obviously revealed my emotion, for the old man was quite moved, pressed my hand and embraced me. He had tears in his eyes." Their intimacy had grown to the point where Sulpiz even ventured to ask Goethe what he had against Friedrich Schlegel, though here there was no question of breaking down the old man's prejudices against a man he considered to be dishonest.

We need not doubt that Sulpiz was right in claiming a personal victory, for Goethe thanked Reinhard with obvious sincerity for having sent him such a "handsome man": "One always fares better with worthy people in their presence than in their absence, for at a distance they usually turn that side towards us which we oppose, but when they are near, one easily finds out how far one may agree."[16]

Reinhard, in his turn, wrote to Sulpiz that he had pleased the old man though he had hardly converted him.[17] He proved to be right.

Their subsequent correspondence shows Sulpiz wooing the old man like a passionate lover, urging him to visit the Rhinelands and their collection: "If ever speech can exert a spell, I hope that heaven will now listen to me kindly and bestow on me the gift to persuade you and to make you proof against all doubts." In the autumn the Rhinelands showed themselves to their best advantage: "Nature herself imposes the law on you that you must visit us, and I count on your honoring a law from that beneficent hand as is your custom."[18]

Since Goethe was not to be moved, Sulpiz suggested they would take the collection to Weimar where it might be displayed: "You see I grasp the hand which you proffered so generously and lovingly with both my hands so that it should be my anchor for my whole life."

But such impetuosity was only too likely to make Goethe withdraw. He warned the young man that it was one thing to come to Weimar as a visitor, when all doors would be open to him, a very different one, however, to try and settle there for a time, which could only lead to disappointment.

Sulpiz was wise enough to take the hint, but he did not allow their friendship to cool during the year 1812, and he had the great satisfaction at the end of that year to find in the recently published installment of Goethe's memoirs that the episode of his early enthusiasm for the Strasbourg minister gave the author the welcome opportunity of referring to the revival of interest in Gothic architecture and to find a few words of praise for Sulpiz in this context. Meanwhile the frame of the collection, now displayed in Heidelberg, had grown, and such eminent visitors as Wilhelm von Humboldt and Jakob Grimm, not to speak of a stream of royalty, reinforced its reputation.

At last, in the autumn of 1814, more than three years after their first meeting in Weimar, Goethe's visit to the spa of Wiesbaden provided a convenient opportunity also for a trip to Heidelberg. He arrived on September 24 and stayed till October 9. The visit appeared to be an unqualified success, and a letter written by Sulpiz a fortnight after Goethe's departure shows that he was under the impression to have fully triumphed at last.

> Now let me tell you about Goethe. You will have heard that he stayed with us for a whole fortnight, but you don't know as yet that being together for this lengthy time, which was in every respect very instructive and profitable for us, we gained his full confidence and established a very close relationship. There is talk of writing a brief account about our collection, our efforts on behalf of old German architecture, and about the way which led us to these studies. "Confound it," he said to me several times, "the world does not yet know what you have and what you want. We intend to tell them, and since it so demands it we shall offer them the golden apples in silver bowls. When I come home I draw up the disposition that I'll send you for your comment and for looking it over to see what I may have missed, you send me all this and I see to the final redaction. It would be strange if we were incapable of achieving a fine result. It is difficult to write something of this kind, but I know my way about, leave it to me, I return at Easter time and bring it along, then we send it for printing to Mohr and Zimmer."[19]
>
> To realize fully what tremendous impression our pictures made on the old but vigorous friend you must know that he had never yet seen a van Eyck and no old German paintings at all except Cranach and a few Dürers. "Oh my dear children," he exclaimed almost every day, "how silly we are, how silly we are. We can't imagine that our grandmother was not also beautiful, those were of a different breed than we are. Yes, by heaven, their merits have to be acknowledged. They deserve it that Princes and Empresses and all Nations come to pay homage to them." Every morning (except when we were busy with architectural matters)

> he arrived in the picture gallery at eight and did not budge till lunchtime, when everything was reviewed and we had to tell him about all the historical evidence and about our opinions, after which he let us hear his own. He was well satisfied with our calm, philosophical and critical approach to the history of art, and I may say that I learned a good deal from him about the course of art history.[20]

A few days later Melchior reports in a letter to a friend that Goethe intends to write about the collection during the winter and then to return at Easter to revise and to get ready for printing.[21]

It cannot come as a surprise to the reader that these high hopes were not and possibly could not be fulfilled. No open breach is noticeable in the correspondence of the following months, but a note of anxiety creeps in when Sulpiz, having described in a letter the visits of the emperor to their gallery, remarks that however much his collection is praised, people are in need of an authority such as Goethe's and that he should therefore make his own opinions about these works known. In his anxiety Sulpiz repeats the appeal: "Carry out your promise of last year, carry out your promise of last year, you can then do something for German antiquities and for us which will offer pleasures to our contemporaries and bear fine fruits for posterity."[22]

But of course it was precisely this type of publicity which Goethe feared. He still disliked the romantic medievalizers, and he surely did not want to appear as a renegade to his old friends in Weimar who firmly believed in the classical principles of art.

Goethe had arranged to combine the second visit to Heidelberg with a tour of the Rhinelands in the company of the former Prussian Minister Freiherr von Stein, an idol of the romantics who had been dismissed from the service as persona non grata to Napoleon. When the two stood in front of the *Dombild* in Cologne Cathedral, the statesman implored the bystander to refrain from any political remark, because unhappily the great man was averse to all that.[23]

Sulpiz Boisserée who was of the party had ample opportunity to witness such manifestations of Goethe's hardening attitudes toward the creations and the taste of German romantic artists. Open and sincere as always, he sought an opportunity for probing the reasons for this bias by submitting some of his own writings on art to his admired friend, but a letter by Sulpiz of 15 September 1815 shows that Goethe refused to be drawn:

> Goethe said he liked my way of describing pictures, only he would not do it that way, because his whole view of art was different. When I asked him what this difference was he first did not want to reply. It was an antimony of their modes of thinking, that could not be helped, it would be useless to try and come to an understanding. We stuck to the subject matter and had to do so, it was right for us, it belonged to our approach, but it was not the ultimate. The minstrel was buried somewhere else [Der Spielmann sey noch irgend anders begraben].[24]

We shall see that Goethe's own account of Boisserée's paintings, on which he was to embark a few months later, can serve to explain this cryptic utterance What he had missed in these enthusiastic descriptions of Christian subjects was the attention to the formal aspects that could be discussed objectively and without gush. No wonder that the second visit to Heidelberg (September 27–October 7), which was to have enabled Goethe to revise his notes and impressions, proved less of a success than the first. There were too many distractions from visitors, and Goethe lapsed into a depression.

Even so he wrote or rather dictated the piece soon after his return to Weimar and had it published in the journal *Aus Kunst und Alterthum,* where it came out in the following spring.

There is an apologetic note in Goethe's letter to his intimate friend Carl Friedrich Zelter, announcing the arrival of the issue on March 11, 1816:

> The little pamphlet "From the Rhine and the Maid, art and antiquities" will reach you soon. I broke it off in the thirteenth sheet, like Sheherazade. Had I recognized the significance of such writings earlier on I would have refused the whole little deal, but I was seduced by and by and so let it flow on. In any case I must gratefully acknowledge the fact that without this urgent compulsion I would never have been able to pay attention to the importance of the preservation of the arts through barbaric ages nor to the peculiarities of their national and provincial restoration. There is much stuff there that resists our sublimated sensuality and that can only be turned into something by means of rational concepts, for the absurd gives us pleasure when we seek to understand it.[25]

If Goethe himself was somewhat noncommittal about his contributions, the Romantics regarded it as contemptible. Thus Dorothea Schlegel, Friedrich's wife, poured out her scorn in a letter on 3 July 1816:

> So this is now the diploma of artistic accolade for the sake of which the Boisserées spent so much time tailwagging to the old pagan. And how superfluous! God knows, whoever sees the collection and whose mind is not wholly closed does not need this stamp of approval to realize that the collection is unique in its way. The Boisserées will hardly be very satisfied with this platitudinous twaddle, but they will surely not omit pretending that they are golden words. The old childish man has tried to minimize Friedrich's merits in relation to the new appreciation of our earliest art by not mentioning him anywhere in this whole work.[26]

It can be safely left to the reader, who must be assumed to have the text of the essay (or its English translation) within reach, to judge how far this intemperate reaction was justified, but anyone who reads the account in its original context must feel sympathy for the two collectors who had pinned such high hopes on this publication. Far from being given pride of place, the section about Heidelberg follows after a survey of a good many other cities in the area from Cologne to Frankfurt and Darmstadt. To be sure a few friendly paragraphs are devoted to the two collectors, their intellectual background, and their achievement, but when the reader then expects to be ushered into the gallery he will be presented with a lengthy digression about the fate of art in the Dark Ages. A few pages are devoted to the *Dombild* (which Goethe had seen in Cologne), but strictly speaking only two of the many paintings in the gallery are singled out for description and appreciation, and even these are not so much discussed for their own sake but to illustrate those "rational concepts" of which Goethe had spoken in his letter to Zelter.

It is true that Sheherazade had promised to continue her story, and the brothers never ceased to urge Goethe to keep his promise. It is also true that a third visit which he planned for the autumn had come to nothing as the axle of the carriage in which he traveled with Heinrich Meyer broke, and the two but narrowly missed serious injury. But it cannot be denied that Goethe's theoretical misgivings had won over his personal sympathies and that he virtually let down his friends. If the essay is still worth reading it is precisely for the sake of those "conceptual constructions" which must have been Goethe's own. Indeed there is every reason to believe that this had been one of the points where Sulpiz acknowledged to have "learned a good deal" from Goethe, without, however, fully understanding what he was driving at.

Having given a conventional account of the rigid and mummified style of Byzantine painting which he knew from a few late Russian icons that he owned, Goethe takes a step back and explains the "great merits" which the style owed to the heritage of the Greeks and the Romans that had been preserved by the guilds.

> For when we referred to this style earlier on as mummified we must not forget that even in hollowed out bodies, dried and resinated muscles, the shape of the skeleton asserts its right. . . .
>
> The highest task of the visual arts is to decorate a particular interior or to create a decoration in an amorphous space. From this demand derives everything that we call an artistic composition, in which the Greeks and Romans were masters.
>
> Whatever is to impress us as a decoration must be articulated, and that in the superior sense so that it should consist of parts which are mutually related to each other. For this to happen it must have a middle, a top and a bottom, a here and a there which first creates that symmetry which can easily be grasped by reason and may be called the lowest degree of decoration. The more manifold, however, the elements become, and the more intricate that initial symmetry, hidden, alternating in contrasts, confronts our eyes as a visible mystery, the more pleasant will the effect of the decoration be, and indeed it will be perfect when we no longer think of these first foundations but are taken by surprise as if we were facing something arbitrary and casual.
>
> It is to this strict and dry symmetry that the Byzantine school always kept and though its pictures become stiff and unpleasant, there still occur cases where the variations in the position of figures confronting each other produces a certain grace . . . this advantage . . . was spread by the Eastern artists and craftsmen over the whole of the converted world.

After mentioning Italian mosaics which he had seen in the "highly esteemed" work of d'Agincourt, Goethe comes to speak of the Netherlands which had equally been dominated by the "Byzantine school."

A general characteristic of the awakening feeling for nature in these regions leads over to what may be called Goethe's masterpiece in Goethe's analytical description, his paragraph on the painting of St. Veronica in the collection (figs. 15.3 and 15.4), "because it can serve in various ways as an illustration of what has been said so far."

> Perhaps it will be found one day that this picture, as far as composition and drawing is concerned, represents a traditional type of Byzantine sacred art. The head of Christ crowned with thorns is dark brown, probably darkened by age, and shows a miraculously noble expression of pain. The corners of the cloth are held by the Saint who, little more than a third of life size, stands behind it and is hidden by it as far as her bust. Features and gestures are extremely graceful. The cloth rests at its lower edge on the indicated floor in whose corners on each side there sit very small singing angels, not taller than one foot if they were standing up; they are so beautifully and skilfully composed in two groups that they completely satisfy the highest demand of the laws of composition. The whole manner of thought at work in this picture points to a traditional well-considered and well-tried-out art. Consider the degree of abstraction necessary to present these fig-

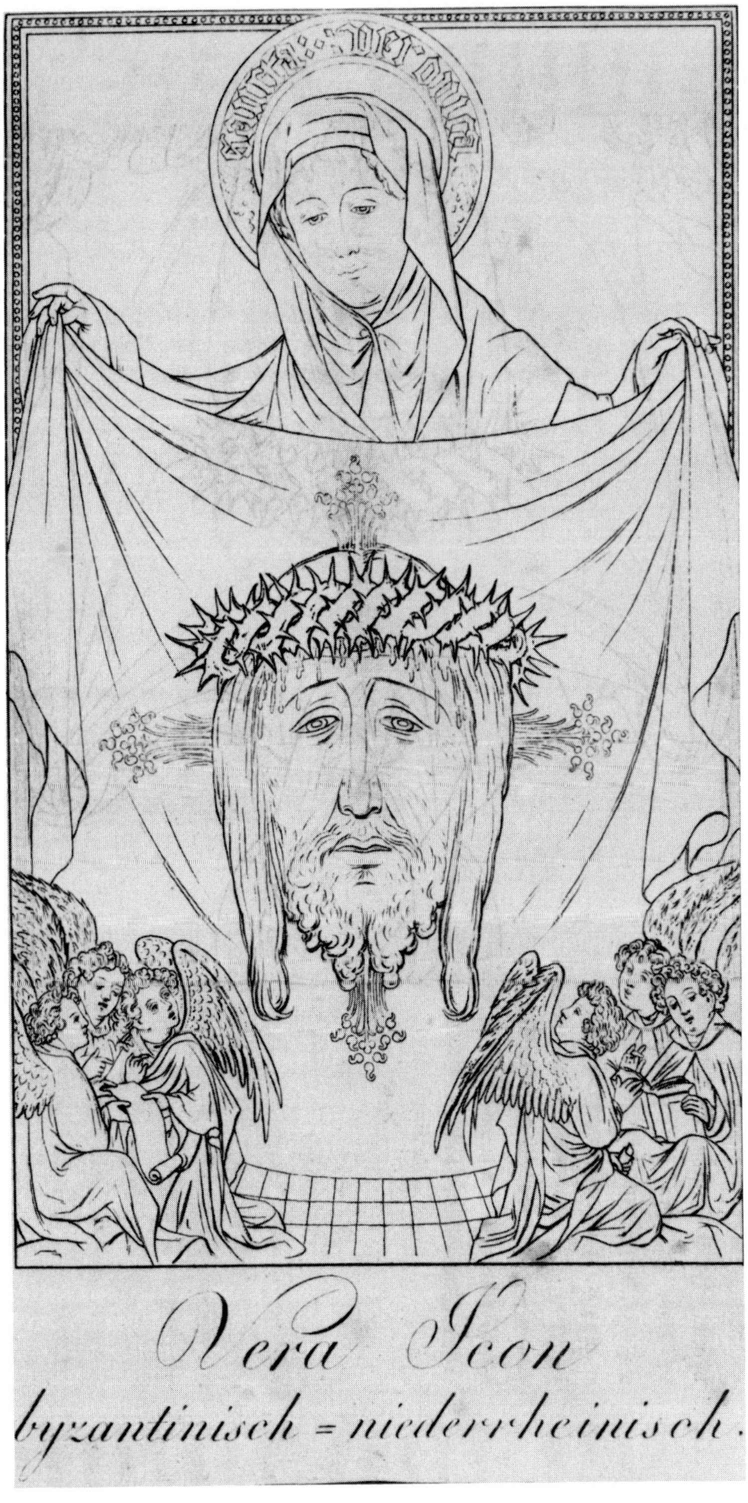

Fig. 15.3. Cologne Master, *St. Veronica*, c. 1410, from Goethe, *Über Kunst und Altertum I*, Stuttgart, 1818. By permission of the British Library.

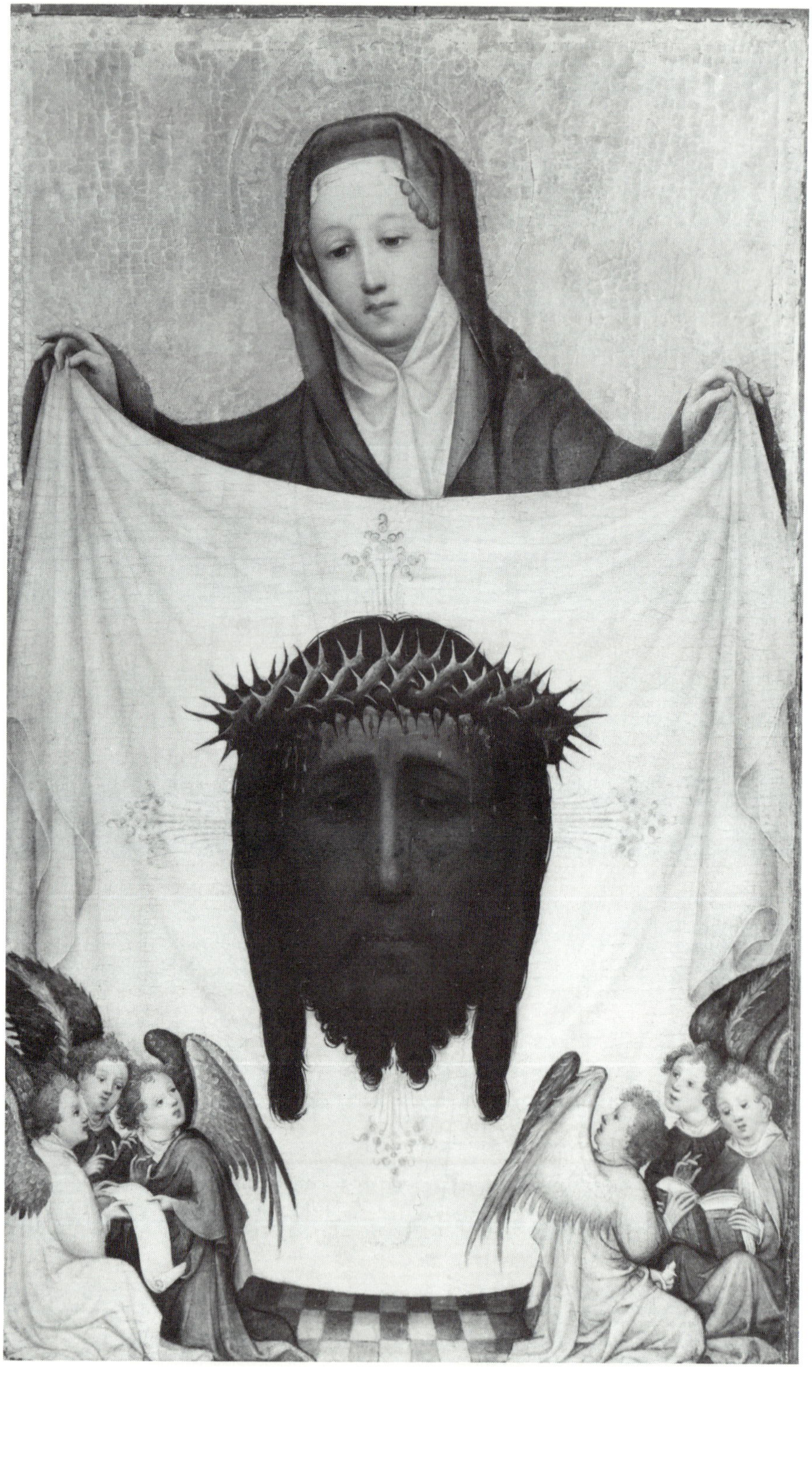

Fig. 15.4. Cologne Master, *St. Veronica*, c. 1410, Munich, Alte Pinakothek.

ures in three dimensions and to symbolize the whole so thoroughly. The little bodies of the angels but most of all their little heads and hands are so beautifully moved and placed in relation to each other that there is nothing to criticize here. If this observation may justify us in deriving the picture from Byzantine art, the charm and the softness with which the Saint is painted and the children are represented demand that we date the execution of the painting into that period of lower Rhenish art which we have already characterized. Combining as it does the twin elements of a strong idea and a pleasing execution it exerts an incredible power over the beholder, an effect to which the contrast between the terrible Medusa-like face and the graceful Virgin with the charming children contributes a great deal.

Turning to the *Dombild*, which, with the brothers Boisserée, he dated a generation too early, Goethe confines himself to the wish that its true merits would be assessed historically and critically, for at present it was "to such extent fumigated with hymns that it is to be feared that it will soon become so obscured to the eyes of the mind as it was when it was darkened by the soot of lamps and candles." In any case he places it in the epoch in which Jan van Eyck had already flourished, and so he comes to the artist to whom the complete revolution of art was to be attributed. The reader need hardly be reminded that the Columba altar, from which the brothers and their visitors derived their ideas of that art, was not by the van Eycks but by Rogier van der Weyden, but at least the painting suggested that one of the revolutionary steps was the discarding of the golden background that had marked the Byzantine tradition. As the passionate investigator of the theory of color, Goethe naturally had something relevant to say about the effects achieved by the "inventor of oil painting." "Even to mention only the rendering of drapery and of rugs he achieves a splendour of the panel that far exceeds the appearance of reality": "Indeed that is the task of real art, for our everyday vision is determined by infinite contingencies both regarding our eyes and the objects themselves, while the painter paints according to laws to show how the objects, separated from each other by light, shadow and colour, should be seen in their perfect visibility by a healthy fresh eye."

In addition van Eyck had mastered the art of perspective and "appropriated the variety of landscape features, especially an infinitude of buildings which meet the eye instead of the meager golden background or cloth."

But Goethe was obviously reluctant to give unqualified praise to an artist of whom he had never heard and who refused to fit into the classical canon of artistic perfection he and the Weimar friends of art had labored so hard to establish in German lands. The time had not yet come for him in which he was ready to proclaim a more latitudinarian attitude in the well known epigram:

But how can ever Jan van Eyck
By Phidias' side be set?
You must, if my advice you like,
Learn each in turn to forget.
For if with One we did remain
How could we fall in love again?
Such is the world, and such is art,
That passions come, as passions part.[27]

Being as yet unwilling to forget Phidias, Goethe proceeds to explain his reservations about the doctrine of progress in art, and in doing so he broke entirely new ground.

> At this point it may sound strange if we say that, in discarding the material and mechanical imperfections of the preceding artistic tradition, van Eyck also threw overboard a technical perfection that had so far been preserved unnoticed, the idea of symmetrical composition. But this also lies in the nature of an extraordinary mind, that in breaking through a material shell he never considers that beyond it there remains an ideal, spiritual limit against which he battles in vain, to which he must submit or which he has to recreate in his own way. Thus van Eyck's compositions exhibit the maximum of truth and loveliness though they fail to satisfy the strict demands of art. . . . In none of his paintings we got to know there is a group that could be set aside those little angels next to St. Veronica.

And so asking for the patience of his readers, he arrives at the formulation we set at the beginning of this essay, that "any progress from a rigid and artificial state toward a free and vital realism also implies a loss which can only be made good by and by, and frequently not before some time has elapsed."

There is a curious irony in the fact that this time had actually arrived with the style of Rogier van der Weyden whose triptych had been presented to Goethe as a work by the revolutionary Jan van Eyck. It is by now a commonplace of art historical studies that Rogier van der Weyden harked back to medieval types of composition. As I put it in my *Story of Art*, without, surely, thinking of Goethe's words, "He saved much of the tradition of lucid design that might otherwise have been lost under the impact of van Eyck's discoveries."

We have seen already that the picture of artistic development in the North worked out by the Boisserée brothers and accepted by Goethe was hopelessly inadequate. But it is precisely for this reason that one must wonder at Goethe's capacity to extract so profound a truth from such garbled information. One factor we have observed in the making—his reluctance to be entirely drawn to the side of the enthusiastic brothers. He did not want to be one of the incense swingers who were about to obscure the real merits of the *Dombild* and would surely also stand in the way of a just appreciation of the Eyckian revolution. It was part of the critical creed he had absorbed from the ancients that perfection was rare in art. Quintilian is typical there in his review of Greek sculptors: Polycletus surpasses the others in care and grace, but though he is accorded the prize by many, to avoid nothing being missed they say that he lacked grandeur; while Demetrius, at the end of Quintilian's list, is blamed for having been more fond of realism than of beauty.[28] The critic's task, therefore, to look for perfection in the Aristotelian mean between the reprehensible extremes was familiar to Goethe, but the way he turned it into a historical theory was his own. How did he come to conceive it?

All worthwhile criticism contains an element of self-criticism, and a case can certainly be made out for Goethe's having derived his critical insight from an examination of his own past. In the company of the Boisserées he had every reason to remember the days of his youth, his passion for Gothic architecture, and his contempt for the classical rules. As a leader of Sturm und Drang, he had thrown the Aristotelian canon to the wind in his play *Goetz von Berlichingen,* which made Herder exclaim, "Shakespeare has quite corrupted you." His slow conversion to classical ideals has been recorded and discussed in innumerable studies. What may not have been stressed, however, is the increasing tolerance he felt for the bugbear of his generation, French classical tragedy. When he went so far, as director of the Weimar theater, as even to stage Voltaire's *Mahomet,* Schiller, who had experienced a similar conversion after the naturalistic excesses of *Die Raueber,* found it necessary to justify this apparent betrayal of earlier ideals in a poem addressed to Goethe.[29] His justification sounds like a pre-echo of Goethe's defense of the Byzantine tradition. At a time of artistic lawlessness, Schiller explains, the French at least held fast to the inherited rules of drama and remained aware of the gulf that separates the realm of nature from the sphere of art. The very artificiality of Voltaire's stilted play could serve as an antidote to artistic anarchy: the value of a tradition, however desiccated, should not be overlooked.

> When real art to die appeared resigned,
> Wild fancy having all the power gained
> The highest and the lowest it combined
> In life and on the stage sheer chaos reigned
> Only among the French could art you find
> Although perfection they had not attained
> They held it tight in the unyielding grip
> Of rigid rules that it should never slip . . .
> To them the stage is always holy ground
> And strictly banished from its festive site
> Is nature's raw and unrefined sound
> Here speech itself is a melodious rite[30]

In other words: better a mummified classicism than none at all. There is no reason to doubt that Goethe here shared Schiller's view.

These speculations about the roots of Goethe's critical insights must of necessity remain conjectural. What can be documented, however, is the influence his analysis had on the budding discipline of art history. In 1827, eleven years after the publication of Goethe's controversial essay, Carl Friedrich Rumohr (1785–1842), an almost exact contemporary of the Boisserée brothers, published his *Italienische Forschungen* which may be called the foundation charter of German art historical studies.[31] There we read that "the highest and most indispensible stylistic law of painting . . . demands that order and internal relations must be observed both in the composition and distribution of representational and of merely decorative and filling forms and configurations."[32] Having adopted this point of view, it is only consistent that Rumohr expresses the same reservations about Giotto that Goethe expressed about van Eyck. True, he must be praised for his cheerful observation of life, but in developing naturalism he "led to the progressive estrangement from the ideals of Christian antiquity."[33]

The extent to which this re-valuation of artistic values affected the course of nineteenth- and twentieth-century art appreciation would have to be the topic of a separate study, to be presented to Elizabeth Holt on her ninetieth birthday.

NOTES

1. *Aus einer Reise am Rhein, Main und Neckar in den Jahren 1814 und 1815. Goethes sämtliche Werke, Jubiläumsausgabe in 40 Bänden* (Stuttgart and Berlin, no date), XXIX, pp. 235–332.

2. *Goethe on Art*, selected, edited and translated by John Gage (London, 1980). See also my review in *Art History*, 2 (June 1982): 237–246. The translations in the text are mine.

3. Eduard Firmenich-Richartz, *Die Brüder Boisserée, I, Sulpiz und Melchior Boisseree als Kunstsammler* (Jena, 1916), henceforward cited as F.-R. The translations in the text are mine.

4. *Friedrich Schlegel, Kritische Gesamtausgabe*, ed. Ernst Behlder, IV (Paderborn etc., 1959).

5. Elizabeth G. Holt, *A Documentary History of Art*, II (New York, 1958), pp. 360–369.

6. F.-R. pp. 63/64. The fragment of an autobiography (undated) was first published by Sulpiz' widow in *Sulpiz Boisserée*, I (Stuttgart, 1862) pp. 15–45. The murals from the church of St. Laurence are lost. A full survey and bibliography of the history of painting in Cologne in the fourteenth and early fifteenth century is to be found in the catalogue of an exhibition at the Wallraf-Richartz Museum, Cologne, March-July 1974, *Vor Stefan Lochner, Die Kölner Maler von 1300 bis 1430* (Cologne, 1974).

7. F.-R., 99–108. The passage quoted is on p. 100.

8. Ibid., 101.

9. Ibid., 61.

10. Ibid., 120.

11. Ibid., 120–21.

12. Ibid., 121–22.

13. Ibid., 122–26.

14. Ibid., 127.

15. For this and the following, ibid., 128–35.

16. Ibid., 144.

17. Ibid.

18. Ibid., 148–50.

19. Ibid., 152.

20. Ibid., 206–207.

21. Ibid., 208.

22. Ibid., 213.

23. Ibid., 217.

24. Ibid., 207.

25. Ibid., 229.

26. Ibid., 242–43.

27. "Modernes." See my review in *Art History* 2 (June 1982), 238.

28. Quintilian, *Institutio Oratoria* 12, x: 9.

29. "An Goethe, als er den Mahomet von Voltaire auf die Bühne brachte." (1800).

30. Es droht die Kunst vom Schauplatz zu verschwinden,
Ihr wildes Reich behauptet Phantasie;
Die Bühne will sie wie die Welt entzünden,
Das Niedrigste und Höchste menget sie.
Nur bei dem Franken war noch Kunst zu finden,
Erschwang er gleich ihr hohes Urbild nie;
Gebannt in unveränderlichen Schranken
Halt er sie fest, und nimmer darf sie wanken.
Ein Heiliger Bezirk ist ihm die Szene;
Verbannt aus ihrem festlichen Gebiet
Sind der Natur nachlässig rohe Töne,
Die Sprache selbst erhebt sich ihm zum Lied
(The translation in the text is mine.)

31. See Julius von Schlosser's introduction to the reprint 1920 (Frankfurt/Main), titled *Carl Friedrich von Rumohr als Begründer der neueren Kunstforschung*.

32. Ibid., 65.

33. Ibid., 273.

16

CHARLES CLÉMENT and the FRENCH LANDSCAPE

HANS LÜTHY

MODERN ART HISTORY has in the past largely overlooked the presence of Charles Clément among the art and cultural critics working primarily during the Second Empire in Paris.[1] Above all, his biography of Théodore Gericault assured Clément of immortality; his catalogue of Gericault's complete works, documenting the paintings, drawings, sculptures, and lithographs, is acknowledged to the present day as an early and classic example of a balanced, art-historically oriented work. (That catalogue appeared originally in the *Gazette des Beaux Arts* and subsequently, in 1868, as the appendix to the biography.) Particularly his rather rational, "scientific" approach, in which the author's presence was secondary to his material, distinguished him clearly from many contemporaries, who brought a more partisan perspective to their texts. Clément, on the other hand, attempted to preserve historical distance even from contemporary art, on which he regularly wrote in the *Journal des Débats* after 1863 as Etienne Delécluze's successor.

By the time Michel Lévy Frères of Paris published an anthology of his essays in 1865, Clément could already look back on a series of publications that were concerned to a great extent with earlier art history (for example, 1861 biographies of Michelangelo, Leonardo da Vinci, and Raphael, as well as the 1862 catalogue of the jewels of the *Musée Napoléon III*). The texts collected in *Etudes sur les Beaux-Arts en France* (1865) begin chronologically, with an article on Nicolas Poussin, which had originally appeared in 1850 in the *Revue des Deux Mondes*. The anthology's essays discuss Alexandre Gabriel Decamps (first published in 1858), Eugène Delacroix (1863), Hippolyte Flandrin (1864), Charles Gleyre (1863), Ernest Meissonier (1863), modern church murals (1864), the Decree on the Académie des Beaux-Arts of 13 November 1864 (1864), and conclude with the study "Les Paysagistes français contemporains" (which will be examined in detail below).

This last, a text of approximately eighty pages, is a reprint of an article originally published in 1853. Clément justified the reprinting of this article, which probably represents his earliest opinion about contemporary art, in an initial footnote as follows: "This study ... is already out of date. Some of our better painters, justifiably celebrated today, are not even mentioned in it. Others who have not fulfilled what their beginnings promised, occupy places of too great importance."[2] Nevertheless, continued Clément, the publication seemed correct to him, because it mirrored the judgments of a particular moment. Clément had at the time lived among a circle of artists whose commentaries, theories, and hopes he had recorded; his aim was to convey (to the reader) the sentiments of a certain period of his youth.

In 1852, Clément was thirty-two years old. After his father, a textile manufacturer in Rouen, died in 1831, Clément spent his childhood with his Swiss mother in the small town of Rolle on Lake Geneva. He studied philosophy and mineralogy in Geneva, Lausanne, Heidelberg, and Tübingen. Midway through the 1840s he established himself in Paris as a private tutor and traveled to London several times between 1848 and 1850. The lengthy article on Poussin, which was first published in several installments in the *Revue des Deux Mondes* in 1850, marked the beginning of Clément's career as an *homme de lettres*. Clément happened onto this path through his friendships with artists, for example (from 1846) with Charles Gleyre, the art critic Gustave Planche, and the young Swiss painter Fritz Berthoud, who at the time was a pupil of Gleyre. Already in his first texts Clément appears well-read, confident and objective. In "Poussin" he already attempted to characterize his own century with the following words:

> This mature century [i.e., the seventeenth century] knew neither this worry, nor this unhealthy sadness which devours us; things which are so intimately part of us, that it seems impossible to discover their origin and to dislodge them: evil inheritance which circulates in our veins and which we have imbibed along with the sustenance from our mothers' breasts.[3]

Elsewhere in the text on Decamps, the reader may discern an equal observation on the perfected times. After establishing Jean-Jacques Rousseau's growing influence, he goes on to describe Rousseau's thought as "un peu maladive." Clément observed that the revival of interest in Rousseau took place for the following reason: "When strong and noble ideas no longer hold up, and human events are such that they create neither the desire to see them nor to paint them, the saddened spirit plunges itself with delight into this source, that vaguely reflects, but not without precision, our sentiments and our passions."[4] Here, Clément referred to the representation of nature by means of landscape painting. It follows logically that landscape painting was, for Clément, the dangerous area in modern art. In "Decamps," as well, Clément again evaluated his own situation:

> But in periods of transition such as ours, nothing which surrounds him helps the poet, and quite to the contrary creates obstacles for him: the confusion of ideas, the ignorance and hostility of some of the public, the passion of materialistic interests, the forgetting and mistrust of the past, the indifference towards the future, convictions treated like chimeras. . . . What can the poet do in the midst of this disorder, and how can he extricate himself from this chaos?[5]

These passages seem, for the present, to offer a somewhat one-sided characterization of Clément; they reflect only one aspect of a world view which was in all probability temporarily influenced by Charles Gleyre's much more fundamental cultural despair. In any case, Clément's friendships and writing demonstrate that he was by no means a revolutionary. "Test carefully the new, acknowledge its advantages, and pronounce a balanced judgment": this philosophy may be said to address the essence of Clément's writings.

The essay "Les paysagistes français contemporains" demonstrates a clear structure. Clément pursued the various aspects of French landscape painting from 1800 to 1850 in its principal and secondary themes, described its rise and fall, attempted to justify, criticize, and praise it; and closed with a discussion of the prospect for a brighter future.

Clément began his essay by considering the succession of painters whose styles derived from Poussin's work—from David, through Pierre-Henri de Valenciennes and Victor Bertin to Achille-Etna Michallon. For Clément, the work of these painters embodied the French classical tradition. Michallon's work heralded the decline of that tradition in a loss of strength, vitality, and meaning. Clément perceived the transition to the *pittoresque* in the work of Jean-Charles-Joseph Rémond, a student of Michallon; this meant for him the end of the *tableau de style*. In Louis-Etienne Watelet's landscapes Clément saw another danger: "He adheres even more closely to nature, but what nature—affected, embellished, diminished." Clément reached a devastating verdict in this context, a verdict which dismisses the audience for such paintings: "They are all cheeky young working girls [*grisettes*] who stopped before these romantic and coquettish landscapes." *Peinture d'histoire*-related landscape painting, on the other hand, has, according to Clément, historical significance of its own. Indeed, it renewed the vitality of landscape painting, albeit by providing an unsuccessful model.[6]

Clément next turned his attention to the origins of the *école moderne*. In his eyes, a second, ever-strengthening genre was developing alongside the Greco-Roman landscape painting inspired by David. Clément recognized its roots in the work of Antoine-Jean Gros and Gericault; with Richard Parkes Bonington and Delacroix, the form developed more fully. Gericault as well as Gros had painted with a feeling for *réalité* which was absent in David's work and which served as the point of departure for the *sentiment moderne*. Bonington was already noted by Clément as one of *la nouvelle école:* "The impression he received substitutes itself for the portrait. . . . The subjective sentiment substitutes itself for tradition. . . . The diffusion, the diversity and the absence of discipline" are further characteristics of the new school.

After 1830, Clément acclaimed a new generation; he named it "first foundlings of paintings." Young, talented artists between sixteen and twenty, who had been trained as craftsmen, formed friendships and on Sundays together they discovered the beauties of the banks of the Seine outside Paris. Their first attempts at painting these landscapes showed "a lively and naive sentiment, sincere in color." Only after the development of a second phase, which grew largely out of independent study in the Louvre, did these artists acquire the techniques of the Dutch painters of the seventeenth century. Clément at this point revealed the identities of this group: Nicolas-Louis Cabat, Jules Dupré, Camille Flers, Narcisse Diaz.

Clément did not bring the chronology of the birth years of these painters into the discussion; his reasons for this omission are not mentioned in his commentary. In any case, he placed Cabat (born 1812) at the head of the group and designated Cabat's painting *L'Etang de Ville d'Avray,* which won a second-place medal at its debut at the Salon of 1834, as the first signal of the group's success. This is reminiscent of Theophile Gautier's enthusiastic review of the sensation Cabat created in 1834.

Clément further described how Cabat had escaped from the outskirts of Paris, which he had found restrictive, to Normandy; and how Flers had discovered Picardy with his paintbrush, while Dupré had depicted isolated areas of Berry and Touraine. Cabat was almost always analyzed as the exception, because he had attempted during the course of his career to progress from the simple landscape *(paysage de genre)* to the classical landscape *(paysage de style)*. This was also the first time that Clément fully presented the theory of the romantic landscape, which focuses on the detail as the central subject of the entire composition: "Monsieur Cabat starts at the small and arrives at the greatest." Or, in a slightly different formulation, "From reality he reaches imagination, from the picturesque he moves on to style." Cabat's work of this time had blurred the distinctions between genre and style: Cabat the philosopher had distorted the view of Cabat the artist. On the other hand, Clément particularly praised Cabat's Italian landscapes because of "a general tinge of melancholy and reverie that belongs to our time."

Clément then went on to discuss Camille Corot, whom he promptly characterized equally an exception. It was impossible to view him as a member of any of these schools. Corot was basically a *peintre de style* who did not make use of the academic apparatus. A few of Clément's key phrases on Corot follow:

> More dreaming than thinking, it is through contemplation that he arrives at Art. ... He is concerned with but one thing: to render his impression simply and naively. It is the improvisation with its charm, the sketch which interests precisely because it is not fixed.... He is a magician. He captures in the rapid sketch, the secret of the fleeting moment, aspects that endure only an instant.

These formulations are above reproach, and for the most part they are still valid today. Clément also recognized the importance of the *valeurs* and in summary characterizes Corot as follows: "the constant elevation of thought and above all, a harmony that results less from its coloration which is very thin and almost monochrome, as from values which are absolutely accurate."[7]

In a minor digression on Corot's technique (faulted time and time again by other critics for being too roughly sketched), Clément sided with Corot, claiming that this point should not be overemphasized. Technique should not be an end in itself and "an excessive technical perfection has always corresponded to decadence in art." Clément followed this sideswipe at the tradition of the Academy with a conclusion about the art of Corot: "Monsieur Corot gives us the impression of a man who would write charming things, but who would never give them this definitive form which imposes them on the spirit." In the same breath Clément acknowledged the exceptional advantages which he recognized in Corot's writing: "Above all the pure, true, heroic, profound sentiment of things." This is also the point at which Clément uses the word *Grec;* his intention is to convey a deep humanism, rising above the differences of the *écoles*.

While Clément had previously addressed the requirements of the *peinture moderne* and discussed its exceptions, he now arrived at the immediate present. He briefly described the significance of Gros, Gericault, and Xavier Sigalon again, invoked, in this respect, Delacroix and Sigalon *("par ses conseils")* and then concluded that it was not really possible to define and classify a truly modern school. The characteristics of contemporary landscape painting were: "No doctrine, no school, no association, but rather the most absolute individualism." The formulas of art of the past were depleted, and painters of the day corresponded to the pioneers of the far West. But—the antithesis appears once again—absolute beauty did not change more or less than the human body.

A long passage follows, which portrays the very best of French art criticism, and follows a digression on seascape painting, concerning "the two inimical brothers," Dupré and Rousseau. They became for Clément the premise upon which the work of the youngest landscape painters was based. Our author now called for the second time upon the "fragment theory": "[That which Rousseau paints,] ... it is not a visage, but a single trait of the countenance, a unique and striking aspect, always true, but ordinarily more curious than beautiful." Then Clément attempted to delineate clear boundaries between Dupré and Rousseau: "Monsieur Rousseau only preoccupies himself with rendering any impression with force and truth." But with respect to Dupré's work he said:

> The subject plays a principal role in his paintings. He searches above all for the appropriateness, the accord of lines; he subordinates accessories and concentrates the interest on the central point of the composition and thus comes closer to a painting of style. . . . Dupré arrives, but through falsification, at that which would appear to us to be the greatest principle of art. The question is this: Should art be exact representation, a close copy of its model, or its interpretation? For us, the response is not in doubt: Art transforms the subject.[8]

Clément is quoted at greater length here because his viewpoint was more clearly expressed than usual. By saying that nature cannot be imitated but only interpreted, Clément consolidated his position. If Dupré had attempted to single out one spot in a painting, to give it a special and particular resemblance to nature, the harmony of the whole would have been lost. The technical means available at the time, specifically the range of the palette, would not permit a representation of the model of nature without a significant loss in value. With the example of *Le Passage du gué,* Clément articulated his reservations and criticisms: the exceptional qualities of even this outstanding painting were contained in the boldness of the execution, rather than in the balance of composition, value, and color which Clément considered so important. In a true *tour de force,* Dupré often overemphasized the most extreme value in a work by structuring the entire painting around it. "Monsieur Dupré often succeeds, but he himself must perceive that he sometimes attempts the impossible." These suggestions seem more like warnings to Dupré that he should not continue on this path. We will not consider, at this moment, whether such recommendations—often pronounced by other art critics of this time as well—were ever taken to heart.

All the same Clément recognized a striving towards the *tableau de style* in Dupré's work; in Rousseau's paintings, to the contrary, the inherent dangers were greater than the pleasure derived from unquestionable talents. First, Clément mentioned Rousseau's tendency towards the roughly sketched. "The works shown to the public are, for the most part, nothing but studies which should keep that name, to receive the praises which they merit." While Clément acknowledged the "textual representation of nature" in Rousseau's work, he nevertheless criticized Rousseau's neglect of beauty. Studying *Bords de l'Oise,* for example, the observer may be baffled by the extraordinary *realité* of the individual elements in the painting, but he would sense, again, the lack of beauty. Rousseau tended above all to the representation of "impressions" in many variations; Rousseau was "a naturalist painter above all, he gives a single cachet of the truth." The execution, though, was undisciplined and insufficient according to Clément. Following this criticism, Clément comments for the very first time on the public and its expectations: "the crowd that cares little about studies or fragments, but that wants paintings, that demands that one present it not with subjective and incomplete impressions, but with general and synthetic impressions, works of art." If art had the goal, namely, to represent nature precisely and literally, continues Clément, then the only art forms could be the daguerrotype and the diorama. Rousseau possessed the ability to reproduce more than mere nature; now, he must continue to pursue that goal. Clément ends this analysis with the hope that "the naturalists are more idealists than they think."[9]

Clément addressed Constant Troyon and François-Louis Français more summarily. He found the following formulation for Troyon's work: "It is nature that the worker loves... covered with herds and harvests... one speaks rural dialect there." On the subject of Français' painting *Novembre* Clément commented "very true, experienced in a lively way, very finely executed." Français however held too closely to the drawing and placed too little emphasis on color: "But the drawing of a picture must not be one of a vignette. Detail is too dominant." In Français' work as well, Clément discovered a tendency toward *style,* but then reprimanded him: "But he will only achieve this superior level of art when he gives his compositions, which are until now more fragments than pictures, greater size and unity."[10]

Following these characterizations of the major contemporary landscape painters, Clément undertook to clarify the relationships between these painters and romanticism in several more general reflections:

> These painters are romantics. They divide the impressions which must produce the object. They throw all the light, all the interest on certain points within their compositions, and, through their search for detail, compromise the general effect. A painting, made thus of fragments, disperses the attention and does not produce a lively and lasting impression.... One doesn't experience the profound emotion which monuments of beauty make one feel.

As though apologizing for the painter as individual, Clément now made several pointed remarks about the background of the artistic scene. He almost abruptly brought up the conflict between science and art. The *métier* was overvalued today: "The vice of that time and also of today. ... The system has always been fatal to the arts." Similar thoughts appeared in Clément's text "L'Académie des Beaux-Arts et le Décret du 13 Novembre" roughly ten years later. Defining romanticism yet again, Clément wrote: "Romanticism divides, takes a trait and exposes it to greater light and gives it a value that it doesn't have. This trait is, above all *singular,* and we understand this word in both its meanings, *unique* and *bizarre.*" For this reason romanticism was an idea gone astray; it was by far too concerned with the examination and analysis of a detail, diverting attention from the whole. Art was however *"ni analytique ni scientifique,"* but rather generalizing. Man had the obligation of applying his intellect to an all-too-diffuse nature to create order from chaos. In a rare flash of humor, Clément then noted that a microscope could more easily be purchased than genius.

In the next section, Clément discussed the orientalists, essentially Alexandre-Gabriel Decamps and Prosper Marilhat. Decamps (to whom Clément was to dedicate a book in 1886) was one of the artists blessed with an original imagination, and was comparable to Sterne or Hoffmann; while Decamps was highly praised by Clément, his many imitators were reprimanded. Marilhat on the other hand showed us the other, more sober aspect of orientalist art: *"peintre exact et naturaliste."* In the picture *Bains de Diane,* the naturalist dominated the dreamer, and in *Arabes syriens en voyage* a very simple and true gift for observation became visible; Marilhat succeeded in rendering his impressions in a vivid and enduring manner. Clément described Eugène Fromentin as Marilhat's best student, although the *pittoresque,* only one aspect of art—and one of the least convincing—still dominated his work. In general, the Orient was an exception, as was the Oriental landscape: "This nature does not talk enough."[11]

Clément then discussed Diaz, whom he considered the last of the orientalists. He once again reproached the unfinished nature of Diaz' works: "His works almost always resemble rough sketches a bit," and found favorable response only because of their sparkle and charm. Clément praised Diaz' *palette féerique* and concluded again with the general: "All the importance of the modern school of landscape is with the colorists, with the naturalists."

For Clément, the only opposition to the romanticists had been offered by a small group "in the name of drawing and of style." Théodore Aligny, an architect of painting, had been the first to take up the gauntlet (Clément cited *Prométhée* and *Le Bon samaritain* as examples); he was joined by Paul Flandrin, Alexandre Desgoffe and Edouard Bertin. Flandrin was apostrophized as a born poet; he was thoroughly Latin, *"du temps d'Auguste et de l'école de Horace."* He was not, however, successful in introducing color and life into his paintings, which combined only balance, harmony, and a rhythmical cadence of line. Desgoffe and Bertin worked to unify *style* and *verité,* and Clément particularly praised Bertin's intentions. However, those intentions were too seldom realized for his success to be fully acknowledged.[12]

In the end, salvation would not come from this group, least of all in the revival of the *peinture de style.* "This abstract and icy nature is not nature... this art of great intentions, but which lacks reality, is not art." Clément further insists: "Nothing breathes, nothing lives in this grandiose and petrified nature, and when life is missing, everything is missing."[13]

The four pages which follow contain Clément's conclusions and a final observation. His discussion of the existential difficulty of the *peinture de style* led him to inquire whether *les naturalistes* are preferable, to which he responds skeptically: "The naturalist school... born of necessity, has thrown itself into an extreme." He very unambiguously declared that the battle over romanticism had taken place and that the romanticists had triumphed; he believed that these soldiers could now, finally, cast off their "habits of violence and exaggeration, taken up in the fight." But landscape painting of all forms led to many bad habits, since precise drawing and the outline had less influence here than in figure painting. The human figure afforded the painter significantly less scope than did interpretation of the landscape: "The inanimate nature has a thousand caprices which imparts a vagueness and gives rise to the most diverse interpretations." Moreover, the landscape painter must resist much greater temptations: "Also, it is less nature than taste, less truth than beauty, with which one must preoccupy oneself in this genre of painting more than in any other."

Since nature gave the artist greater freedom, continued Clément, it was his responsibility to take advantage of that freedom in a way that interpreted the model according to the rules of a strict aesthetic *gout sevère.* Clément postulated that nature was a base from which art may—must—raise itself onto a poetic, even absolute plateau. "In our mediocre century we content ourselves with imperfect works... couldn't modern painting, nonetheless, become greater and above all reach perfection?" Although a *peinture de style proprement dit* could no longer exist, the *style* could only return *along* the circuitous route of *peinture d'histoire.* At present the requirements for this return simply did not exist. Modern painting must command a greater unity and power and a more systematic composition. It must, in other words, emphasize the spirit and the feeling in a work over its *métier* or technique.

Generally speaking, the substantive presence of modern painting could not be denied. "The modern school has rediscovered life which is the first condition of art. In pushing its researches in diverse directions, it has often strayed, but it has enlarged the field of painting."

Clément closed his essay with a call for confirmation: modern painters must bestow art with true monuments once again. Clément regarded the present situation as a compromise between "modern sentiment and composition and the teachings of tradition." His final sentence leaves a conciliatory and hopeful effect: After several pioneers had exhausted themselves in the battle, the future now belonged to the new.

A balanced, fully-detailed tribute to Clément's essay is impossible under the given conditions; the definitions alone of the terms *beauté, realité, verité,* and *style* would exceed the limits of this article. Several highlights must therefore suffice to outline Clément's position. As originally pointed out, Clément has been little noted among the art critics of 1850–80, while his monographs on Gericault and Gleyre are often quoted and remain indispensable tools of art historical research. All the same, he is represented (albeit without the advantage of today's more dependable information) in Joseph C. Sloane's 1951 list of the more important writers on art, which covers the period 1848–70.[14]

What inspired Clément to write the article under examination here? The creation of the Prix de Rome for landscape painting (1817), the official honoring of pure landscape painters, such as Cabat, in the Salons, and finally the decline of the previously influential neoclassical school after 1845 were milestones in the rapid and bewildering development of landscape as subject in the first half of the nineteenth century.[15] The public sought signs and found them in the texts of critics (published in the better periodicals). The journal, *La Revue des Deux-Mondes,* founded in 1829 and edited since 1831 by François Buloz, had a circulation of 16,000 in 1850. Intended for the prosperous, educated reader, this periodical offered a potpourri of political and cultural material that did not attempt to put forward a uniform party line. Gustave Planche, whom Clément had known since 1846 and who probably furnished him access to Buloz, was a regular contributor to this journal. In the 1850 article dedicated to Poussin, Clément already revealed a gift for linking historical thinking with the condition of contemporary artists. Indeed, according to everything we know, Clément turned to art criticism after befriending the painters Gleyre and Berthoud.

Charles Gleyre and (after 1850) Théodore Gericault were for Clément central figures in the art historical development of the first half of the nineteenth century.[16] Again and again, Clément measured other artists against these two, and their names occur in almost every essay in *Etudes sur les Beaux-Arts en France.* Although Gericault had only peripherally touched upon pure landscape painting, his early masterpiece *The Lime Kiln* marks the beginning of the unassuming realism of the simple landscape motif. In the 1830s in the Orient, Gleyre created outstanding landscape sketches and watercolors, but after 1840 he turned instead to the historical landscape and the figure. Clément's fascination with the pure landscape, therefore, is probably based more upon a tangential, theoretical interest than upon a direct desire for the visual. Several pertinent descriptions of landscapes by Dupré and Troyon seem to contradict this belief, but Clément's corresponding passages on figure paintings by Gericault, Leopold Robert, and Gleyre seem even more convincing. It may without question be assumed that Clément was familiar with the two basic treatises on landscape painting by Pierre-Henri de Valenciennes (1800) and Jean-Baptiste Deperthes (1818), and that he himself assumed the same of his readers. Albert Boime has proven how intensively both

Valenciennes and Rodolphe-Léon Deperthes were still read into the second half of the nineteenth century and how great was their influence on several painters. Such important critics as Gustave Planche (born in 1808) and Paul Mantz (born in 1821) represented similar theories, with which Clément does not basically differ; thus he may be associated with a more conservative direction. Charles Baudelaire and Champfleury (both born in 1821) took opposing and, above all, much more aggressive positions. Clément's work is based, from an intellectually historical viewpoint, very clearly on the conceptions of traditional academic painting, applying those theories to measure the value of contemporary painting. On the other hand, paralleling Planche and Mantz, his view remains sufficiently objective to permit him to describe and positively acknowledge new phenomena.

The goal of the critics of this era, however, was as difficult as squaring the circle: how can an author simultaneously call for *beauté* and *style* as the lodestars of painting, while at the same time promoting *verité* and *sentiment moderne* as the greatest advantages of the work of his contemporaries? Valenciennes was the first to admit his inability to resolve these contradictions. Clément entangled himself even deeper in the duality of his theoretical demands on art and his sensitivity to the great painterly qualities of the artists he discusses. Perhaps the problem stems from the difficulty of defining these terms which, as previously mentioned, was an obstacle for Clément and forced theoretical reversals upon him several times. Upon reexamination of Clément's conclusions on Gericault, his ideals together with their contradictions become more evident: although art must return to reflect upon itself and reestablish the relationship with real life, it must also ennoble *réalité,* raising it to a *naturalisme élevé.*[17] This concept contains Clément's basic message to contemporary artists, which is in fact only partially borne out by the future. As a typical example of the discussion prevalent during the beginning of the Second Empire, Clément's work, especially his arguments for and against the landscape painting that developed so magnificently during that period, remains of interest.

NOTES

It was a great pleasure to write this chapter as a Getty Scholar at the Getty Center for the History of Art and the Humanities in Santa Monica, California. I am very much indebted to the staff of the Center's Library and Photo Archive. I especially thank Ingred Globig for her translation; Constance Moffatt, a Center intern, for practical help; Dr. Barbara Gaehtgens for her ideas, and my fellow scholar, Dr. Thomas Gaehtgens, for correcting the text.

1. Cf. Hans A. Lüthy, "Charles Clément, Biographer of Gericault and Gleyre," in *Source,* no. 1 (Fall, 1983) 28–30.

2. Cf. Lorenz Eitner, "Introduction." In Charles Clément, *Gericault,* reimpression de l'édition de 1879 (Paris, 1973).

3. Charles Clément, *Etudes sur les Beaux-Arts en France* (Paris: Michel Lévy Frères, 1865), 3.

4. Ibid., 142.

5. Ibid., 172.

6. Ibid., 322.

7. Ibid., 337.

8. Ibid., 350.

9. Ibid., 358. This is a very important sentence.

10. Ibid., 364.

11. Ibid., 378.

12. Ibid., 386. In 1872 Clément wrote an essay on Bertin, as a note to an exhibition of Bertin's paintings and drawings at the *Ecole des Beaux-Arts* in Paris.

13. Ibid., 389–93.

14. Joseph C. Sloane, *French Painting between the Past and the Present: Artists, Critics and Traditions from 1848 to 1870* (Princeton, N.J., 1951), App. 217–26.

15. The most important publications on the theory and the development of landscape painting are:

—Rosenthal, Leon, *Du Romantisme au Realisme: Essai sur l'évolution de la peinture en France de 1830 à 1848* (Paris, 1914).

—Grate, Pontus, *Deux Critiques d'Art de l'Epoque Romantique: Gustave Planche et Théophile Thoré* (Stockholm, 1959).

—Boime, Alfred, *The Academy and French Painting in the Nineteenth Century* (London, New York, 1971).

—Weisberg, Gabriel P., *The Realist Tradition, French Painting and Drawing 1830–1900* (Cleveland, 1980).

—Herbert, Robert L., *Barbizon Revisited* (Boston, 1962).

—Bouret, Jean, *The Barbizon School and 19th century French Landscape Painting* (Greenwich, Conn., 1973) [lavishly illustrated].

16. Cf. the forthcoming *Catalogue raisonné* by William Hauptman.

17. Clément in his essay on Delacroix, 1863, *Etudes,* 186.

17

FRIEDRICH SCHLEGEL'S RESPONSE to RAPHAEL in PARIS

JANE VAN NIMMEN

AT THE LOUVRE in the summer of 1802 Friedrich Schlegel (1772–1829) sired a new breed of art critic. Undiscovered or neglected paintings of the past became for the first time the quarry of an intellectual effort almost archaeological in impulse. A number of writers would henceforth make it their business to unwrap long-entombed painters, one after another, from shrouds of neglect. As their Lazarus miracles resurrected forgotten or maligned schools, such critics, consciously or unconsciously, consigned others to the attic, where future generations would find and burnish them with renewed esteem. These dialectical pulses of demolition and discovery, reburial and resuscitation, beat in some of the nineteenth century's most distinctive critical hearts: William Hazlitt, Théophile Thoré, John Ruskin, the Goncourts, and, finally, Bernard Berenson, all operated in this new mode. Their work had an expansive effect on taste. The trinity of immortal painters reigning in the late eighteenth century—Raphael, Correggio, and either Titian or Michelangelo—had become by midcentury a gang of forty competing for a foothold in the pantheon of Paul Delaroche's *Hemicycle* (1841) for the Ecole des Beaux Arts, Paris.[1] By the end of the century a character in Emile Zola's *Rome* would spend five hours a day in the Sistine Chapel looking at Botticelli, not Michelangelo.[2] This was the result of a process which began in Paris with Schlegel.

Like the multitude of English tourists pouring into the French capital that summer following the signing of the Peace of Amiens, Schlegel wanted to see the spoils of war enshrined at the Louvre. After the occupation of Italy in 1796, Napoleon had included in his treaty terms the handing over of Italy's true wealth—its art. The Pope saw the *Laocoön* and the *Apollo Belvedere*, along with some eighty other famous works of antique sculpture, seized from their pedestals, sealed into crates, and hauled north on bullock carts. Roman citizens watched the French strip Raphael's *Transfiguration*, then the world's most renowned painting, from the altar where it had stood since shortly after the artist's death and take it to the Vatican for shipment with the marbles. Despite protests by courageous art lovers in France and an outraged public opinion in England and Germany—where every movement of "the kidnapped gods," as Schlegel's brother called the sculpture,[3] was reported in the popular press—the convoy of masterpieces was paraded through the streets of Paris and welcomed at the Louvre in July 1798.

By the time Schlegel reached Paris four years later, eighteen works attributed to Raphael had been brought from Italy to the Louvre, for display with ten others from the former royal collection.[4] In March the museum had opened a temporary exhibition featuring Raphael's *Madonna di Foligno,* newly transposed from its wooden panel to canvas by a surgical process described in hair-raising detail in a brochure on sale to the public. This exhibition of restored Italian works was in place in the Salon Carré until August, when it was taken down to make room for the annual exhibition of living artists. In September and through the fall of 1802, the *Transfiguration* could be seen only by bribing the guardian of the restoration room; it was nevertheless a regular tourist stop. Placed on the floor and in a good light, the famous picture drew a more enthusiastic response under those conditions than after its permanent installation in the Grande Galerie in late December 1802.

Schlegel's description of that installation, written early in 1803, is our principal corroborative record of the new *Transfiguration* bay, designed as a model for the Louvre's progressive policy on the historical, chronological display of paintings. Although Schlegel agreed with other visitors that the long, narrow gallery, lit by a row of windows, was not a suitable place to look at paintings, he gave the museum credit for seeking the most favorable spot and praised the historical arrangement (almost the same as that shown in fig. 17.1):

> The large picture is surrounded by other, smaller pictures of the same painter. On one side, a much-praised Holy Family [the *Holy Family* of Francis I, Paris, Louvre] from his mature period; opposite, a Transfiguration of Mary [the *Coronation of the Virgin* from San Francesco in Perugia, now in the Vatican Pinacoteca, Rome] from his earliest youth, when he was still working in Perugino's style; above, two altarpieces by Perugino; below, the portraits, sketches, and small paintings by Raphael. . . . The Madonna di Foligno [Vatican Pinacoteca, Rome] hangs on the next wall, and on the preceding one the *Jardinière* [Louvre, Paris].
>
> Such a truly instructive assemblage necessarily invites a great many reflections, when one can in this way survey at a glance the gradual development of a great genius from the first, still uncertain, youthful efforts to the last, most elaborate [*ausgearbeitetsten*] work of his life.[5]

Schlegel thus recognized the purpose of the Raphael bay, the first installation opened to the public after the new director of museums, Dominique Vivant Denon, had taken over in November 1802. As Denon told Napoleon, he wanted the *Transfiguration* wall to be a life of the greatest of all painters; Denon would turn a gallery visit into a history course in the art of painting.[6] The true instructor of the Raphael course was Giorgio Vasari; a new French edition of the *Lives* would appear that spring.[7] But the long-accepted three stages described by Vasari—Raphael's journey from the Umbrian *Coronation* to the Roman *Transfiguration,* with a fruitful side trip to Florence—had never before been spelled out on a museum wall. Only in Paris were there both sufficient examples and a strong mandate to educate the public. Schlegel gratefully acknowledged the lesson the Louvre was teaching. He did not, however, accept its basic premise, that the three stages were a one-way road to perfection.

Seeing a large number of Raphael paintings in that didactic, chronological arrangement gave substance and the weight of example to Schlegel's hitherto partially developed theories of painting. He had come to Paris immediately after a stay in Dresden, and his vivid recent experience of the Sistine *Madonna* shaped his response to the dozens of what he considered lesser Raphaels in the French collection. In Dresden,

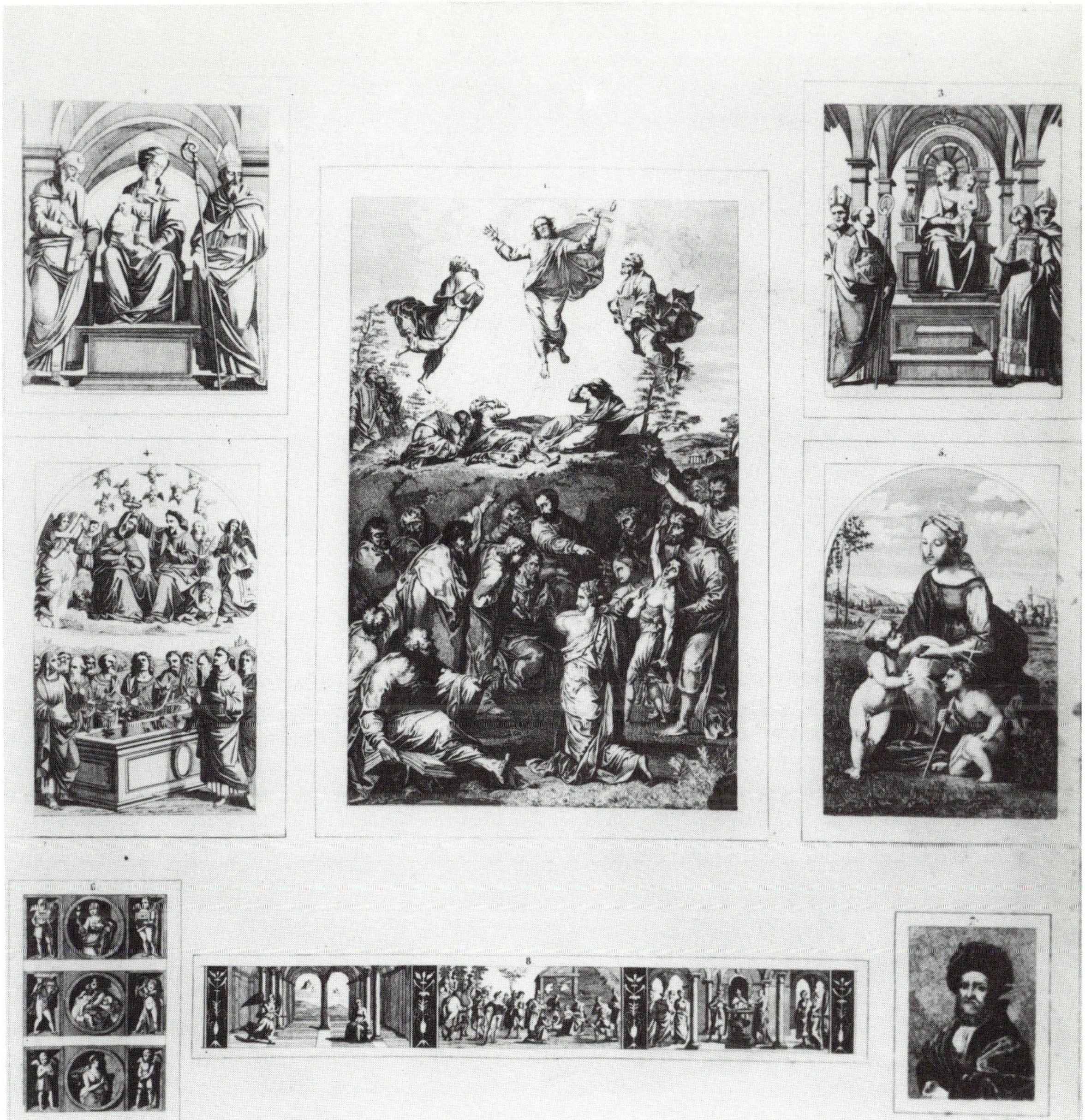

Fig. 17.1. François Couché fils, *Grande Galerie,* 1802. Etching, plate 11, John Griffiths and Maria Cosway, *Collection de gravures à l'eau forte des principaux tableaux d'après l'école italienne, contenus dans le Musée Napoléon* (Paris: Didot Jeune, 1806); original edition, *Galerie du Louvre* (Paris, 1802). Courtesy of the American Philosophical Society Library, Philadelphia.

he had also been in intensive contact with the painter Philipp Otto Runge and the writer Ludwig Tieck. He already shared with them the growing German enthusiasm for the early schools of art. Schlegel's Louvre-born insights concerned the relationship of the modern Italian school—that is, Raphael, Correggio, and Titian—with both its predecessors and successors.

Schlegel moved to Paris for a variety of reasons, including pressing financial need; he also hoped to consolidate there his views on art as he had his views on poetry. Before he left Germany, his most important contribution to European culture had been a single word: the adjective *romantisch*. This label, which he used to describe modern poetry, proved to be a concept so explosive that Schlegel marked with it all future discourse on the literature and art of his period. His pivotal characterization of romantic poetry appeared in a famous passage now called Fragment 116, one of a series of aphorisms, written chiefly by Friedrich Schlegel and his older brother, August Wilhelm (1767–1845), and published in their magazine *Athenäum* in 1798.[8] Schlegel chose the adjective "romantic" to define the rule-breaking, chaotic forms of contemporary poetry in contrast to the rigidity of French classicism. He saw chaos as a positive quality and prophesied that the *roman* or novel—the noun on which his adjective was based—would become the dominant literary form of the nineteenth century.

The Hanover-born pastor's son (fig. 17.2) lived out considerable chaos in his own life during this period. After eloping with the brilliant Dorothea Mendelssohn Veit, a married woman eight years his senior, Schlegel intensified the scandal by publishing a *roman à clé* on the subject *(Lucinde)* in 1799. Fleeing outraged critics, the couple took refuge in Jena that fall with Wilhelm and his wife, Caroline Michaelis Böhmer. This household—laden with genius and run by two ambitious women of thirty-seven—grew increasingly tense in the spring of 1800.[9] The brothers quarreled, their journal foundered, and Wilhelm moved to Berlin, leaving Friedrich in Jena to deliver profound, poorly attended, and allegedly incomprehensible private lectures on philosophy.[10] At a professional impasse, Schlegel left Jena late in 1801 for Berlin. In January 1802 he met Dorothea in Dresden, where they spent the spring. On their way to Paris in May, Schlegel stopped in Weimar to attend the dismal debut of his drama *Alarcos*, a project encouraged by Goethe. He could endure this setback in good spirits, for he had recently made peace with his brother, and at the Leipzig book fair he had found a backer for a new periodical he proposed to edit in Paris under the title *Europa*. The main purposes of the publication were first, to reach a broad public, and, second, to stress a quintessentially romantic quality—diversity *(Mannigfaltigkeit)*.[11] In his own resolve (recorded in notebooks and letters to his brother after he arrived in Paris that June) not only to make a breakthrough as a critic and editor, but to pursue his study of linguistics and to learn to read *Sakuntala* in the original Sanskrit, the thirty-year-old philosopher was a walking example of that romantic quest.

In this state of intense, purposefully chaotic creative ferment, Schlegel went to look at paintings in the Louvre. One of the chief topics of speculation among German intellectuals at this time was the issue of how to talk about paintings. Two Germans before Schlegel had written intensive reports from a picture gallery. Wilhelm Heinse had published his letters from the Düsseldorf gallery in *Der Teutsche Merkur* a few years after Friedrich Schlegel was born.[12] The same Düsseldorf gallery was described in 1790 by the intrepid travel writer Georg Forster, whose art criticism was somewhat crippled by his doubts on the possibility of describing a picture to someone

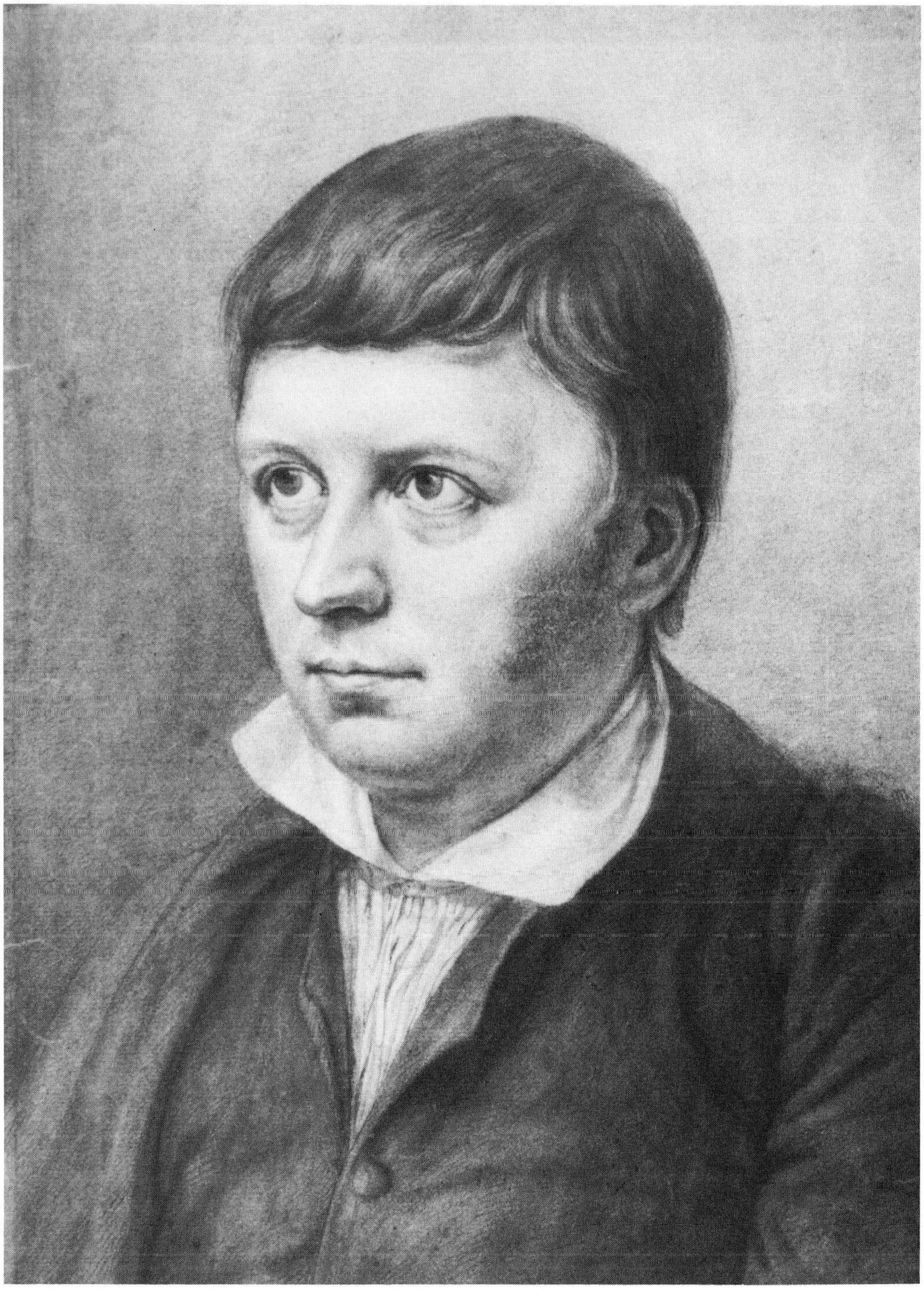

Fig. 17.2. Philipp Veit, *Friedrich Schlegel,* 1810–11. Pastel. Courtesy Freies Deutsches Hochstift Frankfurter Goethemuseum, Frankfurt-am-Main.

who had not seen it.[13] Forster's adventurous spirit (and liberal politics) nevertheless influenced Schlegel, who published a warm defense of the late author in 1797.[14] Schlegel may not have known Heinse's letters (notable for their unusual appreciation of Rubens); Forster's very different response to the Düsseldorf collection, however, was certainly in the back of Schlegel's mind as he set about the same task in Paris.

His own approach to talking about pictures, although he had not yet done so for publication, was presented in the guise of the character of Waller in his brother Wilhelm's widely read *Kunstgespräch* published in the *Athenäum* in 1799.[15] Wilhelm Schlegel's art conversation amply documents the most important influence on all debate, real and fictional, held around 1800 on how one was to look at art. That influence was Denis Diderot.

At the very moment the French began to import art works for their museum, they had exported their first critic. Like other German *litterateurs,* the Schlegels had read Diderot's *Salon of 1765* and his *Essais sur la Peinture* (written in 1766), published together for the first time in December 1795 and translated into German in 1797.[16] The frontispiece to the German edition (fig. 17.3) by Franz Ludwig Catel and Eberhard Henne graphically illustrates the impact of Diderot's criticism on German thought. Entire books on "the beautiful," at that time, might contain no reference at all to any actual works of art, and the leading aesthetic theory of the 1790s had been developed by Kant, a man who had seen only the art treasures of provincial Königsberg. In this environment, Diderot's views bounced from one German mind to another like a lightning bolt, a posthumous charge from the French Enlightenment. His conversational tone, his pointed examples drawn from contemporary art, his takeoff of the traditional academic categories in the saucy chapter headings of his essay on painting—"My Bizarre Thoughts on Drawing" or "Everything I Have Learned in My Life about Chiaroscuro"—cleared the air like a summer storm. One has only to contrast Diderot's essay to the leading German treatise on the same subject written at almost the same time, Anton Raphael Mengs' *Gedanken über die Schönheit und den Geschmack in der Mahlerey* (1762), to appreciate its powerful charm for German readers.[17]

Diderot's *Essai* and particularly his *Salon* (written as a letter to Baron Friedrich Melchior Grimm and circulated to the elite subscribers of his manuscript newsletter, the *Correspondance littéraire*) affected both the form of Friedrich Schlegel's *Gemäldebeschreibungen aus Paris* and his confident and partisan tone.[18] Schlegel, following Heinse and Forster, as well as Diderot, cast his views in the form of long letters, one for each issue of *Europa.*[19] The letters were addressed to an anonymous friend in Dresden; the friend was Tieck, since the revolutionary views they expressed had begun to take shape in conversations with the author of *Franz Sternbalds Wanderungen* (1798) during Schlegel's Dresden stay in the spring of 1802.[20] The traditional form of letters to put across his ideas was an obvious choice for Schlegel. Finding the correct tone of address was more difficult.

His brother had advocated a pragmatic approach to description in an *Athenäum* fragment:

> For the so often unsuccessful art of painting pictures with words, in general no other formula presents itself but to change style according to the subjects. Sometimes the represented moment can be brought to life by a narrative. Other times an almost mathematical precision in local details is necessary. Usually the tone of the description must try to acquaint the reader with the How of it. In this Diderot

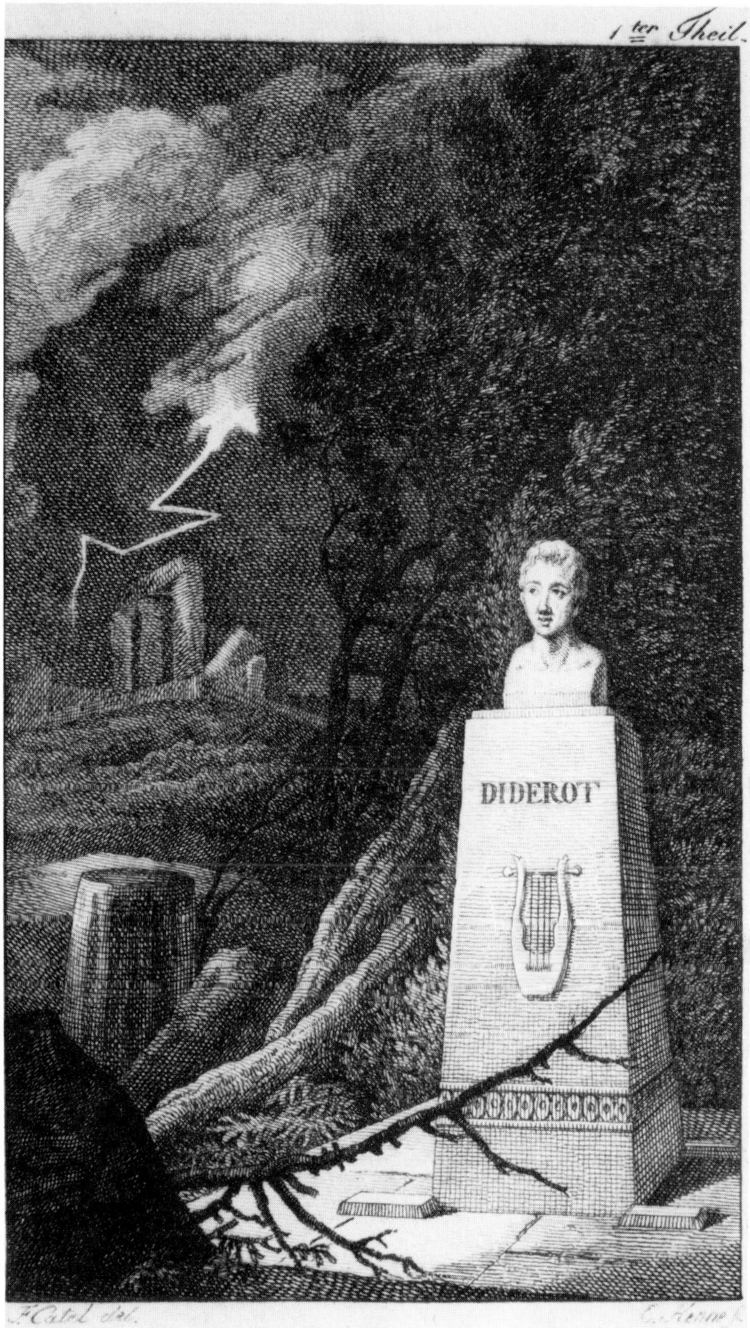

Fig. 17.3. Franz Ludwig Catel and Eberhard Henne, engraved frontispiece for *Sämmtliche Werke von Dionysius Diderot,* trans. Carl Friederich Cramer (Riga: Johann Friedrich Hartknoch, 1797). Courtesy of the Library of Congress, Washington, D.C.

is a master. He makes music of many paintings like Abbot Vogler [George Joseph Vogler, a renowned organ virtuoso and music teacher].[21]

Schlegel, a linguist searching for a tone, would have noticed the advantages in Diderot's lively second person plurals, his switch to a more intimate scolding voice as he began to *tutoyer* François Boucher, his insistent imperative moods. Schlegel's general introduction for the first issue of *Europa* reveals his quest for the right mode of address. To report and disseminate new ideas or useful news, he said, it suffices "to write just as one might speak, if only it is clear." He observed:

> Actually one speaks one way to a friend with similar views, another way to a stranger one wants to approach, and still another in a mixed company. This makes some difference in tone necessary, according to circumstances, each time we address one or the other. With those, however, who consider themselves our adversary, we will not speak at all.[22]

Although *Europa* aimed at diversity and consisted largely of brief, lively reportage on the latest goings-on in Paris, the periodical had a serious side that the mild declaration of its intentions failed to reveal. Schlegel's choice of a frontispiece—Raphael's *St. Michael Vanquishing the Devil* (Louvre, Paris) as drawn by the twenty-two-year-old Ferdinand Jagemann and published in the second volume as an engraving by the better-known contemporary artist Heinrich Lips—offers a strong hint at this more combative aim (fig. 17.4). His final disclaimer in the introduction notwithstanding, Schlegel's major piece of writing for the periodical, the description of the paintings, did address an adversary. The views on art elaborated in the *Europa* letters to Dresden were meant to be a romantic manifesto, and they were recognized as such by the combined opposition forces encamped in Weimar—namely, the self-declared *Kunstfreunde:* Goethe and Heinrich Meyer. As Meyer said himself in 1817:

> In the year 1803 Friedrich Schlegel came forth in his own paper called *Europa,* as the first written instructor of the new archaicizing, Catholic-Christian taste in art, combating the hitherto preserved opinions about true art and the means of fostering it. Religion, mysticism, Christian subjects, or as they are called, symbols, were presented as indispensable requirements for painting and its future thriving. The old school, that is to say, masters and works from the time before Raphael, are granted preference over all later ones; Titian, Correggio, Giulio Romano, del Sarto, etc. are called the last painters.[23]

Schlegel went beyond giving preference to the early Italians, a preference stated baldly in the first letter: "I have a taste only for the old school of painting. I understand and comprehend only this, and only about this can I speak."[24] In the second letter Schlegel published his most far-reaching (and most often quoted) passage on the modern painters:

> This newer school of Italian painting, which is called superior because of Raphael, Titian, Correggio, Giulio Romano, Michelangelo—however many other less epoch-making painters also actually belong to it—is indisputably at the root of the corruption of art.[25]

Apart from heralding opinions that would resound in the work of François Rio and John Ruskin, Schlegel's letters evidence much original thought on that nearly exhausted subject—Raphael. He looked long and respectfully at the *Transfiguration,* although he clearly preferred earlier and smaller works, such as *Silence* or *La Belle Jardinière* (both from the former royal collections). To him Raphael's final painting lacked propriety in expression, the very quality most often lauded by the English and the French. But in writing about the picture, Schlegel did not stop at disputing its

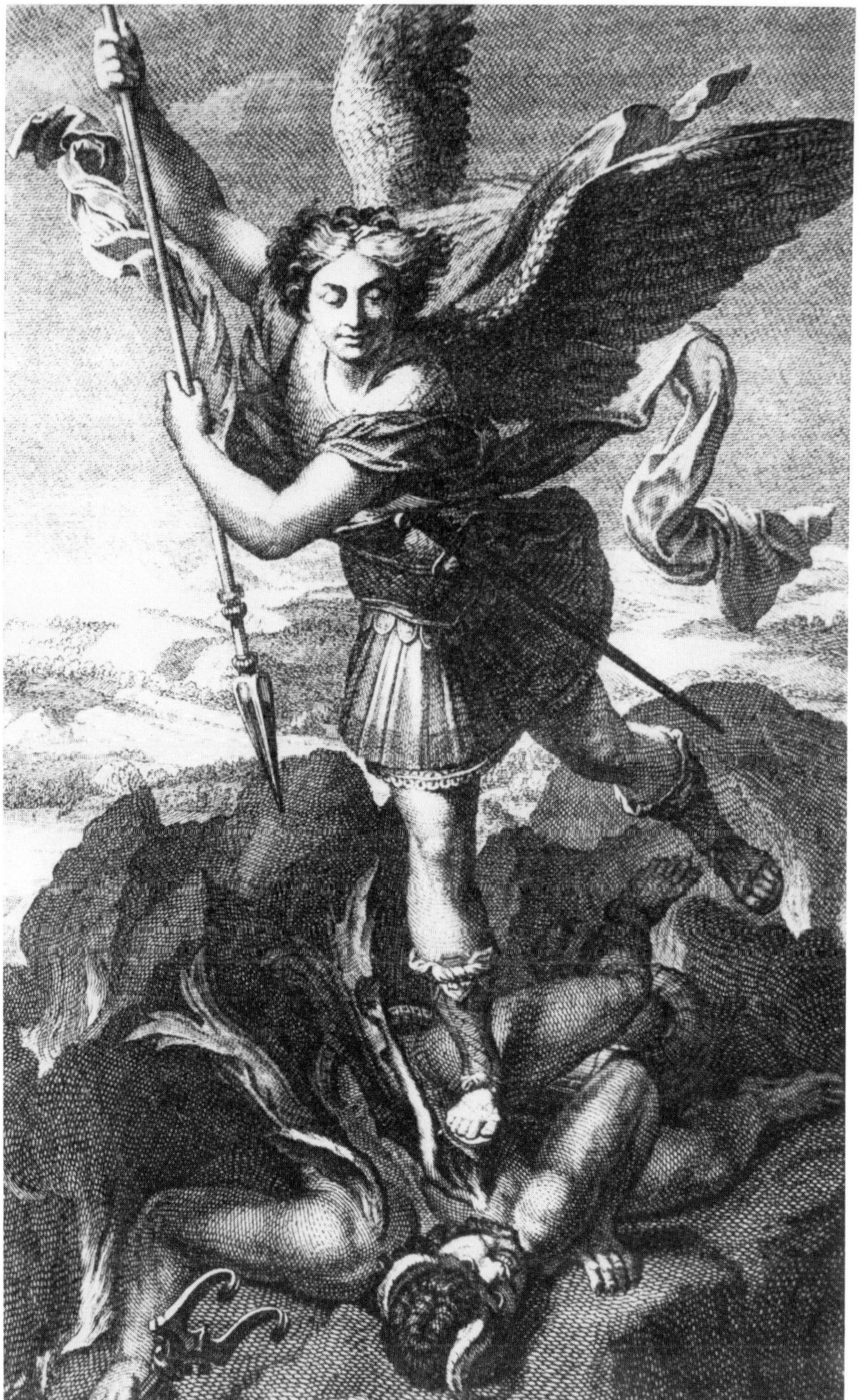

Fig. 17.4. Ferdinand Jagemann and Heinrich Lips, after Raphael, *St. Michael Killing the Dragon* (Louvre, Paris), engraved frontispiece for *Europa* II, 1803. Courtesy of the Universitätsbibliothek, University of Heidelberg.

vaunted propriety. He raised against Raphael a powerful new weapon, one which would eventually come closest to dethroning him. Raphael's reputation had survived both the rivalry with Michelangelo and Sebastiano fostered by his contemporaries and the rivalry with Apelles and the ancients perpetuated by academicians. It was dealt a staggering blow, however, by the rivalry evoked by Schlegel in 1802. For the first time, Raphael faced the hitherto unimaginable competition of his own predecessors—the artists of the *quattrocento*.

Schlegel asserted that people admired the *Transfiguration* (fig. 17.5) more than other works of equal merit because it was much closer and more understandable to painters of the day than that "pure old style" of the early Italians. Admitting that it contained some fine heads, he complained:

> The expression of reproach in the grumblers is quite crude and wild, and the apostles, who cannot aid the boy, appear somewhat foolish, and hardly make a dignified impression. A painter of the olden times would not have painted the subject this way; he would perhaps have let us look much deeper into the abyss of bitter pains, but the rich consolation of the other side would be more sensitive and purer. He would perhaps not have grouped the apostles so artistically, but the strong forms would fill us with respect, the commanding seriousness would silence into submission the loud complaints or soften them in an amiable way with hope, and the feeling of the necessity of suffering and their own limitations would have the dignity of serious grief. This more artistic, if not so deeply beautiful, modern treatment displays itself particularly in the Transfiguration on the mountain. The figure of the Healer floats like a quivering flame over the earth in the air; three apostles blinded from the light lie in theatrical positions on the ground, and also the donatarius in the corner makes an ugly impression. Here also the subject is expressed and executed with only a hasty, superficial enthusiasm which looks above all for a grand effect; not with the unpretentious, strict seriousness, the quiet profundity, with which the deeper religiosity [of earlier masters] would have strived to conceive and express in the subject their reverence and love.[26]

Schlegel was certainly not the first to prefer Raphael's middle or early period to his Roman works; a growing taste for, say, the Borghese *Entombment* is reflected as early as 1797 in Carl Fernow's essay on Raphael's tapestries for *Der Neue Teutsche Merkur.*[27] But his observation that painters and art lovers of his own day felt closer to the late Raphael because of an unbroken line of descent from a work like the *Transfiguration* through the Carracci, Guercino, Albani, and Guido (the favorites, he must have noticed, of the French art commissioners who had selected works from Italy for the Louvre) to Poussin and Mengs, was a sharper distinction of contemporary taste for the past than had yet been voiced in print.[28]

Distancing himself from the prevailing understanding of Raphael was important to Schlegel:

> The modern judgment of art and the traditional opinion of the first of the painters, mimicked often without criticism or distinction and without any personal observation or interpretation, stand in need in many places of a careful correction and a narrower definition. Mengs isolates the character of Raphael in the superiority of his drawing and expression, while more or less denying him chiaroscuro and a gift for color. Not to mention that so many a Raphael painting can be cited with an incomparably beautiful coloring, as, for example, the already

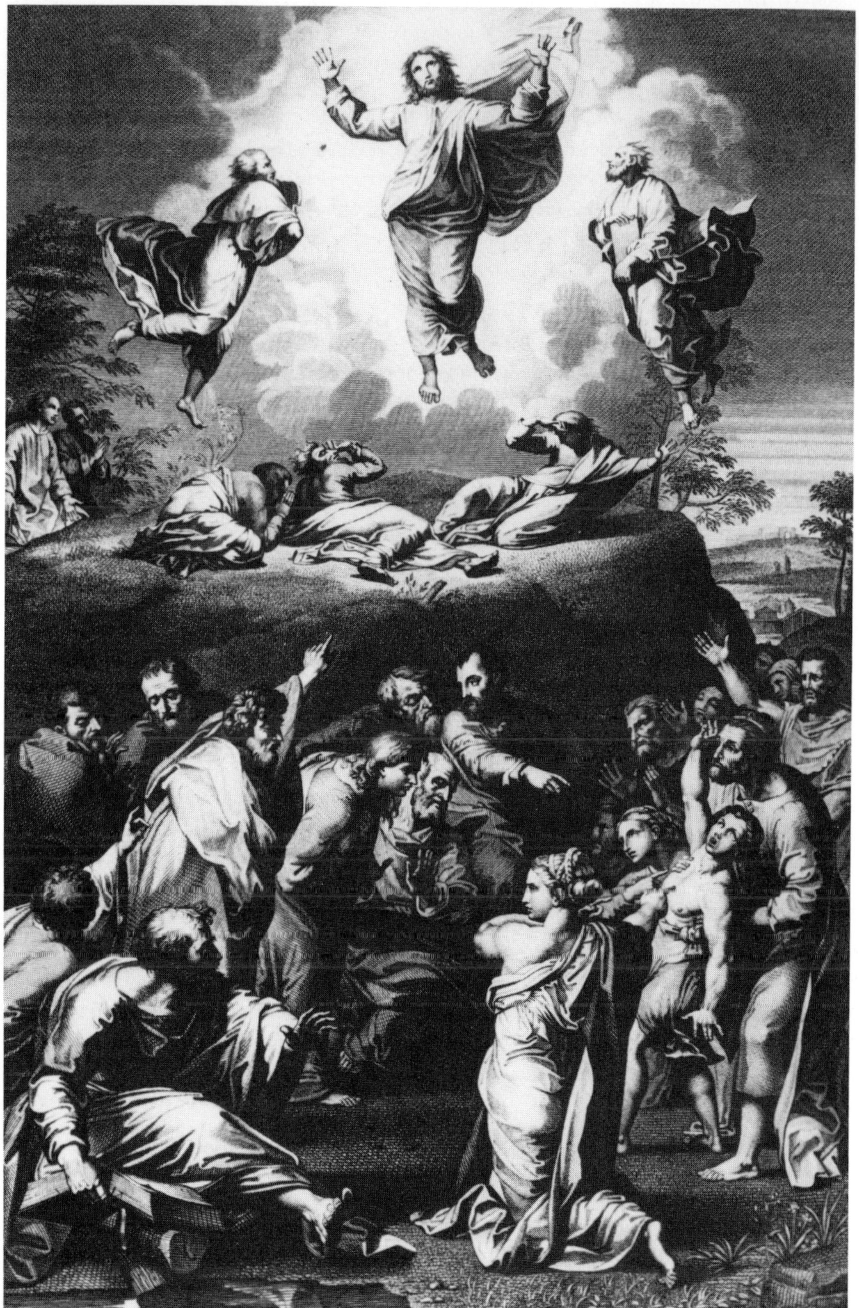

Fig. 17.5. [P. M.?] Bourdon, after Raphael, *The Transfiguration*, etched by L. M. Y. Queverdo and F. Pigeot for Antoine-Michel Filhol, *Galerie du Musée Napoléon publiée par Filhol, et redigé par Lavallée*, 10 vols. (Paris: 1814–15), X (originally published in 1809), Pl. I (No. 715). Courtesy of the Library of Congress, Washington, D.C.

> frequently mentioned *Jardinière;* that whole division is therefore absurd. For don't these qualities determine themselves mutually throughout? Would any other flesh tone be possible with the chiaroscuro of Correggio? Isn't precisely this type of contour appropriate here, as the colors of Raphael actually belong together with his drawing? Isn't drawing and light, character, color, in any good painter an inseparable, harmonious whole? Instead of these vain strivings toward an unsatisfactory classification in order to separate what eternally belongs together and can only operate in unity, one should simply try to fathom, in the most painstaking way, the individual purpose of that work which the artist himself, in that bygone period which thought so very differently from our own, really had in mind.[29]

Rejecting the traditional identification of Raphael with drawing and expression or with a quest for ideal beauty, Schlegel offered instead universality as the essence of his character. He used this seemingly vague word to underline Raphael's role as a transitional figure, who anchored his contemporaries in the rapidly changing art world of the sixteenth century to their sources in the past. Schlegel furthermore defined *Universalität* in Raphael as almost inseparable from "a wonderful flexibility," a "strong talent for assimilation."[30]

His resistance to inherited opinion led Schlegel to look carefully at Raphael's color. Again, he was not the first to recognize its merits. Even Roger de Piles had applauded Raphael's progress in this field late in his career, and Abbé Dubos had praised the color in the Vatican fresco *Mass at Bolsena.*[31] The British, who possessed Raphael's tapestry cartoons in which design and color merged in an "inseparable whole," were even less inclined than the French to mouth the established view that Raphael lost points in this department. While other critics might mourn that Raphael died on the point of of perfecting his single weakness, Schlegel was not eager to see progress in the late Raphael. He therefore looked at color differently, and much more specifically, than writers before him. Speaking of the *Madonna della Sedia,* which he finally saw in Napoleon's suburban villa at St. Cloud late in 1803, Schlegel described a remarkable "weaving" of colors. It was indeed in his use of color that Schlegel felt Raphael most clearly revealed his great diversity and variety.[32]

Another original view of Schlegel's was his insistence that the madonnas be considered as a series, a principle still deemed worthy of emphasis by Heinrick Wölfflin and John Pope-Hennessy.[33] He particularly admired the *Madonna della Sedia,* in which he traced a strong connection with the very earliest madonnas. The picture seemed "to stand on the border between two great periods in the history of Raphael's art," before, "trailing after the dazzling meteor Michelangelo and antiquity, he abandoned the path of innocent love."[34]

Schlegel situated Raphael on a fault line that all future criticism would have to take into account. He located a continental divide within the body of his work and made of the artist a river that flowed both ways. He did not attack the divine Raphael on the vulnerable heel of color or force him into comparisons with Michelangelo or Apelles. Schlegel's attack was aimed at Raphael's reputation and the mistaken ideas about him that veiled his true worth as a link to the past and an embodiment of the diversity and many-sidedness appreciated by the romantics. Yet an assault on the legend inevitably wounded the artist himself. Although Schlegel responded with deep admiration to many of Raphael's works, his indifference to others inflicted on the painter a new kind of injury. The academic approach to Raphael selected certain qualities and rejected others; Schlegel approved of his early works and abandoned him in Rome, at what had always been thought of as the peak of his career. Various artists may have been mauled by critics, but Raphael was the first to be deftly and definitively sliced in two.

Schlegel, loving certain Raphaels, appropriated those works that fit his purposes. The purposes themselves had been clarified on the spot through comparisons made possible by the historical display at the Louvre. Raphael, already a prisoner of war in Paris, became in Schlegel's hands part hostage and part hero to a revolutionary international art movement.

NOTES

1. Francis Haskell pointed out the significance of the Delaroche *Hemicycle* in his opening chapter of *Rediscoveries in Art. Some Aspects of Taste, Fashion and Collecting in England and France* (Ithaca: Cornell University Press, 1976). In this and other works by Professor Haskell I found countless clues to pursue in the course of research for a dissertation, "Responses to Raphael's Works in the Louvre, 1798–1848." The present essay is based on a section of that dissertation, completed in 1986 under the direction of Professor George Levitine, University of Maryland, and David Alan Brown, National Gallery of Art. I am grateful to them for continuing guidance.

2. The significance of Zola's text was first pointed out to me by Elizabeth Gilmore Holt. I am indebted to her for unfailing sustenance and inspiration throughout my study of nineteenth-century European art.

3. August Wilhelm von Schlegel, "Die entführten Götter," *Sämmtliche Werke,* ed. Eduard Böcking, 12 vols. (Leipzig: Weidmann'sche Buchhandlung, 1846–47), I, 61–63; the poem was originally published in *Musenalmanach auf 1798,* 199.

4. Some of the eighteen works were later reattributed to other artists. Another Raphael brought from Italy to Paris at this time was in private hands. Schlegel admired the *Madonna of the Candelabras* (now in the Walters Gallery, Baltimore) before Lucien Bonaparte took it back to Italy in the spring of 1804. The ten works mentioned from the former French royal collection are those in the Louvre during Schlegel's stay; other works attributed to Raphael were still at Versailles.

5. *Kritische Friedrich-Schlegel-Ausgabe,* ed. Ernst Behler, with Jean-Jacques Anstett and Hans Eichner, 35 vols. projected (Munich: Ferdinand Schöningh, 1958–), vol. 4, *Ansichten und Ideen von der christlichen Kunst,* ed. Hans Eichner (Munich: Ferdinand Schöning, 1959), 49; hereafter cited as *KA*, 4. Page references to Schlegel's letters are from Eichner's annotated edition. A reprint edition of *Europa* was published by J. G. Cotta'sche Buchhandlung Nachf., Stuttgart, in 1963, with an afterword by Ernst Behler.

6. Letter from Denon to Napoleon dated *11 nivôse an XI* (1 January 1803), Archives Nationales, AF IV 1049 (dossier catalogued as "2" but marked "B").

7. An announcement appeared in the *Moniteur universel,* no. 206 (*26 germinal an XI* [16 April 1803]), 924; the Raphael biography appeared in the second volume (of three), published in 1804. The French translation was based on the Bottari edition of 1759, with additional footnote references to the new location of paintings brought from Italy to the Louvre. New portraits were etched for the French edition by Guillaume Boichot.

8. *Athenäum,* 1, no. 2 (1798): 28–30.

9. Biographical information on the Schlegels is based on Ernst Behler, *Friedrich Schlegel* (Reinbeck bei Hamburg: Rowohlt, 1966); Hans Eichner, "Introduction" to *KA*, 4, and his biography *Friedrich Schlegel* (New York: Twayne, 1970); and Gisela F. Ritchie, *Caroline Schlegel-Schelling. In Wahrheit und Dichtung* (Bonn: H. Bouvier, 1968). Caroline's fifteen-year-old daughter, Auguste—much loved by her stepfather, Wilhelm, and his brother—died in July 1800; the intricate emotional system of her mourners broke under this additional strain.

10. Wilhelm Schlegel's marriage to Caroline had dissolved during this period; after their divorce in 1803, she would marry the philosopher Friedrich W. J. Schelling. Friedrich Schlegel was further saddened in March 1801 by the death of his friend, the poet Friedrich von Hardenberg (Novalis).

11. Ernst Behler pointed out that this quality, diversity, is a key impulse behind Schlegel's intentions for *Europa;* see Behler's *Die Zeitschriften der Bruder Schlegel: ein Beitrag zur Geschichte der deutschen Romantik* (Darmstadt: Wissenschaftliche Buchgesellschaft, 1983), 63.

12. Heinse's letters appeared under the title "Über einige Gemählde der Düsseldorfer Gallerie" in four parts in *Der Teutsche Merkur,* no. 4 (October and November 1776): 3–46 and 106–19; no. 2 (May 1777): 117–35; and no. 3 (July 1777): 60–60; they were addressed to Heinse's friend and patron Johan Wilhelm Gleim. The letters were reprinted in Wilhelm Heinse, *Sämmtliche Werke,* ed. Carl Schuddekopf, 10 vols. (Leipzig: Insel, 1902–25), vol. 9: 280–323 and 328–63.

13. Georg Forster, *Ansichten vom Niederrhein,* originally published in two volumes in 1791 and 1792, reprinted in *Werke. Sämmtliche Schriften, Tagebücher, Briefe,* 18 vols. (Berlin: Akademie-Verlag, 1958–78), vol. 9. For an illuminating comparison of Heinse and Forster, see Wilhelm Waetzoldt, *Deutsche Kunsthistoriker von Sandrart bis Rumohr* (Leipzig: Seemann, 1921), 205–06.

14. Schlegel's essay, "Georg Forster. Fragment einer Charakteristik der deutschen Klassiker," was originally published in Johan Friedrich Reichardt's paper, *Lyceum der Schönen Künste* (1797); it is reprinted in Friedrich Schlegel, *Kritische Schriften,* ed. Wolfdietrich Rasch (Munich: Carl Hansen Verlag, 1971), 323–45. On Schlegel's connection with Forster, see Marita Gilli, *Georg Forster. l'Oeuvre d'un penseur allemand réaliste et révolutionnaire,* thesis for University of Paris, 1974 (Lille: Atelier réproduction des thèses, 1975).

15. August Wilhelm Schlegel [and Caroline Schlegel], "Die Gemälde," *Athenäum,* 2, no. 1 (1799): 39–151. Hans Eichner has suggested that only the opinions on p. 47 can be firmly attributed to Friedrich Schlegel; see his introduction to *KA,* 4, xiv.

16. Denis Diderot, *Essais sur la peinture* (Paris: Buisson, *an IV* [1795]), and the German translation, *Sämmtliche Werke von Dionysius Diderot,* trans. Carl Friederich Cramer, part 1, *Versuch über die Mahlerey* (Riga: Johann Friedrich Hartknoch, 1797). The best study of Diderot's reception in Germany is still Roland Mortier, *Diderot en Allemagne: 1750–1850* (Paris: Presses Universitaires de France, 1954).

17. Goethe, for example, was both attracted and annoyed by the essay. After reading it in the summer of 1796, he wrote to his friend Heinrich Meyer: "It would really be an agreeable and amusing job, if one had enough courage, to translate the work and continually dispute the text and add examples to illustrate or amplify it" (letter dated 5 August 1796, in *Goethes Briefwechsel mit Heinrich Meyer, Schriften der Goethe Gesellschaft,* 32–35, ed. Max Hecker, 4 vols. [Weimar: Goethe Gesellschaft, 1917–32], 1:310). Goethe found the courage himself to tackle the first and second chapters of Diderot's essay, and published in 1799 an extraordinary dialogue with his departed "friend and adversary" in the second and third numbers of his journal *Propyläen.*

In his stimulating discussion of Diderot, Neil Flax ("Fiction Wars of Art," *Representations* 7 [Summer 1984]: 1–25) comes close to reviving the Catel frontispiece's electrical imagery when he traces a permanent polarization of the methodology of art criticism caused by Goethe's reading of the Salon and the essay. Flax (p. 11) would see Goethe as inventing a formalist position "specifically to counteract the fabulating approach to art" represented by Diderot and his young admirers in Germany. Schlegel, although aligned with the allegorical, fabulating romantics, did not invent stories about paintings at the Louvre. His principal preoccupation was to "place" them—in series, in relationship to one another, in the history of art. Whether his historical, comparative approach means that for Schlegel the influence of Diderot was overruled by a lingering and barely acknowledged influence of Johann Joachim Winckelmann is a question for further study.

18. The Salon appeared in the *Correspondance* in six parts, beginning in January 1766; see Denis Diderot, *Salons,* ed. Jean Seznec and Jean Adhémar, 3 vols. (Oxford: Clarendon Press, 1960), vol. 2. For a modern edition of the essay, see Denis Diderot, *Oeuvres esthétiques,* ed. Paul Vernière (Paris: Garnier, 1959), 659–748.

19. Two letters appeared in the last of *Europa*'s four numbers in 1805; the first issue had been published at the end of February 1803. The letters were: "Nachricht von den Gemälden in Paris," *Europa* 1, Erstes Stuck (1803), 6:108–157; "Vom Raffael," *Europa* 1, Zweites Stuck (1803), 1:3–19; "Nachtrag italiänischer Gemälde," *Europa* 2, Erstes STuck (1803), 2:96–116; "Zweiter Nachtrag alter Gemälde" and "Dritter Nachtrag alter Gemälde," *Europa* 2, Zweites Stuck (1805), 1:1–41, and 6:109–145. Schlegel collected the letters in 1823 under the title *Ansichten der christlichen Kunst* for *Friedrich Schlegel's sämmtliche Werke,* 10 vols. (Vienna: J. Meyer, 1822–25), vol. 6. The only English translation is in the admirable, if not wholly reliable, work of Ellen J. Middleton, *The Aesthetic and Miscellaneous Works of Frederick von Schlegel* (London: Henry G. Bohn, 1849). The second letter, "Vom Raffael," appeared in an Italian transla-

tion by Ursula Vogt and Rosario Assunto, with an introduction and notes by Assunto; see *Pagine su Raffaello*, Collana di Studi e Testi, no. 1 (Urbino: Accademia Raffaello, 1973).

20. Hans Eichner somewhat discounted claims that Tieck and Runge were the originators of Schlegel's views in the *Europa* letters; see his introduction to *KA*, 4, xix, n. 3. After a discussion with Tieck in the fall of 1830 (the year following Schlegel's death), Sulpiz Boisserée noted that Schlegel's ideas on art were half Tieck's (and that Schlegel's ideas on architecture were half his own); Sulpiz Boisserée, *Tagebücher*, ed. Hans-J. Weitz, 3 vols. (Darmstadt: Eduard Roether Verlag, 1981), 2:514. Runge's brother recalled their surprise to see the same ideas expressed by Schlegel in more practical terms; see *Hinterlassene Schriften von Philipp Otto Runge*, 2 vols. (Hamburg: F. Perthes, 1840–41), 47.

21. *Athenäum* 1, Zweites Stuck (1798), 46.

22. Friedrich Schlegel, "Vorrede [zur Europa]," *KA*, 2, *Charakteristiken und Kritiken II (1802–1829)*, ed. Hans Eichner (Munich: Ferdinand Schöningh, 1975), 329.

23. Heinrich Meyer, "Neu-deutsche religiös-patriotische Kunst," *Kunst und Altertum* 1, Heft 2 (1817): 5–62, 133–62; reprinted in Heinrich Meyer, *Kleine Schriften zur Kunst*, Deutsche Litteraturdenkmale des 18. und 19. Jahrhunderts, no. 25, ed. Bernhard Seuffert (Stuttgart: G. J. Göschen'sche Verlagshandlung, 1886), 108.

24. *KA*, 4:13.

25. *KA*, 4:56.

26. *KA*, 4:51.

27. Carl Ludwig Fernow, "Raphaels Tapeten," *Der Neue Teutsche Merkur* 2 (January 1797): 31.

28. *KA*, 4:50.

29. *KA*, 4:53–54.

30. *KA*, 4:49.

31. Roger de Piles, *Abrégé de la Vie des Peintres, avec des réflexions sur leurs ouvrages, et un traité du Peintre Parfait* (Paris: F. Muguet, 1699), 178; Abbé Jean-Baptiste Dubos, *Réflexions critiques sur la poésie et la peinture*, 3 vols. (Paris: J. Mariette, 1719), 48–49. On the changing appreciation of Raphael in the seventeenth and eighteenth century, see the cogent study by Martin Isreal Rosenberg, *Raphael in French Art Theory, Criticism and Practice (1660–1830)*, Ph.D. dissertation for University of Pennsylvania, 1979 (Ann Arbor, Mich.: University Microfilms, 1979).

32. *KA*, 4:98.

33. Heinrich Wölfflin, *Classic Art. An Introduction to the Italian Renaissance*, trans. by Peter and Linda Murray from *Die klassische Kunst* (1899), 3rd ed. (London: Phaidon, 1968), 82–87. While Schlegel's series is not based on the strictly formal analysis of Wölfflin, but rather on an unverifiable scale of earthliness to divinity, he nevertheless comes amazingly close to his successor when he attempts to place works according to their simplicity or complexity, particularly in connection with the *Madonna della Sedia*. See also Sir John Pope-Hennessy's graceful essay, "Rafael of the Dear Madonnas" in *Raphael* (New York: Harper & Row, Icon Editions, 1970), 125–221, for the best recent product of Schlegel's insight that the madonnas were a meaningful series.

34. *KA*, 4:99–100.

VI

Nineteenth-Century Art Historical Implications in Twentieth-Century Context

18

RECONSIDERING WALTER BENJAMIN

"The Age of Mechanical Reproduction" in Retrospect

JACQUELYNN BAAS

In her 1981 essay entitled "The Originality of the Avant-Garde," Rosalind Krauss punctuates a discussion of Rodin and the issue of authenticity by citing what has become the canonical text of poststructuralist art historians: "As we have constantly been reminding ourselves ever since Walter Benjamin's 'Work of Art in the Age of Mechanical Reproduction,' authenticity empties out as a notion as one approaches those mediums which are inherently multiple."[1] Benjamin's essay, uprooted from the politically charged circumstances of its production in the mid-1930s, now figures as the "signifier" of a semiotically-based dichotomy between the photograph as the paradigm of an "age of mechanical reproduction" and the work of art as the fetishized object of a culture that has been surpassed.

While the journal *October* has served as the chief vehicle for the dissemination of this schismatic viewpoint, Douglas Crimp has done the most to amplify its significance. In a 1980 article, "On the Museum's Ruins," Crimp associates Benjamin's argument with Robert Rauschenberg's "flatbed" array of reproduced images. Since I shall be referring to the terms of this reading of Benjamin throughout the following essay, Crimp's formulation is worth quoting:

> No one took seriously the possibility that photography might usurp painting. Less than half a century after photography's invention such a notion was one of those received ideas to be parodied. In our century until recently only Walter Benjamin gave credence to the notion, claiming that inevitably photography would have a truly profound effect upon art, even to the extent that the art of painting might disappear, having lost its all-important aura through mechanical reproduction. . . . But then in the work of Rauschenberg photography began to conspire with painting in its own destruction.[2]

Crimp then turns the Benjamin thesis against the museum, depicting it (á la Foucault) as the institutionalized privileging of the "auratic."

The thrill of belonging to a new era of authenticity and enlightenment, with Benjamin as its quasi-scriptural authority, is even more emphatically evoked four years later. In "The Art of Exhibition," published in the Fall 1984 issue of *October*, Crimp laments that the canonization of the Benjamin thesis by likeminded critics has not produced a comparable dawn of enlightenment at establishment exhibitions of contemporary art:

> If not for Haacke's work [in *documenta 7*], one would hardly have known that photography has recently become an important medium for artists attempting to resist the hegemony of the traditional beaux arts, that Walter Benjamin's classic essay on mechanical reproduction has become central to critical theories of contemporary visual culture. Nor would one have understood that this debate also encompasses a critique of the museum institution in its function of preserving the auratic status of art that was Benjamin's main target.[3]

"The Work of Art in the Age of Mechanical Reproduction," first published without its Marxist prologue in *Zeitschrift für Sozialforschung* in 1936, has indeed become, as Crimp says, a "classic essay . . . central to critical theories of contemporary visual culture." There is some irony in the current privileging of this particular essay as the quasi-scriptural origin of a way of thinking that attacks the mystification of the original work. Is there any more "auratic" text in contemporary criticism than Benjamin's essay? Here I shall argue that the essay requires a more contextual understanding than the poststructuralists have found expedient, and that Benjamin's thesis regarding the impact of technology on visual culture requires a more critical attention than these critics have brought to it.

In fact, the canonization of Benjamin's text provides a useful occasion for reviewing our understanding of the relations between mechanical reproduction, photography, and the history of the print media. In conducting such a review, I believe one is forced to question whether the invention of photography in the first half of the nineteenth century radically changed the nature and the reception of the visual arts, as Benjamin claimed.

In his 1982 study of Benjamin's aesthetic, Richard Wolin suggests that Walter Benjamin's construction of the "crisis" in traditional art forms produced by the advent of photography was primarily motivated by polemical rather than historical goals.

> In 1935 [the year the essay was written] as the Nazis began building up their war machine, whether or not autonomous art could be salvaged seemed to Benjamin an entirely otiose, scholastic question. All prevalent tendencies pointed, in his view, to such art's imminent demise and the incorporation of its dying vestiges into the fascist program of self-glorification. In face of the threat to civilization posed by fascism, bourgeois talk about the preservation of culture seemed reprehensibly self-indulgent. As far as culture was concerned, the only practise that seemed to make sense at the time was to render art serviceable for progressive political ends, for ends that were staunchly opposed to those of fascism: the ends of communism.[4]

In his epilogue, Benjamin described the political context within which his essay emerged.

> The logical result of Fascism is the introduction of aesthetics into political life. The violation of the masses, whom Fascism, with its *Führer* cult, forces to their knees, has its counterpart in the violation of an apparatus which is pressed into the production of ritual values. All efforts to render politics aesthetic culminate in one thing: war.[5]

As we shall see, Benjamin's own interest in a militarized proletarian aesthetic, evident in his Brechtian theory of film, casts an ironic light upon this recoil from the fascist politicization of art. In his prologue, Benjamin outlined the task as he saw it.

> Theses about the art of the proletariat after its assumption of power or about the art of a classless society would have less bearing on these demands than theses about the developmental tendencies of art under present conditions of production. . . . The concepts which are introduced into the theory of art in what follows differ from the more familiar terms in that they are completely useless for the purposes of Fascism. They are, on the other hand, useful for the formulation of revolutionary demands in the politics of art.[6]

For a number of reasons—his friendship with Bertolt Brecht, his intellectual relationship with Theodor Adorno and the Frankfurt School, and above all the desperate political situation—by the 1930s Walter Benjamin was convinced it was essential to think in terms of militancy and sacrifice rather than in terms of cultural balance.[7] In closing his essay, Benjamin writes that since Fascism has made politics "aesthetic," "Communism responds by politicizing art."[8]

Wolin provides a useful analysis of Benjamin's Marxist intentions in the "Work of Art" essay. Benjamin, Wolin writes, "sought to establish the absolute primacy of the forces of *aesthetic* production in the same way Marx attempted to do so for the forces of *economic* production."[9] Like his close friend Bertolt Brecht, Benjamin wanted an activist aesthetic. As Wolin puts it, he was "less concerned with the naive belief that art possessed an independent capacity to change the world than . . . inspired by the possibility of transforming art itself from within, and thus preventing it from degenerating to the level of mere consolation."[10] Essentially, Benjamin's goal was the transformation of art from a humanist individualism to a collective usefulness.

Benjamin's choice of the "age of mechanical reproduction" as the vehicle for his play of historical and aesthetic forces was apparently a secondary idea, a post facto justification for his decision to sacrifice art as he had known it to a higher end without invoking overtly political rationales. In a letter to Max Horkheimer in October 1935, Benjamin called it "the hour of fate" for art:

> It is a question of specifying the precise place in the present which my historical construction will take as its point of departure. . . . The hour of fate of art has, I would . . . like to say, sounded for us, and I have set forth its signature in a series of preliminary reflections which carry the title, "The Work of Art in the Age of Mechanical Reproduction." These reflections make an attempt to give questions about the theory of art a truly contemporary form: and indeed, through avoidance of all *immediate* relation to politics.[11]

Reflecting the engaged stance he had assumed as a Marxist historian, Benjamin commented to Gershom Scholem that his interpretation deliberately incorporated a shared sense of the current "situation": "These reflections anchor the history of art in the nineteenth century in an understanding of the situation of art as it is experienced by us in the present."[12] Benjamin's "age of mechanical reproduction" is thus much less specifiable, at least in chronological terms, than it appears. Admittedly projected upon the nineteenth century, its utopian features appear in the present only in the proleptic sense of its continuity with social revolution.

In appropriating Benjamin's essay for our own theoretical concerns, common sense must be permitted to intervene. Benjamin's perception of the destruction of our experience of authenticity in works of art, and of their loss of "aura" through mechanical reproduction, was hardly self-evident then and is even less so now. On the contrary, modern techniques of reproducing works of art confer a mystical aura upon the "original" that is quantifiably verified in the marketplace. Significantly, however, even Richard Wolin finds nothing worth questioning in Benjamin's thesis. Accepting at face value the claims of "revolutionary" significance for the "new techniques in the production and reception of works of art," Benjamin's theory is taken as the starting point for criticism, rather than being subject to criticism. Wolin's commentary here obviously reflects the impact of the currently fashionable reading, with its ironic displacement of the "auratic" onto Benjamin's own work:

> The entire domain of art is shaken to its innermost core, to the point where it seemingly negates its entire prehistory (i.e., its former auratic or cultic guise). That insight stands as a prerequisite for any informed analysis of art in its present (de-aestheticized) form.[13]

"The Work of Art in the Age of Mechanical Reproduction" contains valuable insights into the present and possible role of art in an age of mass communication. However, a critical glance at Benjamin's contentions, informed by a sense of his polemical context, suggests that Benjamin's historical account has been constructed for ideological purposes. Furthermore, although the spread of photography in its many commercial and artistic applications was an event that had dramatic ramifications for the visual arts,[14] it appears that its impact was largely opposite to the terms of Benjamin's thesis.

Benjamin begins his essay with a disclaimer. "In principle," he states, "a work of art has always been reproducible." However, he pointedly distinguishes between replicas made by hand and "mechanical reproductions" which, he says, "represent something new."[15] But not entirely new, for the Greeks used "two procedures of technically reproducing works of art: founding and stamping. Bronzes, terra cottas, and coins were the only art works which they could produce in quantity."[16] *Quantity* is Benjamin's chief criterion for a medium to qualify as mechanical. He does not explain why the invention of casting or of stamping should not have the historic status he assigns to the woodcut, which is, after all, only an extension of stamping.

> With the woodcut graphic art became mechanically reproducible for the first time, long before script became reproducible by print. The enormous changes which printing the mechanical reproduction of writing, has brought about in literature are a familiar story. However, within the phenomenon which we are here examining from the perspective of world history, print is merely a special, though particularly important, case.[17]

With this statement Benjamin attempts to discount what is generally accepted as the first true revolution in visual communication, at least in European history: the shift in the communication of written knowledge from the copyist's desk to the printer's workshop that occurred during the second half of the fifteenth century. In western Europe the use of the relief block for producing multiple images on paper dates to only a little over fifty years earlier, linked to the expansion of paper production around 1400. Until the development of the printing press, woodblocks were printed by hand through stamping or hand-rubbing—processes that were not essentially different from the founding and stamping techniques of the Greeks.

It is significant that in its earliest years (1400 to 1450) the print remained a secondary artistic medium, useful primarily for the dissemination of popular art in forms like playing cards and religious images. It was only after 1450, when the development of movable metal type, oil-based inks, and wooden hand-presses brought the advent of printing, that the printed image joined the printed word to form a powerful new medium of visual communication.

William Ivins and, more recently, Elizabeth Eisenstein have made us conscious of the revolutionary as opposed to evolutionary nature of this fifteenth-century phenomenon and have alerted us to its immense significance in the development of human culture.[18] Eisenstein's emphasis on the historical link between the printed image and the printed word should be of particular interest to theoreticians who are still trading upon Walter Benjamin's authority concerning the impact of technology on culture. The following two passages fairly represent Eisenstein's position:

> The fact that letters, numbers, and pictures were *all* alike subject to repeatability by the end of the fifteenth century needs more emphasis.
>
> As Dürer's career may suggest, the new arts of printing and engraving, far from reducing the importance of images, increased opportunities for image makers and helped to launch art history down its present path.[19]

One inescapable inference is that the phenomenon described by Benjamin as "the desire of contemporary masses to bring things 'closer' spatially and humanly,"[20] has a more universal application than he wished to entertain.

If we employ Benjamin's own criterion of quantity, we must conclude that the invention of the printing press and related technological advances identify the moment when "graphic art became mechanically reproducible for the first time," not the development of the carved woodblock as a matrix for stamping images. As Marshall McLuhan would later stress, printing "provided the first uniformly repeatable 'commodity,' the first assembly line—mass production."[21]

The linkage between the history of the printed image and that of the printed text requires some technical clarification. The spread of printing and the rise of publishing houses during the second half of the fifteenth century was as crucial for the high-art reproductive medium of engraving (demanding greater skill to make and trouble to print, not type-compatible and thus more costly) as it was for the low-art relief woodcut process (simple, direct, and type-compatible). While the art of engraving on metal goes back to the Greeks and Etruscans, it was not until the 1470s—concurrent with the rise of book production—that the medium was taken up by painters like Martin Schongauer. Again, to quote Eisenstein, "The highly competitive commercial character of the new mode of book production encouraged the relatively rapid adoption of any innovation that commended a given edition to purchasers."[22] This commercial competition carried over into print publishing, where it produced the beginnings of the "star system" of artistic promotion that is such an important aspect of the visual media today.

In order to create new markets and expand old ones, technical innovations in the production of printed images were introduced at a nearly geometrical rate of increase. Variations on the intaglio process developed during the eighteenth century in an effort to duplicate the effects of the drawing media, for instance, are both staggering in quantity and impressive in technical quality. To pose, as Benjamin does, the invention of lithography in Germany at the turn of the nineteenth century as an "essentially new stage" in the development of mechanical reproduction is to be historically misleading.

Although lithography's ease of execution opened up the reproductive media to a wider range of artists, its potential for direct communication was limited by the fact that "fixing" the image on the stone was a complicated and specialized process. Moreover, a heavy press was required to print the stones. Thus, while woodblocks could be inked and printed by hand and it was not uncommon for artists to have their own intaglio presses, lithographic stones had to be prepared and printed by craftsmen-printers in the employ of commercial publishers.

Benjamin, however, used the invention of lithography to introduce a second factor relating to mechanical reproduction: speed. To qualify as an instance of mechanical reproduction in Benjamin's terms, an image needs both to be produced in quantity and to convey its effect rapidly. It must keep pace with modern life. Benjamin's conspicuous preoccupation with quantity and speed helps us understand his rather elusive concept of the "aura" of the traditional work of art.

Following Wolin's analysis, it appears that Benjamin saw his task as applying the Marxist concept of the mode of production to the history of art. Here "the auratic" identified the commodity high art specialized in reproducing for elitist consumption, ironically mystified by associations of originality, difficulty, and strangeness. Benjamin defines the aura as "the unique phenomenon of a distance, however close it may be."[23] An entirely different product, he assumes, should result from combining the Renaissance concept of quantity with the modern concept of speed. Organized into a new mode of production, they have the power to counter the production of auratic distance through the infinite multiplication and rapid dissemination of the formerly unique or rare image. Thus, in art as in life, familiarity can be expected to breed a liberating contempt.

As we have seen, however, the speed with which a lithographic image could be transferred to the stone had nothing to do with its potential as a medium for direct communication with a mass audience. In fact, lithography's advantage in terms of speed was more than offset by its limitation in terms of quantity. Lithographic printing was hampered by the number of good impressions that one stone could produce in comparison with wood-block printing. And since text was printed through the relief letterpress process, lithographs either had to be printed separately and *inserted* into large-circulation journals, or the paper had to be run through two presses.

However, at precisely the same time that lithography was being developed in Germany, the Englishman Thomas Bewick was developing end-grain wood engraving into a medium that was capable of finer detail (that is, denser visual information) than the side-grain woodcut, while retaining the woodcut's traditional advantage as a type-compatible relief printing process. The rapid expansion in the production of illustrated books and periodicals that characterized the nineteenth century was made technically possible through the interdependence of several major developments: smooth machine-made papers, wood engraving capable of great detail, more powerful steam presses, and the invention of a practical stereotype (later electrotype) process for duplicating the surface of set type and relief blocks that was capable of producing infinite editions. For the first time, original images like Bewick's, as well as reproductions of images conceived in other media by other artists, were available to a truly mass audience.[24]

"Lithography enabled graphic art to illustrate everyday life," Walter Benjamin declared, "and it began to keep pace with printing." This is historically inaccurate, I have argued, with regard to both the history of lithography as a medium of visual communication and the relation of the printed image to the printed word. As we have seen, innovations in printing images and text tend to advance together, reflecting the popular desire "to bring things 'closer' spatially and humanly."

By the 1890s technological developments in lithographic printing did achieve the kind of acceleration in the production of imagery that Benjamin attributed to the early years of the medium. This took place, however, over half a century after the moment that Benjamin identified as the most important turning point in the history of the mechanical reproduction of works of art: the development of photography.

> Only a few decades after its invention, lithography was surpassed by photography. For the first time in the process of pictorial reproduction, photography freed the hand of the most important artistic functions which henceforth devolved only upon the eye looking into a lens. . . . The process of pictorial reproduction was accelerated so enormously that it could keep pace with speech.[25]

As with lithography, Benjamin here confounds speed of composition with speed of transmission. Photography itself is a comparatively inefficient reproductive medium. In order to achieve quantity editions it must be linked with one of the traditional print processes. It was not until the second half of the nineteenth century that photography was incorporated into the developing relief printing processes in a manner that suggests analogies with the decisive events of the second half of the fifteenth century. Photorelief printing was perfected between 1875 and 1889, and it was not until the last decade of the century that tonal photographic reproduction was available to a popular audience through mass-circulation journals.[26]

Four centuries after the development of printing, the photorelief process finally eliminated the single advantage the woodcut had maintained over other print media: its type-compatibility. From the beginnings of the printed image in the fifteenth century to the last quarter of the nineteenth century, type-compatible reproductions had been the product of the hand of man. Whether crude or sophisticated, they could lay claim to being works of art. Now, however, the art of reproduction, which in fact had been an art of interpretation, was superseded by information.

This profound cultural shift was effected by two factors: a positivist desire for veracity (as opposed to the traditional concept of authenticity) and economics—photomechanical reproduction eliminated the need for interpretive craftsmen. These were the points emphasized in 1878 by Alfred de Lostalot for the readers of the *Gazette des beaux-arts:*

> Since photography now conveys visual information of almost infallible precision, one cannot help but notice that the wood engraving conceals under the superficial surface seductions of its velvety brilliance a fundamental vice: lack of honesty. It coarsens and distorts the images entrusted to it.

Moreover, de Lostalot goes on to say, "To reproduce well a work characterized by detail and precision, a wood engraving costs as much in both time and money as a good etching, even a copperplate engraving."[27] Over ten years earlier, writing in the *Gazette des beaux-arts* about the prints at the Salon of 1867, the art collector and critic Philippe Burty had complained along similar lines, "The relatively high cost of the wood engraving is the cause of its downfall; it is this which makes publishers want to look for a substitute."[28]

Paradoxically, while advances in photomechanical reproduction during the second half of the nineteenth century destroyed the commercial viability of the traditional reproductive processes, these same advances encouraged a change in thinking about the print as an autonomous medium of expression. In his 1867 Salon review quoted above Philippe Burty wrote:

> Nothing better demonstrates the approaching and irretrievable end of the art of the print than a visit to the fine art galleries of the Exposition Universelle. When one has investigated every nook and cranny . . . it is perfectly clear that the world has lost interest in engraving, that the woodcut is in peril, that "process" engraving promises to put an end to the burin, etching, lithography, and the woodcut, and that the *agent provocateur* in these revolutionary maneuvers is, directly or indirectly, Photography.[29]

However, twenty-two years later, in his catalogue introduction for the 1889 exhibition of the Society of Painter-Printmakers, Burty presented a radically different point of view:

> The photographic reproductive processes, which are improving and bringing about a popularization of information, cannot threaten that which is mediated by the mind, translated by the hand. . . . Nothing which springs from this source of impersonal information has any parallel with the product of human creation. Rather, the two travel toward opposite horizons: Science validates itself in questions of utility; Art nourishes and brings to delicious fruition life itself.[30]

The aggressive aestheticism of Burty's statement conveys a confidence in the future of the print media that proved to be well justified. The 1890s saw an expansion of the visual arts that had its precedent in the time of Dürer. As with the new arts of printing then, the new photographic media that developed in the course of the nineteenth century created new markets and increased opportunities for image makers, opportunities that included the incorporation of photographic imagery into the traditional art media.

But it was not only in the realm of the traditional media that the development of the photomechanical processes brought liberation. These reproductive processes expanded the realm of possibilities for photography as well. As Benjamin points out:

> Around 1900 technical reproduction had reached a standard that not only permitted it to reproduce all transmitted works of art and thus to cause the most profound change in their impact upon the public; it also had captured a place of its own among the artistic processes. For the study of this standard nothing is more revealing than the nature of the repercussions that these two different manifestations—the reproduction of works of art and the art of the film—have had on art in its traditional form.[31]

The distinction between the two aspects of this complex phenomenon—the reproduction of works of art, including photographs, through photomechanical means versus the rise of artistic media like film that are *inherently* directed at a mass audience—is not easily maintained in critical discourse. Benjamin himself wanted to justify an elision of the first into the second category:

> To an ever greater degree, the work of art reproduced becomes the work of art designed for reproducibility. . . . With the different methods of technical repro-

> duction of a work of art, its fitness for exhibition increased to such an extent that the quantitative shift between its two poles turned into a qualitative transformation of its nature.[32]

But within a thriving capitalistic economy, photographic reproductions of traditional works of art have become commodities in themselves. One need only survey the recent history of the art market to discredit the crisis that Benjamin constructed for traditional forms of artistic expression and to construct a crisis of another kind. For reproductions of works of art also have been utilized to promote a fetishism of the original in ways that have not only led to prices that are wildly out of line with the relative value and rarity of art objects, but also to absurdist claims about the inherent value of originality and authenticity. Moreover, the capacity of our society to co-opt unconventional forms of artistic expression (as opposed to unconventional content) would appear to be virtually infinite.

It is finally Benjamin's focus on film that reveals the relentless inertia of his vision. In his view, film must obviously be a privileged medium.

> In the case of films, mechanical reproduction is not, as with literature and painting, an external condition for mass distribution. Mechanical reproduction is inherent in the very technique of film production. This technique not only permits in the most direct way but virtually causes mass distribution.[33]

The effect of this inherent advantage is to endow quantity with the normative status previously assigned to quality.

> The mass is a matrix from which all traditional behavior toward works of art issues today in a new form. Quantity has been transmuted into quality. The greatly increased mass of participants has produced a change in the mode of participation.[34]

Finally (and most revealingly), film is seen as welcoming the "state of distraction" that Benjamin identifies as an essential feature both of the age and of the proletarian destiny of culture. It is a striking measure of his political loyalties that he embraces it with such self-effacing, resolutely anti-elitist earnestness.

> Distraction as provided by art presents a covert control of the extent to which new tasks have become soluble by apperception. Since, moreover, individuals are tempted to avoid such tasks, art will tackle the most difficult and most important ones where it is able to mobilize the masses. Today it does so in the film. Reception in a state of distraction, which is increasing noticeably in all fields of art and is symptomatic of profound changes in apperception, finds in the film its true means of exercise.[35]

This desperate machine-age utopia of what amounts to programmed social responsiveness is what Benjamin's "destruction of the aura" finally intends. There is more than a trace of technological determinism here, which suggests why Benjamin was eager to perceive a technological revolution in the photograph. Film appears to augur its natural evolution toward a controlled environment.

A more realistic view of the role of film within the development of mass communication can perhaps best be elucidated by a passage that Benjamin himself intended in quite the opposite way:

> One of the foremost tasks of art has always been the creation of a demand which could be fully satisfied only later. The history of every art form aspires to effects which could be fully obtained only with a changed technical standard, that is to say, in a new art form.[36]

Benjamin intended to describe developments in the art of the nineteenth century that would lead to the revolutionary triumph of film. From the perspective that half a century gives, however, film in turn can be seen as an aspiration "to effects which could be fully obtained only with a changed technical standard"—the development of the electronic media.[37]

In the final analysis, Benjamin was wrongheaded about the history of mechanical reproduction and wrong in fact about photography as the key to the creation of a mass audience for visual communication. Even from his Marxist standpoint, the relation between photography and art would be seen, not as a prefigurement of the mass communication made possible by the electronic media, but as the final step in the presentation of the art object as commodity. It is ironic that, with the proliferation of video cassette recorders, the perception of film is again becoming a solitary pursuit. At the same time, rising museum attendance would seem to indicate that the traditional forms of painting, sculpture, the graphic arts, and even (perhaps especially) photography have become more, not less, valued by the masses. Contrary to Benjamin's expectations, increasingly refined (and increasingly expensive) art reproductions offered by museums, collectors, even artists themselves, have not lessened the public's interest in the perpetually and mysteriously distant "original" work of art. The aura or perceived potency of presence of the art object is seemingly enhanced, not diminished, in "the age of mechanical reproduction."

NOTES

1. Rosalind E. Krauss, "The Originality of the Avant-Garde," first published in the journal *October* in 1981, republished in *The Originality of the Avant-Garde and Other Modernist Myths* (Cambridge and London: MIT Press, 1985), 152.

2. Douglas Crimp, "On the Museum's Ruins," revised version published in *The Anti-Aesthetic: Essays on Postmodern Culture* (Port Townsend, Wash.: Bay Press, 1983), 52–53.

3. Douglas Crimp, "The Art of Exhibition," *October* 30 (Fall 1984): 56–57.

4. Richard Wolin, *Walter Benjamin: An Aesthetic of Redemption* (New York: Columbia University Press, 1982), 184–85.

5. *Illuminations,* edited and with an introduction by Hannah Arendt, trans. Harry Zohn (New York: Schocken Books, 1969), 241.

6. Ibid., 218.

7. See Wolin, 139–212; and Susan Buck-Morss, *The Origin of Negative Dialectics: Theodor W. Adorno, Walter Benjamin, and the Frankfurt Institute* (New York: The Free Press, 1977), 136–50.

8. Benjamin, *Illuminations,* 242.

9. Wolin, 255.

10. Ibid., 159.

11. Walter Benjamin, *Briefe,* 2 vols., ed. Gershom Scholem and Theodor W. Adorno (Frankfurt: Suhrkamp Verlag, 1966), 2:690, quoted in Wolin, 185–86.

12. Ibid., 695.

13. Wolin, 190.

14. Perhaps most significant within the context in which the present study appears, photography "moved the investigation out of the realm of aesthetic distinctions into that of social functions." Walter Benjamin, from "Walter Benjamin's Short History of Photography," trans. Phil Patton, *Artforum* 15, no. 6 (February 1977): 50.

15. Benjamin, *Illuminations,* 218.

16. Ibid.

17. Ibid., 218–19.

18. William M. Ivins Jr., *Prints and Visual Communication* (Cambridge, Mass.: Harvard University Press, 1953); Elizabeth L. Eisenstein, *The Printing Revolution in Early Modern Europe* (Cambridge: Cambridge University Press, 1983).

19. Eisenstein, 23, 35.

20. Benjamin, *Illuminations,* 223.

21. Marshall McLuhan and Quentin Fiore, *The Medium is the Massage* (New York, London, and Toronto: Bantam Books, 1967), 50.

22. Eisenstein, 21.

23. Benjamin, *Illuminations,* 222.

24. For more information on this subject see my dissertation, "The Artistic Revival of the Woodcut in France, 1875–1894," University of Michigan, 1982, 1–29; and Jacquelynn Baas and Richard S. Field, *The Artistic Revival of the Woodcut in France, 1850–1900* (Ann Arbor, Mich.: University of Michigan Museum of Art, 1984), 14–16.

25. Benjamin, *Illuminations,* 219.

26. Baas and Field, 16–17, 21, n. 20.

27. Alfred de Lostalot, "Exposition Universelle: aquarelles, dessins et gravures," *Gazette des beaux-arts* (November 1878): 726–27.

28. Philippe Burty, "La Gravure et la photographie en 1867," *Gazette des beaux-arts* (September 1867): 262.

29. Ibid., 252.

30. *Exhibitions of the Society of Printmakers 1889–1897* (New York and London: Garland, 1981), p. 8 of the introduction to the catalogue of the 1889 exhibition.

31. Benjamin, *Illuminations,* 219–20.

32. Ibid., 224–25.

33. Ibid., 244, n. 7.

34. Ibid., 239.

35. Ibid., 240.

36. Ibid., 237.

37. Benjamin himself mentions radio in his note 12 (*Illuminations,* p. 247.). That the electronic medium of television was already holding out promise of "perception in a state of distraction" by the time Benjamin wrote his essay is indicated in the contemporary work of the Marxist artist Diego Rivera. Rivera's short-lived mural designed for the RCA Building at Rockefeller Center in 1933, replicated in Mexico the following year, features two gigantic television tubes before which the masses sit mesmerized. See Lucienne Block, "On Location with Diego Rivera," *Art in America* 74, no. 2 (February 1986): 102–23.

19

ART REPRODUCTIONS in the LIBRARY

Notes on their History and Use

WOLFGANG M. FREITAG

> Stendhal: "It is dangerous to buy engravings of paintings one sees on one's travels. Soon the engraving forms the sole recollection and destroys the real memory. So it has happened to me with the Sistine Madonna in Dresden. The beautiful engraving by Müller has destroyed it for me while the bad pastels of Raffael Mengs in the same gallery, of which I have nowhere seen engravings, I still see clearly before me."
>
> This ought to be taken note of by the art historians, whose imaginations are filled with photographs, if not half tones.
>
> Max J. Friedländer[1]

It has always been possible to make copies of works of art. Whatever men have created other men have tried to copy, succeeding more or less. Such copying always was routinely done as exercise by pupils and apprentices as part of their regular training, by master artists as advertisements in order to woo potential clients or to become well-known and famous and naturally also for economic gain, and by third parties who as businessmen were only interested in profits from the sale of reproductions of well-known works.

But until about the year 1400 such reproductions were mostly replicas, i.e., slowly made single copies of the originals and like the originals produced by hand one after another, and no two copies of the same original were ever exactly alike. Due to the slowness of the manual processes, the number of copies that could be made of any given original remained of necessity very small. The ancients knew of only two methods of mechanically reproducing certain types of works of art: casting of sculpture from a mould in bronze or in terra-cotta and the stamping of medals and coins with the aid of a die. With the invention in the West of the woodcut, the first autographic process was developed that was suited to the mass reproduction of line drawings. Art had entered the age of mechanical reproducibility via the printing press. The medium of the woodcut was soon followed by two other mechanical graphic reproduction processes: metal engraving and, much later in the eighteenth century, wood engraving and lithography and certain combinations of these processes that were capable of producing a great variety of pictorial effects.[2]

Thus, beginning with the woodcuts of the fifteenth century, it became possible to make what William M. Ivins has called "exactly repeatable pictorial statements"[3] in large quantities. Such statements could be made either by a creative *inventor* artist *(peintre-graveur)* who drew directly on the woodblock, cut the block himself, or had it cut by a craftsman assistant whose task it was to cut away just the portion of the block not covered with the artist's lines. In this way an artist greatly increased the reach of a direct pictorial statement.

Indirect pictorial statements were all those graphic reproductions through the print medium for which an intermediary, the artisan, was himself responsible for making the repeatable statement after the original statement had been made by the artist. Such copies were mechanically reproducible, but they were not in any sense more "true" than the single replicas of the ancients. They were at best messages about unique original works that had to be seen before they could be understood and appreciated.

The consequences of the invention and perfection of graphic media for the shaping (and warping) of modern man's perception and appreciation of art have been examined by William M. Ivins in his epoch-making work *Prints and Visual Communication*. Ivins was the first to discern that not only verbal languages but also visual languages are subject to the rules of a syntax and that visual statements must be analyzed according to their syntactic structure, which is determined by such factors as the characteristics, i.e., the possibilities and limitations of the materials and tools used, as well as by traditions and conventions of how men see things which, as Ivins discovered, vary greatly among nations:

> Much as he might want to, a German in the fifteenth or sixteenth century could not draw like an Italian, or *vice versa*. We get sharp evidence of this in the copies that each made from the other. . . . Although the specific lines of the original were there before him, the copyist never actually followed them closely in his copy, and rarely made any attempt to do so. . . . Especially was this true when the copy was not only a copy but a translation into another medium. The results of this are perhaps most easily to be seen in the prints after works of art, for in none of them are we able to find the kind of qualitative statement that is necessary for connoisseurship of the work of art itself.[4]

By the turn from the eighteenth to the nineteenth century, the old print media, engraving and etching, were used almost exclusively for purposes of reproduction, and only the new lithographic process, which permitted artists who were no longer adept in using the engraver's burin or the etcher's needle to draw directly on the lithographic stone, became the principal autographic print medium for the creative artist until the revival of the woodcut, which Expressionism brought about.

Photography and the various photochemical and photomechanical printing processes, which were developed to make the positive photographic print compatible with the advanced letterpress technology of the nineteenth century and which soon became the prevalent medium for making reproductions of works of art, were a discovery that to Ivins' mind was even more important for mankind than the invention of printing with movable type. "By the third quarter of the century many experiments had been made towards getting the photograph translated into printer's ink without the intervention of either the draughtsman or the engraver."[5] "Man had at last achieved a way of making visual reports that had no interfering symbolic linear syntax of their own."[6] It took more than twenty years until the above mentioned statement was challenged in a book titled *Visual Communication and the Graphic Arts* by Estelle Jussim.[7] Jussim, borrowing tools from the arsenal of information science and communications theory, proves in her investigation of the channels and codes of the picture language spoken by photographs and disseminated, amplified, and often distorted by the photomechanical print media, "that even today's photographs are simply maps of originals, not duplications of originals."[8] Dr. Jussim devotes one chapter, "The New Technologies and the History of Art,"[9] to the issues of interpretation versus fidelity (after reproductions), the invention and perfection of the making of photographs in the context of an examination of two successive editions of a popular and widely used American art history textbook,[9] and statements by some of the late nineteenth century's most famous print connoisseurs and makers of illustrated books on the problems of reproducing art. Ivins, who had hailed the advent of photography as the great liberating force in art history, pointed out that "it has brought about a very complex restudy and rewriting of the accepted history of the arts of the past," and that "it is interesting to notice how few of the books of connoisseurship published prior to 1880 are still either authoritative or on the shelves for ready reference."[10] And, he further made the observation that the only catalogues raisonnés produced with illustrations in one of the print media that are still useful today are the catalogues raisonnés of prints! All the prephotographic reproductions of works of art have become the object of the student and collector of *prints*. They have not lost their value qua prints. But they are no longer admissible as evidence in the study of the works they depict.

Having learned from Estelle Jussim via Marshall McLuhan and other information theorists that photographic reproductions are not capable of making pictorial statements without syntax and that the photograph as a channel of information transfer is subject to the limitations of a code just as the graphic print media are (even if the photographic code is a subliminal one), we must ask ourselves what kind of art reproductions are likely to of the greatest possible use to the art historian; which are acceptable, which are dangerous, and which ought the art library to consider, and which ought it to reject.

From all that has been said so far, it is clear that all reproductions can only be accepted as messages *about* the originals for which they stand. It is also clear that all messages that have been *twice* encoded and dispatched through channels, as is the case with plates in books or single half-tone or color prints, are less acceptable than direct photographic prints created by a photographer acting as "primary codifier."[11] An art library therefore needs collections of photographs and color transparencies in addition to illustrated books, although the latter may suffice in general, nonspecialized libraries.

The problematic nature of photographic reproductions was recognized by several of the great art historians of the nineteenth century, who each reacted quite differently to the new invention.

Charles Eliot Norton (1827–1908), the first to occupy a chair in the history of art at Harvard, is remembered by his university as the one among its many famous teachers who "taught an unseeing age to see" (inscription on the pedestal of the bust in the vestibule of Norton Lecture Hall, Fogg Art Museum, Cambridge, Massachusetts). But he did so largely without using visual aids. For even though Norton had over the years brought together in the Fogg Art Museum a large if unsystematically gathered collection of illustrative materials—mainly drawings, prints, and small casts—that did include photographs and after 1896 seems to have included some lantern slides, his use of these visual materials actually declined at a time when the technology for making better quality reproductions advanced. That Norton was not unaware of the contribution that good reproductions can make to the study of art and that he had wrestled with the problem in his forties is proven by a note on "The autotype or carbon process in photography," which he published in the *Nation* in 1869.[12]

Rather than confronting them with images, Professor Norton immersed students in the poetry and prose writing of the Renaissance; he endeavored to instill in them through literature the right receptive attitudes, so that the originals which they would see eventually in situ would have a predictable, proper impact upon their minds and aesthetic sensibilities.[13] An interesting contrast is presented in the attitude of one of Norton's European contemporaries, Herman Grimm (1828–1901), art historian at the University of Berlin. As the son of the philologist Wilhelm Grimm and brought up in the ambiance of German classical literature and idealistic philosophy, Grimm had many things in common with Norton (among which was a deep admiration for Ralph Waldo Emerson); the most noteworthy of which in our context, however, was the conviction that art must be experienced emotionally and not only aesthetically and that great poetry and literature are some of the most important conditioners toward that end. Grimm however did not eschew reproductions. He used slides extensively, and he wrote newspaper articles about their revolutionary impact on the teaching of art history. Paradoxically, he used reproductions in order to prepare his students for very much the same experiences of art that Norton had established as his goal in his nonvisual approach to visual art. "The slide projection apparatus," he writes in the *Nationalzeitung,* "enables us to make a clear distinction between that in art which moves the soul and that which is merely of interest from the aspect of art history."[14] Grimm was interested in the aesthetic as well as in the ethical message of art, and he believed that lantern slides were capable of sending these messages.

According to the twentieth century social philosopher Walter Benjamin, any work of art must be considered as having a unique place value depending, of course, which location upon the coordinate value system a dominant culture assigns to it.[15] If the two coordinates are cult-value (vertical) and exhibition-value (horizontal), most of the art of the past that originally possessed high cult-value has moved down the vertical axis and is now chiefly of interest for its exhibit-value.

The art library's visual collection neither is concerned with providing moral or aesthetic uplift nor is it primarily in the business of emulating the museum through holdings of high exhibit-value. The art library's visual collections must contain reproductions that have high *information value,* i.e., data on works of art that can be discussed and interpreted from a variety of scholarly angles. Among those are connoisseurship, history of styles and forms, and iconography. Neither the illustration and documentation of political and social events nor aesthetic goals are to determine the policy of building the collection; only the documentation value in relation to the institution's (academic art department, museum, independent research institute) stated policy objective determines the policy. It has been conservatively estimated that to provide fully adequate visual documentation for study and research in the traditional fields of art history (i.e., the arts of Asia, Europe, and the Americas of historic times, excluding prehistoric art, pre-Columbian art, and the arts of all nonliterate contemporary tribal cultures, which are rapidly emerging as prime areas of art historical investigation) would require a minimum of two million images. From this follows that no art library should attempt to develop collections for multidisciplinary use as long as it is still struggling to satisfy the basic needs of art history. This, however, does not mean that it should not invite scholars from other disciplines to use what it has to offer and to provide subject access to its visual collections from a variety of external (non-art historical) entry points, if it can afford to do so. The problem of the work of art as an object of study or document for the general historian has been discussed by several writers recently.[16]

Considering what has been said so far about the pitfalls of using two-dimensional reproductions of two-dimensional works of art and the danger inherent in such reproductions (that the gullible eye of the beholder is seduced into accepting the message of the medium for the message of the original object, which fails to come through to him), it is not surprising that the use of photography became widespread first in a less problematic area of art history in the documentation of architectural monuments. Here, the enormous difference between the size of the originals and the scale of the reproduction made for perhaps weaker messages but, certainly, also made for messages less in danger of distorting the facts; because here the mental act of distinguishing between the art monument and the message *about* the art monument is more easily performed by the viewer.

Photographs of works of art were made almost immediately after photography was invented, and these photographs were predominantly photos of architectural monuments. (Contrary to the legend that accompanies the serious scientific history of photography, the sixty-six prints supplied by W. H. Fox Talbot to illustrate Sir William Stirlings' *Annals of the Artists of Spain* [1847] which has often been hailed as the first book to use photographs to illustrate an art historical text, the Talbotypes were photographs of reproduction prints, not of the paintings themselves.) The possibilities of photography as an aid to the architectural historian were recognized as early as 1839, i.e., thirteen years after Joseph Nicéphore Niepce had made that famous picture of the inner court of his house, an "architectural photograph," which is considered the first successful photograph from nature.[17]

> Early in November 1839 Horace Vernet, painter of historical battle scenes, who travelled to Egypt with Frederic Goupil Fesquet, reported from Alexandria: "We keep daguerreotyping away like lions."[18]

> The Science Museum, London, possesses 158 wholeplate daguerrotypes of Italian architecture and views taken in 1840 and 1841. . . . They are the earliest surviving photographs of Italy.[19]

In the New World there were related attempts to photograph the architectural past in a series of very successful archaeological photographs. John Lloyd Stephens, an American traveler, and Frederick Catherwood, an English artist, in 1841 revisited the lost cities of Yucatán where they had been two years earlier. The daguerreotypes which they took of the ruined Mayan architecture, supplemented by camera lucida drawings, were published as engravings in *Incidents of Travel in Yucatan* (1843).[20]

The French Commission for Historical Monuments represented by its president, the poet and novelist Prosper Mérimée, recognized early that the best use of photography was to record disintegrating buildings of the past for posterity. In 1842 the architect and *inspecteur* of historic buildings for the City of Paris, Viollet-le-Duc, had daguerreotypes taken of Notre Dame. A photographic chronicle in 1,500 detail photographs of the new wing of the Louvre was made in 1854.

The first major effort to record for archival and registration purposes the holdings of a museum's collection seems to have been undertaken by the English photo-pioneer Roger Fenton when he set out to create a photographic catalogue of the classical sculpture in the British Museum at about 1855 or 1856, shortly after his return from the Crimean War.

Immediately of the greatest importance was the new invention to connoisseurship—that field at the basis of art scholarship that has as its goal the proper attribution of a work of art—in contrast to art history, which is concerned with its interpretation within a historical context. The historian without connoisseurship is on shaky ground. Connoisseurship without thorough grounding in art history is equally suspect but remains at least a possibility. The attribution which the connoisseur makes comes to him spontaneously after looking closely at a work of art; it is a somewhat intuitive discovery. The gift of connoisseurship is not teachable but "trainable," i.e., those who have it instinctively can greatly increase their powers of discrimination by exercising them constantly in front of great art and with the help of photographs. Bernard Berenson (1865–1959), one of the greatest connoisseurs, began his career just at the moment when the photograph had become refined enough to render those tactile properties of paintings that were so important for Berenson's method in determining authenticity. Giovanni Morelli (1816–91), Berenson's revered teacher, already had used the cruder photographs of his day to study the form of details such as ears and fingers on which he based his attribution of schools and "hands," but now it even became possible to make judgments on condition, thickness of paint application (impasto), and other technical properties of a panel or canvas. The collection of photographs that Berenson built and brought together as an adjunct to his library at his Florentine villa I Tatti soon numbered more than 100,000 items, many of them details of larger images, forming a rich visual resource for the study of Italian painting of the late Middle Ages and the Renaissance, each bearing the collector's copious annotations on the verso.[21]

On 14 October 1893, Berenson made the following entry in his notebook that sheds a characteristic light on the way in which he thought photographs should be used by the connoisseur:

> Of the writer on art today we all expect not only that intimate acquaintance with his subject which modern means of conveyance have made possible, but also that patient comparison of a given work with all the other works by the same master which photography has rendered easy. It is not at all difficult to see at any rate nine tenths of a great master's works (Titian's or Tintoretto's, for instance) in such rapid succession that the memory of them will be fresh enough to enable the critic to determine the place and the value of any picture. And when this continuous study of originals is supplemented by isochromatic photographs, such comparison attains almost the accuracy of the physical science.[22]

We have seen from the remark by an equally famous connoisseur of the twentieth century, Max J. Friedländer, which is quoted at the head of this paper, that Berenson's enthusiasm for photographs as an aid in the task of connoisseurship was not shared by all workers in the field.

The reception of the new tool by art historians who were not primarily connoisseurs or museum officials was even more mixed. Jacob Burckhardt (1818–97), the great Swiss master historian and author of the *Cicerone* (1855), appreciated and used photographs (the little man and his big portfolio of photographs were a familiar sight in the streets of Basel, where he lived and taught at the university). On his travels he took great pains to find photographers in Florence, Rome, and in other Italian cities that he visited who were capable of producing reproductions that would lend themselves to his interpretation of the works they represented. "Since we have photography," he writes to Heinrich Wölfflin in a letter dated 24 September 1896, "I cannot believe in the possibility that that which is great in art can ever go under or lose its power."[23] Wölfflin could not have disagreed more as can be seen from portions of the correspondence with his teacher concerning the progress of his great work on the Renaissance, *Die Klassische Kunst,* which appeared in 1899: "To illustrate your book with good photographs in a sensible format—I know—is not your cup of tea," writes Burckhardt on 29 August 1896.[24] And Wölfflin, who had such a horror of distortion by all reproductions but especially photographs—so much so that he had originally considered publishing his book without any illustrations at all—replies from Italy after looking at art in situ:

> From day to day I become more convinced that it is absolutely futile to try to understand monumental art on the basis of what we can learn from photographs. I have to strike out more and more of the notes I made in Basel. But, of course, nobody will in the least appreciate what I am doing because today people want to have only photographs explained. (23 May 1897)[25]

Burckhardt was far from being uncritical in his use of art reproductions. He was well aware that photographing the work of art meant the intraposition of an external interpreting intelligence between the work of art and its viewer. Wölfflin, by insisting that the students were all able to draw reasonably well so that they could make their own sketches of the works they studied in his seminar, made sure that at least one intermediary step in the transmission of the visual data was eliminated.

A long time before the tremendous power of the photographic enlargement to alter the meaning of the original was realized, again by such writers as Jussim, Burckhardt had asked himself questions about the harmful effects that the change of scale from the original to reproduction might have on the beholder. Burckhardt thought that the change of the dimensions that occurs in reproductions was something that must always be kept in mind, and he was perfectly aware that it greatly modifies the message the viewer receives; but, like Hans Tietze (1880–1954) after him, he felt that reductions in format distorted much less than enlargements. And here the projected photograph, the slide, was the greatest offender. Tietze had dealt with other aspects of reproductions in a chapter of his *Methode der Kunstgeschichte*[26] in which he attempts a classification of art historical sources:

> The change of scale relationships is only one change of many caused by photography. Obviously, the choice of the view point is also of the greatest importance. Anyone who has ever photographed a building has consciously influenced the psychological impact of the object, be it through a foreshortening of some unsightly lines, through a loss of depth and the apparent crossing of architectural lines or through the inclusion of "mood inducing" elements such as foreground detail, etc. Clearly, our innate artistic preferences often get the upper hand when we have set out to take a documentary picture of a piece of architecture. These interpretative manipulations can, if worst comes to worst, result in the complete falsification of the artistic message of the original. A sculpture photographed from a wrong angle can be distorted beyond recognition, and the photograph of

> a painting which has been darkened or lightened too much in the process of being developed and printed, in which all original tonal values have been changed, certainly is a source that we must approach with a most critical attitude.[27]

Clarence Kennedy, whose 1924 Harvard Ph.D. dissertation appears to be the very first doctoral thesis dealing with the problem of photographing art accepted by a major American university[28] and whose whole career was shaped by the dichotomy of objective versus subjective values in interpretation, had become aware of the vexing fact that photography of sculpture can be explanation, criticism, interpretation. The photographer of any work of art has several alternatives. He may attempt to photograph in an objective way, or he may use the work of art as a motif or a kind of light-modulating device to create an image for personal expression.[29]

The skepticism with which a Wölfflin regarded all photographs, the warning note that Burckhardt sounded to be on the alert for possible distortions caused by changes of scale and choice of point of view, is still echoed by today's art historians' great mistrust of color reproductions and rightly so. Color fidelity to the original is extremely important for the reproduction as document, and it is very difficult—almost impossible—to obtain; it is logical that faithful reproductions in color are impossible to produce unless the dimensions of the reproductions correspond exactly to those of the originals. But even these are likely to disappoint, as anyone knows who has looked at framed 1:1 reproductions for sale in a museum shop. Since most colored art photographs and slides are either reductions or enlargements, they distort the originals; the most that can be expected of them is that the shades, intensities, and the color temperatures of the pigments on the print or slide reproduction correspond at least in degree to the tonal values of the original. As we have noted when considering distortions of scale, slides have the greatest potential for transmitting misinformation on original color. Even the best color slides, even if projected from a correct distance so that the projected image on the screen is neither larger nor smaller than the original, will falsify the message of the original because they are transparent, and this adds the luminosity of a stained glass window indiscriminately to a fresco, to a wooden panel, or to a canvas. Such an intensification, which eclipses the exhibit-value but not the information-value of the original, will have the dangerous consequence of making the original appear flat to the student who must learn art history from slides if he happens to live far distant from the site of the originals. Edgar Wind in a footnote to his essay on "The Mechanization of Art" likens the good black-and-white photograph of an oil painting to a conscientious piano transcription of an orchestral score where all sounds of the full orchestra are given their reduced equivalents on the "grey scale" of the piano keyboard. Color prints he compares to the sound of a reduced orchestra in which, moreover, "all instruments play out of tune."[30]

Thus for study, teaching, and serious critical scholarship in most fields of art there is still nothing better to take the place of the black-and-white photograph, where with careful printing one can at least control the tonal contrasts.

Today even the purists among art historians will of course use color slides for lecture demonstrations simply because their students have become conditioned all through their lives by the mass media, especially magazines and color television, to a coarseness of art perception that they cannot simply shed. Visual education or re-education, which must precede or accompany art historical education, should attempt first to teach students how to find a personal relationship to the originals and then how to read messages about these works in monochrome.

After what has been said until now, it will come as a surprise that there is a place for the color photograph, the color slide, and even certain types of photomechanical and electronic analog color and digital reproductions in the arsenal of the art historian at all. But this is definitely the case, because, in order to study modern painting, especially of certain schools (beginning with the Impressionists perhaps but certainly with the Fauves and continuing through the Cubist and Expressionist painting between the two world wars), one needs color reproductions for archival, study, and teaching purposes. Color becomes even more of a necessity to give an idea of post-World War II developments. Black-and-white reproductions are not adequate for works by Tachists; the chromatic complexities of Abstract Expressionists, Action Painters, minimal art and conceptual art practitioners; nor such representational art movements as pop art and photo-realism.

Some modern two-dimensional art (but not abstract expressionism which is the most difficult to reproduce in any medium) suffers surprisingly little distortion of its message when it is reproduced photographically or photomechanically. (Such obvious works, like Roy Lichtenstein's Mickey Mouse serigraphs and Andy Warhol's Campbell Soup cans, that are conceived to be manufactured as multiples regardless whether they were originally executed in the medium of oil, silk-screen, or lithography, are not meant here.) It has been suggested by writers such as Benjamin and Wind that the modern painter, knowingly or unknowingly, has been influenced by the color photography of our day and by the color printing processes surrounding him to produce works that are no longer intended to exert their greatest impact in the "here and now" of their singular existence in a unique location; instead, they are meant to be disseminated and are most effective in mass reproductions of various sorts. Wind maintains that this subconscious reorientation began as early as in the days of van Gogh and the Douanier Rousseau.[31]

Be that as it may, there is a need for color photographs and slides in the art library to document modern and contemporary movements of painting and other two-dimensional art, but they should only be substituted for black and white after it has been ascertained that the almost infinite range of shades of grey in which the monochrome photograph is capable of producing tonal values is not better suited for documenting the particular art work.

The contributions that analog videodisks and optical digital disks can make to the study of the visual arts will do much to bring the universe of images within reach of every scholar. Up to 54,000 separate images in black and white or in color can be stored on one side of a single twelve-inch videodisk. They can be scanned at various speeds or studied one by one in frozen motion on the screen of a monitor connected to a videodisk player. The player contains a microprocessor that enables the user to call up specific images or sequences of pictures; the videodisk can also be connected to more sophisticated microcomputers and to large mainframes as well. If properly programmed, this electronic image storage and delivery system is capable of supplying answers to many old iconographic, historical, and stylistic questions that have defied scholarly effort so far. The machine will also prompt scholars to ask new questions and posit theorems which grow out of the occupation with it. The intellectual level of inquiry will, of course, entirely depend on the level of sophistication of the computer programs that future generations of art historians will be able to write. The possibilities are endless, and they are daunting.

For the individual art library, the new technology opens up the prospect of becoming able to provide universal availability of art reproductions. Every art library can now, at least theoretically, provide in addition to its own visual resources, access to other visual resources collections, even those that reside in geographically remote repositories if it has them recorded on videodisks. And a "jukebox" holding 100 videodisks which can store more than ten million art reproductions takes up only about fifteen square feet of library space. The process of systematically recording several of the world's great image collections—not only photographic archives and historic print collections but also whole museum collections are being put to disk—is well under way; and the museum without walls, or rather the world museum within the walls of every art library, is no longer an impossible dream.

But a word of caution is appropriate here. Image banks, whether on videodisks or on microfiche, have a great future in art libraries as cataloguing and inventory devices. They will also help to preserve deterioriating originals by making out of unique items renewable resources. We are confident that they will also stimulate entirely new forms of scholarly inquiry, because scanning of great masses of images in a sequential mode may reveal relationships between works of art that have gone unrecognized before. Nevertheless it would be a matter for regret and, I believe, a great mistake if art librarians concluded that, because images can be put on microfiche and laser disks, they can now dispose of their traditional photograph collections or cease to develop them further. They must realize that the new technologies, although they do permit the harnessing of the ever increasing masses of graphic records that are available, do also bring risks of constraints along with promises of greater efficiency.

Although the quality of the images of works of art that can be generated electronically on the analog videodisk has significantly improved during the decade during which this technology has been used, and although in good time even better results in true-to-life fidelity may be expected from the newer optical digital disk which has much less storage capacity yet offers greater resolution and sharpness, the fact remains that in the presentations of works of art through these media the previously lamented stained-glass-window effect has not disappeared. It is also well to remember that the fidelity of the color reproduced is only as good as that of the slide from which the disk was mastered—or rather the filmstrip made from the slide from which the videotape was made from which the master was cut from which the disk that results was pressed! The videodisk image, it must be realized, is a fifth- or at best a fourth-generation image—a sobering thought.

Another even more serious argument against the exclusive reliance upon video or optical digital recordings as reproductions that can serve as stand-ins for the original works of art is the today often overlooked fact that all the electronic storage and display media allow consultation of the file only sequentially, one image at a time, or at best under exceptionally favorable conditions when two monitors are placed side by side, also the viewing of two images simultaneously like in the typical art history classroom. The euphoria with which the new electronic image bank is greeted by the library profession must be tempered. Too little attention is being paid to the fact that the videodisk, like all electronic storage systems and learning devices, reduces a simultaneously existing theoretically infinite reality of images—sophisticated computer programs for access notwithstanding—to a closed logical system in which the scholar as end user is in danger of becoming a mere link in a closed circuit of information.

It therefore appears to this writer that the old-fashioned black-and-white photograph is for teaching and research and for many other scholarly purposes still the best medium of reproduction, not because it necessarily contains the most complete information about the original but because it allows us to distinguish clearly between medium and message, reproduction and original; precisely because its code is recognizable and easy to understand.

Art librarians must continue to collect photographic prints with discrimination and with great care must preserve photographic collections entrusted to them. Future generations of art scholars should not be deprived of the instrument that the greatest of their spiritual ancestors have used with such virtuosity. Art historians must, no matter what different approaches electronic media may make possible, still be able to spread quantities of photographs out on their work table or to pin them up in changing juxtapositions on the wall of their study, to shuffle and reorder them under different aspects in search of new meanings. The serendipitous art historical research process that, when practised by men like Berenson, Warburg, Panofsky, and Gombrich and many art scholars before and after them, has led to such great advances in scholarship is too precious to jeopardize it by abandoning the collecting of photographs. This 150-year-old technology that is as old as our discipline and which, for the intellectual stimulation it provides and the ability to keep a faithful record of the past, has become its principal tool, will very likely remain unchallenged in that role.

Only recently an entirely new method for making full color, exact size reproductions of paintings and other two-dimensional art has been perfected by the Polaroid Corporation using its famous patented instant direct photograph process in a specially constructed room-sized camera. The reproductions obtained are true replicas, offering excellent color fidelity and capable of rendering every surface detail. There is no doubt that these Polaroid Replicas® are the most exciting advance in reprographic technology. But because they must be painstakingly produced one at a time, they have more in common with the manual methods for making replicas than with the photographic processes that produce multiple copies of images. And because the process is costly and commands prices of hundreds of dollars per picture, the use of Polaroid Replicas® in art history study and teaching remains, at least for the time being and for the foreseeable future, limited to didactic applications where single major works are studied. It will be a long time before the replicas produced by the Polaroid process will enter art library collections. It remains to be seen if they will ever replace the traditional photograph.

Today a new and revolutionary means for presenting three-dimensional views of small sculpture and objects is available through holography.[32] It is a triumph of the combination of modern optics and laser technology resulting in true color and original scale projected images not on a screen, but in a clear, free-standing plastic cube. Placed in a darkened room, the image of the object can be viewed "in the round" from all sides, and the only element that distinguishes it in its physical presence from the original is that it cannot be touched and handled. With the invention of holography, the "museum without walls" of which Malraux spoke has come one step closer to realization and has, although the application of the new medium remains for the time being limited to relatively small originals, eliminated one severe drawback of the photograph and the slide which substitute two-dimensional images for a three-dimensional reality.

All art begins with a concept in the artist's mind that triggers the process of creation and usually ends with the realization of the concept in a permanently fixed image or work that is subject to being replicated or reproduced by the technologies reviewed in the preceding paragraphs. In a negative sense, this is possible even with regard to concepts that result only in "minimal art," i.e., shapes or objects that are banal if taken by themselves and which evoke the intended associations in the beholder (the realization of the artistic concept) only in their interactions (either clash or unexpected harmony) with their environment. But still photography is not capable at all of capturing the essence of artistic concepts that find their realization in *processes*, natural or staged, and that thus stand at the borderline of the traditional visual and the performing arts. It also must fail in the interpretation of kinetic art concepts, no matter whether these appear in the form of seventeenth-century fountains as in the gardens of Versailles with their magnificent combination of "living" jets of water with sculpture; as the gently moving "mobiles" of the twentieth-century sculptor Alexander Calder; or as today's motor-driven, machine-like animated sculptures of Jean Tinguely, some of which are meant to give their ultimate artistic message to the world in the final moment of their self-destruction. For this art as well as for "light art," "earth art," certain other types of "environmental art," "happenings," and other "performance and action" arts, the motion picture film and the videotape are the only means of recording and reproducing the unique event. For it can be assumed that, although these art forms do not result in a durable work in the traditional sense, the perishable work is important enough to remember and to study. It is under this latter documentary aspect that the art library must concern itself with the media of film and video. But it should limit its professional responsibility to providing reproductions as records of works, whether static objects or events, executed in other media.

Since the librarian's responsibility includes the furnishing of biographical information on artists and since this comprises individual as well as collective biography, it can be argued that the many films being made that show artists in the act of creating art or interviews with artists conducted by critics, studio visits, or filmed gallery talks at exhibition openings do belong within the purview of the art library's activities. Whether a library should engage in building a collection of such films and tapes must be carefully weighed in each individual case. The answer will be yes or no depending on a number of factors. Among these are the availability of acquisitions funds, assurance of continued strong budgets to maintain and service the collections (which includes considerable funds for the operation of projection and related equipment), and, above all, a clear and unambiguous policy statement from the institutional leadership that the film and videotape activities are indeed a legitimate and wanted library function. The traditional art historical research library, serving a typical academic constituency of students and professors, certainly has no business spending its limited resources on films of conventional artistic actions if it has not already achieved completeness in its photographic archives. Materials that can be used in the typical art historical study process of rapid comparisons in conjunction with books and periodicals have priority over materials that cannot be used at a moment's notice and which have to be programmed. Programming the showing of films or videotapes always involves delays. And, since delays are expected and accepted by the users of these materials with little or no complaint, the question must be asked whether it is worth the expense to shorten the waiting period by having a collection on the premises of one's own library. Or, is borrowing or renting such materials from institutions that specialize in this kind of art documentation, including educational film libraries and even commercial film distributors, not a more economical solution? Here opens certainly a very promising field of cooperation between traditional academic art libraries and institutions dedicated to the documentation of modern and contemporary art movements. Not only museums and archives of modern art but also art schools and academies, their financial resources permitting, are likely to take on the collecting of films and videotapes, often specializing in the documentation of a particular area, national or geographic, medium or movement. These resources should be shared as widely as possible.

In an entirely different category are motion pictures and video presentations made not *about* but *by* artists—films not made by artists or others with a documentary invention but film art and video art as products of the creative imagination. Granted that the distinction between the documentary mode and the artistic mode, i.e., film or videotape as medium, is not always easy to make, films and tapes as artistic creations belong in the museum or a separate film archive, not in the general art library. The justification for this opinion rests on the analogy that can be drawn to the print. Although some art libraries still administer a print collection that contains both reproduction prints and original, creative first statements made by an artist in one of the print media (the terms "fine prints" or "masterprints" which are sometimes used in the names of library print departments serve only to confuse), nonreproductive graphic art belongs in the print room of a museum. The library should at the most be expected to collect reproduction prints of the prephotographic era if the reproduced works of art have been lost or destroyed or are, for other reasons, not accessible to the photographic camera. As more and more museums recognize the presence of film and video art as legitimate media of aesthetic expression for the modern visual artist and show this in their administrative structure by adding separate curatorial departments for videotape and film or by creating appropriate subdivisions in their prints and photographs departments, it will become easier for the art library to draw the line that separates it from the museum. Museum and library have each their own share of the responsibility in the preservation and transmission of our artistic heritage. The task that they share is so huge that only a clear understanding of the different roles they must play with regard to visual resources documentation can avoid most undesirable duplication of effort and waste.

As far as the art library of today and tomorrow is concerned, its principal mission is not different from that of other libraries in this age of transition: to preserve the past and the present for the future. The task is as difficult and as complex as the charge sounds simple. It has been so well expressed in the brief remarks that the Deputy Librarian of Congress made recently when addressing an international meeting of librarians that it may be permitted to end this paper on the note he sounded.

> It is, in fact, a curious position the library world finds itself in today. We are looking backwards to preserve the record of our past, and to the future, with its myriad new technologies. The decisions we are making today will effectively preserve or obliterate the memory of the past, since the future generations will have no communal memory of the past save what we are able to preserve. . . . Likewise, decisions we are making today will shape the future.[33]

NOTES

1. Max J. Friedländer, *Reminiscences and Reflections* (Greenwich, Conn.: New York Graphic Society, 1969), 33.

2. William M. Ivins, Jr., *Prints and Visual Communication* (Cambridge, Mass.: Harvard University Press, 1953).

3. Ibid., 3.

4. Ibid., 164–65.

5. Ibid., 176.

6. Ibid., 177.

7. Estelle Jussim, *Visual Communication and the Graphic Arts* (New York, London: R. R. Bowker, 1974).

8. Ibid., 274.

9. Ibid., 237–78.

10. Ivins, *Prints,* 177.

11. Jussim, *Visual Communication,* 345.

12. Charles Eliot Norton, "The Autotype or Carbon Process in Photography," *The Nation* (21 January 1869): 47.

13. The lecture notes of three Harvard undergraduates, Charles Rathbone Ballou, James Duncan Phillips (Class of 1897), and Charles Chauncey Stillman (Class of 1898), that are preserved in the Harvard University Archives indicate that in his famous survey courses on medieval art and history (Fine Arts-4 and Italian-4) Norton did regularly use floor plans and architectural elevation drawings, that "views" were only shown occasionally and that so-called viewing assignments were mostly directed to illustrations in published works. For example, one of the students notes that for his next class he must "look at sculpture in Viollet-le-Duc."

14. "Die Umgestaltung der Universitätsvorlesungen über neuere Kunstgeschichte durch das Skioptikon," *Nationalzeitung* (Berlin, 1892).

15. Walter Benjamin, "The Work of Art in the Age of Mechanical Reproduction," *Illuminations,* ed. Hannah Arendt, trans. Harry Zohn (New York: Schocken Books, 1969).

16. Cf. Günther Bandmann, "Das Kunstwerk als Gegenstand der Universalgeschichte," *Jahrbuch für Ästhetik und allgemeine Kunstwissenschaft* 7 (1962): 146–66; John Hale, "What Help from Art," *Times Literary Supplement* (7 April 1966); and Leopold D. Ettlinger, "Kunstgeschichte als Geschichte," *Jahrbuch der Hamburger Kunstsammlungen* 16 (1971): 7–19.

17. Helmut and Alison Gernsheim, *A Concise History of Photography* (New York: Grosset and Dunlap, 1965).

18. Ibid., 72.

19. Ibid., 68.

20. Ibid., 72.

21. Martin Faigel, "Berenson Library," *Encyclopedia of Library and Information Science,* ed. Allen Kent and Harold Lancour, vol. 2 (1969).

22. Hanna Kiel, ed., *The Berenson Treasury; A Selection from the Works, Unpublished Writings, Letters, Diaries, and Journals: 1887–1958* (London: Methuen & Co., 1964), 69–70.

23. Joseph Gantner, ed., *Jacob Burckhardt und Heinrich Wölfflin: Briefwechsel und andere Dokumente ihrer Begegnung 1882–1897* (Basel: Benno Schwabe, 1948), 114.

24. Ibid., 111.

25. Ibid., 122.

26. Hans Tietze, *Die Methode der Kunstgeschichte. Ein Versuch* (Leipzig: Carl Seemann, 1913).

27. Ibid., 302–303.

28. Clarence Kennedy, "Light and Shade and the Point of View in the Study of Greek Sculpture." Ph.D. diss., Harvard University, 1924.

29. Ibid., ch. 2, "Light," 33–87, passim.

30. Edgar Wind, "The Mechanization of Art," *Art and Anarchy* (London: Faber and Faber, 1963), 165–66.

31. Ibid., 77.

32. *Holography* is a means of recording (usually on film) the interference pattern of the two halves of a split coherent wave source (such as a laser beam). One half of the beam goes directly to the film, and the other half is reflected from the subject being holographed onto the film. When a laser beam is directed back through the resultant *hologram* the interference pattern of the film distorts the light so that it forms a wave front nearly equivalent to that coming from the original subject, Holograms are therefore three dimensional.

Definition from Monty M. Maxwell, "Unconventional Photographic Systems; How Will They Change Your Library?" *Wilson Library Bulletin* 46 (February 1972): 521.

33. William B. Welsh, "The Role of the Library of Congress in Transition," from an address given at the 51st Council and General Conference, IFLA (International Federation of Library Associations and Institutions) Chicago, 21 August 1985.

ELIZABETH GILMORE HOLT

A Bibliography of Her Work

ANTJE BULTMANN LEMKE

"I HAVE to find out what went on in Zola's mind." This perceptive comment reflected Elizabeth Holt's motivation as she selected the material for her *Documentary History of Art*. How did artists respond to each other's work? Who were the critics that reviewed the exhibitions, and who promoted and sponsored artists and exhibitions? To shed light on such questions, Elizabeth Holt gathered sources from disparate periods, from the Middle Ages to the dawn of the twentieth century.

About the conception of the series she stated, "When I received the appointment as instructor at Duke University [1934], I was confronted by Helen Gardner's formidable volume *Art Through the Ages* [1926]. A totally erroneous impression of Abbot Suger was presented to the beginning student by the inclusion of a few lines of his writing, excerpted from Kingsley Porter's translated section in *Medieval Architecture* [1912]. I learned no translation existed of the constantly cited Ghiberti *Commentarii* (even the Schlosser German edition of 1911 was out of print). Few undergraduates could read a foreign language and were thus deprived of the pleasure and stimulation of reading 'how it really was' in ages past."

To open the door to the riches of Italian, French, and other foreign sources that had been largely unavailable to the majority of most English-speaking students, Elizabeth Holt set out to search for and to translate original documents. While intended for the student and the interested amateur, the *Documentary History* became an indispensable source for many scholars, while helping to democratize and popularize the discipline of art history.

In retrospect, the significance of the gathered texts was that they provided a methodological foundation that has influenced later generations in the field. In addition to selections from traditional art history sources, Holt's work included documents from literary and popular magazines, the daily press, correspondence, and from novels. Whenever possible, Holt provided the entire document rather than excerpts. Thus many selections include comments related to a specific art work or event, or contain other observations and reflections that increase the reader's understanding of the intellectual climate in which works were created or exhibited. Holt's introductions to the volumes, to the various chapters, and to the statements of individual artists and critics reflect an assimilation of ideas and themes based upon scholarly documentation and intuition. Concisely presented, these prefatory texts prepare the foundation for reading the full document.

Underlying her decisions was Elizabeth Holt's belief that the materials selected should not be presented according to the philosophy or ideology of a given compiler. Rather, she remained true to her historical inclinations noting that "to be faithful to the sources is my only command." She wanted every reader of her books to form his own opinion without intervention or manipulation by commentators or interpretors.

While Elizabeth Holt's main contributions are found in the volumes in the *Documentary History* series and in her new publications, not all fully published, she did make other contributions to the field. These are listed below.

BIBLIOGRAPHY

ARTICLES

"The Documentation for the Contribution of Three Mid-Nineteenth-Century Exhibitions to the Popularization of Japanese Art," in *Art the Ape of Nature: Studies in Honor of W. H. Janson,* Moshe Barasch, Lucy Feeman Sandler, Patricia Egan, eds. New York: Abrams; Englewood Cliffs, N.J.: Prentice-Hall, 1981.

"Revivalist Themes in American Prints and Folksongs, 1830–50." *American Printmaking Before 1876, Fact, Fiction, and Fantasy.* Washington, D.C.: Library of Congress, 1975.

MONOGRAPHS

"Die Augsburger Andachts-Epitaphien im Zusammenhang mit der Monumentalen Plastik." Munich, 1934. Dissertation.

Literary Sources of Art History: An Anthology of Texts from Theophilus to Goethe. Princeton, N.J.: Princeton University Press, 1947. Reprinted Oxford: Oxford University Press, 1947.

AAUW Looks at Social Security. Washington, D.C.: American Association of University Women, Status of Women Committee, 1956.

A Documentary History of Art, vol. 1: The Middle Ages and the Renaissance. Garden City, N.Y.: Doubleday, 1957. Reprinted Princeton, N.J.: Princeton University Press, 1981.

A Documentary History of Art, vol. 2: Michelangelo and the Mannerists: The Baroque and the Eighteenth Century. Garden City, N.Y.: Doubleday, 1958. Reprinted Princeton, N.J.: Princeton University Press, 1982.

From the Classicists to the Impressionists: A Documentary History of Art and Architecture in the 19th Century. (DHA vol. 3) Garden City, N.Y.: Doubleday, 1966. Reprinted London: University of London Press, 1966. Reprinted New York: New York University Press, 1966.

Storia Documentaria dell'arte dall medioevo al XVIII secolo. Milan: Feltrinelli, 1972. Italian edition of *Literary Sources of Art History.*

The Triumph of Art for the Public: The Emerging Role of Exhibitions and Critics (1785–1848). Garden City, N.Y.: Anchor Press, 1979. Reprinted Washington, D.C.: Decatur House Press, 1981.

The Art of All Nations, 1850–1873: The Emerging Role of Exhibitions and Critics. Garden City, N.Y.: Anchor Press, 1981. Reprinted Princeton, N.J.: Princeton University Press, 1981.

The Expanding World of Art: Premonitions of the 20th Century, 1873–1900. New Haven: Yale University Press, 1986.

REVIEW

"Theories of Modern Art." *Art Bulletin* 54, no. 2 (June 1972): 229–31.

FILM

Pictures to Serve the People: American Lithography, 1830–1855. American Antiquarian Society. Released by ACI Films, 1975.

INDEX

Page numbers in italics refer to illustrations.

THE DOCUMENTED IMAGE

was composed in 10 on 12 Sabon on a Mergenthaler Linotron 202
by Partners Composition;
with display type set in Weiss
by Dix Type Inc.;
printed by sheet-fed offset on 60-pound, acid-free Glatco Smooth white,
Smyth sewn and bound over binder's boards in Joanna Arrestox B
by Maple-Vail Book Manufacturing Group, Inc.;
with dust jackets printed in two colors
by Niles & Phipps Lithographers;
designed by Sara L. Eddy;
and published by

SYRACUSE UNIVERSITY PRESS
SYRACUSE, NEW YORK 13244-5160